Intravenous Anaesthesia

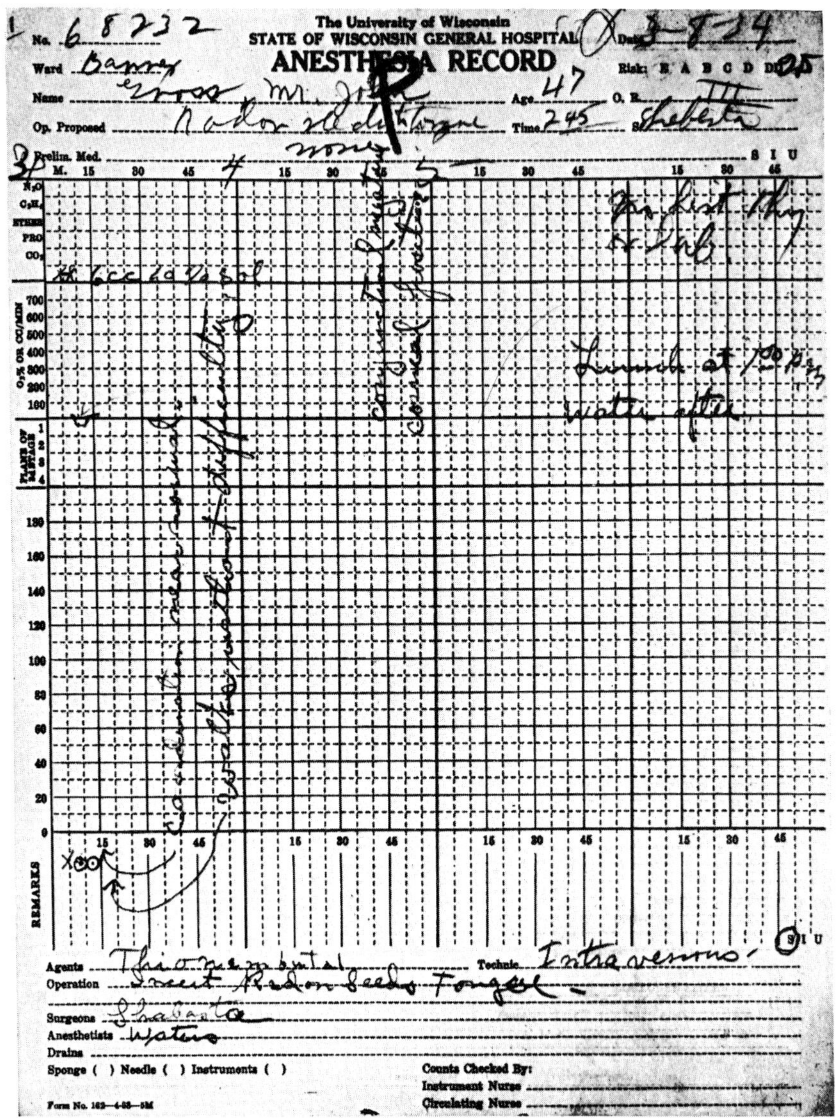

The University of Wisconsin
STATE OF WISCONSIN GENERAL HOSPITAL

ANESTHESIA RECORD

No. 68232 Date 3-8-34
Ward
Name Age 47 O. R.
Op. Proposed Time 245
Prelim. Med. none
Risk: E A B C D DE
S I U

N₂O
C₂H₄
ETHER
PRO
CO₂

O₂% OR CC/MIN 700 600 500 400 300 200 100

PLANE OF 3d STAGE 1 2 3 4

180 160 140 120 100 80 60 40 20 0

REMARKS

Lunch at 1:00 P.M. water after

Agents Thiopentobarbital Technic Intravenous
Operation Insert Radon Seeds Tongue
Surgeons
Anesthetists Waters
Drains
Sponge ( ) Needle ( ) Instruments ( )
Counts Checked By:
Instrument Nurse
Circulating Nurse
Form No. 163—4-33—5M

Reproduction of the anaesthetic record of the first administration of thiopentone for clinical anaesthesia. This was given by Dr R.M. Waters at the University of Wisconsin Hospital, Madison, on 8th March 1934.

Intravenous Anaesthesia

John W Dundee
MD PhD FRCP FFARCS
Professor of Anaesthetics, The Queen's University of Belfast; Consultant Anaesthetist, Belfast Teaching Hospitals, Northern Ireland

Gordon M Wyant
CD MD FRCP(C) FFARCS
Professor Emeritus of Anaesthesia, University of Saskatchewan, Saskatoon, Canada

With contributions by

Richard S J Clarke
MD PhD FFARCS
Professor of Clinical Anaesthesia, The Queen's University of Belfast; Consultant Anaesthetist, Belfast Teaching Hospitals, Northern Ireland

Alan C McKay
MD FFARCS
Consultant Anaesthetist, Belfast City and Musgrave Park Hospitals, Northern Ireland

James G Bovill
MD FFARCSI
Professor of Experimental Anaesthesia, Department of Anaesthesiology, University of Leiden Hospital, The Netherlands

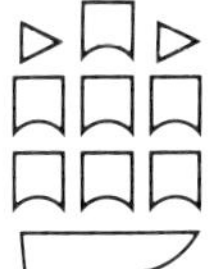

CHURCHILL LIVINGSTONE
EDINBURGH LONDON MELBOURNE AND NEW YORK 1988

CHURCHILL LIVINGSTONE
Medical Division of Longman Group UK Limited

Distributed in the United States of America by Churchill Livingstone Inc., 1560 Broadway, New York, N.Y. 10036, and by associated companies, branches and representatives throughout the world.

First edition 1974
Reprinted 1977
Second edition 1988

ISBN 0-443-02072-8

British Library Cataloguing in Publication Data

Dundee, John W.
Intravenous anaesthesia. — 2nd ed.
1. Intravenous anesthesia
I. Title II. Wyant, Gordon M.
617'.962 RD85.I6

Library of Congress Cataloging in Publication Data

Dundee, John W. (John Wharry)
Intravenous anaesthesia.

[Includes bibliographies and index.
1. Intravenous anesthesia.] I. Wyant, Gordon M. (Gordon Michael), 1914- . II. Title. [DNLM: 1. Anesthesia, Intravenous. WO 285 D914i]
RD85.I6D85 1987 617'.962 87-8022

Produced by Longman Group (FE) Limited
Printed in Hong Kong

Preface to second edition

It has been 11 years since the first edition of this book was published and, although it was reprinted three years later, it has long since been out of print. While it is regrettable that so many years had to elapse before a second edition could be prepared there are hidden benefits in this delay. A number of intravenous anaesthetic agents have come and gone, Althesin being the most prominent of these. Despite its early promise and wide distribution throughout the world, it eventually had to be withdrawn. However, it made us conscious of the importance of hypersensitivity reactions and this finds expression in the fact that an entire chapter is now being given over to this subject. Many other significant changes have been made in this edition to bring it up to current knowledge and practice. The authors welcome new contributors. Alan McKay has written the chapter on mode of action of barbiturates while James Bovill has taken over the chapter on neurolept analgesia: Richard Clarke who wrote on eugenols in the first edition has here written the chapter on hypersensitivity. Peter Howard, William Toner and Elizabeth McClean have contributed to the appendices.

The first edition of this book had the fortune of being favourably received by our colleagues. We have tried to keep the same basic format and have attempted to give an overview of the field without losing ourselves in confusing detail. We hope that we have once again succeeded in this endeavour. The success of the first edition of this book is attested by its translation into an Italian and Spanish edition.

Again much work has been done by our various secretaries. Special mention must be made of Mrs Noelle Collins (Belfast) and Miss Noella Mailhot (Saskatoon). Special recognition is due to the publishers who have demonstrated formidable patience and forbearance when one deadline after the other has come and gone without tangible results.

Belfast and Saskatoon
1988

J. W. D.
G. M. W.

Preface to first edition

It is more than four years ago that the decision was made to write this book on *Intravenous Anaesthesia*. Only two books on this subject had been available at one time or another, both of them out of print. The one by the late Dr Charles Adams of Rochester, Minnesota, had originally been published in 1944 and Dundee's book entitled *Thiopentone and Other Thiobarbiturates* in 1956.

When the decision to cooperate on this book first was made, one of us (J. W. D.) was being urged to undertake the writing of a second edition of *Thiopentone and Other Thiobarbiturates* and the other (G. M. W.) was already under contract to produce a comprehensive review of intravenous anaesthesia. It was logical therefore that we should combine our efforts rather than duplicating each other's work, each perhaps with more limited objectives. Such a joint authorship presented no mean challenge in view of the considerable difficulties inherent in intercontinental cooperation of this kind. For instance, the writing of the manuscript spanned three postal strikes, one in the United Kingdom and two in Canada, not to mention a number of 'work-to-rule' slow-downs by Canadian postal workers, all of which certainly did not contribute to the simplification of the task. After preliminary discussions in San Francisco, four editorial meetings took place, one in Belfast, one in Saskatoon, one in Kyoto, Japan, and the final one in London.

The field of intravenous anaesthesia has developed rapidly over the last several years, well beyond the scope of the barbiturates. If for no other reason this alone would seem to require a comprehensive review of its present state. Dissociative, neurolept and steroid anaesthesia have opened up new vistas, and developments in this field are so rapid that some chapters will be lacking the latest information by the time the book appears in print. This unfortunately is unavoidable but we have tried to complete the available information up to the end of March 1973. On occasions it has been possible to insert more new data at proof stage and there will be a few more recent references.

An attempt has been made to produce a comprehensive review of the entire field of intravenous anaesthesia, but we have stopped short of the encyclopaedic recital of every available report on every pertinent subject in the world literature. We must leave it to the reader to decide whether our objective has been reached.

One of the basic decisions which had to be made at the outset was that of spelling, names of drugs and arrangements of references. Since the book is being printed in the United Kingdom and since moreover Canada uses the *British Pharmacopoeia*, the usage of Great Britain have been followed. However, U.S.P. equivalents as well as trade names for all drugs are listed in a glossary.

In two areas, namely the eugenols and neurolept analgesia we have had the good fortune of enlisting the cooperation of Drs Richard S. J. Clarke and James D. Morrison respectively and we wish to record our appreciation to them for having made available their very specialised knowledge in these fields.

As is usual, many people have contributed both directly and indirectly to the completion of this work. Our colleagues and residents have been a constant intellectual stimulus and have assisted us with valuable advice by scrutinising the text and making suggestions for changes. Our special thanks go to our secretaries, Mrs Noelle Collins

(Belfast) and Mrs Lois Poole (Saskatoon) who have spent many hours typing and retyping manuscripts. We are grateful to the publishers Messrs Churchill Livingstone for their cooperation. Mr Peter S. Wyant, BSc, and later Mr Raymond E. Wyant, BA were engaged as summer students in assembling some of the background information from the world literature.

Last, but by no means least, we must mention our long-suffering families who may not have assisted in the writing of the manuscript but without whose understanding and sacrifice we could not have found the time and inspiration to accumulate over many years the background knowledge and experience which finally led to the production of this book.

Belfast and Saskatoon
January 1974

J. W. D.
G. M. W.

Acknowledgements

Royal College of Physicians of Edinburgh for permission to reproduce Fig. 1. Department of Anaesthetics, University of Wisconsin Hospital and the late R M Waters for permission to reproduce the Frontispiece. To all staff of the University Department of Belfast for their patient proof-reading; to the Medical Photography units of Belfast City Hospital for many of the illustrations.

Our thanks are due to the editors and publishers of the following journals and books for permission to reproduce the tables and figures listed below:

Anaesthesia: Tables 4.6, 11.1; Figures 8.2, 11.3, 12.12, 14.5

Anaesthesia and Intensive Care: Figure 4.6

Anesthesia and Analgesia: Figures 13.15, 13.16

Anesthesiology: Tables 6.3, 6.5, 8.2, 9.1; Figures 6.6, 6.10, 9.1, 13.8, 13.9, 13.10, 13.12

Brain Research: Table 7.1

British Journal of Anaesthesia: Table 16.1; Figures 8.3, 11.2, 12.7, 12.11, 13.11, 13.14, 17.2, 17.3

British Journal of Clinical Pharmacology: Figures 12.8, 12.12

British Journal of Obstetrics and Gynaecology: Table 4.8

Clinical Pharmacology and Therapeutics: Figure 13.6

European Journal of Pharmacology: Figure 13.2

International Anesthesiology Clinics: Table 14.4

Journal of the Royal Society of Medicine: Figure 17.1

Lancet: Figure 12.5

Postgraduate Medical Journal: Tables 11.1, 11.2, 15.5; Figures 11.3, 11.4

Adverse response to intravenous drugs. Academic Press, London 1978. Fig. 14.4

Current topics in anaesthesia. Series 1: Intravenous anaesthetic agents. Edited by J W Dundee. Edward Arnold, London, 1979. Figures 8.1, 16.2

Drug disposition in anaesthesia. Edited by D R Stanski and W D Watkins. Grune & Stratton, New York, 1982. Figure 6.3

Molecular mechanisms in general anaesthesia. Edited by M J Halsey, R A Millar and J A Sutton. Churchill Livingstone, Edinburgh, 1974. Table 5.2

Pharmacological basis of therapeutics, 3rd edn. Edited by L S Goodman and A Gilman. Macmillan, New York, 1965. Figure 4.1

Pharmacokinetics of anaesthesia. Edited by C Prys-Roberts and C C Hug, 1984. Blackwell, Oxford, 1984. Figure 6.4

Scientific Foundations of Anaesthesia, 3rd edn. Edited by C. Scurr and S Feldman. Heinemann, London, 1982. Table 4.4, 4.7; Figure 6.5

Glaxo Laboratories Ltd: for data in Table 14.7

The following tables and figures were acknowledged in the 1st edition:
Tables 4.4, 4.5, 6.2, 8.4, 8.5; Figures 1.3, 2.1, 2.3, 2.6, 4.5, 5.2, 6.1, 6.2, 6.8, 6.9, 6.10, 8.1, 8.3, 8.5, 8.6, 8.7, 8.8, 8.9, 8.10, 9.3

Contents

1

History

Our story begins in the year 1628. This was the year in which William Harvey published his epoch-making treatise *Exercitalio Anatomica De Motu Cordis Et Sanguinis In Animalibus.* True, his work has been preceded by the studies of the 15th and 16th century renaissance anatomists, foremost of whom were Leonardo, Michael Servetus, Realdo Colombo and Andrea Cesalpino, who had speculated on the functional significance of the heart and blood vessels, but it needed the genius of Harvey to grasp and prove by experiment their true physiological significance.

Twenty-eight years after Harvey's monumental discovery and following experiments in animals, the first attempt at an intravenous injection in man was made by Christopher Wren, the famous English architect who at that time was Savillian Professor of Astronomy at Oxford University. His intravenous injection of opium by means of a quill and bladder resulted in the incidental production of unconsciousness, but it is doubtful whether Wren was aware that he had in fact produced a form of anaesthesia.

The first deliberate attempt at intravenous anaesthesia must be attributed to Sigismund Elsholtz, who in 1665 injected the solution of an opiate with the avowed purpose of producing insensibility. It would appear, however, that his work was largely ignored since almost 200 years were to elapse before the production of insensibility to pain by means of intravenous injections was taken up again.

Without the syringe, intravenous anaesthesia could not have developed. Credit for its perfection must go to Alexander Wood of Edinburgh (Fig. 1.1) However, not even he had any concept of drugs being given intravenously. His paper published in 1855 was entitled: 'A new method of treating painful neuralgias by the direct application of opiates to painful points'. In it he suggested that the beneficial effects of injected morphine were due to a local action on the painful spots — an idea with which pharmacologists would have very little sympathy for many years. At no time does he ever mention absorption of and a general analgesic action from the injected opiate. However, perhaps there was some truth in his original suggestion, for we are now becoming aware of the direct analgesic effect of opiates, particularly in the extradural apace.

The hollow needle was perfected by Francis Rynd, a Dublin surgeon, around 1845. His paper

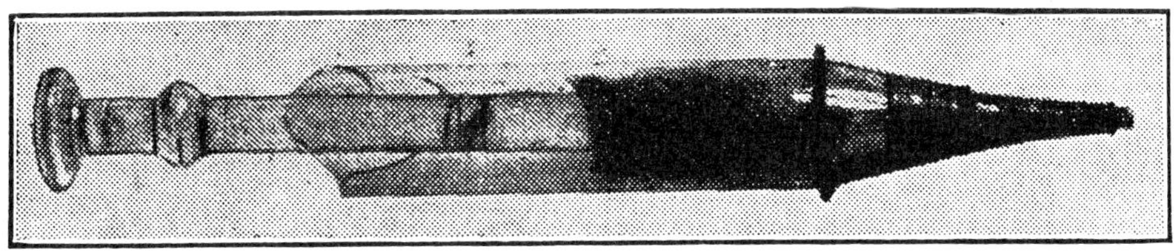

Fig. 1.1 Alexander Wood's syringe (displayed in the Royal College of Physicians of Edinburgh).

entitled: 'Neuralgia — introduction of fluid to the nerve', like that of Wood, deals with the local injection of morphine.

However, it was not until 1872 that Pierre Cyprian Oré of Lyons availed himself of these new tools for the purpose of producing anaesthesia by injecting chloral hydrate intravenously. Several unfortunate postoperative deaths conspired against acceptance of this method.

There followed another hiatus of 33 years until rediscovery of the intravenous route for the production of anaesthesia and, although somewhat haltingly at first because of the lack of truly suitable drugs, intravenous anaesthesia from then on progressed at an uninterrupted and continuously accelerating pace, the culmination of which probably has not been reached even today. The process was started in 1905 by Krawkow in St Petersburg. He injected Hedonal (methyl-propyl-carbinol-urethane) which gained a measure of popularity in Russia and in other parts of Europe. Four years later Burkhardt popularised the intravenous use of diethyl ether and chloroform. Of these, diethyl ether in 5 per cent normal saline proved to be the more satisfactory of the two but, despite good reports from many countries, the method never gained widespread acceptance. In the same year the German surgeon August Bier described intravenous regional analgesia with procaine, a technique which after half a century of oblivion has been reintroduced into clinical practice in recent years with a considerable measure of success. Parenthetically, Bier's discovery was followed three years later by the intra-arterial injection of procaine, advocated by Goyanes of Madrid.

In 1913 Noel and Souttar reported the intravenous use of paraldehyde followed in 1916 by magnesium sulphate by Peck and Meltzer.

BARBITURATES

Meanwhile the barbiturates had made their appearance. Barbituric acid, alternatively known as malonyl urea, had been prepared in 1864 by Adolf von Baeyer. Berlin-born Baeyer was to achieve fame in 1905 by the award of the Nobel prize for chemistry, but this was unconnected with his work on the barbiturates. There are several versions of the origin of the word *Barbiturate* which all are agreed is a combination of the name *Barbara* with *urea*. It has been suggested that Barbara was either his mother or a girlfriend — his wife's name was not Barbara and he was not married until several years later (Carter, 1951). An alternative attractive story for which there is, however, no foundation (Kendall, 1946) suggests that Baeyer celebrated the discovery of the drug by visiting a nearby tavern frequented by artillery officers on St Barbara's Day, Barbara being the patron saint of artillery officers, and in the ensuing festivities Barbara was amalgamated with urea to give the new compound its name. In 1903 Fischer & von Mering synthesised barbitone (the sodium salt of barbituric acid) which was given the trade name of Veronal. It has been suggested that the name is derived from Verona, Italy where Fischer had spent a recent holiday. Later in 1921 they introduced Somnifen, a combination of the diethyl amines of diethyl barbituric acid and diallyl barbituric acid, which achieved some popularity in continental Europe. Its pharmacology has been described by Redonnet in 1920 and credit for its introduction must go to Bardet (1921) and Bardet & Bardet (1921). There are few clinical data on its use and the lack of scientific interest in this field is shown by the formulation of the drug being changed from a diallyl to allypropyl side chain without any record of it in the available literature.

At about the same time a number of workers reported good results from the intravenous administration of ethyl alcohol, and in 1929 Kirschner described intravenous tribromethanol (Avertin); but none of these could withstand the onslaught of the barbiturates. A re-evaluation of tribromethanol by Dwyer, Strout and Thomas (1953) found this anaesthetic unsatisfactory, while intravenous ethyl alcohol since has regained a limited place as a supplement to general anaesthesia.

By and large the epoch until 1932 was characterised by a profusion of new barbiturates, many of which were adapted for intravenous anaesthesia. The German obstetrician, R. Bumm, first introduced Pernoston (sodium 2-butyl-β-bromallyl barbiturate) in 1927 and this achieved a measure of popularity. Zerfas and McCallum reported in 1929 on the intravenous use of the sodium salt of amylobarbitone (Amytal) and this was widely accepted in the English-speaking world, having been popularised particularly by Lundy of the Mayo Clinic. The popularity of amylobarbitone was rivalled only by sodium pentobarbitone (Nembutal), introduced in 1930 by Fitch, Waters and Tatum.

Intravenous anaesthesia truly came of age in 1932 with the first published report by Weese and Scharpff of hexobarbitone (Evipal or Evipan). This drug more closely had the characteristics of an intravenous anaesthetic as set forth elsewhere in this book, and hence its acceptance was widespread and enthusiastic. Adams estimated that within the first 12 years some 10 million administrations of the drug had taken place (Fig. 1.2).

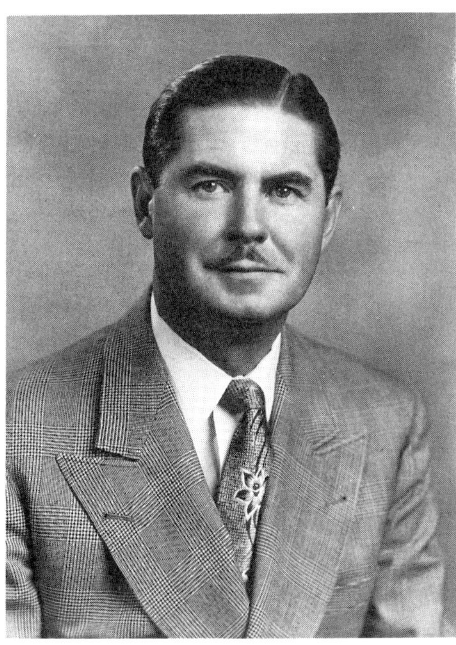

Fig. 1.2 R Charles Adams, 1906–56. A member of the staff of the Mayo Clinic, and author of the book *Intravenous Anaesthesia* published in 1944. This 700 page volume covered the development of intravenous anaesthesia from its beginnings in 1872 to its year of publication and represented one of the big steps in the advancement of this method from an art to a science.

In contrast to previous barbiturates, adequate doses of hexobarbitone would induce anaesthesia in one arm–brain circulation time. This allowed a flexibility of dosage comparable with the inhalational agents. The age of the *rapid acting* induction agent had arrived.

In 1934 a few lesser barbiturates made their appearance, all at approximately the same time, but none of them could compete with hexobarbitone. A few more prominent examples of these drugs were butobarbitone (Neonal; Soneryl) and ethyl Soneryl. Another was Eunarcon (sodium isopropyl-β-bromallyl-N-methyl barbiturate) and Narconumal or methyl Numal (sodium methylallyl isopropyl barbiturate). None of these was rapidly acting.

Thiopentone

However, the intravenous anaesthetic which was to displace them all, which would dwarf all newcomers and which even today, after more than 50 years, still reigns supreme, was yet to come. Research had been progressing with a new group of hypnotically active thiobarbiturates (Tabern & Volwiler, 1935). In 1934 John S Lundy in Rochester, Minnesota and Ralph M Waters in Madison, Wisconsin, started clinical trials of thiopentone (Compound 8064, Pentothal). Although both men carried out their work simultaneously, and Lundy published the first report (Lundy & Tovell, 1934), it seems clear now that to Waters belongs the distinction of the first clinical administration of thiopentone in humans (Pratt et al, 1936). A copy of the anaesthesia record of this first administration of thiopentone, which took place on 8 March 1934, is reproduced as the Frontispiece of this book. When Waters was approached by one of the authors (JWD) to authenticate and give approval for publication of this record, he showed a degree of modesty which is a mark of greatness. In a prolonged conversation he insisted that "John Lundy deserves the credit . . . I only happened to give it first . . . . what is the importance of priority?". To seal matters there was a firm request (in writing) that the record should not appear in public until after his (Waters's) death. Meanwhile, the more outgoing Lundy was unaware of this and one was politely requested not to inform him (Dundee, 1984). The first report on the use of thiopentone in Britain was published by Jarman & Abel in 1936.

Acceptance of intravenous barbiturates

Acceptance of intravenous barbiturates has varied somewhat from country to country. In an attempt to examine this in more detail the incidence of its use has been analysed in a number of civilian hospitals in Britain and the United States (Fig. 1.3). While these figures might not represent fully the practices in the countries concerned, they show some distinct trends. The early popularity of this form of induction was greater in the United States than elsewhere, but showed a distinct falling off in the 1942–46 period, and even 10 years later it was not used nearly as frequently as in Britain. By contrast, induction of anaesthesia by intravenous agents in Britain was limited until 1944–45, after which it grew rapidly and by 1955 it was used in about 90 per cent of all anaesthetics.

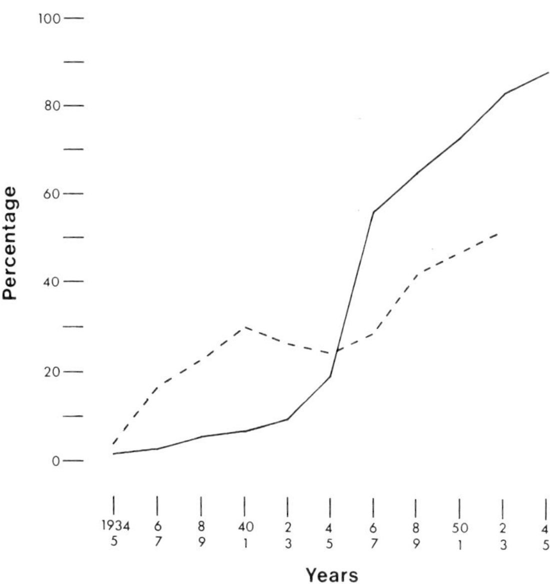

Fig. 1.3 Percentage incidence of use of intravenous anaesthetics in a selected number of hospitals in the UK ——, and the US – – – – –, in the first two decades after this introduction (Dundee 1956)

The early popularity of intravenous anaesthesia outside the United Kingdom might be due to the fact that hexobarbitone was of German origin while thiopentone was an American product. The disastrous results which followed the administration of hexobarbitone and thiopentone at Pearl Harbour in December 1941 might have been responsible for the decrease of their popularity in the United States during the later war years. Following these events, Halford (1943) quoted intravenous anaesthesia as 'an ideal method of euthanasia' in war surgery. One wonders what the present status of these agents would have been had the issue of *Anesthesiology* that reported the Pearl Harbour disasters not also contained a paper by Adams and Gray (1943) describing the successful administration of thiopentone to a patient in deep shock, and an Editorial pointing out that possibly the faults lay with the administration rather than with the drug. Credit must go to Henry S Ruth from the Hahnemann Hospital, Philadephia, the first editor of 'Anaesthesiology', for his foresight in preparing this historic issue of the Journal.

Not only were hexobarbitone and thiopentone new drugs, but they heralded a new concept of anaesthesia. For almost a century anaesthetists had employed one agent only, or two at the most; anaesthesia was usually induced with ether or chloroform and maintained with the same agent, with the occasional use of nitrous oxide-oxygen. There was no reason to believe that thiopentone or hexobarbitone, with their more rapid and pleasant induction could not be used in the same way, as substitutes for the inhalation agents. The early anaesthetic literature contains many references to the use of thiopentone as the sole agent, often in quite large doses. Looking back, we were fortunate that there were not more 'Pearl Harbour' type disasters before the toxicity of large doses was appreciated; yet there might have been many which were not reported. It was simply not appreciated that anaesthetic vapours somewhat limit their own toxicity in spontaneously breathing patients by controlling their uptake (Chapter 2). Furthermore they all had some analgesic action and deep anaesthesia was not necessary to obtund a physical response from a skin incision or other painful stimulus.

In contrast to the United States, the use of thiopentone in British civilian hospitals during the war years was limited by the lack of trained anaesthetists. However, when these experienced specialists returned, the popularity of intravenous anaesthesia increased enormously and even today this form of induction appears to be used more widely in the United Kingdom than in the United States or in some European countries.

The demonstration of the synergistic action of thiopentone with nitrous oxide and oxygen was first described by Organe & Broad from the Westminster Hospital, London in 1938. This is an almost forgotten, or at least underestimated landmark in the development of its clinical use. It might be looked upon as the forerunner of our present day 'balanced techniques' and it undoubtedly played a major part in the universal acceptance of thiopentone as an induction agent. Although the thiopentone–nitrous oxide combination was described before the Pearl Harbour incident its significance could not have been appreciated at the time. We have since seen the development of the analgesic component in intravenous anaesthesia with the use of parenteral analgesics and more recently with the neurolept techniques or large doses of fentanyl (q.v.).

For the sake of clarity a comprehensive list of drugs which are currently in use, or have been used in the past, is given in Table 1.1.

Other barbiturates

In the early studies of thiopentone (which he refers to as Barbiturate A), Lundy included another drug 'sodium allyl secondary butyl thiobarbituric acid' to which he refers as Barbiturate B (Lundy, 1935). This is the sulphur analogue of amylobarbitone, later known as *thioethamyl*, which was available for a short time as Venesetic. He equated it in potency to hexobarbitone and as less potent than thiopentone. On this basis he preferred thiopentone "for the same reason that I prefer pentobarbital to sodium amytal for surgical cases, I wish to use a minimal amount of drug to produce a given effect, anticipating that, at least in the average patient, the effect will be characteristic and that in the unusual case fewer variations will be noted than if a larger quantity of another drug had been given."

Despite some competition from other barbiturates, thiopentone has remained essentially unchallenged among the intravenous anaesthetics. Anaesthetists are indeed fortunate that this was chosen for clinical trials out of the many thiobarbiturates synthesised at the time by Tabern & Volwiler. *Thiamylal*, an equally good agent, was passed over for another 15 years (Dornette, 1954) and today remains a comparatively little used but very acceptable substitute for thiopentone. In fact one large multicentre 'double blind' comparison

Table 1.1·Names of many of the drugs used in intravenous anaesthesia. Those in brackets are rarely used or *completely abandoned.

Rapidly acting induction agents	
Barbiturates:	Thiobarbiturates: thiopentone, thiamylal, thiobutobarbitone (buthalitone*, methitural*, thialbarbitone*, thioethamyl*) Oxybarbiturates: methohexitone (hexobarbitone, enibomal)
*Eugenols**:	Propanidid (G 29505, Propinal)
*Steroids**:	(Althesin/Alfathesin/Alfatesin/Alphadione**) (minaxolone*)
Imidazoles:	Etomidate
Hindered phenols:	Propofol (Disoprofol; ICI 35868)
Slower acting drugs (basal hypnotics)	
Barbiturates:	Pentobarbitone, amylobarbitone
Phencyclidines:	Ketamine
Benzodiazepines:	Diazepam, flunitrazepam, midazolam
Neurolept drug combinations:	Various analgesic-tranquillizer combinations
Opioids:	Large doses of morphine, phenoperidine, fentanyl etc
Others	(Dolitrone*) (Alcohol*) (Sodium oxybutyrate/Gamma-OH*) (Chlormethiazole, SCTZ*)

** No generic name: Althesin (UK) and Alfathesin/Alfatesin (Europe and Canada) are trade names, while Alphadione is the name used in Japan.

showed the two drugs to be indistinguishable in their clinical action (Tovell et al, 1955). It was known commercially as Surital, although some of the British studies were with a preparation known as Thioseconal, indicating its relationship to quinalbarbitone (Secobarbital or Seconal). Despite some early trials (Barran & Wylie, 1951; Dundee & Riding, 1955; Jolly & Lederer, 1955) the drug was never available commercially in Britain. *Thialbarbitone*, the use of which was first reported by Carrington & Raventos in 1946, was another very acceptable alternative to thiopentone. Its main field of use was in Britain (Kemithal) and South America (Kemithene). However it never achieved great popularity and is now no longer commercially available. Another similar drug is *thiobutobarbitone* (or Inactin) which was described in 1935 in the same publication as thiopentone by Tabern & Volwiler; it was not introduced into clinical practice until 1952 by Horatz and Sturtzbecher and its pharmacology was described by Nieschultz in 1953. It enjoys a considerable popularity in Germany. Apart from a difference in potency it is also virtually indistinguishable from thiopentone (Dundee & Riding, 1960).

These four drugs (thiopentone, thiamylal, thialbarbitone and thiobutobarbitone) all had similar action and all were thiobarbiturates (Chapter 5), whereas hexobarbitone was a methylated barbiturate. The next advance came in this latter group with the synthesis of methohexitone, known originally as Lilly 25 398 (Stoelting, 1957). A similar compound (Lilly 22 451) had been studied by Chernish et al (1956) and although it was more potent than thiopentone and was followed by a more rapid recovery, it had convulsive properties. It was then fractioned into low and high melting point isomers, the latter being methohexitone (Redish et al, 1958). It is the only member of the barbiturate series which offers any real competition to thiopentone, although now in a rather different field. This includes outpatient operations, dental procedures and electroconvulsive therapy (Wyant & Barr, 1960). Its more rapid recovery, as compared with thiopentone, has been convincingly confirmed (Breimer, 1976; Carson et al, 1975; Whitwam, 1976) and it is particularly interesting to note that the incidence of induction complications, such as abnormal movements and hiccough (Wyant & Chang, 1959) is much less with the present day drug than with that introduced into Britain around 1960 (Dundee & Moore, 1961); this is due to greater purity attained by the manufacturers.

Two other thiobarbiturates were later introduced into anaesthesia but abandoned after a time because of the high incidence of induction complications. Buthalitone, which had been synthesised by Miller et al (1936) was 'rediscovered' about 20 years later and introduced by Helmuth Weese, who had been involved with hexobarbitone (Weese & Koss, 1954). It was marketed for a short time under the names of Baytinal and Ulbreval in Germany and as Transithal in Britain. Although shorter acting than thiopentone, induction complications were unacceptably high. The other drug, methitural, embraced an interesting concept in its formulation by including a sulphur atom in the thioethyl side chain in the hope that this would accelerate its breakdown and at the same time liberate methionine, which would protect the liver from the toxic effects of the barbiturates (Zima et al, 1954; Dietmann, 1954; Reifferscheid & Dietmann, 1954). Its more rapid recovery, compared with thiopentone, was not confirmed (Wyant et al, 1958). After a brief period of clinical use in North America (as Neraval) and Germany (as Thiogenal), it was abandoned mainly because of the very turbulent induction.

Other avenues were explored unsuccessfully to find more acceptable barbiturates. These included the spirobarbiturates and spirothiobarbiturates (Swanson et al, 1950; Volpitto, 1951) in North America and the JL compounds in France (Buchel & Levy, 1951; 1953). Certain N-methyl and N-ethyl thiobarbiturates were described by Peel et al (1959) in Britain, but subsequently proved unacceptable in clinical use (Barron et al, 1961), as had other methyl thiobarbiturates (Stoelting, 1953).

NON-BARBITURATES

It had gradually become evident that further advances in intravenous anaesthetics were unlikely to come from the barbiturate (or thiobarbiturate) series of compounds. These drugs carry certain inherent disadvantages and research chemists have sought out non-barbiturate induction agents. One such drug was *Dolitrone*; early reports by Thompson et al (1954) and by Lundy (1954, 1955, 1956) suggested that it was primarily an analgesic, although anaesthesia could be produced with large doses. He even suggested that dolitrone might open up 'an era of general analgesia' and described its successful use in subhypnotic doses for such painful procedures as dressing of burns, haemorrhoidectomies and dental extractions. Subsequent studies by Tait and his colleagues (1956) did not confirm Lundy's favourable impression of dolitrone; analgesia was inconsistent and although induction was smooth and pleasant, recovery was delayed and coughing and laryngospasm occurred more frequently than with equivalent doses of thiopentone. Despite this outcome, tribute must be paid to Lundy for his prophetic vision of the role of analgesia in anaesthesia.

As the result of an investigation into shock caused by intravenous thiamine chlorhydrate, French workers identified an injectable derivative of the thiazole fraction with hypnotic and sedative properties (Charonnat et al, 1957). A clinical study of this compound, known as *SCTZ* was reported by Laborit and his colleagues from Paris in 1957; they found that although the drug would rapidiy produce sleep, the patient would continue to react to stimuli, no matter how deeply anaesthetised. An annotation (1957) in the British Medical Journal referred to SCTZ as "producing sleep without any degree of analgesia or anaesthesia". This description is fully borne out by the experience of Dundee (1958) who used it as an induction agent in 40 patients. He found that it was unbelievably difficult to produce any semblance to surgical anaesthesia in some of the patients, although they were undoubtedly asleep. Part of the difficulty miqht have been due to the very dilute solution (2%) and the need for large volumes, coupled with a prolonged induction time, but the lack of any element of analgesia was very apparent. More recently a more dilute (0.8%) solution has been introduced as *chlormethiazole*, and it is used as an anticonvulsant and in the treatment of alcoholism and psychosis. Its trade name, Heminevrin is indicative of its derivation from the Vitamin B molecule.

Eugenols

Eugenol, a phenoxyacetic acid derivative, is one of the chief constituents of oil of cloves and cinnamon leaf oil; it has been a domestic toothache remedy for many years. Workers at Geigy Laboratories in Basle (Switzerland) investigating several derivatives of eugenol during the 1950s found that some of them had general anaesthetic properties, but differed in effect from thiopentone. In particular, they stimulated respiration rather than depressed it, and recovery was very rapid due to enzymatic breakdown (Thuillier & Domenjoz, 1957). Their principal disadvantage was lack of stability in water.

The first clinically used eugenol was known principally as G 29 505, although one preparation named Estil was marketed for a short time in Germany (Simmer et al, 1960). The rapidity of recovery was confirmed (Feuerstein, 1957; Just et al, 1961; Swerdlow, 1961) and this suggested its potential use in outpatient anaesthesia. The problem of lack of solubility was never solved and available preparations caused an unacceptably high incidence of venous thrombosis. Even the use of an emulsion with a specially prepared lecithin was not acceptable. It was this, rather than the incidence of involuntary muscle movements (Dundee & Rajagopalan, 1962; Wright & Payne, 1962), which led to its abandonment.

A second eugenol, Propinol, was described by Nishimura in one Japanese publication in 1962 but did not warrant further study.

Research with the eugenols started at the Bayer Laboratories, Elberfeld, W. Germany in 1954 (Hiltmann et al, 1965); some 37 derivatives of phenoxyacetic acid were studied for brevity of action and lack of toxicity. As with the barbiturates, very slight modification resulted in compounds which caused convulsions. However, the outcome of this search was the drug known as propanidid (FBA 1340, Epontol, Fabontal) which was the first really acceptable non-barbiturate intravenous anaesthetic.

Over the years anaesthetists had built their induction techniques on the expected duration of action of thiopentone, and when propanidid was introduced its shorter action often led to problems. When the duration of action was extended by increasing the dose, the result was an increased incidence of hypotension. Furthermore a solubilizing agent, Cremophor EL, was required, giving a viscid sticky frothy solution. Despite these problems, propanidid enjoyed considerable success and perhaps this might have continued had Althesin not come on to the scene. Initially, propanidid was only used in Europe, but later its use spread to most of the world, except North America. A second problem was the occasional occurrence of profound cardiovascular depression. This might have been due to hypersensitivity or might simply have been dose-related toxicity in poor-risk patients (Chapters 14 and 18). As the shortest-acting of the available induction agents, it enjoyed limited popularity, particularly in outpatients, but it was withdrawn from use in 1983.

The eugenols introduced anaesthetists to solubilizing agents, made one aware of the possibility of hypersensitivity reactions and above all brought on the realisation of just how good an agent thiopentone is. Propanidid, however, did show that it was possible to find acceptable non-barbiturate induction agents.

Steroids

The hypnotic properties of steroids have been known for over 30 years since Hans Selye (1941) reported the occurrence of reversible unconsciousness in rats following the intraperitoneal injection of large quantities of several steroid hormones. He was favourably impressed by their lack of toxicity and in 1942 reported the results of a study of the anaesthetic properties of 75 different steroids. Pregnanedione, the most potent of these, was devoid of hormonal activity.

More than a decade was to pass before any practical development of this work emerged when P'An et al (1955) reported their animal experiments with *hydroxydione*. This anaesthetic was known as Viadril in North America and Britain, and as Presuren in Europe. Although it had a wider safety margin than thiopentone, there was a delay in onset of action, it was rather too long-lasting and followed by an unacceptably high incidence of thrombophlebitis (Murphy et al, 1955; Galley & Rooms, 1956; Lerman, 1956; Taylor & Shearer, 1956): the combination of these properties led to its abandonment in clinical practice.

Nevertheless hydroxydione possessed several good features which were sufficient for the pharmaceutical industry to retain some interest in steroid anaesthesia although it was obvious that the delayed onset of action would have to be overcome. Robertson & Wynn-Williams (1961) suggested that some metabolites of hydroxydione might be responsible for its anaesthetic activity, and although its major breakdown product, pregnanediolone, had anaesthetic properties it was too toxic for human use. A similar substituted water-soluble compound, GR 2/146, produced satisfactory anaesthesia in animals (Atkinson et al, 1965; Cocker et al, 1965), but on clinical trials many patients experienced disturbing paraesthesias which precluded its further clinical use (Sutton, 1972).

The lessons learnt from this experience were not lost, as workers at Glaxo Research Laboratories in England now understood the relationship between structure and anaesthetic activity of the steroids. Rapid onset and high anaesthetic, potency were associated with the presence of a free 3 α-hydroxyl group, but this posed problems of water solubility (Davis & Pearce, 1972). In continuing research alphaxalone (GR 2/234) showed promise as a safe, potent, rapidly-acting anaesthetic agent, but even the use of the non-ionic surface-active agent Cremophor EL did not solve the solubility problems. Fortunately the addition of a small amount of another steroid, alphadolone acetate (GR 2/1574), increased the solubility of alphaxalone more then threefold. Alphadolone is itself half as potent as alphaxalone as an anaesthetic and its action is additive in the mixture originally known as CT 1341 or commercially as Althesin or Alfathesin. It does not have an official name and is known either as aphaxalone/alphadolone or simply, as in this book, by its trade name, Althesin.

Althesin was an entirely British product, its pharmacological properties in animals having been described by workers from Glaxo Research Laboratories. Child and his colleagues (1971; 1972) found in mice that, like hydroxydione, it had a remarkably high therapeutic index compared with thiopentone. The initial clinical evaluation was carried out in Glasgow by Campbell and his colleagues (1971) and in Belfast (Clarke et al, 1971; Montgomery et al. 1971; Carson, 1972; Clarke et al, 1973). Althesin had proved to be a most acceptable induction agent, despite the use of a solvent, and it heralded the use of continuous infusion techniques which were later to be employed with other agents. Ramsay and colleagues (1974) from the London Hospital used it as a controllable sedative in an intensive therapy unit, while Savege et al (1975) from the same institution explored its potential in anaesthesia. This was the result of concern over pollution of the operating area atmosphere with anaesthetic gases and vapours.

The progress of Althesin was not without its difficulties. It has not been used in the USA presumably because of problems with the solvent. More seriously, it has been followed by a spate of reports of hypersensitivity reactions, which although not exclusively due to Althesin are more common with this agent than with thiopentone (Chapter 14). The first of these was by Horton from Cardiff in 1973, followed by a report of five cases by Avery & Evans in Southampton in the same year. It was obvious that a rapidly-acting, water-soluble steroid would be welcomed.

Tribute must be paid to the perseverance of the pharmaceutical industry in continuing the search for steroid anaesthetics. The seeming incompatibility of water-solubility and rapid onset of action was eventually overcome with minaxolone, which, in comparison to Althesin, was a single steroid (Davis et al, 1979). Its clinical evaluation was first carried out in a three centre collaborative study involving the London Hospital, Bristol Royal Infirmary and the Royal Infirmary, Glasgow (Aveling et al 1979a, b), but subsequent clinical use revealed certain problems during induction and recovery (McNeill et al, 1979; 1981). Research with minaxolone was discontinued for equivocal toxicological reasons after about 1200 administrations. Although we do not have a new intravenous steroid anaesthetic there are many lessons to be learnt from the minaxolone studies and these may eventually play their part in the search for the ideal intravenous anaesthetic (Dundee, 1981). The withdrawal of Althesin from clinical use in 1984, although regretted by many (Morgan & Whitwam, 1985) was not unexpected, but the drug continues to be used in veterinary practice.

Ketamine

Ketamine is the foremost of a group of drugs which produce of state quite different from conventional anaesthesia, characterized by hypertonus, light sedation, amnesia and marked analgesia, and in some ways resembles the effects of the neurolept drugs.

The drugs used in dissociative anaesthesia belong to the phenyl cyclohexamine group. It is not possible to discuss these independently from the development of the concept of dissociative anaesthesia as the history of each of them is intimately intertwined. There have been few branches of anaesthesia which have caused as much controversy as this concept and the drugs associated with it, and it has been difficult at times to separate fact from fiction. The search for an injectable water-soluble compound, stable in solution, with a long shelf-life, non-irritant on intravenous or intramuscular administration and producing smooth, rapid onset of action with minimal depressant effects on the cardiovascular and respiratory systems led to an investigation of the phencyclidine (CI 395, PCP sernyl) and its cognate CI 400, cyclohexamine. Studies in North America (Greifenstein et al, 1958; Collins et al, 1960) and in Britain (Johnstone et al, 1959) showed that though these drugs produced adequate anaesthesia they were followed by long-lasting psychomimetic activity which precluded their widespread clinical use.

Continuing research at the pharmacology laboratory of Parke Davis in Ann Arbor later led to the introduction of ketamine, its pharmacology first being reported by Graham Chen (1965) and Duncan A McCarthy and associates (1965). Their first description was that of a compound with a cataleptic, analgesic and anaesthetic action but without hypnotic properties. In 1969 Chen defined catalepsy as a "kinetic state with the loss of orthostatic reflexes without impairment of consciousness, in which the extremities appeared to be paralysed by motor and sensory failure". From this description one can see the problems which were involved in the introduction not only of a new drug but of a new concept. It was continuing pharmacological studies by Domino and his colleagues (1965) from Ann Arbor which led to ketamine being used in anaesthesia, while Corssen & Domino (1966) first coined the term 'dissociative anaesthesia' to describe a state characterised by complete analgesia combined with only superficial sleep (Corssen 1969). About the same time both the drug ketamine and the term 'dissociative anaesthesia' were used by European workers (Langrehr, 1969). There was much controversy before ketamine was introduced commercially in North America in 1970 and even more controversy when it was introduced into Britain in the same year without any preliminary clinical studies in that country. This was probably due to the manufacturer's description as a "rapidly-acting, non-barbiturate general anaesthetic" and suggestion that it would be useful for short procedures. This gave the impression that it was suitable in every way as a substitute for the well-established thiopentone and it was in this context that it underwent its first investigations in Britain. It soon became apparent that it was quite unacceptable as a routine substitute for the established drugs and that it was followed by an unacceptably high incidence of emergence delirium. We now know that this is partly due to the different regimens of premedication and the different duration of a 'short' operation in the two countries, and by an unfortunate coincidence its almost exclusive use was in unpremedicated women who would appear to be more than usually susceptible to disturbing emergence sequelae. One of the authors (JWD) was involved in this early study (Dundee et al, 1970) and this was an experience that he would never want to repeat. Undoubtedly this influenced the introduction of ketamine in Britain and it has taken many years before ketamine found an established, although limited place in anaesthetic practice.

It had taken most of a decade to appreciate that ketamine is not a drug which can be used routinely but which should be limited to conditions for which it is of specific benefit. Other avenues which have been explored for its use include continuous infusion of high (Lilburn et al, 1978) and low (Pandit et al, 1980) dosage.

Workers from the Department of Anesthesia and Pharmacology at the University of California in San Francisco have investigated the use of ketamine isomers in animals (Marietta et al, 1977; Ryder et al, 1978) and in man (White et al, 1980). This approach would seem to be worthy of further study.

Etomidate

Chemically this is a completely different compound from other intravenous anaesthetics which was developed in the research laboratories of Janssen Pharmaceutica at Beerse in Belgium and reported by Janssen and his colleagues in 1971. Known initially as R 26 490 (and subsequently given the trade name of Hypnomidate), its experimental pharmacology was described by Reneman & Janssen (1977).

The first clinical report on its use was by Doenicke and his colleagues from the surgical polyclinic in Munich in 1973 who described it as a pure hypnotic without analgesic activity. After several years of continuing experimental and clinical research this 'barbiturate-free' hypnotic was 'launched' at a Symposium at the 4th European Congress of Anaesthesiology in Madrid, in September 1974.

Early Continental European studies revealed two major disadvantages of etomidate — pain on intravenous injection and involuntary muscle movements (Doenicke, 1977a, b) and these have influenced its subsequent development. A multinational evaluation (Schuermans et al, 1978) described these as inconvenient, but not harmful, but despite claims of lesser cardiovascular toxicity, most anaesthetists would not equate it favourably with thiopentone as an induction agent (Dundee & Zacharias, 1979). Kalenda (1977) from Utrecht gave it in combination with fentanyl, actually referring to its use as " . . . an induction agent in fentanyl anaesthesia", and this has set the pattern for its use as an induction agent. Pretreatment with this short-acting opioid is now fairly standard practice with etomidate and is recommended in the promotional literature on the drug.

A continuous infusion, also known as total intravenous anaesthesia, is the alternative approach to the use of etomidate, and this eliminates the pain on administration. It appears to have been first used by Kay & Rolly at the University of Ghent (Belgium) in 1977. The first studies were in children (Kay, 1976; 1977a, b) but later were extended to adults (Kay & Rolly, 1977c). Here again it can be combined with fentanyl (Lees et al, 1981). Hitherto undescribed toxicological problems have arisen from the prolonged use of etomidate, particularly as a sedative-hypnotic in intensive therapy units, and the licencing authorities have withdrawn approval for this use in some countries.

Propofol

Propofol is the result of systematic investigation by the Department of Clinical Research at the laboratories of ICI Pharmaceuticals, who were looking for an agent which would produce rapid, smooth induction of anaesthesia with rapid metabolism, which would allow it to be used for maintenance of anaesthesia and which was free of the risk of anaphylactoid reaction (Stark, 1985). The discovery of anaesthetic activity of the alkyl phenols was described by James & Glen (1980) and from that research emerged the hindered phenol, 2-, 6 di-isopropyl phenol which was first known as ICI 35 868. This drug was first mentioned in the literature by Rhodes & Longshaw (1977) in their report of a study presented at a conference at Uppsala University, Sweden, in May 1977. A subsequent paper by Ian Glen (1980b) from ICI reported its pharmacology in detail while Adam et al (1980) described its pharmacokinetics in animals.

The first clinical trials of propofol were carried out in Belgium and reported by Kay & Rolly (1977a, b). This showed it to be a promising induction agent but with a problem relating to pain on injection. The Autumn 1979 meeting of the Anaesthetic Research Society had two British papers on the drug: its animal pharmacology (Glen, 1980a) and preliminary clinical results (Rogers et al, 1980a). This latter was a collaborative multicentre trial involving 20 patients from the Western Infirmary, Glasgow and the University Hospital of South Manchester. It supported the Belgian view that propofol is a promising compound, as did a further report by Rogers et al (1980b). These were subsequently confirmed by a number of clinical reports from Belfast (Briggs et al 1981a, b; 1982 a, c).

However, propofol is not soluble in water and the clinical trial preparation was solubilized with Cremophor EL. In the light of experience with Althesin and to a lesser extent with propanidid, it was not surprising that Briggs et al (1982b) reported a severe anaphylactic reaction following its use. Two subsequent reports led to the drug being withdrawn from clinical use in its original form. The drug has now been reformulated in an emulsion form and, at the time of writing, has undergone extensive clinical trials. It offers an alternative to thiopentone in a ready made solution.

CONTINUOUS INTRAVENOUS ANAESTHESIA

Despite the disastrous results when thiopentone had originally been used as the sole anaesthetic agent, infusions of it have been used off and on, mainly as anticonvulsants. In 1950 O'Donel Browne reported its use in eclampsia, but even then the toxicity of thiopentone was not fully appreciated: though the incidence of convulsions was markedly reduced, mortality was not lowered as barbiturate toxicity became the main cause of death. Grant & McNeilly (1953) have also described thiopentone infusions to control the convulsions of tetanus.

Concern over pollution of the operating room atmosphere with anaesthetic gas or vapours led Savege and his colleagues (1975) to explore the potential use of continuous infusions of Althesin as a means of maintaining sleep. Other workers from the same Institution — The London Hospital — had previously reported its use as a sedative in the intensive therapy unit (Ramsay et al, 1974) and in their hands it allowed rapid and excellent control of the level of sedation. This is an interesting concept and while it was made safer by the substitution of Althesin for thiopentone, nevertheless the lessons which have been learnt over many years will have to be borne in mind. Dechene (1977) added a new concept by combining the infusions with parenteral analgesics and this is evoking much interest at present. Knell

(1983) has shown that good results can be obtained by intermittent injection of methohexitone, ketamine and a relaxant, and techniques similar to this are widely used.

Interest continues in the use of barbiturate infusions for head injuries, although their efficacy is much in doubt. It was hoped that etomidate would prove to be the most suitable drug in this field, particularly after withdrawal of Althesin, but recent work throws doubt on this. Propofol may well fill this gap. The development of sophisticated infusion equipment may open up new vistas in this field which has not progressed as far as the original investigations would have led one to expect.

MORPHINE AND SIMILAR DRUGS

The anaesthetic and analgesic properties of opium have been recognized and utilized by the medical profession for more than 2000 years. Opium is obtained from the juice of the unripe seed head of the poppy plant, *Papaver somniferum*, the word opium being derived from the Greek word for juice. Opium contains at least 25 active alkaloids, of which only three, morphine, codeine and papaverine, remain in clinical use. The isolation by Sertümer in 1803 of morphine, which he named after Morpheus, the Greek god of dreams, and the subsequent discovery by Robiquet of codeine in 1832 and papaverine in 1848 paved the way for the controlled administration of opiates.

In the late 19th century morphine was frequently given intramuscularly for preoperative medication, as a supplement to ether or chloroform anaesthesia or for postoperative pain relief. One technique, popularised by Schneiderlin and others in Europe and the USA, involved intermittent intramuscular administration of large doses of morphine (up to 70 mg) and scopolamine as a complete anaesthetic. Not surprisingly, in view of the facilities and knowledge of resuscitation available at that time, several deaths occurred and the technique fell into deserved disrepute. Apart from the safety aspect, it fell far short of the standards of anaesthesia expected by modern surgeons; it was reported that only 70% of patients so treated needed restraint during surgery.

The use of morphine-like drugs virtually disappeared from anaesthetic practice for some 30 years. It was not until the 1940s that they again established an important role, with the introduction of the rapid acting barbiturates, which although inducing unconsciousness did not provide analgesia. An important development was the introduction of pethidine supplementation of nitrous oxide anaesthesia (Neff, Mayer and Perales, 1947; Mushin and Rendell-Baker, 1949). This may have stemmed from the concept of barbiturate–analgesic combination (thiopentone–nitrous oxide) as reported by Organe and Broad in 1938. Balanced anaesthesia as we know it today involving the use of an induction agent, a myoneural blocking drug and an opioid was probably first described by Mushin & Rendell-Baker (1949).

Pethidine, the first synthetic opioid, was synthetized by Eisleb and Schaumann in 1939. Since then many synthetic and semi-synthetic compounds have been produced. The most popular of these are the phenylpiperidine derivatives that include fentanyl and phenoperidine.

Workers in continental Europe advocated a state known as *artificial hiberation* produced by the lytic cocktail of Laborit & Huguenard in 1954. This lytic cocktail was a mixture of analgesics and tranquillizers and, although looked on at the time as something revolutionary, was really one of the many variations of balanced anaesthesia. This introduced the then new drug chlorpromazine and the allied phenothiazine, promethazine, into anaesthetic practice; the artificial hiberation technique enjoyed a considerable popularity in the 1954–1960 era. The mixture of chlorpromazine, pethidine and promethazine was used for intravenous induction of anaesthesia on occasions as sole anaesthetic but, while the concept remains, these drugs were replaced by more rapid and shorter-acting compounds and the term 'artificial hiberation' has been replaced by that of 'neurolept anaesthesia'.

The term '*neurolept analgesia*', indicating a state of apparent indifference to pain produced by a combination of a potent analgesic in neuroleptic or tranquilliser drugs, was first described by de Castro & Mundeleer in 1959. This varies from artificial hibernation in that the patient remains conscious but assumes a trance-like demeanour. It was possible for patients to undergo major operations without the need of any other form of anaesthesia; Nilsson & Janssen (1961) offered this as an alternative to general anaesthesia.

Tribute must be paid to Paul Janssen, who in 1966 had described the structure–activity relationships of neurolept drugs. Earlier on he had synthesized droperidol (Janssen et al, 1963) and this was the neurolept drug which was most popular in this technique. Larson & Duhr (1963) had pointed out that droperidol, if given alone, resulted in a patient indifferent to his environment, and apparently placid and drowsy although readily rousable. However there appeared to be a paradox, for although the subject seemed placid his or her subjective experience might have been one of agitation and apprehension (Hider, 1964) and may have included feelings of restlessness. This necessitated the concomitant use of analgesic drugs, hence the term 'neurolept analgesia'.

Around the same time the Janssen Laboratories had produced the potent narcotic, phenoperidine, and the even more potent fentanyl, and the scene was set for a useful combination of these in anaesthesia (Janssen, 1962). Since both droperidol and fentanyl (and phenoperidine) were manufactured by the same company it was not long before they were being marketed in a fixed combination under the trade name of Innovar (Thalamonal in Britain).

Neurolept analgesia eventually became neurolept anaesthesia, either by the use of larger doses of the drugs or by the concomitant use of inhalation agents and the next logical step was the addition of myoneural blocking drugs, making neurolept anaesthesia simply another form of balanced anaesthesia, differing little from that described by Gray & Rees (1952).

Myriads of drugs have been used in the various neurolept techniques and some of these will be described in Chapter 13. It suffices here to mention that the neurolept concept was first popularised in continental Europe — presumably because Janssen Laboratories is a Belgian firm. It was then introduced into North America where workers at the University of Pennsylvania did a comparative study of its safety and efficacy (Holderness et al, 1963). Except in some centres, its popularisation in Britain was slower, probably because the concept of balanced anaesthesia was already more firmly established there than in either Continental Europe or North America, and to many people the neurolept techniques seemed like a variation on a theme. In fact many now use small doses of droperidol or fentanyl as part of a balanced technique in which other established drugs are also used.

It is not surprising that the next step in this sequence was to use larger doses of narcotics as complete anaesthetics. The introduction of this concept can be attributed to a report by Lowenstein and his colleagues in 1969 in which they described the cardiovascular effects of doses of up to 1 mg kg^{-1} morphine in patients with severe heart disease, oxygen being used as carrier gas (Lowenstein et al, 1969). Stanley (1980) has pointed out that in fact morphine in doses of 1–3 mg kg^{-1} together with hyoscine 1–2 mg, given with oxygen, were used as a complete anaesthetic in the last two decades of the 19th Century. However a number of deaths caused most anaesthetists and surgeons to abandon the technique (Babcock, 1905; Van Hoosen, 1915; Boit, 1934).

The continued evaluation of large-dose narcotic techniques owes much to the enthusiasm of Ted Stanley from the University of Utah, who not only pioneered the clinical use of fentanyl as an alternative to morphine but also investigated the pharmacology of large doses of both morphine and fentanyl. These techniques have proved most useful in cardiac operations on poor risk patients. They have furthermore led to the concept of 'stress-free anaesthesia' which has certainly aroused much interest both among clinicians and pharmacologists. This emphasises the fundamental need for a narcotic element in clinical anaesthesia and the possible advantages from suppressing the normal humoral and cardiovascular effects to stress by the use of large doses of opioids. This would appear to be one of the fields in which intravenous anaesthesia is likely to develop in the future. Such advances are also tied up with the interest in continuous intravenous anaesthesia and the need to reduce pollution in the operating room atmosphere from gaseous or volatile agents.

TRANQUILLISERS AS INTRAVENOUS ANAESTHETICS/HYPNOTICS

The first use of these drugs was as preanaesthetic medication; in this capacity chlorpromazine and later other phenothiazines enjoyed a period of popularity in the late 1950s. The advent of chlordiazepoxide (Librium) followed by diazepam (Valium) gave fresh impetus to this concept and it is not surprising that diazepam was evaluated as a possible induction agent and as a parenteral hypnotic.

Much of the early work with diazepam was carried out in continental Europe (Randall et al, 1961) particularly with reference to its uses in psychiatry. Chlordiazepoxide had been discovered during a systematic search for an orally active muscle relaxant with mephenesin-like properties (Randall, 1982). It had been synthesized by Leo H. Sternbach of Hoffman-La Roche Laboratories, and it was a search for a similar compound with a less bitter taste that led to the synthesis of diazepam (Randall et al, 1961; Sternbach, 1982) which was first known as RO 52807.

As long ago as 1964 du Cailar et al and Aguado-Matorras & Aquerreta, both from France, reported their experience with a combination of diazepam and dextromoramide in what they termed 'neurolept analgesia' and in the same year Huguenard & Margelidon had emphasised the part that diazepam could play in this state (*induction de la neuroplégie — complement de l'analgésie periphérique*).

Diazepam was made available in parenteral injectable form in 1960. European studies by Campan & Espagno (1964) and by Blondeau (1965) suggested its value as an induction agent. The first reported use appears to have been by Farb (1963) who gave it as pre-interview medication in psychiatry. In 1965, Hendrickse & Sherman, working in Ibadan, Nigeria, and Kazim, working in Port of Spain, Trinidad, described its efficacy in relieving spasm in tetanus. The rapid muscle relaxation reported by the latter workers prompted Stovner & Endresen (1965) from Oslo to use it as an intravenous anaesthetic. They reported their findings in more detail in the following year and it was in 1966 that du Cailar and his colleagues studied *Utilisation du diazepam (Valium) comme agent narcotique d'induction au cours de narco-ataralgésie*. While these workers and McClish (1966) from Canada were very enthusiastic about its value, this was not shared by Cushman (1966) or by Brown & Dundee (1968), who found that it was probably too unreliable to replace orthodox intravenous anaesthetics. This controversy still persists more than a decade later.

It is in the field of sedation, particularly in dental practice, that intravenous diazepam would seem to have its main place. David Main and Ian Murray-Lawson from Dundee pioneered this work: they first used it for this purpose in 1966, giving it to the apprehensive wife of an anaesthetist (Main, 1968). This was followed by Keilty & Blackwood (1969) who emphasised its amnesic action.

It has also been used for cardioversion (Nutter & Massumi, 1965; Kernohan, 1966; Vinge, et al, 1971) and, not surprisingly, in labour (Bepko et al, 1965). Not only was its sedative and tranquillising effect beneficial here; but its anticonvulsant action was also put to use in the management of eclampsia (Lean & Ratnam, 1968). Unfortunately enthusiasm often outstripped knowledge of the basic pharmacology of the drug by obstetricians and there are many reports of depressed babies following the use of excessive doses: what might have been a useful technique has now fallen into disrepute.

There are few injectable benzodiazepines among the many compounds which have been synthesised. Lorazepam has too slow an onset and possibly too prolonged an action to be of value in the field of intravenous anaesthesia. The compound flunitrazepam was also developed by Roche Products and has had considerable clinical use. The early reports on its use in intravenous anaesthesia are difficult to interpret as in some studies other drugs have also been given (de Castro, 1972) or the reports are incomplete, inconclusive or based on too small a number of observations (Ungerer & Erasmus, 1973; Villand et al, 1973).

In general these reports showed a great similarity between the actions of diazepam and flunitrazepam (de Oliviera et al, 1973; Stovner et al, 1973). Dundee and his colleagues studied it as sole induction agent in 220 subjects in 1976 and convincingly concluded that flunitrazepam is not a very satisfactory drug for the induction of anaesthesia because, like diazepam, it is unreliable in use and recovery is too prolonged for routine use. Subsequent papers have often disagreed with this study but it has not always been clear whether these have included other drugs. A subsequent paper from the same Department (Clarke & Lyons, 1977) compared equipotent doses of induction agents for heavily premedicated patients having cardiac operations and could find no difference between the action of diazepam and flunitrazepam.

One of the more recent studies by Mattilla et al (1977) from Kuobio University Centre in Finland compares flunitrazepam with Althesin as induction agents in balanced anaesthesia and shows that when analgesics and other drugs are given then the benzodiazepines and orthodox induction agents are very similar, particularly in long operations. This point has not always been appreciated and might explain many of the apparently contradictory statements which have appeared in the literature.

There has been one crossover trial of comparison between flunitrazepam and diazepam in conservative dentistry (Dixon et al, 1980) carried out at University of Sheffield Medical School and this has shown no real difference between the two benzodiazepines. With the advent of a water-soluble benzodiazepine it is unlikely that flunitrazepam will play any further part in intravenous anaesthesia except in countries where it is already established.

The benzodiazepine which is likely to replace all others in anaesthetic practice is the water-soluble midazolam. This is also a product of Roche Research which was introduced around 1978 as RO 21–3981 (Conner et al, 1978). The first clinical report of its use was by Reves and his colleagues from Birmingham, Alabama (1978). Its evaluation in Britain was slightly delayed and the first report was from Belfast by Dundee and colleagues (1980).

The drug is now commercially available in Europe and Britain and reports suggest that it can rival diazepam in its versatility. Some workers recommend it as an induction agent, while others feel that it should be reserved for sedation. Early reports in this latter field are particularly promising. Kawar et al (1982) and McGimpsey et al (1983) found it very satisfactory in dental practice, and its use as sedative for endoscopy has been studied by Kawar et al (1983).

Others

A few other drugs such as *sodium gamma-hydroxybutyrate* (Gamma-OH) have been used as have some of the newer volatile inhalational agents, but these have played little or no part in the development of intravenous anaesthesia. A detailed discussion of the history of intravenous *alcohol* appeared in the first edition of this book: this drug played no part in the development of modern intravenous anaesthesia as in a subsequent re-evaluation it was 'weighed in the balance and found wanting'.

In prospect

The administration of suitable drugs by the intravenous route has played a very major part in making anaesthesia more acceptable to patients. Some feel that it might have lowered the standing of the administrator in the estimation of the patient as "anyone could give a simple injection". Compactness and simplicity of equipment were reasons given for its popularity in emergency situations and, as pointed out above, tragedies followed this use by untrained personnel. Certainly the appearance of an advertisement for trainee anesthesiologists in the US forces in the same issue of *Anesthesiology* as the Pearl Harbour reports suggests that intravenous anaesthesia showed the need for specialist anaesthetists and might have played a major part in the development of the specialty in North America.

At a conference on History of Modern Anaesthesia (Rotterdam, May 1982) Professor Emeritus Sir Robert Macintosh recalled the part it played in establishing academic anaesthesia in Britain. William Morris (later Lord Nuffield) was so impressed by his personal experience of an intravenous induction, as compared with a previous inhalation anaesthetic, that he insisted that his endowments to the University of Oxford should include a Chair in Anaesthetics. This was an unheard of precedent, but his persistence led to the establishment of the first academic Department of Anaesthesia in Britain.

REFERENCES

Adam H K Glen J B Hoyle P A 1980 Pharmacokinetics in laboratory animals of IC 35 868, a new i.v. anaesthetic agent. British Journal of Anaesthesia 52: 743–746

Adams R C, Gray H K 1943 Intravenous anesthesia with pentothal sodium in the case of gunshot wound associated with accompanying severe traumatic shock and loss of blood: report of a case. Anesthesiology 4: 70–73

Aguada-Matorras A, Aquerreta Mtz-Lagos E 1964 Neuroleptanalgésie avec Valium-Palfium (Neuroleptanalgésie with Valium plus Dextromoramide). Annales de l'anesthésiologie Française 5: 722–726

Annotation 1957 New cerebral depressant. British Medical Journal 2:152

Atkinson R M, Davis B, Bratt M A, Sharpe H M, Tomich E G 1965 Action of some steroids on the central nervous system of the mouse. II: Pharmacology. Journal of Medical Chemistry 8: 426–432

Aveling W, Chang H, Clements E, Waters A, Savege T M, Campbell D, Fitch W, Prys-Roberts C, Sear J W, Simpson P 1979a Early clinical evaluation of minaxolone, a new steroid intravenous anaesthetic agent. British Journal of Anaesthesia 5:564P

Aveling W, Sear J W, Fitch W, Chang H, Waters A, Cooper P, Simpson P, Savege T M, Prys-Roberts C, Campbell D 1979b Early clinical evaluation of minaxolone: a new intravenous steroid anaesthetic agent. Lancet 2: 71–73

Avery A F, Evans A 1973 Reactions to Althesin. British Journal of Anaesthesia 45: 301–303

Babcock W W 1905 A new method of surgical anesthesia. Proceedings of Philadelphia County Medical Society 26: 347–351

Bardet D 1921 Sur l'utilisation comme anésthésique générale, d'un produit nouveau, le diéthyl-diallyl-barbiturate de diéthylamine. Bulletin Général de Thérapeutique Médicale, Chirurgicale, Obstétricale et Pharmaceutique, 172: 27–33

Bardet D, Bardet G 1921 Contribution a l'étude des hypnotiques ureiques; action et utilisation du diéthyl-diallyl barbiturate de diéthylamine. Bullétin Général de Thérapeutique Médicale, Chircugicale, Obstétricale et Pharmaceutique 172: 173–205

Barran D A N, Wylie W D 1951 A clinical trial of sodium thioquinalbarbitone, a new barbiturate. Anaesthesia 6: 202–205

Barron D W, Dundee J W, King R 1961 Experiences with a new methyl-thiobarbiturate (B 137). Anesthesia and Analgesia . . . Current Researches 40:491

Behan R J 1920 Ethyl alcohol intravenously as postoperative sedative. American Journal of Surgery 69: 227–229

Bepko F, Lowe E, Waxman B 1965 Relief of the emotional factor in labor with parenterally administered diazepam. Obstetrics-Gynecology 26: 852–857

Bier A 1908 Ueber einen neuen Weg Localanaesthesia an den Gliedmassen zu erzeugen. Archiv fur Klinische Chirurgie, vereinigt mit Deutsche Zeitschrift fur Chirurgie 86:1007

Blondeau P 1965 Diazepam et anésthesie génerale. Cahiers d'Anesthesiologie 13: 207–217

Boit H 1934 Die Kombination von Skopolamin-Dilaudid mit ortlicher Betaubung und mit Evipankurznarkose bie mittleren und grossen Operationen. Zentralblatt fur Chirurgie 61: 1662–1664

Breimer D D 1976 Pharmacokinetics of methohexitone following intravenous infusion in humans. British Journal of Anaesthesia 48: 643–649

Briggs L P, Bahar M, Beers H T B, Clarke R S J, Dundee J W, Wright P J. McAuley D M, O'Neill M P 1982a Effect of preanaesthetic medication on anaesthesia with ICI 35 868. British Journal of Anaesthesia 54: 303–306

Briggs L P, Clarke R S J, Dundee J W, Moore J, Bahar M, Wright P J 1981 a Use of di-isopropyl phenol as main agent for short procedures. British Journal of Anaesthesia 53: 1197–1202

Briggs L P, Clarke R S J, Watkins J 1982b An adverse reaction to the administration of ICI 35 868 (Diprivan). Anaesthesia 37: 1099–1101

Briggs L P, Dundee J W, Bahar M, Clarke R S J 1982c Comparison of the effect of di-isopropyl phenol (ICI 35 868) and thiopentone on response to somatic pain. British Journal of Anaesthesia 54: 307–311

Briggs, L P, Dundee J W, Clarke R S J 1981b Some observations with di-isopropyl phenol (ICI 35 868). British Journal of Anaesthesia 53: 183P–184P

Brown S S, Dundee J W 1968 Clinical studies of induction agents. XXV: Diazepam. British Journal of Anaesthesia 40: 108–112

Buchel L, Levy J 1951 Sur deux nouvelles substances de la série des barbituriques et thiobarbituriques. Anesthésie et analgésie 8: 433–437

Buchel L, Levy J 1953 Sur un barbiturique à courte durée d'action. Anesthésie et Analgésie 10: 351–357

Bumm R 1927 Intravenous Narkosen mit Barbitursaurederivaten. Klinische Wochenschrift 6: 725–726

Burkhardt L 1909 Die intravenose Narkose mit Aether und Chloroform. Munchener medizinische Wochenschrift 2: 2365–2369

Campan L, Espagno, M-Th 1964 Note sur le diazepam en anesthésiologie. Annales de l'anesthésiologie Française 5: 711–720

Campbell D, Forrester A C, Miller D C, Hutton I, Kennedy J A, Lawrie, T D V, Lorimer A R, McCall D 1971 A preliminary clinical study of CT 1341 — a steroid Anaesthetic agent. British Journal of Anaesthesia 43: 14–24

Carrington H C, Raventos J 1946 Kemithal: a new intravenous anaesthetic. British Journal of Pharmacology 1: 215–224

Carson I W 1972 Group trial of Althesin as an intravenous anaesthetic. Postgraduate Medical Journal 48: 108–111

Carson I W, Graham J, Dundee J W 1975 Clinical studies of induction agents. XLIII: Recovery from Althesin — a comparative study with thiopentone and methohexitone. British Journal of Anaesthesia 47: 358–364

Carter M K 1951 The history of barbituric acid. Journal of Chemical Education 28: 524–526

Charonnat R, Lechat P, Chareton J 1957 Sur les propriétés

pharmacodynamiques d'un dérivé thiazolique l'ère note. Thérapie 12: 68–71

Chen G 1965 Evaluation of phencyclidine-type cataleptic activity. Archives Internationales de Pharmacodynamie et de Thérapie 157: 193–201

Chen G 1969 Pharmacology of ketamine. Anaesthesist 18:4

Chernish S M, Gruber C M, Demeyer M, Littlefield S, Stoelting V K 1956 Double blind comparison of compound 22451, pentothal and surital. Federation Proceedings 15:409

Child K J, Currie J P, Davis B, Dodds M G, Pearce D R, Twissell D F 1971 The pharmacological properties in animals of CT 1341 — a new steroid anaesthetic agent. British Journal of Anaesthesia 43: 2–13

Child K J, Davis B, Dodds M G and Twissell D J 1972 Anaesthetic, cardiovascular and respiratory effects of the new steroidal agent CT 1341: a comparison with other i.v. anaesthetic drugs in the unrestrained cat. British Journal of Pharmacology 46: 189–200

Clarke R S J, Dundee J W, Carson I W 1973 A new steroid anaesthetic — Althesin. Proceedings of the Royal Society of Medicine 66: 1027–1029

Clarke R S J, Lyons S M 1977 Diazepam and flunitrazepam as induction agents for cardiac general surgical operations. Acta Anaesthesiologica Scandinavica 21: 282–292

Clarke R S J, Montgomery S J, Dundee J W, Bovill J G 1971 Clinical studies of induction agents. XXIX: CT 1341, a new steroid anaesthetic. British Journal of Anaesthesia 43: 947–952

Cocker J D, Elks J, May P J, Nice F A, Phillips G H, Wall W F 1965 Action of some steroids on the central nervous system of the mouse. I: Synthetic methods. Journal of Medical Chemistry 8: 417–425

Collins V J, Gorospe C A, Rovenstine C A 1960 Intravenous non-barbiturate, non-narcotic analgesics. Preliminary studies 1: cyclohexyl amines. Current Researches in Anesthesia 39: 302–306

Conner J T, Katz R L, Pagano R R, Graham C W 1978 Ro 21–3981 for intravenous surgical premedication and induction of anaesthesia. Anesthesia and Analgesia . . . Current Researches 57: 1–5

Corssen G 1969 Allgemeine klinische Erfahrungen mit Ketamine bei mehr als 1500 Fällen. Anaesthesist 18:25

Corssen G, Domino E F 1966 Dissociative anesthesia: further pharmacologic studies and first clinical experience with the phencyclidine derivative CI 581. Anesthesia and Analgesia . . . Current Researches 45: 29

Cushman R P A 1966 Diazepam in intravenous anaesthesia. Lancet 1: 1042

Davis B, Dodds M C, Dolamore P G, Gardner C J, Sawyer P R, Twissell D J, Vallance D K 1979 Minaxolone: a new water-soluble steroid anaesthetic. British Journal of Anaesthesia 51: 564P

Davis B, Pearce D R 1972 An introduction to Althesin (CT 1341). Postgraduate Medical Journal 48: 13–17

De Castro J 1972 L'utilisation de la ketamine et du Ro 5–4200: 1/100 en anesthésie i.v. subvigile. Ars medici 27: 1286–1306

De Castro J, Mundeleer P 1959 Anesthésie sans sommeil 'La neuroleptanalgésie'. Acta Chirurgie Belgica 58:689

Dechene J P 1977 Alfathesin by continuous infusion supplemented with intermittent pentazocine. Canadian Anaesthetists' Society Journal 24: 702

De Oliviera A A M, Duarte D F, Gesser N, Linhares S 1973 Ro 5–4200 — Emprego em inducao anestesica. Revista Brasileira de Anestesiologia 23: 72–78

Dietmann K 1954 Uber die moderne Thiobarbiturat-Kurz-Narkese Weiterer Bericht über Thiogenal. Deutsche Medizinische Wochenschrift 79:1748

Dixon R A, Bennett N R, Harrison M J, Kenyon C, Thornton J A 1980 I.v. flunitrazepam and i.v. diazepam in conservative dentistry. British Journal of Anaesthesia 52: 517–525

Doenicke A 1977a Etomidate, a new hypnotic agent for intravenous application. In: Etomidate, an intravenous hypnotic agent. Springer, Berlin, p 25–30

Doenicke A 1977b Etomidate as a 'new drug in intravenous anaesthesia' (conclusion). In: Etomidate, an intravenous hypnotic agent. Springer, Berlin, p 152–155

Doenicke A, Kugler J, Penzel G, Laub M, Kalmar L, Killian I, Bezecny H 1973 Hirnfunktion und Toleranzbreite nach Etomidate einem neuen barbituratfreien i.v. applizierbaren Hypnoticum. Anaesthesist 22: 357–366

Domino E F, Chodoff P, Corssen G 1965 Pharmacologic effects of CI 581, a new dissociative anesthetic in man. Clinical Pharmacology and Therapeutics 6: 279–290

Dornette W H L 1954 From ampoule to beaker. Current Researches in Anesthesia 33:38

Du Cailar J, Gestin Y, Galibert A M 1966 Utilisation du diazepam (Valium) comme agent narcotique d'induction au cours de narco-ataralgésie. Annales de l'Anesthésiologie Française 7:203

Du Cailar J, Rioux J, Bellanger A, Grolleau D 1964 Utilisation du diazepam (Valium) en prémédication. Annales de l'anesthésiologie française 5:706

Dundee J W 1958 SCTZ — a new intravenous anaesthetic? British Journal of Anaesthesia 30:409

Dundee J W 1981 Editorial. Minaxolone and beyond. Anaesthesia 36: 579–581

Dundee J W 1984 Editorial. Fifty years of thiopentone. British Journal of Anaesthesia 56: 211–213

Dundee J W, George K A, Varadarajan C R, Clarke R S J, Nair S G 1976 Anaesthesia and amnesia with flunitrazepam. British Journal of Anaesthesia 48:266

Dundee J W, Knox J W D, Black G W, Moore J, Pandit S K, Bovill J G, Clarke R S J, Love S H S, Elliott J, Coppel D L 1970 Ketamine as an induction agent in anaesthetics. Lancet 1: 1370–1371

Dundee J W, Moore J 1961 Thiopentone and Methohexital. A comparison as main anaesthetic agents for a standard operation. Anaesthesia 16: 50–60

Dundee J W, Rajagopalan M S 1962 Clinical studies of induction agents. IV: A comparison of G 29505 and thiopentone as main anaesthetic agents for a standard operation. British Journal of Anaesthesia 34: 869–874

Dundee J W, Riding J E 1955 A clinical trial of thiamylal as an intravenous anaesthetic in 1750 cases. British Journal of Anaesthesia 27: 381–388

Dundee J W, Riding J E 1960 A comparison of Inactin and thiopentone as intravenous anaesthetics. British Journal of Anaesthesia 32: 206–218

Dundee J W, Samuel I 0, Wilson D B, Toner W, Howard P J 1980 Midazolam maleate: a water-soluble benzodiazepine: preliminary results. British Journal of Clinical Pharmacology 9: 305P–306P

Dundee J W, Zacharias M 1979 Etomidate. In: Dundee J W (ed) Current topics in anaesthesia. 1: Intravenous Anaesthetic Agents. Arnold, London, ch 6, p 46–66

Dwyer C S, Strout W G, Thomas B P 1953 Intravenous Avertin anesthesia. Anesthesiology 14: 291–298

Editorial 1943 The question of intravenous anesthesia in war surgery. Anesthesiology 4: 67–69
Eisleb O, Schaumann O 1939 Dolantin, ein neuartiges Spasmolytikum und Analgetikum (Chemisches und Pharmakologisches). Deutsche medizinische Wochenschrift 65: 967–968
Farb H H 1963 Intravenous diazepam as pre-interview medication. Diseases of the Nervous System 24: 233–236
Feuerstein V 1957 The intravenous anaesthetic G 29505: preliminary clinical notes. Anaesthesist 6:177
Fischer E, von Mering J 1903 Ueber eine neue Klasse vonSchlafmitteln. Therapie der Gegenwart 5: 97–101
Fitch R H, Waters R M, Tatum A L 1930 The intravenous use of the barbituric acid hypnotics in surgery. American Journal of Surgery 9: 110–114
Galley A H, Rooms M 1956 Intravenous steroid anaesthetic: experiences with Viadril. Lancet 1: 990–994
Glen J B 1980a The animal pharmacology of ICI 35868: a new i.v. anaesthetic agent. British Journal of Anaesthesia 52:230P
Glen J B 1980b Animal studies of the anaesthetic activity of ICI 35868. British Journal of Anaesthesia 52: 731–742
Goyanes J 1912 La anestesia per la via arterial. Revista de Clinica de Madrid 8: 401–422
Grant A P, McNeilly J W 1953 Treatment of tetanus with intravenous thiopentone and pethidine. Irish Journal of Medical Science, 6th series, 212–217
Gray T C, Rees G J 1952 The role of apnoea in anaesthesia for major surgery. British Medical Journal 2: 891–892
Greifenstein F E, Devault M, Voshitake J, Grejewski J E 1958 A study of l-aryl cyclohexylamine for anesthesia. Anesthesia and Analgesia . . . Current Researches 37:283
Halford F J 1943 A critique of intravenous anesthesia in war surgery. Anesthesiology 4: 67–69
Hendrickse R G, Sherman P M 1965 Therapeutic trial of diazepam in tetanus. Lancet 1: 737–738
Hider C F 1964 In: Shepherd N W (ed). The application of neuroleptanalgesia in anaesthetic and other practice. Pergamon Press, London, p.87
Hiltmann R, Wollweber H, Wirth W, Hoffmeister F 1965 Neue estergruppenhaltige Phenoxyessigsaüreamide mit narkotischer Wirksamkeit. In: Horatz K, Frey R, Zindler M (eds) Die intravenöse Kurznarkose mit dem neuen Phenoxyessigsaürederivat Propanidid (Epontol). Springer, Berlin, p 1–17
Holderness M C, Chase P E, Dripps R D 1963 A narcotic analgesic and a butyrophenone with nitrous oxide for general anaesthesia. Anesthesiology 24: 336
Horatz K, Sturtzbecher F 1952 Neue Hilfsmitel in der Anaestesie. Anaesthesist 1:149
Horton J N 1973 Adverse reaction to Althesin. Anaesthesia 28: 182–183
Huguenard J, Margelidon J B 1964 Deux indications particulieres du diazepam injectable. (Induction de la neuroplégie — complement de l'analgésie periphérique Annales de l'anesthésiologie francaise 5:731
James R, Glen J B 1980 Synthesis, biological evaluation and preliminary structure-activity considerations of a series of alkyphenols as intravenous anaesthetic agents. Journal of Medicinal Chemistry 23:1350
Janssen P A J 1962 A review of the chemical features associated with strong morphine-like activity. British Journal of Anaesthesia 34: 260–268
Janssen P A J 1966 The chemical anatomy of neuroleptic drugs. Sartryck ur Farmacevtisk Revy 65: 272–295
Janssen P A J, Niemegeers C J E, Schellekens K H L, Lenaerts F M 1971 Etomidate, R-(+)-l (α-methyl-benzyl) imidazole-5-carboxylate (R 16659), a potent short-acting and relatively atoxic intravenous hypnotic agent in rats. Arzneimittel-Forschung 21: 1234–43
Janssen P A J, Niemegeers C J E, Schellekens K H L, Verbruggen F J, Van Nueten J M 1963 The pharmacology of dehydrobenzperidol, a new potent and short-acting neuroleptic agent chemically related to haloperidol. Arzneimittel-Forschung 13: 205–211
Jarman R, Abel A L 1936 Intravenous anaesthesia with pentothal sodium. Lancet 1:230, 422–423.
Johnston M, Evans V, Baigel S 1959 Sernyl (CI-395) in clinical anaesthesia. British Journal of Anaesthesia 31: 433–439
Jolly C R, Lederer J 1955 Thioquinalbarbitone sodium. A clinical trial. Anaesthesia 10: 292–294
Just 0, Henschel W F, Nussgen W, Paul F 1961 Estil (2-methoxy-4-allylphenoxyacetic acid-N-N-diethylamide) a new type of non-barbiturate short-acting anaesthetic for intravenous use. Chirurgica 32:121
Kalenda Z 1977 The use of etomidate as an induction agent in fentanyl analgesia. In: Doenicke A (ed). Etomidate, an intravenous hypnotic agent. Springer, Berlin, p 130–139
Kawar P, McGimpsey J G, Gamble J A S, Browne E S, Dundee J W 1982 Midazolam as a sedative in dentistry. British Journal of Anaesthesia 54: 1137–1139
Kawar P, Porter K G, Hunter E K, McLaughlin J, Dundee J W 1983 Midazolam for upper gastrointestinal endoscopy. Annals of the Royal College of Surgeons of England 65: 283–285
Kay B 1976 A clinical assessment of the use of etomidate in children. British Journal of Anaesthesia 48: 207–211
Kay B 1977a Total intravenous anesthesia with etomidate. 1. A trial in children. Acta Anaesthesiologica Belgica 28: 107–113
Kay B 1977b Total intravenous anesthesia with etomidate. II: Evaluation of a practical technique for children. Acta Anaesthesiologica Belgica 28: 115–121
Kay B, Rolly G 1977a ICI 35 868, a new intravenous induction agent. Acta Anaesthesiologica Belgica 28: 303–316
Kay B, Rolly G 1977b ICI 35868 — the effect of a change of formulation on pain after intravenous injection. Acta Anaesthesiologica Belgica 28: 317–322
Kay B, Rolly G 1977c Total intravenous anesthesia with etomidate. III: Some observations in adults. Acta Anaesthesiologica Belgica 28: 157–164
Kazim E 1965 Diazepam in tetanus. Lancet 1:1162
Keilty S R, Blackwood S 1969 Sedation for conservative dentistry. British Journal of Clinical Practice 23: 365–357
Kendall J 1946 Barbituric acid. Journal of Chemical Education 23:2
Kernohan R J 1966 Diazepam in cardioversion. Lancet 1:718
Kirschner M 1929 Eine psycheschonende und steuerbare Form der Allgemeinbetaübung. Chirurgica 1: 673–682
Knell P J W 1983 Total intravenous anaesthesia by an intermittent technique. Use of methohexitone, ketamine and a muscle relaxant. Anaesthesia 38: 586–587
Krawkow N F 1908 Ueber die Hedonal-Chloroform-Narkose. Naunyn-Schmiedeberg's Archiv für experimentelle Pathologie and Pharmakologie, Suppl, 317–326
Laborit H, Coirault R, Damasio R, Gaujard R G, Laborit G, Fabrizy P, Charonnat R, Lechat P, Chareton J 1957 Sur un type nouveau d'anesthésie chirurgicale et sur l'emploi en thérapeutique d'un depresseur du cortex cerebral. Anesthésie, Analgésie, Réanimation 14: 384–411

Laborit H, Huguenard P 1954 Pratique de l'hibernothérapie en chirurgie et en medécine. Masson, Paris
Langrehr D 1969 Dissoziative anasthesie dürch Ketamine. Actuelle Chirurgie 4: 71–78
Larson A G, Duhr M B 1963 A new technique for inducing controlled hypotension. Lancet 1: 128–131
Lean T H, Ratnam S S 1968 The use of chlordiazepoxide in patients with severe pregnancy toxaemia (a preliminary study of effects on the newborn infant). Journal of Obstetrics and Gynaecology of the British Commonwealth 75: 853–855
Lees N W, Glasser J, McGroarty F J, Miller B M 1981 Etomidate and fentanyl for maintenance of anaesthesia. British Journal of Anaesthesia 53: 959–961
Lerman L H 1956 Viadril: new steroid anaesthetic. Preliminary Communication. British Medical Journal 2: 129–132
Lilburn J K, Moore J, Dundee J W 1978 Attempts to attenuate the cardio-stimulatory effects of ketamine. Anaesthesia 33: 499–505
Lowenstein E, Hallowell P, Levine F H, Daggett W M, Austen W G, Laver M B 1969 Cardiovascular response to large doses of intravenous morphine in man. New England Journal of Medicine 281: 1389–1393
Lundy J S 1935 Intravenous anesthesia: preliminary report of the use of two new thiobarbiturates. Proceedings of Staff Meetings of the Mayo Clinic 10: 534–543
Lundy J S 1954 Hope for an era of analgesia. Journal of the American Nurse Anesthetist 22:25
Lundy J S 1955 Development of analgesia after a century of anesthesia. Journal of the American Medical Association 157:1399
Lundy J S 1956 New drugs and an era of analgesia and amnesia. Journal of the American Medical Association 162:97
Lundy J S, Tovell R M 1934 Some of the newer local and general anesthetic agents. Methods of their administration. Northwest Medicine (Seattle) 33: 308–311
McCarthy D A, Chen G, Laump D H, Ensor C 1965 General anesthetic and other pharmacological properties of 2-(0-chlorophenyl)-2-methylamino cyclohexanone HCl (C1-581). Journal of New Drugs 5: 21–33
McClish A 1966 Diazepam as an intravenous induction agent for general anaesthesia. Canadian Anaesthetists' Society Journal 13: 562–575
McGimpsey J G, Kawar P, Gamble J A S, Browne E S, Dundee J W 1983 Midazolam in dentistry. British Dental Journal 155: 47–50
McNeill H G, Clarke R S J, Dundee J W, Briggs L P 1979 The influence of dosage and premedication on induction of anaesthesia with minaxolone. Acta Anaesthesiologica Belgica 30: 169–173
McNeill H G, Clarke R S J, Dundee J W, Briggs L P 1981 Minaxolone: an evaluation with and without premedication. Anaesthesia 36: 592–596
Main D M G 1968 The use of diazepam in dental anaesthetics. In: Knight P J, Burgess C G (eds). Diazepam in Anaesthesia, Wright, Bristol. pp. 85–87
Marietta M P, Way W L, Castagnoli N, Trevor A J 1977 On the pharmacology of the ketamine enantimorphs in the rat. Journal of Pharmacology and Experimental Therapeutics 202: 157–165
Mattila M A K, Martigainen P, Saila K 1977 Flunitrazepam compared with Althesin as an induction agent in balanced anaesthesia. British Journal of Anaesthesia 48: 1041–1046
Miller E, Munch J C, Crossley F S, Hartung W H 1936 Thiobarbiturates. Journal of the American Chemical Society 58: 1090–1091
Montgomery S J, Clarke R S J, Dundee J W, Bovill J G 1971 Clinical studies with a new steroid anaesthetic CT 1341. British Journal of Anaesthesia 43:718
Morgan M (ed) 1983 Total Intravenous Anaesthesia. Anaesthesia 38 suppl: 1–72
Morgan M, Whitwam J C 1985 Editorial: Althesin. Anaesthesia 40: 12–123
Murphy F J, Guadagni N P, De Bon F 1955 Use of steroid anesthesia in surgery. Journal of the American Medical Association 158: 1412–1414
Mushin W W, Rendell-Baker L 1949 Pethidine as a supplement to nitrous oxide anaesthesia. British Medical Journal 2:472
Neff W, Mayer E C, Perales M 1947 Nitrous oxide and oxygen anaesthesia with curare relaxation. California Medicine 66: 67–69
Nieschultz O 1953 Narkotische Wirkungen einiger Thiobarbitursauren. Arsneimittel-Forschung 4:411
Nilsson E, Janssen P 1961 Neuroleptanalgesia, an alternative to general anaesthesia. Acta Anaesthesiologica Scandinavica 5:73
Nishimura N 1962 On Propinal (2-M-4-P) a new intravenous, nonbarbiturate anesthetic agent. Anesthesia and Analgesia . . . Current Researches 41: 265–271
Noel H, Souttar H S 1913 The anaesthetic effects of the intravenous injection of paraldehyde. Annals of Surgery 57: 64–67.
Nutter D 0, Massumi R A 1965 Diazepam in cardioversion. New England Journal of Medicine 273: 650–651
O'Donel Browne 1950 The treatment of eclampsia. Journal of Obstetrics and Gynaecology of the British Empire 57: 773–582
Oré P C 1874 De l'anesthésie produite chez l'homme par les injections de chloral dans les veines. Comptes rendus des séances de l'Académie des sciences 78: 515–517; 651–654
Organe G S W, Broad R J B 1938 Pentothal with nitrous oxide and oxygen. Lancet 2: 1170–1172
P'An S Y, Gardocki J E, Hutcheon D E, Rudel H, Kodet M J, Laubach G D 1955 General anesthetic and other pharmacological properties of a soluble steroid, 21-hydroxypregnanedione sodium succinate. Journal of Pharmacology and Experimental Therapeutics 115: 432–441
Pandit S K, Kothary S P, Kumar S M 1980 Low-dose intravenous infusion technique with ketamine. Anesthesia 35: 669–675
Peck C H, Meltzer S J 1916 Anesthesia in human beings by intravenous injection of magnesium sulphate. Journal of the American Medical Association 67: 1131–1133
Peel M E, Macauley B, Collier H O, Hurst J H, Robinson F A, Taylor E P 1959 A new short-acting thiobarbiturate. Nature 183:1443
Pratt T W, Tatum A L, Hathaway H R, Waters R M 1936 Sodium ethyl (l-methyl butyl) thiobarbiturate: preliminary experimental and clinical study. American Journal of Surgery 31:464
Ramsay M A E, Savege T M, Simpson B R J, Goodwin R 1974 Controlled sedation with alphaxalone-alphadolone. British Medical Journal ii: 656–659
Randall L O 1982 Discovery of benzodiazepines. In: Usdin E, Skolnick P, Tallman J F Jr, Greenblatt D, Paul S M (eds). Pharmacology of Benzodiazepines. Macmillan, London, pp. 15–22

Randall L O, Heise G A, Schallek W, Bagdon R E, Banziger R, Boris A, Moe R A, Abrams A B 1961 Pharmacological and clinical studies on Valium, a new psychotherapeutic agent of the benzodiazepine class. Current Therapeutic Research, Clinical and Experimental 3: 405–425

Redish C H, Vore R E, Chernish S M, Gruber C M 1958 A comparison of thiopental sodium, methitural sodium and methohexital sodium in oral surgery patients. Oral Surgery 11: 603–616

Redonnet T A 1920 Recherches comparatives sur l'action pharmaco-dynamique des derives de l'acide barbiturique. Archives Internationales de Pharmacodynamie et de Therapie 25: 241–253

Rees G J, Gray T C 1950 Methyl-n-propyl ether. British Journal of Anaesthesia 22: 83–91

Reifferscheid M, Dietmann K 1954 Vorlaufige experimentell-klinische Untersuchungsergebnisse mit einem neuen kurzwirkenden Barbiturat. Deutzche Medizinische Wochenschrift 79:638

Reneman R S, Janssen P A J 1977 The experimental pharmacology of etomidate, a new potent, short-acting intravenous hypnotic. In: Doenicke A (ed) Etomidate, an intravenous hypnotic agent. Springer, Berlin, p 1–5

Reves J G, Corssen G, Holcomb C 1978 Comparison of two benzodiazepines for anaesthesia induction: midazolam and diazepam. Canadian Anaesthetists' Society Journal 25: 211–214.

Rhodes C, Longshaw S 1977 Autoradiographic distribution study of a short-acting anaesthetic ICI 35868. Acta pharmacologica et toxicologica 41: 132–3

Robertson J D, Wynn-Williams A 1961 Studies on clinical and pathological effects of hydroxydione. Anaesthesia 16: 389–409

Rogers K M, Adam H K, Dewar K M S, Kay B, McCubbin T D, Spence A A, Stephenson D 1980a ICI 35868, a new i.v. anaesthetic: preliminary findings in 20 patients. British Journal of Anaesthesia 52:230P

Rogers K M, Dewar K M S, McCubbin T D, Spence A A 1980b Preliminary experience with ICI 35868 as an i.v. induction agent: comparison with Althesin. British Journal of Anaesthesia 52: 807–810

Ryder S, Way W L, Trevor A J 1978 Comparative pharmacology of the optical isomers of ketamine in mice. European Journal of Pharmacology 49: 15–23

Rynd F 1845 Neuralgia — introduction of fluid to the nerve. Dublin Medical Press 13: 167–168

Savege T H, Ramsay M A E, Curran J P J, Cotter J, Walling P T, Simpson B R 1975 Intravenous anaesthesia by infusion. A technique using alphaxalone/alphadolone (Althesin). Anaesthesia 30: 757–764

Schuermans V, Dom J, Dony J, Scheijgrond H, Brugmans J 1978 Multinational evaluation of etomidate for anesthesia induction. Conclusions and consequences. Anaesthesist 27: 52–59

Selye H 1941 Anaesthetic effects of steroid hormones. Proceedings of the Society of Experimental Biology and Medicine 46:116

Selye H 1942 Studies concerning the correlation between anesthetic potency, hormonal activity and chemical structure among steroid compounds. Anesthesia and Analgesia . . . Current Researches 21: 41–47

Simmer H, Simmer I, Beck H 1960 Zum Nachweis des 2-Methoxy-4-allylphenoxyessigsau N,N-diathylamid in menschlichen substraten. Arzneimittel-Forschung 10:153

Stanley T H 1980 Narcotics as complete anesthetics. In: Aldrete J A and Stanley T H (eds). Trends in intravenous anesthesia. Year Book Medical Publishers, Chicago. p 367–384

Stark R D 1985 Opening remarks. Postgraduate Medical Journal 61 (Suppl 3):1

Sternbach L H 1982 The discovery of CNS active 1,4-benzodiazepines (chemistry) In: Usdin E, Skolnick P, Tallman J F Jr, Greenblatt D, Paul S M (eds) Pharmacology of Benzodiazepines, Macmillan, London, p 7–14

Stoelting V K 1953 Clinical use of newer intravenous barbiturates in anesthesiology. Current Researches in Anesthesia 32:270

Stoelting V K 1957 Use of a new intravenous oxygen barbiturate 25 398 for intravenous anesthesia. Anesthesia and Analgesia . . . Current Researches 36: 49–51

Stovner J, Endresen R 1965 Diazepam in intravenous anaesthesia. Lancet 2:1298

Stovner J, Endresen R 1966 Intravenous anaesthesia with diazepam. Proceedings of the 2nd European Congress of Anaesthesiology. Acta Anaesthesiologica Scandinavica, Supplement 24: 223–226

Stovner J, Endresen R, Osterud A 1973 Intravenous anaesthesia with a new benzodiazepine RO 5–4200. Acta anaesthesiologica Scandinavica 17: 163–169

Sutton J A 1972 A brief history of steroid anaesthesia before Althesin (CT 1341). Postgraduate Medical Journal, Supplement 2, 48: 9–13

Swanson E E, Mueller L B, Henderson F G, Chen K K 1950 Pharmacology of spiro-barbituric and spiro-thiobarbituric acids. Current Researches in Anesthesia 29: 89–96

Swerdlow M 1961 A new intravenous anaesthetic G 29 505. British Journal of Anaesthesia 33: 104–108

Tabern D L, Volwiler E H 1935 Sulfur-containing barbiturate hypnotics. Journal of the American Chemical Society 57: 1961–1963

Tait C A, Davis D A , Grosskreutz D C, Boniface K F 1956 A new intravenous anesthetic — Dolitrone. Anesthesiology 17: 536–546

Taylor N, Shearer W M 1956 The anaesthetic properties of 21-hydroxy pregnanedione sodium hemisuccinate (hydroxydione). British Journal of Anaesthesia 28: 67–69

Thompson G R, Smith J K, Werner H W 1954 Pharmacology of 5-ethyl-6-phenyl-m-thiazene-2-4-dione. Federation Proceedings 13:411

Thuillier M J, Domenjoz R 1957 Pharmacological aspects of intravenous anesthesia with 2-methoxy-4-allylphenoxyacetic acid (G 29 505). Anaesthesist 6: 163–167

Tovell R M, Anderson C C, Sadove M S, Artusio J F Jr, Papper E M, Coakley C S, Hudon F, Smith S M, Thomas G J 1955 A comparative clinical and statistical study of thiopental and thiamylal in human anesthesia. Anesthesiology 16: 910–926

Ungerer M J, Erasmus F R 1973 Evaluation of a new benzodiazepine, flunitrazepam (RO 5–4200) as an anaesthetic induction agents. South African Medical Journal 47: 787–790

Van Hoosen B 1915 Scopolamine-morphine anesthesia. House of Manz, Chicago, p 15–18

Villand J, Carli H, Klepping C 1973 Emergency oesophageal and gastric fibroscopy in 102 cases of upper gastro-intestinal haemorrhaging. Revue Française de Gastroenterologie 87: 77–85

Vinge L N, Wyant G M, Lopez J F 1971 Diazepam in

cardioversion. Canadian Anaesthetists' Society Journal 18: 166–171

Volpitto P P 1951 Experiences with ultra short-acting intravenous barbiturates combined with decamethonium bromide for endotracheal intubation. Anesthesiology 12: 648–655

Weese H, Koss F H 1954 A new ultra short-acting anaesthetic. Deutsche Medizinische Wochenschrift 79:601

Weese H, Scharpff W 1932 Evipan, ein neuartiges Einschlafmittel. Deutsche Medizinische Wochenschrift 58: 1205–1207

White P F, Ham J, Way W L, Trevor A J 1980 Pharmacology of ketamine isomers in surgical patients. Anesthesiology 52: 231–239

Whitwam J G 1976 Methohexitone. British Journal of Anaesthesia 48: 617–619

Wood A 1855 A new method of treating neuralgia by the direct application of opiates to the painful points. Edinburgh Medical and Surgical Journal 82: 265–281

Wren C 1665 An account of the rise and attempts of a way to convey liquors immediately into the mass of blood. Philosophical Transactions of the Royal Society of London 1: 128–130

Wright D A, Payne J P 1962 A clinical study of intravenous anaesthesia with a eugenol derivative G 29 505. British Journal of Anaesthesia 34: 379–385

Wyant G M, Chang C A 1959 Sodium methohexital: a clinical study. Canadian Anaesthetists' Society Journal 6: 40–50

Wyant G M, Chang C A, Aasheim G M 1958 Sodium methitural, a clinical study. Canadian Anaesthetists' Society Journal 5:262

Wyant G M, Barr J S 1980 Further comparative studies of sodium methohexital. Canadian Anaesthetists' Society Journal 7: 127–135

Zerfas L G, McCallum J T C 1929 Analgesic and anaesthetic properties of sodium isoamylethyl barbiturate: preliminary report. Journal of Indiana Medical Association 22: 47–50

Zima 0, von Werder F, Hotovy R 1954 Methylthioathyl 2 phenyl thiobarbitursaures natrium (Thiogenal) ein neues Kurznarcoticum. Anaesthesist 3: 244–245

ADDITIONAL READING

Adams R C 1944 Intravenous anesthesia. Hoeber, New York and London

Dundee J W, McIlroy P D A 1982 The history of the barbiturates. Anaesthesia 37: 726–734

Vandam L P 1982 The history of anesthesiology. Reprint series, part 12. Intravenous Anesthesia. Wood Library-Museum of Anesthesiology. American Society of Anesthesiologists

2

The intravenous route

The popularity of the intravenous route might be traced to two sources. First there is the patient who likes the pleasantness and speed of induction when compared to the application of a face mask and the inhalation of gases or vapours which might or might not have a distinctive odour, interpreted by him as pleasant or otherwise. Then there is the physician. With him the popularity of intravenous anaesthesia stems to a large extent from the apparent simplicity of the method and from the fact that a minimum of equipment and complicated apparatus is required to administer the anaesthetic. However, both these arguments are fallacious to a degree and indeed are not devoid of danger.

As far as the patient is concerned, a well-administered inhalation induction with a non-irritating drug can be a good deal more pleasant than innumerable unsuccessful attempts at venipuncture. Many intravenous anaesthetics are irritants to the subcutaneous tissues and extravasation therefore is painful: post-injection haematomata might develop, needles might break, and an intra-arterial injection even can place the limb in jeopardy, if not promptly and competently treated.

From the physician's point of view, the ease with which an intravenous drug can be introduced into the patient's circulation really constitutes one of its greatest hazards. The process of transfer of a gas or vapour from a reservoir bag to the brain via the airways, the alveolar membrane and the bloodstream with the complex mechanisms of diffusion gradients, distribution, solubility and so forth is bypassed when the intravenous route is used. Plasma levels of the drug are established with great rapidity, so that high concentrations of the drug suddenly exert their impact on the heart, the vasomotor, the respiratory and other vital centres. Though these effects tend to be transient where the systems are normal, in less than fit patients a vicious circle might be entered. Decreased venous return leads to a further fall in cardiac output, which in turn decreases coronary blood flow causing more hypotension with a fall in venous return, and so on.

Any overdose administered by the inhalation route can be corrected with relative ease by the simple expedient of ventilating the patient's lungs with gases not containing the offending anaesthetic, thus reversing the concentration gradient. No such mechanism within his immediate control is available to the anaesthetist in the case of parenterally administered drugs. Only after they have been redistributed or are broken down will the effect of an overdose or of any other untoward event be dissipated.

While the concentration of inhalation agents is adjusted as indicated by the clinical response, no such fine adjustment is available for intravenously administered agents. The time of onset of anaesthesia after an effective dose of an intravenous anaesthetic is roughly that of the arm-brain circulation. This rapid establishment of equilibrium between blood and brain is a pharmacological characteristic of intravenous anaesthetics almost as essential as short duration of action if intravenous anaesthesia is to be controllable (Butler, 1950). Even in fit patients, however, there is a wide variation in the arm-brain circulation time and therefore injection at a fixed rate is fraught with danger. The only safe procedure is to inject an initial small dose and to observe what time elapses before its effects are apparent, a similar interval being allowed for the appearance of action of subsequent doses. Repeated injections lead to an abrupt stepping up of the plasma level each time an injection is made. In this respect, too, intravenous anaesthesia differs from inhalation anaesthesia. A further safeguard of inhalation anaesthesia, not available in intravenous anaesthesia, is that undue depth of anaesthesia is associated with a diminished volume of respiration and with circulatory impairment which, at least in the presence of spontaneous respiration, will limit the amount of anaesthetic which can be taken up.

As far as simplicity of equipment is concerned, no intravenous anaesthetic should be administered without adequate facilities being available for access to the airway and for artificial ventilation. This in itself increases the need for apparatus beyond that of a mere syringe and a needle.

The advantage of the lack of irritation to the respiratory mucosa by intravenous anaesthetics also probably is more apparent than real, for the kind of patient in whom one fears unfavourable reaction to inhalation anaesthetics is the same who often produces problems with laryngospasm, bronchospasm, hiccup and coughing following injection of intravenous drugs.

Finally, the problem of cumulative action of intravenously administered anaesthetics and their breakdown products has to be considered as well as a greater likelihood that pathological conditions might interfere with redistribution and breakdown.

The rapid onset of anaesthesia with some intravenous agents leads to a more complete and sudden relaxation of the cardiac sphincter and loss of the protective reflexes. Thus the dangers of regurgitation and aspiration of intestinal contents might be enhanced when compared with conventional inhalation techniques.

NON-DRUG FACTORS INFLUENCING ONSET

Non-drug factors governing the onset of intravenous anaesthetics are of vital importance when rapidly acting drugs are used, particularly if intermittent injection techniques are employed. With adequate doses the all-important factor is the forearm blood flow, which depends on the cardiac output and the state of the peripheral circulation.

Cardiac output is decreased in cardiac disease and in circulatory failure, and it is well known that the onset of action of thiopentone is slower than normal in subjects with these conditions. Although it will be increased in thyrotoxicosis and severe anaemia, as well as after exercise, these are not likely to noticeably affect the rate of onset of intravenous drugs.

Pathological narrowing of vessels is a less likely cause of delay in onset of action of drugs than inadvertent partial occlusion of blood flow by tight clothing or an improperly released tourniquet. In clinical practice the effect of the environmental temperature is of great importance and is often forgotten. Studies carried out by Dundee (1957) in two adjoining hospitals, one with and one without air conditioning, during a hot Philadelphia summer illustrate this point. Injections were given over two to three seconds and the time noted from the end of injection until the patient stopped counting. Average times (in seconds) for doses in excess of 3.5 mg per kg, which would be expected to produce sleep consistently with both thiopentone and pentobarbitone were as shown in Table 2.1.

Table 2.1 Average time (seconds) for onset of action of drugs

Room temperature	*Thiopentone*	*Pentobarbitone*
22–23°C	19.7	33.2
29–32°C	14.9	21.2

Tests carried out on the scatter of readings showed that temperature differences of this order produced a statistically significant effect on the onset of action of both drugs. That this was due to peripheral vasodilatation was demonstrated by injecting thiopentone at the lower environmental temperature during the period of reactive hyperaemia which follows release of an arterial tourniquet. As shown in Figure 2.1 this reduces the rate of onset to that found at the higher temperatures.

As a side issue, it is worth noting the short time of onset of methohexitone and thiopentone following rapid injection of varying doses during the period of post-tourniquet reactive hyperaemia (Clarke *et al.*, 1968). The data in Table 2.1 show what might be expected at high environmental

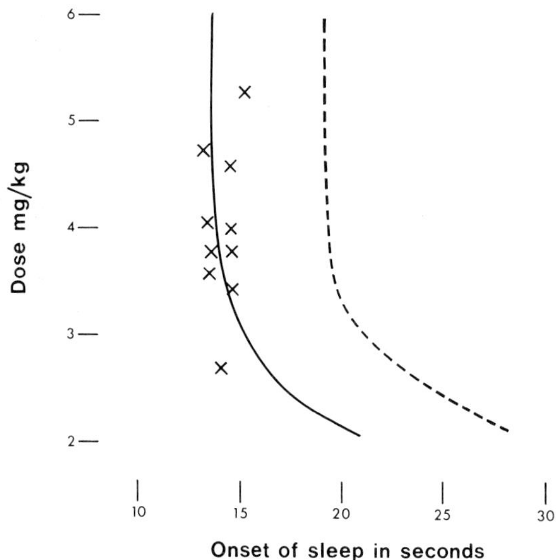

Fig. 2.1 Time of onset action — as judged by patient stopping counting — of varying doses of thiopentone at two environmental temperatures. Solid line = 29 to 32°C. Broken line = 22 to 23°C. X = times recorded during the period of reactive hyperaemia which followed release of an arterial tourniquet; environmental temperature 22 to 23°C. (Dundee, 1957)

temperatures and demonstrate that these drugs are truly rapidly acting.

ANATOMY

The veins of the upper extremity

We shall concern ourselves here only with those veins which are of importance to the anaesthetist in relation to the administration of intravenous anaesthetics and other drugs. For all practical purposes, we shall therefore consider the cephalic and basilic systems, and the subclavian vein.

The cephalic vein arises from the dorsal venous network of the hand which in turn collects blood from the digital veins. The dorsal venous network is arranged in an irregular fashion and drains into both the cephalic and basilic veins. The cephalic vein originates at the radial border of the wrist and winds around the radial border of the forearm. It crosses in the groove between the biceps and the brachioradialis muscles, to ascend along the lateral border of the biceps until it pierces the clavipectoral fascia between the pectoralis major and deltoid muscles. It then joins the axillary vein.

The basilic vein originates from the ulnar portion of the dorsal venous network and, ascending on the posterior surface of the ulnar side of the forearm, winds around the ulna to the anterior surface of the elbow, where it ascends between the biceps and pronator teres muscles and crosses the brachial artery superficial to the lacertus fibrosus or bicipital aponeurosis. Thence it runs upward along the medial border of the biceps to perforate the deep fascia just distal to the middle of the arm. At the lower border of the teres major muscle it forms the axillary vein by merging with the brachial vein.

The median antebrachial vein drains the volar venous plexus of the hand, ascends on the ulnar side of the forearm to enter either the basilic or the *median cubital vein*, which is a branch of the cephalic vein crossing in front of the elbow to join the basilic vein.

All anatomical relations of these veins important to the anaesthetist occur in front of the elbow joint where the cephalic vein crosses superficial to the musculocutaneous nerve, while the basilic vein and median cubital veins relate to the brachial artery which is immediately deep but separated from them by the lacertus fibrosus. In this location also filaments of the medial antebrachial cutaneous nerve pass both in front and behind the basilic vein.

The subclavian vein is a continuation of the axillary vein and extends from the border of the first rib to the sternal end of the clavicle. There it unites with the internal jugular vein to form the innominate vein. It has the clavicle and subclavius muscle in front and the subclavian artery behind and above. The scalenus anterior muscle and the phrenic nerve are interposed between artery and vein. Below it are the first rib and the pleura.

No attempt is made in this short description to detail the tributaries to the system nor any other anatomical relationships not of direct interest to the anaesthetist.

The antecubital fossa (Figs 2.2, 2.3)

Some of the important anatomical relations of the superficial veins with other structures have already been sketched, but because of their complexity and special interest to the anaesthetist they will be

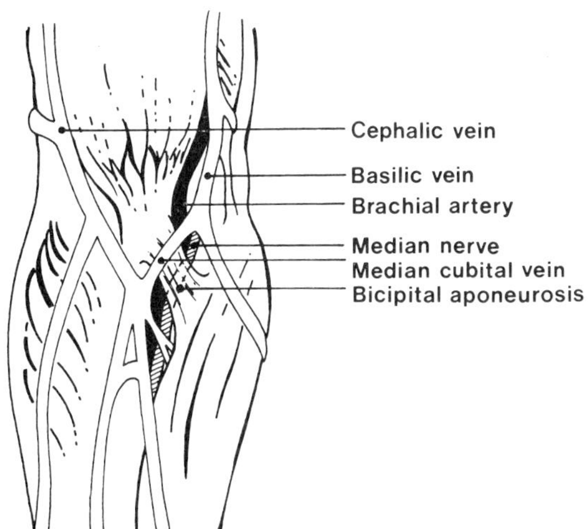

Fig. 2.2 Superficial veins in the right antecubital fossa.

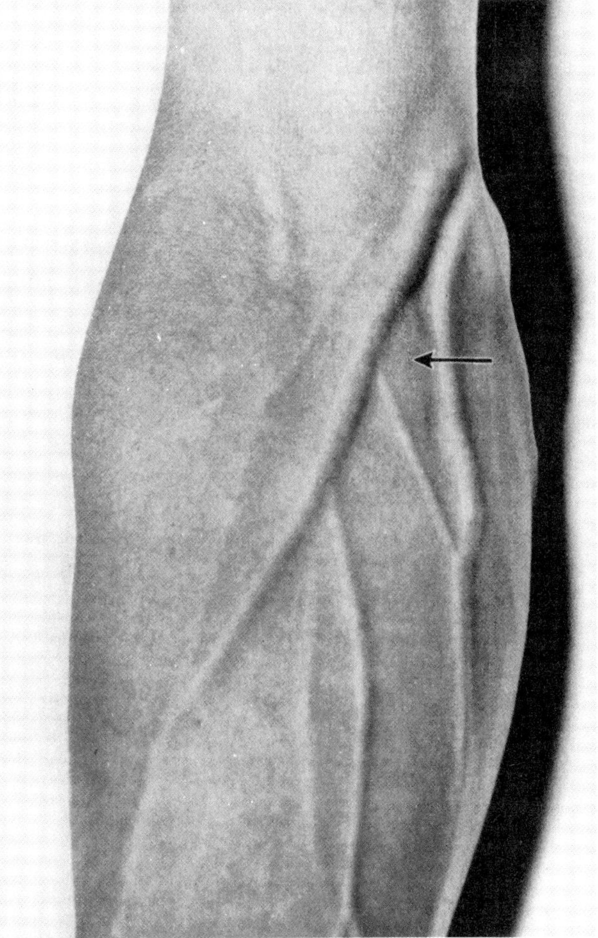

Fig. 2.3 Antecubital fossa showing veins distended by rubber band. Arrow indicates superficial ulnar artery. Gliding of needle to enter medial basilic vein may lead to puncture of the artery. (Cohen, 1948)

considered now in the context of the antecubital fossa.

The antecubital fossa at the bend of the elbow is a triangular space with the base proximal and coinciding with a line connecting the epicondyles of the humerus. The lateral side of the triangle is formed by the brachioradialis and the medial border by the pronator teres. The floor of the space is formed by the brachialis and supinator muscles. The brachial artery, accompanied by its veins, occupies the middle of the space and at the level of the neck of the radius divides into radial and ulnar arteries. The median nerve lies close to the artery on its medial side in the proximal part of the space but is separated from it distally by the ulnar head of the pronator teres. The biceps tendon is situated lateral to the artery. Overlying the artery is the median cubital vein which is separated from it by the lacertus fibrosus. While the vicinity of the median cubital vein and the basilic vein to the brachial artery and median nerve constitutes a hazard, even more important is the occasional occurrence of a superficial ulnar artery, arising higher in the upper arm, which on occasion penetrates the deep fascia, coming to lie subcutaneously in the region of the antecubital fossa (Cohen, 1948). This abnormality, when it exists, constitutes a major hazard to the use of the antecubital fossa for the injection of drugs, since the anomalous ulnar artery is situated immediately beneath the median cubital vein and above the lacertus fibrosus and thus unprotected by it (Fig. 2.3). When therefore the antecubital fossa is chosen for injection, the basilic or median cubital veins should be avoided because of their vicinity to these important structures.

TECHNIQUE

Any vein which happens to be accessible can be used for the administration of intravenous anaesthetics. However, when a choice presents itself, a number of factors should be taken into consideration in selecting the actual site for injection. Some such factors are anatomical ones, particularly the presence of other structures which might be injured by the venipuncture, the size of the vein, its support by surrounding connective tissue, the ability or otherwise to immobilise the part without undue discomfort to the patient, the different degrees of pain engendered by needle puncture in different areas, etc. Some agents, such as diazepam, cause pain on injection unless this is made into a fairly large vein. Others tend to sclerose small veins and again the injection should be made into a more proximal large vein. As pointed out previously, the antecubital fossa, which is so often used for the purpose, is in reality a relatively unsuitable site because of the vicinity of the median nerve and brachial artery and the possibility of the presence of an anomalous ulnar artery which, with the application of a tourniquet, might cease to pulsate. Also, if a needle is used rather than a plastic catheter and is left in place, the arm must be immobilised for long periods of time. Venipuncture at the dorsum of the hand is painful and the injection of irritating substances such as thiopentone might lead to fibrosis of the small muscles of the hand. This complication has been attributed also to retrograde distribution into the arterial system caused by the damming-back effect of the tourniquet. Baillie (1958) has described the accidental intra-arterial injection of thiopentone on the back of the hand, and in one instance arterial blood, as determined by blood gas measurements, has been obtained from a puncture at the dorsum of the hand by Ready (1972) in one of our Departments.

The sites of choice, provided adequate superficial veins are available, are the veins in the forearm where flow is good and immobilisation is not required. However, the danger of accidental arterial injection must be kept in mind even in this situation, where it has occurred into a duplicated radial artery (Deshpande, 1967). The use of veins of the foot and leg is discouraged because of their susceptibility to phlebitis and they should not be used unless this is the only avenue to the venous system which is available. Other sites of injection which may be used are the superficial jugular and the subclavian vein. The latter can be entered frequently when no other veins are available since it does not collapse when flow is reduced. However, puncture of this vein might lead to complications specific to its anatomical relationship. Pneumothorax is one such complication and we have seen one case of hydrothorax where the contents of an entire intravenous infusion of 1000 ml had been deposited *in toto* into the ipsilateral pleural space.

Venipuncture for the purpose of injecting substances differs from that done merely to remove a sample of blood. In the latter case entry into the vein is maintained only momentarily and it matters little if part of the bevel of the needle rests outside the vein as long as sufficient blood can be aspirated into the sampling syringe. In contrast, the same situation during injection would lead to extravasation and must be avoided at all cost. In order to achieve this end the puncture is made at a more acute angle to the skin and as much in line as possible with the general direction of the vein. After entry into the vein has been made, the needle or plastic cannula is advanced gently within its lumen for some distance. This manœuvre can be facilitated by the simultaneous injection of saline in order to dilate the vein just ahead of the advancing point. Active spasm can be overcome by substituting small amounts of local anaesthetic for the saline. There is not only increased stability assured by advancing the needle or cannula within the vein, but also the likelihood of leakage of solution back past the hole in the vein alongside the needle is minimised.

Where the external diameter of the needle tends to approach that of the vein, partial extrusion of the bevel can be prevented by entering the vein with the bevel downwards, that is parallel to the wall of the vein, and then rotating it back into the usual position while dilating the vein from within by the injection of saline against a lightly applied tourniquet (Fig. 2.4).

Finally, in securing the needle or cannula to the skin, a figure-of-eight sling of narrow adhesive tape applied around the hub will lend stability to the system and will limit lateral mobility.

DELIVERY SYSTEMS

Many different systems of delivering intravenous anaesthetics and supplemental drugs have been

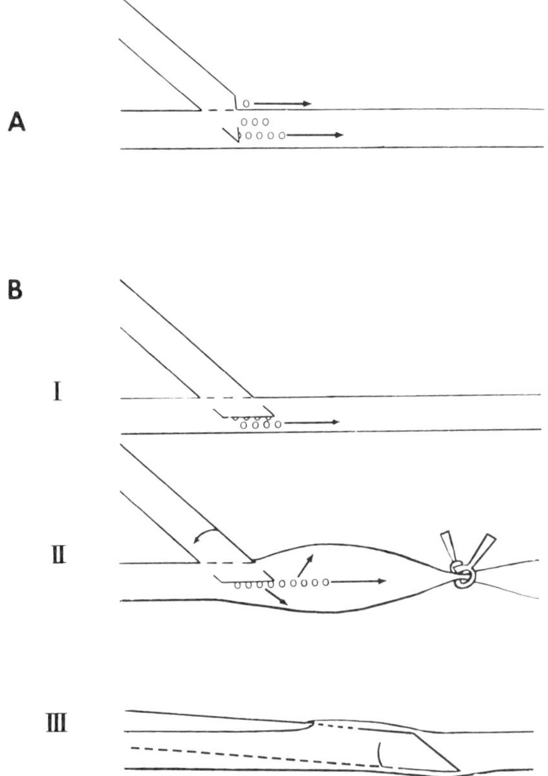

Fig. 2.4 A. Partial extrusion of the bevel of a needle the size of which approaches the diameter of the vein.
B. I. With the bevel pointing downward — no difficulty is experienced placing it entirely within the lumen of the vein.
B. II. With a tourniquet applied and simultaneous injection through the needle, the vein is being distended to allow rotation of the needle into the 'bevel-up' position.
B. III. The needle is lying bevel-up within the lumen of the vein which is stretched over it.

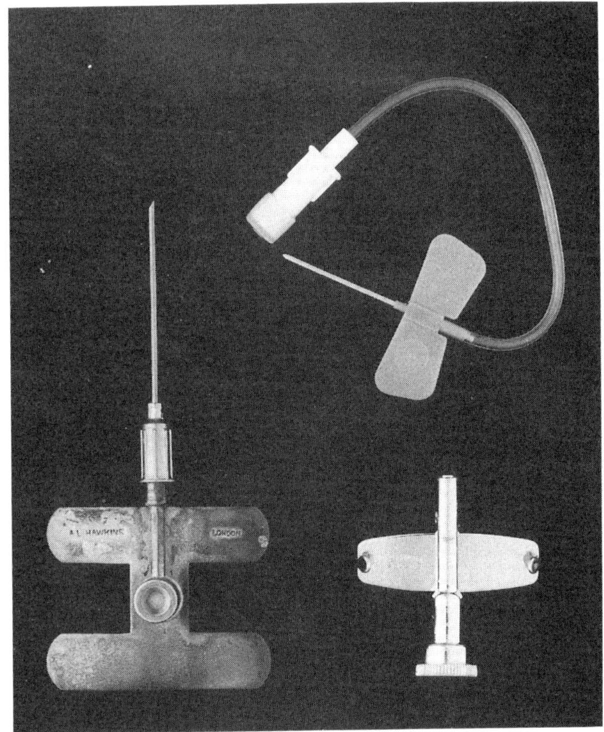

Fig. 2.5 Various modifications of the Gordh principle, including a butterfly (Abbott) intermittent injection needle.

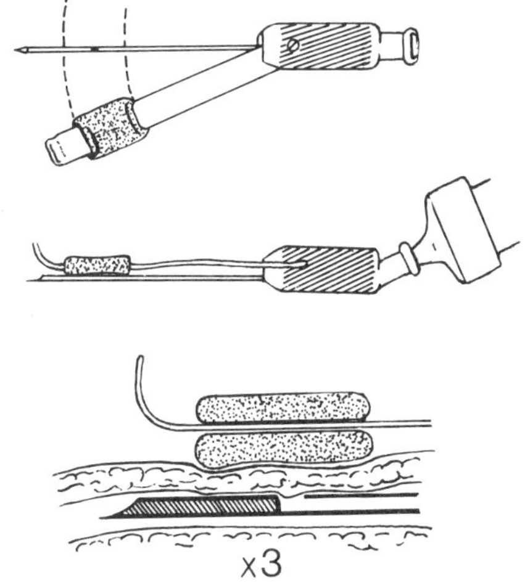

Fig. 2.6 The Mitchell self-sealing needle. (Mitchell, 1952).

developed and have been described in the literature over the years. Many of these have proven rather too complicated for what is, in the last analysis, a relatively simple situation.

By and large the delivery of intravenous drugs can be divided into single injections in which a needle, attached to a syringe, is inserted into a vein, the injection made and the needle then withdrawn. An alternative to this is the establishment of a more lasting avenue into the venous system either by means of an indwelling needle or cannula which remains *in situ* until the need for intravenous medication of any kind no longer exists. Whenever possible this is achieved by percutaneous puncture, rather than by venous cutdown. Continuous or intermittent injection can be accomplished in one of two different ways. It may consist of an intravenous drip infusion of either the dilute anaesthetic itself or some non-anaesthetic substance such as a crystalloid solution. Most infusion sets are provided with special injection sites into which supplemental injections of drugs may be made. The other system of establishing and retaining entry into the veins is that of using a needle closed off when not in use and into which injections can be made from time to time if and when required. Such systems are represented by the types of needles described by Gordh (1945) and by Mitchell (1952) as illustrated in Figures 2.5 and 2.6.

In recent years the steel needle has been largely replaced by the intravenous plastic catheter of which many diverse models are available (Figs 2.7 and 2.8). They are particularly useful when infusions are maintained over any period of time

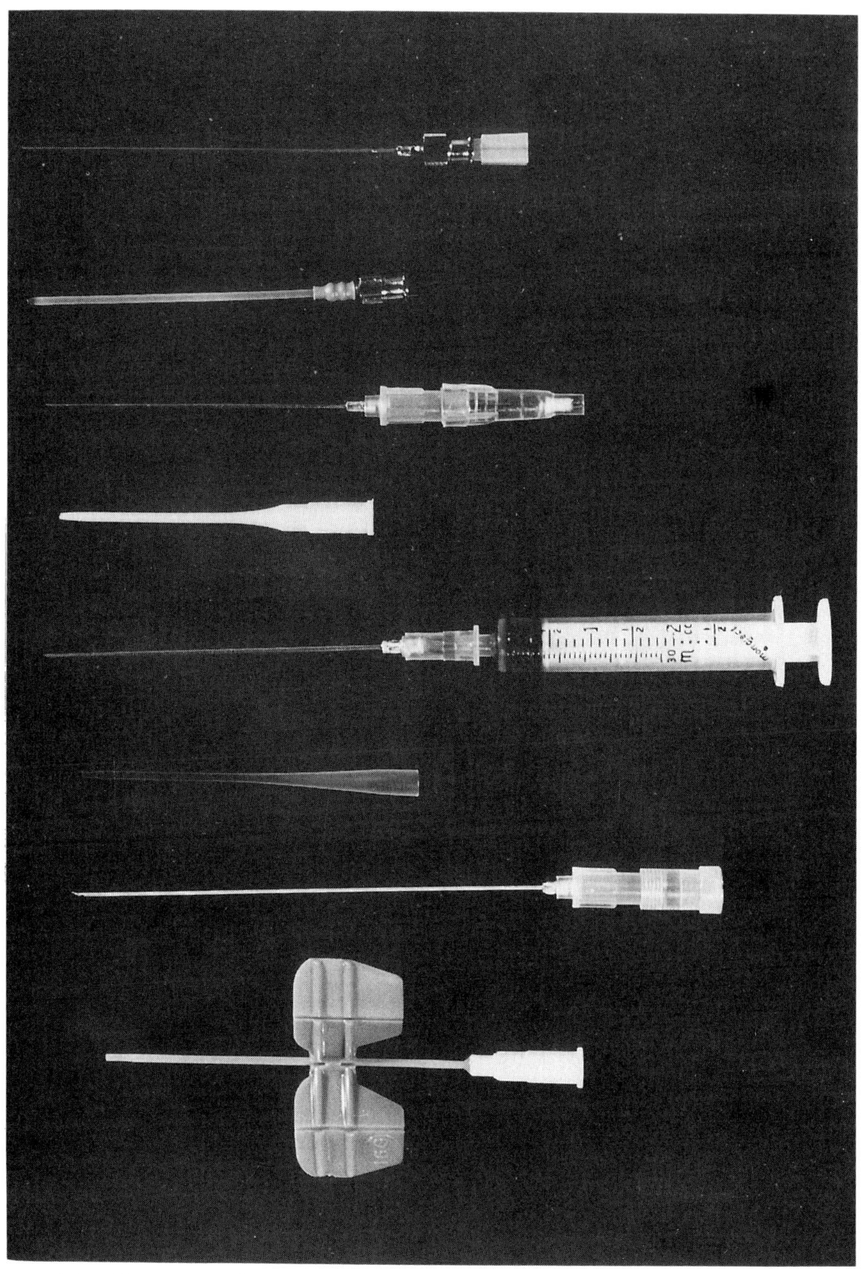

Fig. 2.7. Various models of intravenous plastic cannulae, showing the plastic sheaths removed from their respective introducers.

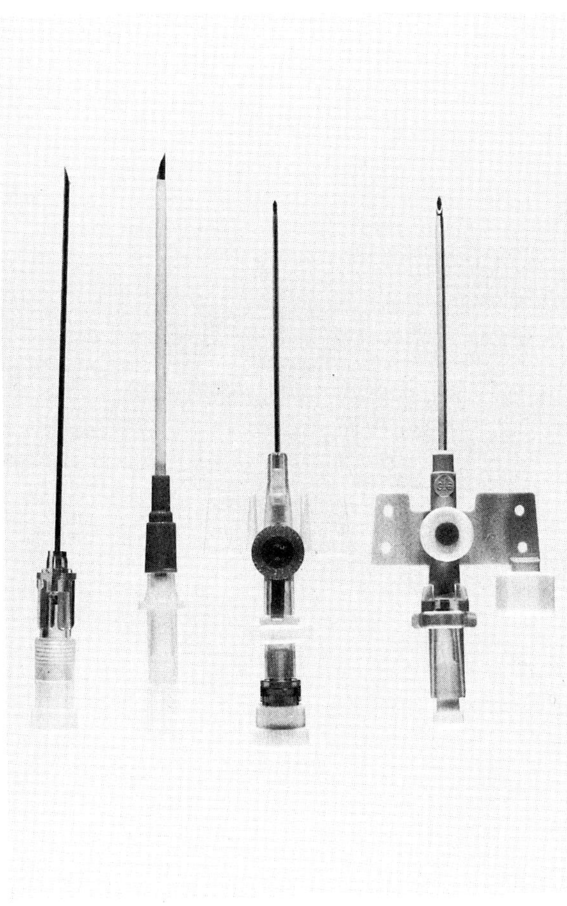

Fig. 2.8 Other intravenous plastic cannulae.

or where the infusion site cannot be kept under constant observation, as for instance during operations with the arm at the patient's side and covered by drapes. Of all the models available, the 'Butterfly' has proven the most popular over the years.

While no doubt many of these catheters are more irritating to veins than their counterparts (Thomas, Evers and Racz, 1970), once introduced, they have the principal advantage over the needle that interstitial infiltration is not likely to occur. There is evidence that the duration of infusion (Medical Research Council Report, 1957) and the site of placement of the catheter (Fonkalsrud *et al.*, 1968) are factors which influence the degree of venous irritation. Although Jones and Craig (1972) found that the highest incidence of venous reaction occurred with polyvinylchloride and less with the use of either polypropylene, TFE-Teflon or FEP-Teflon, they concluded that differences were clinically not important. It is of course well known that agents administered intravenously play as major part in the causation of local venous reactions, irrespective of any factors relating to either needle or cannula (Hästbacka *et al.*, 1965; Thomas *et al.*, 1970). There is a remote possibility of breakage of plastic cannulae and to facilitate their location in the body a radio-opaque strip is incorporated into the wall of most of these. There is also a risk of shearing off part of a cannula by reinserting the introducing needle through the lumen and this practice should be avoided.

In selecting needles or catheters, cognisance must be taken of the fact that they invariably are the narrowest parts of any infusion systems and thus determine the resistance to flow in the entire system by the power of four of the internal radius. Therefore, if administration of a substance of higher viscosity is contemplated, an attempt must be made not to impede unduly its flow by choosing a needle or cannula of too narrow a gauge. The more complex delivery systems used in continuous intravenous anaesthesia will be discussed in Chapter 17.

REFERENCES

Baillie T W 1958 Accidental intra-arterial administration of thiopentone on the back of the hand. British Journal of Anaesthesia 30: 373–374

Butler T C 1950 The rate of penetration of barbituric acid derivatives into the brain. Journal of Pharmacology and Experimental Therapeutics 100: 219–226

Clarke R S J, Dundee J W, Barron D W, McArdle L, Howard P J 1968 Clinical studies of induction agents. XXVI: The relative potencies of thiopentone, methohexitone and propanidid. British Journal of Anaesthesia 40: 593–601

Cohen S M 1948 Accidental intra-arterial injection of drugs. Lancet ii: 409–416

Deshpande A M 1967 Accidental injection of thialbarbitone into an anomalous radial artery. British Journal of Anaesthesia 39: 83–85

Dundee J W 1957 Abnormal responses to barbiturates. British Journal of Anaesthesia 29: 440–446

Fonkalsrud E W, Pederson B M, Murphy J, Beckerman J H 1968 Reduction of infusion thrombophlebitis with buffered glucose solutions. Surgery 63: 280–284

Gordh T 1945 A new, simple and practical needle for intravenous anesthesia. Anesthesiology 6: 258–260

Hästbacka J, Tammisto T, Elfving G, Tiitinen P 1965 Infusion thrombophlebitis. Acta anaesthesiologica scandinavica 10: 9–30

Jones M V, Craig, Douglas B 1972 Venous reaction to plastic intravenous cannulas: Influence of cannula composition. Canadian Anaesthetists' Society Journal 19: 491–497

Medical Research Council Report 1957 Thrombophlebitis following intravenous infusions: A trial of plastic and rubber giving sets. Lancet i: 595–597

Mitchell J W 1952 Self-sealing intravenous needle. Anesthesia 7: 258–259

Ready L B 1972 An unusual site of injection of intra-arterial thiopentone. Canadian Anaesthetists' Society Journal 19: 657–658

Thomas E T, Evers W, Racz G B 1970 Post-infusion phlebitis. Anaesthesia and Analgesia, Current Researches 49: 150–159

3

Intravenous anaesthetics

Only a relatively few years ago there would have been no problem answering the question: *what is an intravenous anaesthetic*? The definition then was 'a drug that, in adequate doses, would safely and reversibly produce loss of consciousness, preferably in one arm–brain circulation time'. Such an agent could be given either in a single dose, by intermittent injection, or by infusion. A number of easily identifiable drugs, such as thiopentone, fell into this category. Other agents such as diazepam could be given to produce a light level of sedation or basal narcosis in larger doses, but there was no suggestion that they would replace conventional drugs.

This definition has become less clear with the increasing popularity of the opioids. The combination of a potent analgesic and a less potent hypnotic can be used to induce anaesthesia — albeit more slowly than with orthodox drugs. The preliminary administration of fentanyl, or other potent opioid, has made 'induction' possible with what would normally be subhypnotic doses of induction agents. Large doses of opioids have themselves been used for induction and maintenance of anaesthesia, although this is reserved for specific indications (Chapter 13). By reducing the frequency of side effects, such as spontaneous muscle movements, the opioids have also made possible the safe use of otherwise unacceptable drugs as induction agents.

The current definition for an intravenous anaesthetic should be 'a drug, or a mixture of drugs, which will induce anaesthesia when injected in sufficient doses and which could possibly be given intermittently or by infusion for maintenance'. The term 'total intravenous anaesthesia' indicates a state in which an induction agent with or without an opioid is used as the main anaesthetic agent. Strictly speaking this involves no inhalational agents, but in practice nitrous oxide and oxygen are often used.

CLASSIFICATION

Intravenous anaesthetics can be classified according to their chemistry, their speed of onset of action, or their clinical acceptability. A classification based on the duration of action is unsatisfactory, although important in relation to the fields of usefulness of individual agents. The terms 'ultra-short' and 'short' acting are often used indiscriminately and can be both confusing and misleading to those who are unaware of the pharmacokinetics of these drugs.

Table 3.1 classifies available drugs according to their speed of onset and chemistry. Two of the groups listed have been withdrawn from clinical use, but are included here to put the subject into perspective as intravenous anaesthesia has benefitted from the knowledge accrued from their use. An

Table 3.1 A classification of intravenous anaesthetics

Rapidly-acting (induction agents)
Thiobarbiturates, methylbarbiturates
Eugenols
Steroids
Imidazole derivatives
Hindered phenols
Slower-acting (basal hypnotics; sedatives)
Phenylcyclohexamines
Benzodiazepines
(Oxy) barbiturates
Opioid-neuroleptic/tranquilliser combination
Large doses of opioids
Others Chlormethiazole, hydroxybutyrate, alcohol.

updated (December 1986) classification is given in Table 15.1. Dividing drugs into *rapidly acting* and *slowly acting* identifies those which one would class as *primary induction agents* and those which one would consider as *basal hypnotics* and sedatives.

When an intravenous anaesthetic drug is to be given intermittently to maintain a desired level of anaesthesia it is important that it should produce its desired effect in one arm–brain circulation time; thus fluctuations of depth will be minimal. This is less important when the agent is used primarily for induction, although it is still desirable, particularly in patients who are either unusually sensitive or resistant to anaesthetics. Rapidly acting drugs will in effective doses produce loss of consciousness in one arm–brain circulation time.

The rapidly acting drugs are primarily induction agents which can also be used for maintenance of anaesthesia, either alone or preferably with an analgesic, be it by parenteral administration or by inhalation of nitrous oxide and oxygen. Within this group, the rapidly metabolized eugenols which are no longer available for clinical use, could justifiably have been termed ultra-short acting and the alphaxalone-alphadolone mixture (Althesin) which depends on both translocation and detoxication for recovery referred to as 'short acting'. When given by intermittent administration or by infusion they have a less cumulative effect than the barbiturates. The same might also apply to etomidate and propofol.

Generally speaking, drugs which have a rapid onset of action will act for a shorter time than more slowly acting compounds. In normal induction doses, the benzodiazepine and the neurolept combination are much longer acting than either thiopentone or etomidate. Because of this it is easier to use the longer-acting drugs or basal hypnotics to produce a light level of sedation.

The rapidly-acting drugs have more 'instant toxicity' or are more prone to cause a 'bolus effect', with more profound cardiovascular and respiratory depression than the slower-acting compounds. In contrast the latter have a toxic effect which is usually specific for the individual drugs. This varies from emergence delirium with ketamine to respiratory depression with fentanyl. Sometimes such side effects can be used to advantage, for instance the amnesia from injectable benzodiazepines can be advantageous when using the drug for dentistry or endoscopy.

INDIVIDUAL DRUGS

As an alternative, drugs could be classified according to their clinical acceptability.

Barbiturates: Table 3.2 gives such a classification for the barbiturates. With increasing competition from new drugs, all unsatisfactory barbiturates have been withdrawn from clinical use in most countries and are only included here to illustrate the classification.

The early water-soluble steroid *hydroxydione* (Viadril, Presuren) was slowly-acting and is no longer used. *Althesin*, a mixture of two steroids, and the water-soluble *minaxolone* have been withdrawn from use.

Etomidate (Hypnomidate) is the only imidazole derivative which has been used clinically.

Propofol (Diprivan), formerly known as disoprofol and ICI 35868) is the only substituted phenol which has been studied in man. The term 'hindered phenol' refers to stereochemistry of the compound in which two isopropyl side chains 'protect' the hydroxyl group.

Ketamine (Ketalar, Ketaject) is the sole representative of the phenyl cyclohexamines in clinical use.

Table 3.2 Classification of barbiturates according to clinical acceptability

Very satisfactory and equally acceptable (differing only in potency):	thiopentone, thiamylal, thiobutobarbitone, thialbarbitone⁺
Unsatisfactory: too high an incidence of side effects:	buthalitone⁺, methitural⁺, hexobarbitone★ methyl thiopentone⁺
Difficult to categorize: unique advantages, side effects:	methohexitone★ enibomal★

⁺ withdrawn from clinical use
All are thiobarbiturates except those marked ★, which are methyl oxybarbiturates

Benzodiazepines: only a very small number of the available bendodiazepines has been prepared in a solution and of these *diazepam* (Valium, Diazemuls), *flunitrazepam* and *midazolam* (Hypnovel) have been used in anaesthesia.

Pentobarbitone is the only injectable barbiturate in clinical use in Britain, although *quinalbarbitone* (Secobarbital) and *amylobarbitone* (Amytal) are used elsewhere.

Opioids: a large number of *neurolept* combinations are in current use but the only opioids to enjoy widespread popularity are fentanyl, alfentanil and morphine. The use of the latter is generally limited to prolonged operations or circumstances where patients are ventilated into the postoperative period. A number of fentanyl derivatives are under investigation for their potential use in anaesthesia (Chapter 13).

Miscellaneous

Not included above are a number of compounds that are rarely, if ever, given as intravenous anaesthetics. Some of these have been tried and abandoned while other are used occasionally; in most instances they are given as an infusion. Such drugs include dilute solutions of alcohol, procaine, paraldehyde, bromethol, chlormethiazole and hydroxybutyrate (Gamma OH).

SOLUTIONS

An alternative, and clinically important classification would be according to solubility, or the means used to make an injectable preparation (Table 3.3). Individual drugs in some of the groups are made up commercially in different forms and one preparation (diazepam) has been commercially available in three forms.

Table 3.3 Classification of intravenous anaesthetics according to their solvents or means used to prepare injectable solutions

Aqueous
Thiobarbiturates and Methylbarbiturates
Minaxolone (steroid)
Etomidate†
Ketamine
Midazolam (benzodiazepine)
Opioids
Organic solvents
Etomidate
Diazepam and Flunitrazepam (benzodiazepines)
*Solubilizing agents**
Epontol (eugenol)
Althesin (steroid)
Propofol (ICI 35868)
Emulsions
Early eugenol (G 29505)
Diazepam
Propofol

* All preparations solubilised in Cremophor have been withdrawn from clinical use
† Not marketed in aqueous solution

Aqueous

The simplest form of solution is aqueous, but some drugs are insoluble in water and others are unstable in aqueous solution. Major examples of the latter are thiopentone and related drugs which are prepared for clinical use as sodium salts to be dissolved in water or saline before use. These salts are readily soluble in water and the commercial preparations normally contain a mixture of six parts of anhydrous sodium carbonate and 100 parts (w/w) of barbiturate. This prevents precipitation of the insoluble free acid by atmospheric carbon dioxide and makes an alkaline solution (pH 10–11), which is irritant on extravenous injection. By contrast, ketamine forms an acid aqueous solution (pH 3.5–5.5); and some preparations contain a preservative. It is non-irritant on either intramuscular or intravenous injection.

Although the salt of etomidate is very soluble in water, the aqueous solution, containing a phosphate buffer (pH 3.5), is unstable and the drug is marketed in an organic solvent.

The opioids are all soluble in water. The stability of the aqueous solution varies from drug to drug and some commercial preparations contain stabilising agents.

Midazolam is available as a buffered aqueous solution and solubility is achieved by opening of the benzodiazepine ring which occurs reversibly below pH 4.0. The ring closes immediately in the plasma and thereafter it behaves as any other benzodiazepine.

The original steroid anaesthetic, hydroxydione,

was soluble in water, but had a long onset time. Althesin, which is rapidly acting, is insoluble, being dispensed in cremophor. For some time it seemed that as far as steroid anaesthesia was concerned it would not be possible to combine rapidity of onset with water solubility. However, this was overcome with minaxolone which had a different side chain configuration.

Organic solvents

These consist mainly of various combinations of glycols — polyethylene or propylene, alcohol, sodium benzoate or benzoic acid. The solutions, although stable, are slightly viscid and a wide bore needle is required for rapid intravenous injection. They are not miscible with water or saline and mixing with these will produce a slightly cloudy emulsion.

Pain on injection and venous thrombosis are the main problems with organic solutions such as Valium brand of diazepam or etomidate. Even though only veins of larger calibre are used and variations made in the solvents, the incidence of neither complication can be brought down to acceptable limits.

Normal doses of organic solvents appear to be devoid of toxic effects when given intravenously (Morris, Nelson and Calvey, 1942) but large doses can cause intravascular haemolysis. This was reported when very large doses were given with mephenesin at a time when it was used as a muscle relaxant during general anaesthesia.

Solubilising agents

Solubilising agents include various hydrophobic forms of polyoxylated castor oil, consisting of esters of ricinolinic acid and glycerine-polyglycol esters. They act by incorporating drugs into micelles or globules to form a colloidal solution. The result is a slightly viscid solution which is miscible with water. The solubilising agents used in anaesthesia are Cremophor EL and Tensid. The molecular weight of Tensid is 3000 at 20°C and 3170 at 37°C (Scholtan and Lie, 1966).

These agents were used to solubilise propanidid, Althesin and propofol. Many of the toxic properties of Epontol (propanidid solution) were attributed to Cremophor EL but this is unlikely. The solubilising agent has been studied thoroughly in both animals and humans by Doenicke (1965), who showed that it did not cause either the cardiovascular depression, or the respiratory stimulation seen with propanidid. It is quickly eliminated from the body, mainly by the kidneys (Duhm et al, 1965), with 50–75% excretion within two hours of administration of very large doses.

There is, however, good evidence to incriminate Cremophor and allied drugs with the hypersensitivity reactions seen with the cremophor preparations of Althesin and propofol. This is discussed in detail in Chapter 14.

Emulsions

One of the earliest eugenol preparations (G 29 505) was for a time studied in emulsion form. This reduced the incidence of injection pain and phlebitis. More recently an emulsion of diazepam in soya bean oil (Diazemuls) has become available and this likewise has reduced the incidence of these complications. After early use of propofol in a solubilising agent it is now reformulated as an emulsion and this is free-flowing and very easy to inject.

USES

Bearing in mind the above, most intravenous anaesthetics can be used for the following purposes:

- As induction agents for general anaesthesia
- As sole or main anaesthetics for brief surgical procedures
- As an infusion
- To supplement an inhalation agent of low potency or in combination with analgesics
- In conjunction with regional analgesia
- To relieve certain pathological states of central nervous stimulation.

ADVANTAGES

These are many advantages to be gained from the use of intravenous anaesthetics and some of these have already been dealt with. It bears repeating that rapidity of onset, pleasantness of induction, the absence of irritation of the respiratory tract and the absence of cumbersome equipment are cases in point. All intravenous anaesthetics may be used safely in the presence of cautery and electrical equipment, and none is incompatible with catecholamines when these are infiltrated to produce haemostasis. Unless large doses have been used, recovery from intravenous anaesthesia usually is rapid, but the rapidity or otherwise of emergence varies from drug to drug, as does the degree of hangover, if any. Indeed, the last two considerations are the ones which frequently are among the determining factors in the selection of one rather than the other intravenous anaesthetic. Emergence from anaesthesia is smooth as a rule and is not accompanied by undue excitement, nausea or vomiting. All these advantages however are in general terms and specific drugs vary in one respect or another. This will become clear when individual drugs are considered in later chapters.

DOSAGE

Unlike the inhalation anaesthetics, which can be titrated to the requirements of the individual patient until the desired response has been obtained, the dose of an intravenously administered agent must be predetermined, largely on the basis of experience. There is no definite dosage that will suit all patients and the requirements of each must be individually assessed. This is best done by the injection of a test dose which will give some indication of the particular patient's response to the drug at that particular time. It is then possible to assess more accurately the amount required to be both safe and adequate for the desired purpose. Requirements are roughly related to body weight and, as a rule, males tolerate larger doses than females. Also, young patients require relatively larger amounts than the more elderly, in whom, in particular, cognisance must be taken of the slower circulation time, which in turn delays the manifestations of the maximum effect of the drug. If this particular point is not realised, a marked overdose may result from the subsequent injection of supplemental doses on the mistaken assumption that the initial injection was inadequate. Resistance to thiobarbiturates and a number of other intravenous anaesthetics may be encountered in persons who have acquired a tolerance to narcotic and analgesic drugs, but occasionally one may encounter a case of 'idiopathic resistance'.

Sensitivity to intravenous anaesthetics may occur in many pathological conditions, the most commonly encountered ones being shock, severe anaemia and uraemia. A combination of one or more of these is often found in ulcerative colitis, malnutrition, intestinal obstruction, severe burns, advanced malignant disease, and in malaria. Under these circumstances a marked reduction in the amount of drugs injected is imperative and in some instances it may be advisable to avoid some of them altogether for induction of anaesthesia, as, for instance, the thiobarbiturates. In the case of drugs which rely on detoxication by the liver, hepatic dysfunction may lead to delay of recovery although the degree of liver damage must be severe before such a response is seen. Prolonged narcosis also results from the administration of large doses of drugs either singly or by repeated or continuous injection. This is especially so for those agents whose action depends largely on redistribution rather than breakdown, as is the case with the thiobarbiturates. Obviously in determining the dosage of intravenous anaesthetics, one must bear in mind also the preoperative administration of sedative, hypnotic and analgesic drugs and any other intravenous supplement which it may be proposed to administer in the course of anaesthesia.

A number of intravenously administered agents, in particular barbiturates, exert a depressant effect on the myocardium as well as producing peripheral vosadilation. A composition of these two factors may lead to severe hypotension which in turn reduces coronary blood flow to a precarious level. This is especially dangerous in patients with pre-existing cardiac disease. The compensatory vasoconstriction which occurs early in the 'shock state' can be broken down by the vasodilation which follows the injection of barbiturates and result in unexpected profound hypotension. In constrast with the effect of many inhalation anaesthetics catecholamine release is not a general property of intravenous anaesthetics and this may also contribute to the marked cardiovascular reactions which can occur, particularly following a rapid injection. Hypertensive patients may experience severe falls in blood pressure following intravenous induction, particularly with barbiturates. Patients receiving phenothiazines or other vasodilators may react similarly.

In obstetrics the dose of barbiturate administered to the mother should be kept to a minimum since these drugs cross the placental barrier and thus exercise the same depressive effect on the fetus as they do on the mother. If doses are kept small, the effects of redistribution as well as the further dilution inherent in the peculiarity of the fetal circulation, make it possible to administer the drugs with safety, even if the infant is born within minutes of the induction. However, the possibility of the mother recalling events occurring soon after induction must be appreciated.

CONTRAINDICATIONS

The absolute contraindications to intravenous anaesthesia by and large do not differ from those which apply to all general anaesthesia. They include the unavailability of means to inflate the lungs, pre-existing mechanical interference with the airway, potential interference with the patency of the airway or lack of access to it during the operation. It goes without saying that the absence of suitable veins is a barrier to intravenous anaesthesia especially if this involves repeated attempts at venipuncture. There are many alternatives and equally pleasant means of inducing anaesthesia and indeed repeated attempts to insert a needle defeat the very purpose of a pleasant induction. Frequently veins become apparent once anaesthesia has been induced and suitable steps can then be taken to assure the subsequent administration of supplementary intravenous agents if required.

General anaesthesia including intravenous anaesthesia should not be administered to outpatients unless suitable arrangements exist for them to be accompanied after release from hospital. Normal mental faculties return faster with some agents than with others; nevertheless we must assume that after none of them are patients fully capable of making fine judgements for varying periods of time even after full consciousness has returned.

There are many other contraindications to the use of intravenous anaesthesia but these can more properly be discussed with the various agents. As a generality, however, it can be said that drugs which cause a sudden peripheral vasodilation are contraindicated in states of fixed cardiac output or cardiac decompensation. The inability of these patients to adjust cardiac output leads to a precipitous fall of mean aortic pressure with consequent cessation of coronary perfusion and the inevitable fatal consequence arising from this combination.

ABUSES

There are many ways in which drugs can be misused in clinical anaesthesia. Among the intravenous agents the most frequently abused one undoubtedly is thiopentone, if for no other reason than that it is the most commonly used one.

The prolonged administration of most intravenous anaesthetics as sole agent should be limited to the planned use of infusions, rather than continuously 'topping up', and should include an analgesic element in the technique. Low dose techniques have been used to provide 'sedation' for conservative dentistry but there is the risk of inadvertently deepening anaesthesia without proper airway control. Rapid administration of intravenous anaesthetics might well accentuate to an unacceptable degree some otherwise relatively minor side effects. These considerations, however, do not apply to the same degree to the judicious supplementation of inhalation anaesthetic agents, such as nitrous oxide-oxygen, provided doses are kept within acceptable limits, just sufficient to prevent awareness during anaesthesia.

Few, if any, intravenous anaesthetics are suitable to permit tracheal intubation and this is especially true for the thiobarbiturates, which do not depress laryngeal reflexes. However, small intravenous doses of narcotic analgesics may be administered for purposes of sedation and to ensure patient cooperation if preinduction tracheal intubation is desired.

DANGERS

Every intravenous injection carries the danger of infection, breakage of needles, and haematoma formation. In recent years the dangers of *infection* have been greatly reduced by the widespread use of disposable needles and syringes, but where non-disposable material is being used, cross-infection must be prevented by proper cleaning of equipment, followed by boiling in alkaline water and autoclaving or steam sterilisation. The skin is not a likely source of infection although it should be cleaned by the application of a suitable antiseptic. *Breakage of needles* is most likely to result from movement of the limb during or after induction of anaesthesia. This complication is greatly reduced by the increased use of plastic intravenous cannulae. *Haematoma formation* after withdrawal of the needle is commonly the result of an inadequately released torniquet or constriction of the limb by clothing. Application of digital pressure to the site of needle puncture should do much to prevent this occurrence, which is especially prone to occur if superficial veins have been used in patients with deficient supportive connective tissue.

The *local irritant* effect of agents such as thiopentone may result in tissue necrosis if large amounts of a concentrated solution have been deposited in the subcutaneous tissue. Likewise intra-arterial injection may lead to serious complications, including gangrene. These complications will be discussed in detail elsewhere (pages 121–124).

In relation to thiopentone, Michael D Nosworthy has stated that one of the dangers of the agent is that it is *fatally easy to give*. This usually is due to a lack of appreciation of the limitations or contraindications of this or any other drug. This is especially true in states of hypovolaemia, where even relatively small doses may markedly depress vital systems, and in old age when the full impact of the drug may not become evident for much longer than one might be led to expect from previous experience. This being so, a supplemental injection may be made which in time will prove to have been an overdose. Only occasionally is an overdose caused by a technical misadventure, such as a tight constriction about the site of injection, and consequent release of large amounts of the drug when the constriction is removed.

Cardiovascular collapse is the most serious of the many effects of intravenous anaesthetics and is the one that is the most difficult to treat. Elevation of the feet may be all that is required, but failure of the patient to improve may be an indication for the use of suitable drug therapy or even for major resuscitative measures.

Since apnoea, or *respiratory depression*, frequently accompanies cardiovascular collapse, artificial respiration should be carried out with oxygen for as long as is necessary. Carbon dioxide administration plays *no part* in the treatment of respiratory depression, while analeptics may be harmful by virtue of increasing the cerebral oxygen consumption. If apnoea is prolonged, the adequacy of artificial ventilation should be monitored by means of blood-gas determinations wherever such facilities are available. This may avoid also an undue prolongation of the apnoea due to hyperventilation with consequent hypocarbia.

Damage to the brachial plexus by stretching or, more commonly, rotator cuff strains of the shoulder joint, may result from abduction and extension of the arm. The danger is increased by external rotation of the forearm, by the use of a shoulder rest, and by allowing the arm to fall behind the coronal plane. If intravenous supplementation of anaesthesia is required with the patient in this position, the arm can be placed across the chest, or better still, an intravenous infusion system can be set up and the arm placed at the side of the patient. When the arm is by the side and covered by drapes, the use of a plastic catheter rather than a needle is preferred in order to reduce the risk of interstitial infusion due to inadvertent perforation of the vein. The use of veins in the foot is not recommended except in the rare circumstances in which these are the only veins available. The venous circulation in the legs is impaired in many surgical patients and any additional trauma to the intima resulting from the infusion of extraneous material may aggravate the danger of venous thrombosis.

BALANCED ANAESTHESIA

The term 'balanced anaesthesia' is applied to the

combination of two or more drugs, each given for a specific purpose, with the object of thereby avoiding the toxic effects of one single agent required in relatively large doses. The term was applied originally to the combination of general anaesthesia with local anaesthesia to produce muscular relaxation. Now it is generally taken to include the administration of drugs which produce (1) sleep; (2) analgesia or reflex depression and (3) muscle relaxation when required.

In the present-day context the earliest type of 'balanced anaesthesia' probably was the combination of thiopentone with nitrous oxide and oxygen reported by Organe and Broad in 1938. This resulted in much superior anaesthesia to that obtained with thiopentone alone, the analgesic action of the nitrous oxide permitting a marked reduction of the amount of barbiturate needed with consequently a quicker return of consciousness. This synergism between the two drugs has been further demonstrated by Paulson (1952); his average requirement of thiopentone for stripping of varicose veins was 21.7 mg min^{-1} when given alone as compared with 14.4 mg min^{-1} when combined with 66 per cent nitrous oxide in oxygen.

The thiopentone-nitrous oxide-oxygen technique is very widely practised now and opiate premedication further enhances the effectiveness of the barbiturate, which provides the 'sleep' component of the triad. Analgesia can also be provided during anaesthesia by the intravenous injection of opioids. The drugs used in neurolept anaesthesia do themselves produce balanced anaesthesia (sleep or tranquillity with analgesia), with or without nitrous oxide, as does ketamine.

A muscle relaxant can be added to these combinations, with or without hyperventilation, to allow for light anaesthesia for major abdominal or thoracic operations and this is a widely practised technique (Gray & Rees, 1952), in which any of the intravenous anaesthetics may be employed. A single 'sleep' dose of an induction agent is usually all that is required, with analgesic supplementation during the actual operation (Dundee et al, 1969). Others prefer low concentrations of inhalation agents to contribute both to the 'sleep' and 'reflex suppression' components of the triad. Dilute, intravenous infusions of local anaesthetics can also be used for this purpose and appear to be popular in Third World countries or where nitrous oxide is not readily available.

'Crash induction'

This is a variation of balanced anaesthesia in which sleep and relaxation are produced rapidly to facilitate tracheal intubation, the subsequent anaesthesia being continued with any appropriate drug or drugs. When used for the routine induction of balanced anesthesia, any combination of intravenous anaesthetics and relaxants may be used. However, when quick tracheal intubation is essential because of a risk of aspiration of gastric contents, and it is decided that induction of anaesthesia should precede intubation, a rapidly acting intravenous agent (barbiturate or propofol) should be used, preferably followed by a rapidly acting relaxant.

Situations arise where there exists a need for very brief anaesthesia and relaxation alone, and where the solution may well be in a technique akin to the crash induction. An example for this are the conditions necessary for the safe performance of electroconvulsive (electroshock) therapy. Here the combination of a short-acting intravenous anaesthetic such as methohexitone with suxamethonium allows the procedure to be carried out, followed by fast recovery from anaesthesia.

Sedation techniques

These are used to make patients less aware of procedures being carried out under local analgesia. This includes operations under topical (such as endoscopy), infiltration (such as dental procedures) or extradural or subarachnoid techniques (more major abdominal procedures). A very light level of sedation is all that is needed and while this can be provided by intermittent injections (or even infusions) of rapidly-acting induction agents, the use of small doses of basal hypnotics is preferred.

REFERENCES

Doenicke A 1965 General pharmacology of propanidid. Acta Anaesthesiologica Scandinavica 17: 21–26

Duhm B, Maul W, Medenward H, Patzschke K, Wegner L A 1965 Tierexperimentelle Untersuchungen mit Propanidid-^{14}C. In: Horatz K, Frey R, Zindler M (eds) Die intravenose Kurznarkose mit dem neuen Phenoxyessigsaurederivat, Propanidid (Epontol). Springer, Berlin, p 78

Dundee J W, Brown S S, Hamilton R C, McDowell S A 1969 Analgesic supplementation of light general anaesthesia: a study of its advantages using sequential analysis. Anaesthesia 24: 52–61

Gray T C, Rees G J 1952 The role of apnoea in anaesthesia for major surgery. British Medical Journal 2: 891–892

Morris H J, Nelson A A, Calvery H O 1942 Observations on the chronic toxicities of propylene glycol, ethylene glycol, diethylene glycol, ethylene glycol mono-ethyl-ether and diethylene glycol mono-ethyl-ether. Journal of Pharmacology and Experimental Therapeutics 74:266

Organe G S W, Broad R J B 1938 Pentothal with nitrous oxide and oxygen. Lancet 2: 1170–1172

Paulson J A 1952 Thiopental sodium and ether anesthesia. Journal of the American Medical Association 150: 983–987

Scholtan W, Lie S Y 1966 Kolloid-chemische Eigenschaften eines neuen Kurznarkoticums. Arzneimittel-Forschung 16:679

4

Pharmacokinetics of intravenous anaesthetics

The ultimate objective in administering a drug is to achieve a concentration at its site of action which is sufficient to produce the desired pharmacological effect. Drugs are carried in plasma water and this is the medium through which they reach their site of action at the tissue receptor. Only a very small proportion of administered drug reaches the site of action and the factors which determine this must be understood. Pharmacokinetics, the movement of drugs, is the quantitative study of the disposition of a drug in the body: this includes absorption from the site of administration, distribution to body tissues and fluids, including sites of action, biotransformation to pharmacologically inactive or active metabolites and excretion of drug and/or its metabolites from the body.

In general there is a direct relationship between the drug concentrations at the site of action and its effect. In practice one usually measures the plasma concentration of a drug but this might not reflect accurately the concentration at the receptor; thus, plasma concentration is not necessarily a reflection of drug activity. This is further complicated by varying sensitivity to the drug at the receptor, particularly after prolonged administration. However, a basic premise of pharmacokinetic studies is that by measuring concentration in plasma it is usually possible to predict concentrations at the receptor or at least to follow the rise and fall of drug concentration at this site (Hug, 1978).

In this chapter are outlined some of the pharmacokinetic principles which apply to intravenous anaesthetics. It is not a detailed discussion of the topic; instead is it intended to simplify understanding of subsequent chapters and the principles of drug action. Apart from the rapid attainment of an initial high blood concentration and the need for metabolism in the body, intravenous anaesthetics have pharmacokinetic profiles similar to inhalational drugs or those given by other routes.

PHARMACOKINETICS

Broadly speaking there are two approaches to this subject — descriptive and mathematical. Though this chapter concentrates on the former, the latter cannot be entirely ignored. Both physiologically based or perfusion models (which depend on perfusion rates and solubility coefficients) and pharmacokinetic models (based on plasma and tissue concentrations) have been used to study this subject. For a fuller description of some aspects of this, readers are referred to the additional sources given at the end of the chapter.

Pharmacokinetics must not be confused with *pharmacodynamics*, which refers to the effect of drugs on the body. Their differences can be rather simplistically demonstrated by considering pharmacokinetics as 'the effect of the body on drugs' and pharmacodynamics as 'the effect of drugs on the body'.

The term kinetic implies movement and force and one must envisage pharmacokinetics as applying to a constantly changing state governed in the main by tissue gradients. The two-way arrows in Figure 4.1 indicate a constantly changing state of drug distribution. Once a drug reaches the blood stream a certain amount is bound reversibly to plasma proteins and rendered pharmacologically inactive. It is only the 'free' or unbound drug which is available for transport and

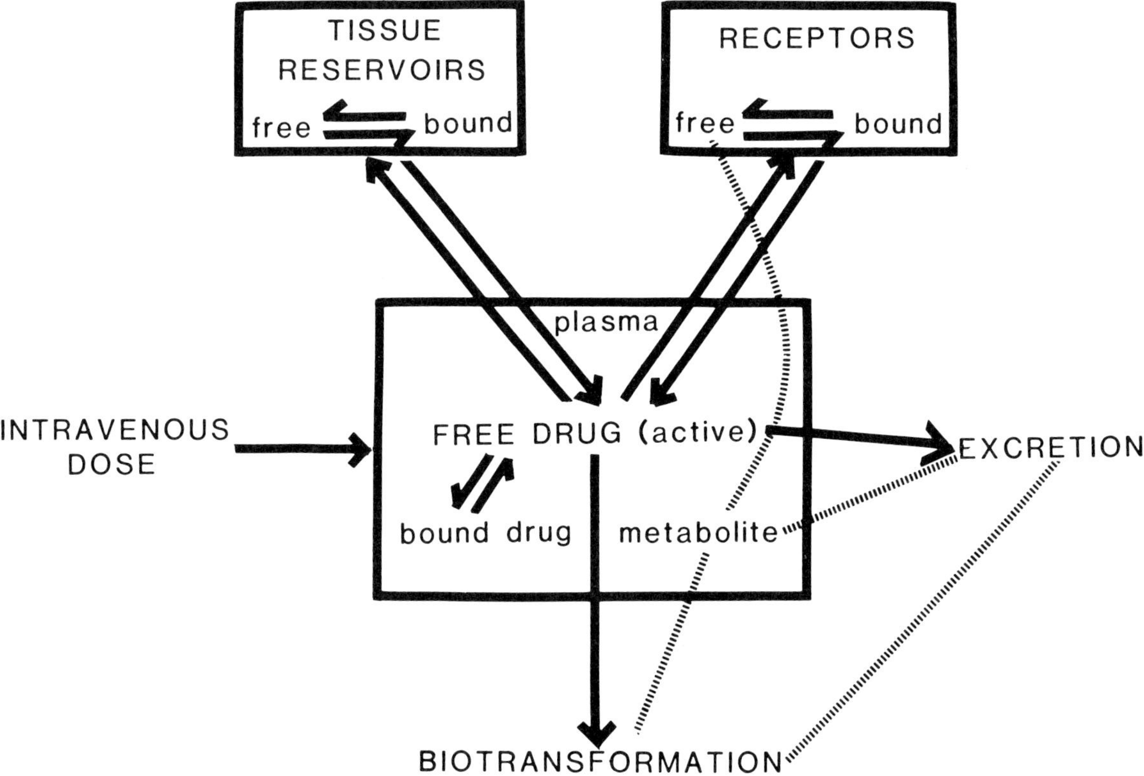

Fig. 4.1 Schematic representation of the inter-relationship of the distribution, binding, biotransformation and excretion of a drug given by the intravenous route and its concentration at its locus of action (Modified from Fingl and Woodbury, 1965).

distribution to tissue receptors and to other tissues. Further binding of drugs to tissues takes place in proportion to the particular affinity of that tissue for the drug and also in proportion to its blood supply.

Broadly speaking tissues can be divided into those where the main action of a drug is desirable and those where it has no therapeutic action. In practice only a very small amount of active drug reaches its primary locus of action.

Drugs can be excreted unchanged, rendered pharmacologically inert by processes such as conjugation, or metabolised, and excreted in the urine or faeces. The metabolite itself might have some pharmacological activity. In many cases two or more of these processes occur together. Conjugation changes the relative water/fat solubility or affects ionisation in such a way as to promote excretion.

Intravenous route of administration

By virtue of the fact that a drug is injected directly into the blood stream it bypasses the problems of volatilisation and distribution in the lung inherent in inhalation anaesthetics. While the same principles apply to the distribution of all drugs in the body, there are some peculiarities of intravenous drugs.

- They will reach the desired locus of action more quickly than drugs which have to be volatilised and absorbed from alveoli or others which have to be absorbed from an injection site. For this reason they are likely to have a more rapid onset of action.
- In contrast to the inhalation agents which are largely excreted unchanged, intravenous drugs cannot be removed from the body by their route of administration. They are dependent on

redistribution and metabolism for reduction of their concentration in the brain.

- The cardiovascular effects of an intravenous anaesthetic or any intravenously administered drug might affect the pattern of distribution to 'non-essential' depot tissues and intensify and prolong its own action.

DRUG DISTRIBUTION

Distribution

Distribution is a term which implies dispersion in the body. Functionally the body is a multicompartment organ, the different tissues or functional compartments differing with respect to:
a) blood supply
b) size of tissue
c) tissue/blood partition coefficients in relation to drugs

Table 4.1 is a simplification of the concept of pharmacokinetic compartments, the figures being for a 70 kg subject in the 30–39 age group with a surface area of 1.83 m^2.

Redistribution to a poorly perfused organ will take longer than to a well perfused one: a tissue with high affinity for a drug will take it up more quickly than one which has a low affinity. This introduces the concept of *time constant*, i.e. the relative rate at which each tissue will equilibrate with a drug. This is related to the capacity of the tissue for the drug in relation to tissue perfusion. The capacity of a tissue for a drug is the product of tissue volume and the tissue/blood partition coefficient. A large, well perfused organ can hold a great deal of drug, particularly one for which it has a high partition coefficient.

Tension

Drug *tension* or *partial pressure* depends on the tendency for molecules to move from blood to tissue or from tissue to blood until tissue–blood coefficients are satisfied. This depends on tissue gradients with drug passing from one tissue to another until the balance is restored.

Extent of distribution

Extent of distribution depends on a number of factors, i.e.

1. Physicochemical properties of the drug, particularly its lipid solubility.
2. Regional blood flow to various tissues and organs.
3. Binding to plasma proteins and to other body constituents: drug bound to plasma proteins is no longer easily diffusible.
4. Transport across membranes. This is a passive process, as active transport across cell membranes plays no known part in the distribution of intravenous anaesthetics.

Most acidic drugs are confined to the extracellular space but most basic drugs are distributed throughout the body.

Equilibrium

The circulating drug is in a state of dynamic equilibrium in which these various processes all play a part; there is a constant interchange of free drug from plasma to specific receptor sites as equilibrium is continually disturbed by excretion or biotransformation. While the rate of diffusion across a membrane is proportional to the concentration gradient of the drug across the membrane in keeping with Fick's law, molecular size, spatial configuration, the degree of ionisation of an electrolyte and lipid solubility are all important. As molecular size increases lipid solubility becomes more important.

Table 4.1 Concept of pharmacokinetic tissue compartments with different perfusion rates

Perfusion	*Tissue*	*% body mass*	*% cardiac output*	*Blood flow/weight**
High (vessel-rich tissues)	Brain, heart, viscera	9	75	75
Moderate	Skeletal muscle	50	18	3.3
Poor	Fat	19	5	2.2

* l 100 kg tissue^{-1} min^{-1}
(modified from Ghoneim and Spector, 1981)

Lipid solubility

In practice, lipid solubility is a major determinant in the ability of a drug to penetrate a cell membrane and this is particularly important in relation to drugs which undergo partial ionization at body pH. Membrane permeability to the non-ionised form is much greater than to the ionic one. The cell membrane is thus preferentially permeable to the lipid soluble non-ionised drugs, but resists penetration of the water-soluble ionised form.

Lipid-soluble drugs,which cross the blood brain and other barriers, will also readily cross the placenta. A build up of concentration is enhanced by the large placental blood flow. However, since the maternal arterial concentration will be reduced by dilution with the infant's blood, the peak level of drug in the fetus is unlikely to reach that in the mother.

Ionisation

The extent of ionisation of a drug is a function of its dissociation constant and the pH of the surrounding tissues. pKa is a term used to express the negative logarithm of the *dissociation constant*. This is a useful way of comparing the strengths of acids and bases: the stronger an acid, the lower is its pKa, the stronger a base, the higher is its pKa, although acids and bases cannot be identified by the pKa value. It is helpful to remember that at 50 per cent ionisation the pH is the same as the pKa. This is of great clinical importance in drugs with a pKa near the pH of plasma; here a small change in pH can make a large change in the degree of ionisation, and in time in the distribution in the body. As an example, thiopentone (a weak acid) has a pKa of 7.6, approximately 60 per cent of drug being non-ionised at blood pH and thus its distribution can be affected by clinical changes in blood pH.

Plasma protein binding

Most drugs are reversibly bound to the non-diffusible constituents of plasma, mostly albumin, the extent varying with the affinity of the individual drug, available binding sites and the drug concentration. Plasma binding is primarily a method for transport of drugs to their site of action. The binding of extremely lipid-soluble compounds might in part be essential for their transport in plasma due to their low solubility in plasma water. Binding appears to occur immediately on injection but the limited blood volume to which the initial bolus is exposed might have inadequate binding capacity until adequate mixing occurs in the body.

Chemical configuration affects binding, as is demonstrated by the fact that thiobarbiturates are bound to a greater extent than their oxygen analogues: roughly twice as much thiopentone is bound to protein than pentobarbitone (Goldbaum & Smith, 1954). The difference probably relates to the effect of the sulphur substitution on the affinity for a hydrophobic portion of the protein. In the case of both of these drugs the bound fraction increases with pH to maximum around pH 8.0.

An increase in plasma binding (similar to increase in blood solubility) results in a decrease in the tissue/blood partition coefficient, thus lowering partial pressure or activity. Binding can therefore increase the disappearance of drugs like barbiturates from the blood, provided there is not a corresponding change in tissue binding.

Since binding sites might be saturated at high drug concentrations, resulting in a relatively low bound fraction, and likewise low concentrations result in a relatively high bound fraction, values for protein binding are only useful if they are measured at therapeutic concentrations.

METABOLISM AND EXCRETION

Metabolism is the process by which the body changes a drug to render it pharmacologically inactive. Alternative terms are *detoxication* and *biotransformation*. *Excretion* is removal from the body, usually by the kidney or in the bile. The molecular weight of a drug and its metabolites is important in determining the route of excretion; those above 400–500 are usually excreted in the bile while those with lower molecular weights appear in the urine.

To be excreted unchanged by the kidney a drug must be relatively insoluble in lipids, and ionised. By virtue of their requirements to produce anaesthesia, it is obvious that this does not apply to intravenous anaesthetics. These highly lipid soluble non-ionised compounds will diffuse from the glomerular filtrates into the blood (reabsorption) and theoretically could remain permanently in the body unless converted into lipid insoluble ionised metabolites.

Drug metabolism occurs chiefly in the liver, although other tissues such as lung, kidney and blood might be involved. The metabolite is generally pharmacologically inactive but some have hypnotic activity. The chemical changes involved are:

1. Non-synthetic: oxidation, reduction, hydrolysis.
2. Synthetic: conjugation with other substances such as glycuronic acid (glycuronidation), acetic acid (acetylation) or sulphate ester (etheral sulphate formation).

These metabolites fulfil the criteria for renal excretion with respect to water solubility and ionisation. Some drugs, or possibly their hypnotically active metabolites, are excreted into the bile and pass into the intestine, where a portion is reabsorbed, a process referred to as entero-hepatic recirculation or biliary recycling, and thus their stay in the body is prolonged.

The extraction ratio of drugs is important in relation to their hepatic clearance as they pass through the liver. The removal of drugs with a high clearance (70 per cent and over) is dependent on the hepatic blood flow: conversely the removal of those with a clearance of 30 per cent and under is dependent on microsomal enzyme activity and is affected by enzyme induction or inhibition (Wilkinson & Shand, 1975; Sear, 1983).

DEFINITIONS

For an understanding of the pharmacokinetic profile of individual drugs a number of terms must be defined.

Compartment models

Compartmental analysis conceives the body as consisting of distinct compartments interconnected by first-order mass transfer constants. The simplest is a *one-compartment open model* in which the drug is distributed and eliminated on an exponential basis. More relevant to the present topic is a *two-compartment open model*, a small central compartment roughly equivalent to the plasma volume and the richly perfused tissues and a larger peripheral compartment which is in equilibrium with this. Reversible transfer occurs between the central and peripheral compartments in proportion to relative drug concentrations and rate constants are designated as k_{12}, k_{21}, k_{el}.

Partition coefficients

This is the relative affinity of two immiscible media for a drug. The tissue/blood partition coefficient is of great importance in determining the rate of transfer of a drug from blood and its excretion or metabolism. A high partition coefficient slows elimination by limiting the delivery of the drug to the site of metabolism or excretion.

Volume of distribution

V_d or apparent volume of distribution, is the volume of fluid into which the drug appears to distribute with a concentration equal to that in plasma. This expresses the extent to which a drug passes from plasma to peripheral tissues. V_d can only be estimated if the drug is given intravenously or if its systemic bioavailability is known.

Clearance

This is the concept used to describe the removal of a drug from a biological system. Clearance is measured as the apparent volume from which a drug is removed in a given period of time and is usually expressed as ml min ^{1}.

Area under the curve (AUC)

The profile of time-related plasma concentrations expressed in units of concentration X time. $AUC_{0 \rightarrow \infty}$ may be used to determine V_d of a drug following intravenous administration.

Half-life

The mathematical representation of the term for

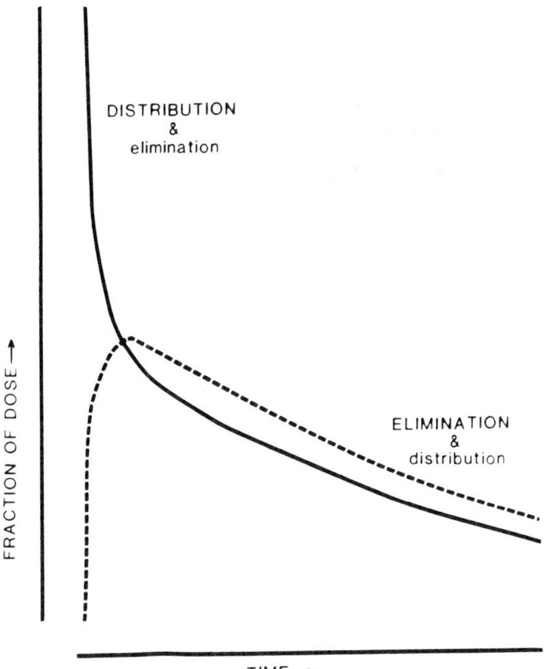

Fig. 4.2 Concept of initial redistribution and elimination of intravenous drugs in a two compartment open model —— plasma (central pool) – – – well perfused peripheral compartment.

the initial distribution ($t\frac{1}{2}\alpha$) and final elimination ($t\frac{1}{2}\beta$) of a drug (Fig. 4.2). These are calculated from the rate of decline of the plasma concentration. The rapid initial fall represents the distribution of the drug from the central to the peripheral compartments. Elimination half-life (usually referred to simply as the half-life) is the more important parameter and usually increases with age.

As the term implies, the distribution half-life depends on rate of dispersion of the drug throughout the body, while the elimination (or terminal) half-life is mainly related to inactivation.

First-order kinetics

This refers to the transfer (or metabolism) of a constant fraction of drug per unit time. The passive processes of absorption and glomerular filtration are examples where the rate of transfer of drug is directly proportional to the amount to be moved. The absolute rate of this process diminishes with time as concentration decreases.

Zero-order (or dose-dependent) *kinetics*

Here the body's ability to remove a drug is limited (or the processes might become saturated) and the reaction proceeds at a fixed rate irrespective of concentration.

Elimination

Elimination is the sum of all the processes that remove the drug from the body (excretion and metabolism). It is usually quantified by the elimination rate constant (K or K_{el}) which is the sum of all the metabolic or excretory processes in the body. It is related to the elimination half-life ($t\frac{1}{2}\beta$) as follows:

$$K_{el} = 0.693/t\tfrac{1}{2}$$

These are usually calculated from a semi-logarithmic plot of serum concentration against time preferably after intravenous injection.

INFUSION PHARMACOKINETICS

Although continuous infusion of intravenous anaesthetics has been used off and on for many years it is only very recently that an attempt has been made to understand their pharmacokinetics when given by this route. Generally speaking one aims to attain a constant plasma level (SS) of the infused drug adequate to produce the desired level of anaesthesia. This can be achieved in three ways, as illustrated in Figure 4.3.

1 Continuous infusion rate: A delay will always occur between the start of the infusion and the establishment of a steady state plateau. The rate at which this plateau is achieved depends upon the distribution (α) and elimination (β) half-lives of the drugs used (Table 4.2). As the initial distribution (α) is usually much faster than β it can be ignored. Thus for practical purposes the rate of attainment of steady state during continuous intravenous infusion is related to the elimination half-life ($t\frac{1}{2}\beta$). The magnitude of this steady state concentration (C_{ss}) is related to both the infusion rate and clearance (Q/V,β). Doubling the infusion rate doubles the steady state concentration but does not influence the rate at which steady state is achieved.

2 Two stage infusion rate: The delay in achieving

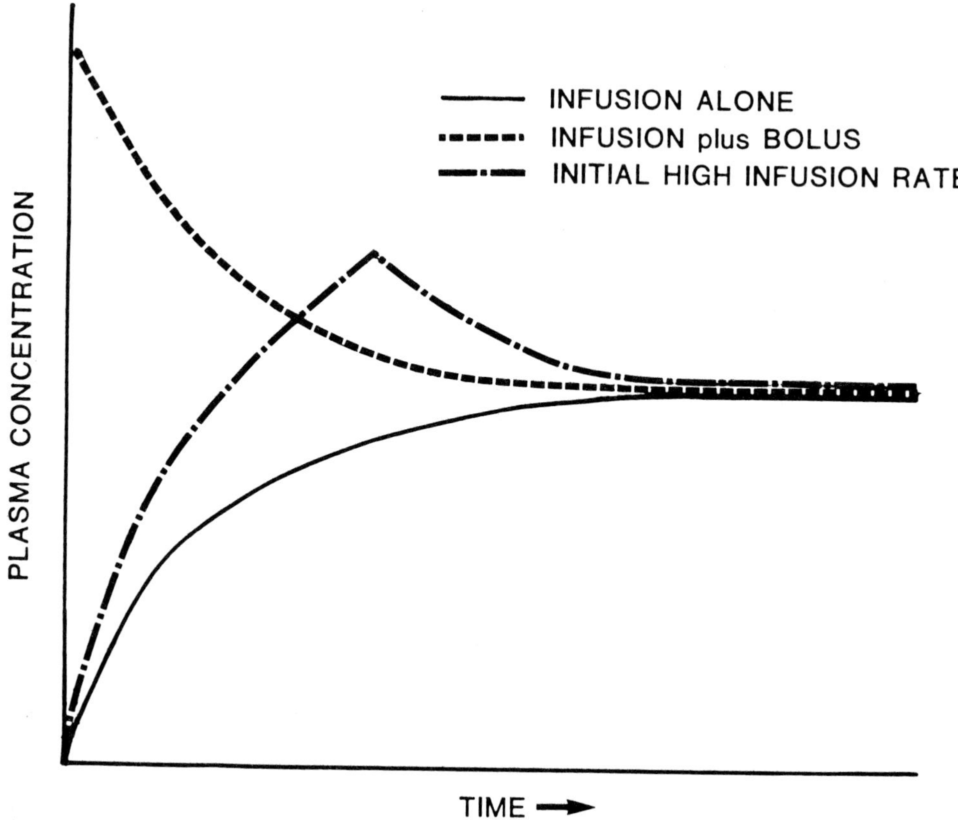

Fig. 4.3 Alternative approaches to achieving a steady plasma concentration of an intravenous anaesthetic given by dilute infusion
——— infusion alone
– – – – initial bolus followed by infusion
–·–·–· initial high infusion rate.

Table 4.2 Duration of drug infusion and approach to steady state

Time (multiples of $t\frac{1}{2}\beta$)	*Percentage of steady state achieved*
0.5	29
1	50
2	75
3	88
3.3	90
4	94
5	97
6	98
7	99

(from data of Greenblatt & Koch-Weser (1975) and Hug (1978)).

a steady state level can be shortened by using an initial fast infusion rate and reducing it once the desired degree of depression is achieved. This is more difficult to achieve in practice than in theory and one usually reduces the infusion rate gradually until the desired level is reached.

3 Initial bolus followed by infusion: It might be difficult, or even impossible, to avoid a 'dip' in the plasma level as initial distribution of the bolus can occur faster than the rise due to the infusion. In practice one may give small incremental doses to 'cover' this period.

Elimination pharmacokinetics are similar for infusion techniques as for single doses, except that the total amount of the drug in the body will be greater and some might be sequestrated in poorly perfused tissues.

CLINICAL SIGNIFICANCE OF PHARMACOKINETICS

Aspects of intravenous anaesthetics which are dependent on their pharmacokinetic profile will be discussed here, with particular reference to clinical practice. Of necessity most examples will relate to thiopentone, although other drugs will be mentioned if data are available.

Onset of action

Onset of action depends on an adequate concentration of active drug being delivered to the cerebral cells. Rapidly acting drugs are those which, in adequate concentrations, will induce loss of consciousness in one arm-brain circulation time (Table 3.1). This can vary from 10 to 30 seconds dependinq on the condition of the patient and the state of the peripheral circulation. Slower acting drugs might take 30 to 120 seconds and they never act in one circulation time. The differences can be explained as follows:

slow onset — dissociation characteristics delay transfer across the 'blood-brain' barrier
— breakdown occurs to hypnotically active drug in the body

rapid onset — non-ionised: no blood-brain barrier
— high lipid-solubility

The differences between these two groups can be illustrated by comparing the onset of action of thiopentone with its oxygen analogue, pentobarbitone. It will be recalled (Chapter 1) that rapidity of action was one of the factors which led to the eclipse of pentobarbitone as an intravenous anaesthetic by its sulphur analogue, thiopentone. Figure 4.4 shows the time of onset of action of varying doses of these drugs, measured from the end of a rapid injection into large antecubital veins in fit adults. At all doses the activity of thiopentone occurred earlier than that of pentobarbitone, as judged by the first detectable change in the eeg pattern.

Using stopping of counting as a simpler endpoint one could still detect a significantly earlier onset of action of thiopentone as compared with pentobarbitone (Table 2.1).

These drug differences can be explained by some physical characteristics as shown in Table 4.4. The all-important difference is in the partition coefficient of the non-ionised form of the drug which is 60 times higher with thiopentone than with pentobarbitone. There are small differences in the pKa of the two compounds which are reflected by the fraction of the non-ionised form at the pH of blood and there is also more plasma binding of thiopentone which should make pentobarbitone a slightly more potent drug on a weight basis. The more rapid onset is undoubtedly due to the greater affinity of brain tissue for thiopentone as compared with pentobarbitone.

It is interesting to note that a similar relationship exists with a large number of barbiturates in animals (Table 4.4). Here again the lipid solubility of unionised drug is shown to be all-important.

Also of clinical significance is the effect of the

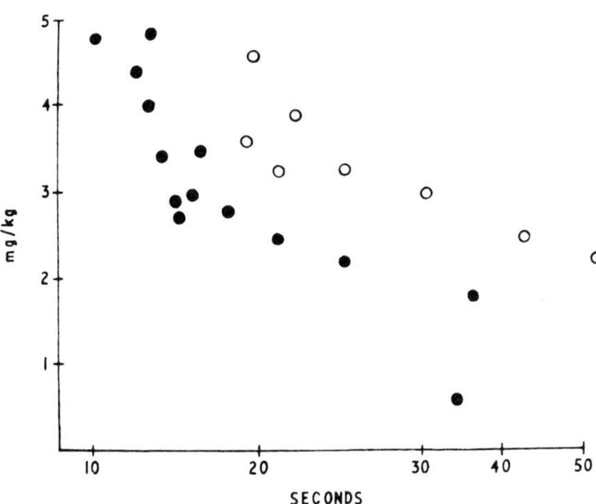

Fig. 4.4 Time to onset of action, as judged by first changes in EEG pattern of thiopentone ● and pentobarbitone ○.

Table 4.3 Some physical properties of thiopentone and pentobarbitone*

	Thiopentone	*Pentobarbitone*
pKa	7.6	8.1
Fraction non-ionized at pH 7.4	0.61	0.83
Fraction bound to plasma protein at pH 7.4	0.75	0.40
Partition coefficient (n-heptane/water) of non-ionized form	3.30	0.05

* Taken from the survey by Lant (1982) and based on the work of Brodie & Hogben (1957) and Hogben et al (1959). The different figures given for the same physical property of a drug are due to differences in methodology of individual workers. It has been necessary to give strictly comparable data for two or more drugs in each comparison and the apparent discrepancies are unavoidable.

environmental temperature as shown in Table 2.1. This emphasises the 'delivery' aspect of pharmacokinetics. A high environmental temperature is associated with forearm vasodilatation and possibly a greater cardiac output than at lower temperatures. This is confirmed by the ability to reproduce the effects of high temperature by injecting during a period of forearm hyperaemia following release of an arterial tourniquet (Fig. 2.1).

At present we have no intravenous anaesthetics which we know for certain to be pro-drugs, i.e. agents converted to pharmacologically active drugs in the body. Hydroxydione, the early water-soluble steroid, might have been such a drug, since the delay in onset of action was in the region of 3–5 minutes. This was even further prolonged in unfit patients and was particularly noticeable in those with jaundice or other evidence of liver dysfunction. In that case the onset time might have been as long as 5–10 minutes and to explain this one could invoke delay in conversion to the hypnotically active metabolite.

All injectable benzodiazepines have a slower onset of action than thiopentone. Clinically this is in the 60–90 second range with diazepam but it might extent to 10 minutes with lorazepam. Under controlled conditions, Dundee and Kawar (1982) found,that, on the average, loss of consciousness occurred 11 s after rapid injection of thiopentone compared with 38 s with midazolam. All of the fit young patients lost consciousness with 4+ mg kg^{-1} thiopentone as compared with 40 per cent with 0.3 mg kg^{-1} midazolam.

Unlike the standard induction agents, some patients given seemingly adequate doses of diazepam, midazolam or flunitrazepam do not lose consciousness within 3 minutes even when the injection is given rapidly during forearm reactive hyperaemia (Dundee and Kawar, 1982): the consistency of action is more marked and the onset time is shorter in the elderly. This is in general agreement with other clinical observations on the use of these drugs: the elderly are generally considered to be more sensitive to normal doses of diazepam and more prone to side effects (Greenblatt & Koch-Weser, 1974).

As a group, the benzodiazepines are more highly bound to plasma proteins than the barbiturates, the figures for diazepam and midazolam being in the 95–99 per cent range. This might explain the variability in response as compared with thiopentone. For highly albumen-bound drugs the free concentration in the serum is only a small percentage of the total concentration. Small changes in serum albumen levels will result in relatively large alterations in the amount of free, pharmacologically active drug and thus in variation of clinical response. Differing responses to intravenous benzodiazepines might be due to normal individual variations in plasma proteins or to pathological processes which result in hypo-albuminaemia as in malnutrition, liver or kidney disease. Koch-Weser and Sellers (1976) point out that even mild hypoalbuminaemia might double the free serum concentration of highly bound drugs. Although one cannot generalise about the

Table 4.4 Relationship between certain physico-chemical properties and onset of action of five barbiturates in mice (from Sharpless, 1970).

	*Partition coefficient**	*Protein binding*** *Plasma*	*Brain*	*Onset of action in mice†* *(min)*	pKa°
Barbitone	1	0.05	0.06	22.0	7.8
Phenobarbitone	3	0.20	0.19	12.0	7.3
Pentobarbitone	39	0.35	0.29	0.1	8.0
Quinalbarbitone	52	0.44	0.39	0.1	7.9
Thiopentone	580	0.65	0.50	0	7.4

* Methylene chloride/water coefficient of nonionized form at 25°C (Bush, 1963).
** 0.001 M barbiturate acids by 1% brain serum albumen in M/15 phosphate buffer at pH 7.4, and by rabbit brain homogenetics (Goldbaum & Smith, 1954).
† Butler (1942)
° Ionization exponent at 25°C (Bush, 1963).

effects of ageing, a number of workers have investigated its influence on the proportion of drug bound to plasma protein and found a significant reduction of bound drug in the elderly (Mitchard, 1977).

While variations in binding might explain the variation in response to drugs it does not explain their slow onset. With clinically tolerable doses injected rapidly, it has not been possible to 'beat' the 25–30 second onset time. Diazepam has a pKa of 3.5 and relatively low fat solubility, the octanol/water partition coefficient being 2.79 and heptane/water 1.68 (Curry & Whelpton, 1979) which offers an adequate explanation for the delay in onset compared with the rapidly acting induction agents.

Potency

As already mentioned, all intravenous anaesthetics have a physicochemical affinity for plasma protein, mainly albumen, and exist in the blood in either the free or bound form.

Plasma proteins can be looked upon as non-specific receptors, which act as a store for some drugs. Where the level is abnormally low, storage will be reduced and a higher than normal concentration of free drug will be available to exert its action, both therapeutic and toxic. Thus the clinical potency of the highly bound drug is affected and this is a contributory cause of increased sensitivity in poor risk patients.

The speed of injection can also affect the potency by virtue of saturation of binding sites. With rapid intravenous injection the binding capacity of the albumen molecules in the limited blood volume available for mixing with the drug might well be exceeded. The rapid introduction of highly bound drugs into the circulation produces very much higher concentrations of free drug than when the administration is slow enough to allow mixing with the entire blood volume during injection (Koch-Weser & Sellers, 1976). The higher level of free drug in the serum might be reflected in a greater drug concentration at the sites of action in highly perfused tissues.

A significant reduction in the ED50, and thus greater potency, was observed when thiopentone, methohexitone and Althesin were injected over 5 s as compared with administration over 15 s (Aveling, Bradshaw & Crankshaw, 1978). No difference was noted with infusion times of 15, 30, and 60 s, nor was there a demonstrable effect of injection speed on the potency of propanidid.

These findings are in keeping with clinical impressions of the effect of rapid injection and 'normal doses' are sometimes given rapidly to produce transient muscle relaxation. One forms the impression that recovery is also more rapid after fast injection, but this has not been substantiated in clinical studies with thiopentone, methohexitone and propofol (Bahar et al, 1982). In practice it is possible that the amount of drug given by rapid injection might be reduced subconsciously, thus leading to a more rapid recovery. It is with the highly bound benzodiazepines, rather than with thiopentone, that one might expect increased potency following rapid injection but this is difficult to quantitate clinically.

The most important clinical application of this variable potency is the oft-repeated advice to inject drugs slowly in poor-risk patients. Target organs, which are probably already sensitive to their depressant effects, should be exposed to as low an active drug concentration as is compatible with a therapeutic effect.

Non-pharmacokinetic alterations in potency of intravenous anaesthetics also occur, the most common example being the effects of opioid premedicants, particularly when large doses are combined with hyoscine or a phenothiazine. Here the effect in reducing the induction dose of thiopentone — calculated by a standard clinical method (Dundee et al, 1982) — is greater than when benzodiazepine or 'light opioid' premedication is given: these latter reduced the dose as compared with that required by unpremedicated patients. These changes are independent of the degree of apprehension and must represent a cerebral effect of the premedicant. Different groups of drugs contribute in different ways to the state of clinical anaesthesia, particularly the combination of a hypnotic induction agent and an analgesic. In a study with intravenous premedication, Dundee et al (1985) found a significant reduction in the induction dose of thiopentone following 50 to 100 μg fentanyl. The clinical importance of this is well established in the technique of balanced anaesthesia.

The lower average induction dose and hence greater potency of thiopentone for women as compared with men (Dundee et al, 1982) can also be explained on a pharmacokinetic basis (Christensen, Andreasen & Janssen, 1980; 1981). Based on the relationship between the rate constant (k_{12}) and the initial venous blood concentration with sampling at 40 s after the end of injection of thiopentone, Christensen and his colleagues concluded that it is the initial rate constant (k_{12}) that determines the dose necessary for induction. They found a significantly higher initial concentration at 40 s in venous blood in males, as compared with female subjects, pointing to a higher k_{12}. There was also a relatively larger apparent initial volume of distribution in women, as compared with men.

The same group ef Scandinavian workers (Christensen, Andreasen and Janssen, 1982) found a smaller redistribution rate constant (k_{12}) in elderly as compared with young subjects. This is in keeping with the lower induction dose that they (1983) and others (Dundee et al, 1982) found in elderly patients.

The sensitivity to thiopentone, as manifested by a lower induction dose, found by Edwards and Ellis (1973) and Dundee and Hassard (1983) in patients with a low haemoglobin could be multifactorial in origin. Low plasma proteins would be part of the general 'poor condition' of anaemic patients, who might well have other metabolic or nutritional problems.

Displacement

Displacement from binding sites is another way in which potency of drugs could be altered, although there is little evidence to suggest that this is important in relation to the induction dose of intravenous anaesthetics. Theoretically this effect should be more marked with highly bound drugs but in practice sudden increases in free drug would lead to a bodywide change in distribution and thus minimise the clinical effects.

Interference with plasma binding might be the explanation of why pre-treatment with probencidid 0.5–1.0 g given 3 hours before induction can prolong the action of thiopentone to a statistically significant degree (Kaukinen, Eerola and Ylipalo, 1980). The prolongation of action was similar with one and two doses of probencidid; apnoea or other untoward complications was no more common in pretreated patients. Pretreatment with probencidid also reduces the induction dose of thiopentone (McMurray, Dundee & Henshaw, 1984). There have been no reports of unexpected overaction of induction agents in patients who were receiving therapeutic doses of probencidid.

Aspirin might be an important drug as far as binding to albumen is concerned as it affects this in a complicated manner involving acetylation of a lysine residue within the peptic region of the albumen molecule (Pickard, Hawkins & Farr, 1973). It is surprising that overaction of diazepam or midazolam has not been reported in patients on aspirin therapy. One is a basic and the other is an acidic drug, and the two might interact with different fractions of plasma protein. Perhaps the combination of the two drugs given in the correct time sequence to produce an interaction has not occurred or alternatively, the effect of clinical doses of aspirin in plasma binding might be too small to detect clinically.

Other non-steroidal anti-inflammatory drugs such as phenylbutazone and naproxen have been shown to produce a similar effect in animals (Chaplin, Roszkowski & Richards, 1973), but there are no clinical reports of their importance in man.

Distribution in the body

The 'classical' picture of the distribution of thiopentone in the body, as calculated by Price (1960), is shown in Figure 4.5. This shows the concept of injection into a central pool of blood and rapid uptake by highly perfused organs. Within one minute after injection the blood has given up 90 per cent of the injected dose, principally to the central nervous system, heart, liver and other well-perfused viscera. During the subsequent 15–30 minutes these viscera and the brain are in turn depleted because of further redistribution.

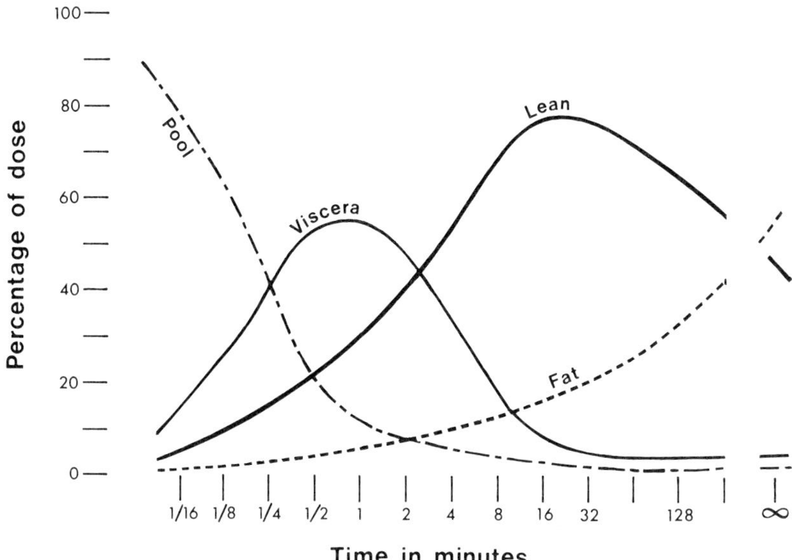

Fig. 4.5 Calculated distribution of drug in various tissues following a single injection of thiopentone (Price, 1960).

About 80 per cent of the thiopentone given up by the richly perfused viscera is distributed to the other aqueous tissues of the body (lean tissues in Fig. 4.5) with a small amount entering the fat. All of this is in keeping with the principles set out in Tables 4.1, 4.3 and 4.5. There is general agreement about this profile, although opinions and findings are at variance with respect to the degree of uptake by fat and the role of detoxication in the early pharmacokinetics of thiopentone. These will be discussed in the appropriate chapter.

Any factor which alters the profile of Fig. 4.5 or the dynamic balance of Figure 4.1 will affect the clinical action of an intravenous anaesthetic.

The first, and probably the most important of these, is the volume of the central pool into which the drug is initially distributed. Hypovolaemia will increase the circulatory concentration and possibly increase the amount of free drug and, since this is often accompanied by vasoconstriction or other derangements of circulatory dynamics, the perfusion of non-essential tissues will be affected. Anaesthetists are acutely aware of the lowered tolerance of the shocked patient to thiopentone and similar drugs and tend to reduce dosage accordingly.

In addition, because of their adverse haemodynamic effects, the action of intravenous anaesthetics can be prolonged in patients in whom they have caused hypotension. It is not possible to prove this point experimentally but it is in agreement with clinical impressions.

Body size, particularly lean body mass, is another factor which can affect the course of clinical anaesthesia. The initial dose of intravenous anaesthetics is often calculated on a weight basis as mg kg^{-1}, or less commonly on a weight per body surface (mg m^{-2}) basis. Although there is an enormous range of dosage in any patient population, it is more marked in the obese who, on a weight basis, require less than other body types. This is shown in the case of thiopentone on data obtained from about 600 fit unpremedicated adults (Table 4.5). Here the average dose required for the obese was significantly less ($P < 0.001$) than for other physical types, while the differences between requirements in the other groups did not reach statistical significance.

Table 4.5 Average dose of thiopentone (mg kg^{-1}) required to induce anaesthesia in healthy unpremedicated subjects when given under standard conditions. (from Dundee et al, 1982)

Build	— average	3.58
	— thin	3.69
	— muscular	3.78
	— obese	3.21

Body size, and particularly lean body mass, is less in the young adult than in the elderly and this could be another factor contributing to the known sensitivity of this age group to intravenous anaesthetics. Here again one can infer a smaller blood volume with which the initial dose is mixed. This is not to be confused with the V_d which is often increased in the elderly.

Acid-base changes

These should be considered in relation to the distribution of drugs in the body for while they have an effect on plasma binding their principal action is on the wider distribution of drugs. This effect varies from drug to drug but it is best illustrated by reference to thiopentone.

Table 4.6, calculated by Ghoneim and Spector (1982), shows the effect of changes in plasma pH on a weakly acidic drug. A high plasma pH favours ionisation so that less will cross membranes, such as the blood–brain barrier. Thus, although the total amount of drug in the plasma will increase, the effective intracellular concentration is reduced. The opposite occurs with acidosis. In Table 4.6 the ratio of non-ionised to ionised is 0.6 at normal plasma pH and only 0.25 at pH 8.1. While this is an extreme example it does emphasise the danger of overdose in acidotic patients. Furthermore it is usually poor risk patients who present with acidosis and this is another reason for care in their handling.

Table 4.6 Distribution of thiopentone (pKa 7.6) in plasma and cells under normal physiological conditions (A) and with varied plasma pH (B) (Ghoneim & Spector, 1982).

A

	Plasma (pH 7.4)	Cell (pH 7.1)	
(1.6)	Nonionized drug ⟷	Nonionized drug	(1.6)
	⇅	⇅	
(1.0)	Ionized drug	Ionized drug	(0.5)
(2.6)	Total drug	Total drug	(2.1)

B

	Plasma (pH 8.1)	Cell (pH 7.1)	
(1)	Nonionized drug ⟷	Nonionized drug	(1)
	⇅	⇅	
(3.1)	Ionized drug	Ionized drug	(0.3)
(4.1)	Total drug	Total drug	(1.3)

Changes in pregnancy

Plasma volume might be increased by as much as 50 per cent in pregnancy and this is accompanied by a decrease in concentration of plasma proteins. Together they tend to reduce the total concentration of drugs that are normally highly protein bound, thus increasing the fraction of free drug. There is also an increase in total body water, which is greater when oedema is present, but this primarily affects the polar drugs with a small V_D rather than the lipophilic intravenous anaesthetics. The increase in renal blood flow which occurs during pregnancy is unlikely to affect the pharmacokinetics of intravenous anaesthetics, nor does the metabolic activity of the fetal liver (Woods et al, 1982).

The haemodynamic changes are probably, on the other hand, of some practical importance as greater cardiac output and a shorter circulation time tend to enhance any deleterious effects of a bolus administration. This is particularly important near term when maternal hypotension can have an adverse effect on the fetus. Maternal acidosis which can result from prolonged labour, particularly when the mother is starved or vomiting, will affect the action of drugs in the manner described above, thus increasing the potential toxicity of intravenous anaesthetics.

Placental transfer

Placental transfer is also part of the larger picture of distribution of drugs in the body — the placenta and fetus can simply be looked upon as a deep pharmacokinetic compartment with its own constants (k_{13}).

Uterine contractions which affect placental blood flow can influence transfer of drugs to the fetus. If the peak maternal concentration occurs during a contraction, theoretically the accompanying reduction in intravillous blood flow will reduce placental transmission. This has been demonstrated with diazepam (Haram et al, 1978) and theoretically it could be important with induction doses of thiopentone and similar drugs. However, one cannot envisage a technique which would reliably ensure the arrival of the bolus at the placenta at the appropriate moment to minimise placental transfer, yet with normal techniques of administration one would expect the fetus of a mother in labour to receive less drug than that of a non-labouring mother.

Keeping the peak maternal concentration low might be important in elective Caesarean section operation particularly where this is carried out because of concern for the fetus. With prolonged or slow administration, this effect is unlikely to be important but with infusions there is a likelihood of a drug accumulating in the fetus.

Drugs mainly cross the placenta by passive diffusion, the placenta behaving like any other lipid membrane. Lipid-soluble drugs with a molecular weight of 600–1000 diffuse with ease, and water-soluble substances of molecular weights up to 100 cross the placenta readily if non-ionised (Reynolds, 1982). The barbiturates and other induction agents and the benzodiazepines are all sufficiently lipid-soluble to cross the placenta readily. However the large maternal binding of drugs will reduce the amount that the baby receives over a limited period of time, particularly if the maternal bolus coincides with a uterine contraction. Because of a small pH gradient across the placenta and possible different protein binding properties of maternal and fetal plasma, equilibrium between maternal and fetal concentrations does not necessarily occur at equal total concentrations. Once equilibrium has occurred the fetal concentration is likely to fall at a slower rate than that of the mother and eventually placental transfer will be reversed. The degree and duration of placental transfer can be determined by measuring drug concentration in umbilical artery and vein. When the arterial concentration is the higher of the two the drug then passes from fetus to mother.

The ability of the fetus to conjugate or metabolise drugs is less than that of the mother and most drugs are eliminated by transfer back to the maternal circulation. Hydrophobic metabolites cannot be readily excreted, and accumulate in the amniotic fluid.

Diazepam is a good example of a drug which tends to accumulate in the fetus and which is removed from the neonate at a slower rate than from the mother. In patients who had received 10 mg intravenously at varying times during labour, Gamble et al (1977) measured venous concentrations in the mother and neonate (Table 4.7). The average values show an infant: maternal ratio of approximately 1.4:1 at delivery and 1.6:1 one day later. The importance of this is obvious when large doses of diazepam are given as an anticonvulsant in eclampsia.

Enzyme induction

Enzyme induction refers to stimulation of metabolising enzymes in liver microsomes, either by drugs given previously, or on occasions by the continuous or repeated administration of the same drug; this is referred to as self-induction. Experimental evidence indicates that the mechanism of this effect involves synthesis of more microsomal drug-metabolising enzymes, including cytochrome P450. This might take a number of days to develop and although the phenomenon is reversible some time will elapse before enzyme activity returns to pretreatment levels.

A large number of drugs are involved in this, and relevant 'enzyme inducers' include barbiturates and other hypnotics, anticonvulsants, phenothiazines, antidepressants and mild analgesics. Development of tolerance to barbiturates might be related to self-induced acceleration of their own hepatic microsomal metabolism, but adaptive change at the drug receptor is also a cause; this is acquired cellular tolerance (Remmer, 1962).

Enzyme induction is of little clinical importance in relation to normal doses of intravenous anaesthetics. The adaptive cellular changes from long-term administration are more likely to lead to resistance to induction doses. Its importance in continuous intravenous administration has not

Table 4.7 Plasma diazepam levels (mean ± SEM) in 10 mothers and infants at delivery and 24 hr later following 10 mg intravenously given to mothers in labour. (from Gamble et al, 1977)

	Mean plasma diazepam (ng ml⁻¹) *Delivery*	*24 hr*
Mother	134 ± 17.6	46 ± 1.2
Infant	196 ± 21.1	75 ± 8.4

been evaluated. If one likens this situation to that following intraperitoneal administration in animals (Quinn, Axelrod & Brodie, 1958) then the duration of action might be markedly affected by enzyme activity (Table 4.8). The likelihood of self-induction occurring during infusions of thiopentone and similar drugs remains a possibility.

Table 4.8 Duration of action of 100 mg kg^{-1} hexobarbitone intraperitoneally (except dog, 50 mg kg^{-1} i.v.) in different species related to liver microsomal enzyme activity. (from Quinn, Axelrod & Brodie, 1958)

Species	*Duration of action (min)*	*Hexobarbitone half- life (min)*	*Enzyme activity (ug g^{-1} hr^{-1})*
Mouse	12 ± 8	19 ± 7	598 ± 184
Rabbit	49 ± 12	60 ± 11	196 ± 28
Rat	90 ± 15	140 ± 54	134 ± 51
Dog	315 ± 105	260 ± 20	36 ± 30

In practice the dangers of enzyme induction are associated with oral anticoagulants and anticonvulsants. Serious consequences can result from changing the hypnotic used by patients in common therapy from an inducer (pentobarbitone or phenobarbitone) to a non-inducer. We now know that a single administration of thiopentone, propofol or midazolam has no such effect, although Nimmo, Thompson and Prescott (1981) have implicated halothane as a possible cause of enzyme induction; in their patients, anaesthesia was induced by thiopentone.

RECOVERY

The rapid injection of a bolus of 2.5 mg kg^{-1} thiopentone over 5, 10, 15 and 30 s in the dog produces curves for the arterial concentration shown in Fig. 4.6. The peak concentrations for 5 s

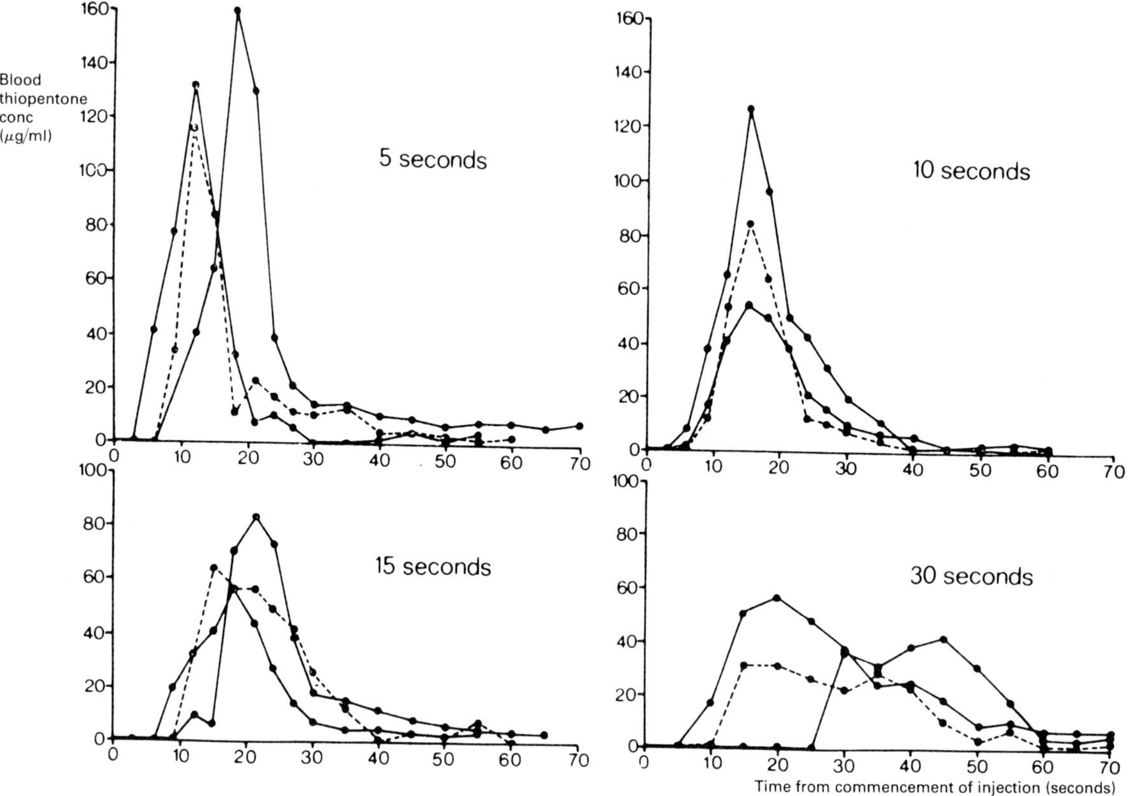

Fig. 4.6 Plasma concentration in arterial blood following 2.5 mg kg^{-1} thiopentone in the dog, given intravenously at the rates shown. (Aveling, Bradshaw and Crankshaw, 1978).

injections are at least twice those for doses given over 15 s (Crankshaw, Rosler & Ware, 1979). However the AUC and equilibrium plasma concentrations are similar at the four injection speeds. This is in keeping with the clinical observations of Bahar and his colleagues (1982) who found that, within the usual clinical range of injection times, the speed of administration did not affect recovery with 4 mg kg^{-1} thiopentone, 1.5 mg kg^{-1} methohexitone and 2 mg kg^{-1} propofol.

Recovery from anaesthesia is a complex event, involving factors other than the brain or plasma level of drug. Since most intravenous anaesthetics follow the course shown in Figure 4.5 for thiopentone, any factor which alters this will affect recovery. The early distribution phase can account for recovery from normal induction doses of rapidly acting drugs. Factors such as blood volume and body mass have already been discussed; they are less important with the conventional induction agents.

The *elimination* or *terminal half-life* is only important with large doses of rapidly acting, and thus rapidly diffusible drugs, most often given by infusion, or with the slower acting basal hypnotics such as the benzodiazepines. Christensen, Andreasen & Janssen (1981; 1982) found an increase in terminal half-life of thiopentone with advancing years, with larger V_d (V_2, V_3) in the elderly, but emphasized that the distribution rate constant (k_{12}) is the predominant factor in the pharmacokinetic profile of a dose sufficient to obtund the lash reflex.

A prolongation of $t_{\frac{1}{2}}\beta$ with age has been demonstrated convincingly with diazepam (Klotz et al, 1975; Breimer, 1979; Greenblatt et al, 1980) and with midazolam (Collier et al, 1982; Harper et al, 1985). This is of clinical importance and is a reason for reducing the dosage in the elderly. It is likely that these generalisations with respect to age apply to all intravenous anaesthetics.

There has been much speculation on the importance of liver dysfunction in prolonging thiopentone narcosis, but one should note that most of the literature on this subject is 30 to 35 years old (Scheifley & Higgins, 1940; Masson & Beland, 1945; Shideman et al, 1947; 1949; Walker & Wynn Parry, 1949; Dundee, 1956). It is worth noting that in early studies it was with doses of 1.0 g thiopentone that Dundee (1952) demonstrated a prolongation of action of thiopentone with induced liver dysfunction. While the liver can remove up to 50 per cent of the drug from the hepatic blood flow, even in patients with liver disease, it is only with very large doses which 'saturate' the early redistribution process that the influence of detoxication on recovery can be detected.

Drugs which affect plasma binding can delay recovery from highly bound drugs. In the field of anaesthesia, synergism with other drugs must be remembered as a cause of delayed recovery, particularly if there are analgesics which contribute in a different manner to the production of surgical anaesthesia. They act in a manner similar to 'increasing the threshold' for noxious stimuli or, to put it in the reverse manner, they decrease the cerebral and plasma concentrations at which patients react to stimuli. Minor degrees of persistent curarisation can have a similar effect.

All of this assumes that the response of patients to drugs is reproducible and consistent, but this is not so. Even allowing for the effects of other drugs and certain pathological conditions there is the phenomenon of *tolerance* (referred to elsewhere as *adaptive cellular* changes) which, in the present context, is clinically seen as resistance to the hypnotic effects of drugs. Acquired tolerance to one hypnotic, and even to alcohol, can lead to cross tolerance to others with a similar clinical effect, even though of a different chemical group. The phenomenon of acute cerebral tolerance to thiopentone has been recognised for many years both in animals (Shideman et al, 1948) and humans (Mark et al, 1949; Brodie et al, 1951; Dundee 1956; Dundee et al, 1956). One important feature is the return of consciousness at higher plasma concentrations following single large doses of thiopentone than after smaller doses (Dundee et al, 1956). These findings have been confirmed by Toner et al (1980) and although the underlying mechanism has been doubted by Hudson et al (1982) it is clear that with different doses the same person can react very differently to thiopentone.

Given over a period of time, the plasma level required to maintain a given level of anaesthesia gradually increases. Most important, the plasma level at which consciousness is regained increases with the dose given as a bolus. Brand and his colleagues (1961) could not correlate the depth of thiopentone anaesthesia, as shown by the electroencephalogram, with plasma levels and clearly there are a number of non-pharmacokinetic factors which can affect recovery from anaesthesia. The extent to which this applies to other intravenous anaesthetics is not known but it is likely that the same cellular adaptive changes occur.

OPIOIDS

These drugs often play an important part in intravenous anaesthesia, even to the extent of being the sole agents. More commonly they are given in single or repeated doses or, in the case of the shorter-acting drugs, as a continuous infusion. Total intravenous anaesthesia can be produced by an infusion of an opiate (usually fentanyl) with an orthodox induction agent (Major et al, 1982; Jones et al, 1983). Their pharmacokinetic pattern is similar to that of other intravenous agents, namely distribution to a two, or sometimes three, compartment model (Bovill et al, 1981; Bower & Hull, 1983).

The onset of action of all drugs in this group is slower than that of thiopentone, varying from 1–3 min after normal intravenous doses. Comparing the properties of morphine with the more rapidly acting pethidine the delay in effect of the latter could be correlated with its lower lipid solubility and with a greater portion of ionised drug in the relatively acidic brain (Oldendorf. et al, 1972). Hug and colleagues (1981), who studied the pharmacokinetics of morphine in the dog, found a rapid clearance from the plasma but a delay of 15–30 minutes before the peak concentration occurred in the cerebrospinal fluid. The ventilatory depressant effects of the morphine could not be correlated with either plasma or cerebrospinal fluid levels.

The more rapid onset of the new drugs fentanyl and alfentanil can be correlated with their lipid solubility which makes them more suitable for use in a continuous infusion.

Entero-hepatic recirculation, as described for the basic drugs such as opioids has been demonstrated also for pethidine and methadone (Lynn et al, 1976; Stoeckel, Hengstmann & Schuttler, 1979). Fentanyl is excreted in the gastric juice and reabsorbed from the alkaline small intestine. The storage capacity of the stomach wall can account for about 20 per cent of injected fentanyl and this could explain the unexpected occurrence of late respiratory depression (Adams & Pybus, 1978); it could also explain the secondary peaks in plasma concentration frequently observed 20 to 50 minutes after administration (McQuay et al, 1979). One might expect these peaks to be reduced or even eliminated by administering alkalis and this has been shown for phenoperidine (Calvey, Milne & Williams, 1983).

The influence of age on pharmacokinetics has been clearly demonstrated for morphine; the plasma half-life in young adults of about three hours (Stanski, Greenblatt & Lowenstein, 1978) can be prolonged in older patients (Jaffe & Martin, 1980). This has also been demonstrated for pethidine (Chan et al, 1975) and fentanyl (Bentley et al, 1982) and probably applies to all opioids.

From the clinician's point of view it is important to realise that the pharmacokinetics of opioids can be influenced by the presence of certain anaesthetics; while only a clinical impression for most drugs, it has been substantiated in the case of fentanyl (Murphy & Hug, 1982). The dose administered also affects the pharmacokinetic profile and particularly the toxicity of drugs of the fentanyl type. Fentanyl is highly bound to plasma protein (Bower, 1981), variation of which can also affect the pharmacokinetics and clinical effects of this potent drug.

It is not always appreciated that morphine has an active metabolite (morphine glucuronide) which can produce respiratory depression (Sassajima, 1970), but this has not been demonstrated with the newer drugs. However a toxic excitatory metabolite of pethidine has been described and can explain the rare case of 'convulsion' after large doses in patients with liver disease.

This brief survey highlights both similarities and differences between the pharmacokinetics of the opioids and the other drugs used in intravenous anaesthesia. These should be understood before large doses of these agents are administered simultaneously.

REFERENCES

Adams A P, Pybus D A 1978 Delayed respiratory depression after use of fentanyl during anaesthesia. British Medical Journal 1: 278–279

Aveling W, Bradshaw A D, Crankshaw D P 1978 The effect of speed of injection on the potency of anaesthetic induction agents. Anaesthesia and Intensive Care 6: 116–119

Bahar M, Dundee J W, O'Neill M P, Briggs L P, Moore J, Merrett J D 1982 Recovery from intravenous anaesthesia. Comparison of disoprofol with thiopentone and methohexitone. Anaesthesia 37: 1171–1175

Bentley J B, Borel J D, Nenad R E, Gillespie T J 1982 Age and fentanyl pharmacokinetics. Anesthesia and Analgesia 61: 968–971

Bovill J G, Sebel P S, Blackburn C L, Heykants J 1981 The pharmacokinetics of alfentanil. Anesthesiology 55:A 174

Bower S 1981 Plasma protein binding of fentanyl. Journal of Pharmacy and Pharmacology 33: 507–513

Bower S, Hull C J 1983 Comparative pharmacokinetics of fentanyl and alfentanil. British Journal of Anaesthesia 54: 871–877

Brand L, Mazzia V D B, van Poznak A, Burns J J, Mark L C 1961 Lack of correlation between electroencephalographic effects and plasma concentrations of thiopentone. British Journal of Anaesthesia 33: 92–96

Breimer D D 1979 Pharmacokinetics and metabolism of various benzodiazepines used as hypnotics. British Journal of Clinical Pharmacology 8: 75–135

Brodie B B, Hogben C A M 1957 Some physico-chemical factors in drug action. Journal of Pharmacy and Pharmacology 9: 345–380

Brodie B B, Mark L C, Lief P A, Bernstein E, Papper E M 1951 Acute tolerance to thiopentone. Journal of Pharmacology and Experimental Therapeutics 102: 215–218

Bush M T 1963 Sedatives and hypnotics 1: Absorption, fate and excretion. In: Root W S, Hofmann F G (eds) Physiological pharmacology: a comprehensive treatise, Part A, 1st ed. Academic Press, London

Butler T C 1942 The delay in onset of action of intravenously injected anesthetics. Journal of Pharmacology and Experimental Therapeutics 74: 118–128

Calvey T N, Milne I A, Williams N E 1983 Effect of antacids on the plasma concentration of phenoperidine. British Journal of Anaesthesia 55: 535–539

Chan K, Kendall M J, Mitchard M, Well W D E 1975 The effect of ageing on plasma pethidine concentration. British Journal of Clinical Pharmacology 2: 297–302

Chaplin M D, Roszkowski A P, Richards R K 1973 Displacement of thiopental from plasma proteins by nonsteroidal anti-inflammatory agents. Proceedings of Society of Experimental Biology and Medicine 143: 667–671

Christensen J H, Andreasen F, Janssen J A 1980 Pharmacokinetics of thiopentone in 'a group of young women and a group of young men. British Journal of Anaesthesia 52: 913–918

Christensen J H, Andreasen F, Janssen J A 1981 Influence of age and sex on the pharmacokinetics of thiopentone. British Journal of Anaesthesia 53: 1189–1196

Christensen J H, Andreasen F, Janssen J A 1982 Pharmacokinetics and pharmacodynamics of thiopentone — acomparison between young and elderly patients. Anaesthesia 37: 398–404

Christensen J H, Andreasen F, Janssen J A 1983 Thiopentone sensitivity in young and elderly women. British Journal of Anaesthesia 55: 33–39

Collier P S, Kawar P, Gamble J A S, Dundee J W 1982 Influence of age on pharmacokinetics of midazolam. British Journal of Clinical Pharmacology 13: 602P

Crankshaw D P, Rosler A, Ware M 1979 The short term distribution of thiopentone in the dog. Anaesthesia and Intensive Care 7: 148–151

Curry S H, Whelpton R 1979 Pharmacokinetics of closely related benzodiazepines. British Journal of Clinical Pharmacology 8: 155–215

Dundee J W 1952 Thiopentone narcosis in the presence of hepatic dysfunction. British Journal of Anaesthesia 24: 81–100

Dundee J W 1956 Thiopentone and other thiobarbiturates. Livingstone, Edinburgh

Dundee J W, Halliday N J, McMurray T J, Harper K W 1985 Pretreatment with opioids. The effect on thiopentone induction requirements and on the onset of action of midazolam. Anaesthesia 41: 159–161

Dundee J W, Hassard T H 1983 The influence of haemoglobin and plasma urea levels on the induction dose of thiopentone. Anaesthesia 38: 26–28

Dundee J W, Hassard T H, McGowan W A W, Henshaw J 1982 The 'induction' dose of thiopentone. A method of study and preliminary illustrative results. Anaesthesia 37: 1176–1184

Dundee J W, Kawar P 1982 Letter to the Editor: Consistency of action of midazolam. Anesthesia and Analgesia 61: 544–545

Dundee J W, Price H L, Dripps R D 1956 Acute tolerance to thiopentone in man. British Journal of Anaesthesia 28: 344–352

Edwards R, Ellis F R 1973 Clinical significance of thiopentone binding to haemoglobin and plasma protein. British Journal of Anaesthesia 45: 891–893

Fingl E, Woodbury D M 1965 General principles. In: Goodman L S, Gilman A (eds) The pharmacological basis of therapeutics, 6th edn. Macmillan, New York

Gamble J A S, Moore J, Lamki H, Howard P J 1977 A study of plasma diazepam levels in mother and infant. British Journal of Obstetrics and Gynaecology 84: 588–591

Ghoneim M, Spector R 1982 Pharmacokinetics of drugs administered intravenously. In: Scurr C, Feldman S (eds) Scientific foundations of anaesthesia, 3rd edn. Heinemann Medical, London. p.425–424

Goldbaum L R, Smith T K 1954 The interaction of barbiturates with serum albumin and its possible relation to their disposition and pharmacological actions. Journal of Pharmacology and Experimental Therapeutics 111: 197–209

Greenblatt D J, Allen M D, Harmatz J S, Shader R I 1980 Diazepam disposition determinants. Clinical Pharmacology and Therapeutics 27: 301–311

Greenblatt D J, Koch-Weser J 1974 Clinical toxicity of chlordiazepoxide and diazepam in relation to serum albumin concentration: a report from the Boston Collaborative Drug Surveillance Program. European Journal of Clinical Pharmacology 7: 259–262

Greenblatt D J, Koch-Weser J 1975 Drug therapy : clinical pharmacokinetics. New England Journal of Medicine 293: 702–705, 964–970

Haram K, Bakke O M, Johannessen K H, Lund T 1978 Transplacental passage of diazepam during labor: influence of uterine contractions. Clinical Pharmacology and Therapeutics 24: 590–599

Harper K W, Collier P S, Dundee J W, Elliott P, Halliday N J, Lowry K G 1985 Age and nature of operation influence the pharmacokinetics of midazolam. British Journal of Anaesthesia 57: 866–871

Hogben C A M, Tocco D J, Brodie B B, Schanker L S 1959 On the mechanism of intestinal absorption of drugs. Journal of Pharmacology and Experimental Therapeutics 125: 275–282

Hudson R J, Stanski D R, Meathe E, Saidman L J 1982 Does acute tolerance to thiopental exist? Anesthesiology 57:A501

Hug C C 1978 Pharmacokinetics of drugs administered intravenously. Anesthesia and Analgesia 57: 704–728

Hug C C, Murphy M R, Rigel D P, Olson W A 1981 Pharmacokinetics of morphine injected intravenously into the anaesthetised dog. Anesthesiology 54: 38–47

Jaffe J H, Martin W R 1980 Opioid analgesics and antagonists. In: Gilman A G, Goodman L S, Gilman A (eds) The pharmacological basis of therapeutics. 1985, Macmillan, New York

Jones D, Laurence A S, Thornton J A 1983 Total intravenous anaesthesia with etomidate-fentanyl: use in general and gynaecological surgery. Anaesthesia 38: 29–34

Kaukinen S, Eerola M, Ylipalo P 1980 Prolongation of thiopentone anaesthesia by probenecid. British Journal of Anaesthesia 52: 603–607

Klotz U, Avant G R, Hoyumpa A, Schenker S, Wilkinson G R 1975 The effects of age and liver disease on the disposition and elimination of diazepam in adult man. Journal of Clinical Investigation 55: 347–359

Koch-Weser J, Sellers E M 1976 Drug therapy: binding of drugs to serum albumin. New England Journal of Medicine 294: 311–316, 526–531

Lant A F 1982 Factors affecting the action of drugs. In: Scurr C, Feldman S (eds) Scientific foundations of anaesthesia, 3rd edn. Heinemann, London

Lynn R K, Olsen G D, Leger R M, Gordon E P, Smith R G, Gerber N 1976 The secretion of methadone and its major metabolite in the gastric juice of humans. Drug Metabolism and Disposition 4: 504

Major E, Verniquet A J W, Yate P M, Waddell T K 1982 Disoprofol and fentanyl for total intravenous anaesthesia. Anaesthesia 37: 541–547

Mark L C, Papper E M, Brodie B B, Rovenstine E A 1949 Quantitative pharmacologic studies with Pentothal. New York State Journal of Medicine 49:1546

Masson G M C, Beland E 1945 Influence of the liver and the kidney on the duration of anaesthesia produced by barbiturates. Anesthesiology 6: 483–491

Mitchard M 1977 Drug distribution in the elderly. In: Crooks J, Stevenson I H (eds) Drugs and the elderly. Macmillan, London

Murphy M R, Hug C C 1982 Dose-dependent pharmacokinetics of fentanyl. Anesthesiology 57:A347

McMurray T J, Dundee J W, Henshaw J S 1984 The influence of probenecid on the induction dose of thiopentone. British Journal of Clinical Pharmacology 17:224P

McQuay H J, Moore R A, Paterson G M C, Adams A P 1979 Plasma fentanyl concentrations and clinical observations during and after operation. British Journal of Anaesthesia 51:741

Nimmo W S, Thompson P G, Prescott L F 1981 Microsomal enzyme induction after halothane anaesthesia. British Journal of Clinical Pharmacology 12: 433–434

Oldendorf W H, Hyman S, Braun L, Oldendorf S Z 1972 Blood-brain barrier: penetration of morphine, codeine, heroin and metadone after carotid injection. Science 178: 984–986

Pickard R N, Hawkins D, Farr R S 1973 The influence of acetylsalicylic acid on the binding of acetnozate to human albumin. Annals of the New York Academy of Science 226: 341–354

Price H L 1960 A dynamic concept of the distribution of thiopental in the human body. Anesthesiology 21: 40–45

Quinn G P, Axelrod J, Brodie B B 1958 Species, strain and sex differences in metabolism of hexobarbitone, amidopyrine, antipyrine and aniline. Biochemical Pharmacology 1: 152–159

Remmer H 1962 Drug tolerance. In: Mongar J L, de Reuck A U S (eds) Enzymes and drug action. Churchill, London

Reynolds F 1982 The placenta: structure, physiology and pharmacokinetics. In: Scurr C, Feldman S (eds) Scientific foundations of anaesthesia, 3rd edn. Heinemann, London

Sassajima M 1970 Analgesic effects of morphine-3-monoglucuronide. Keio Gaku 47: 421–526

Scheifley C H, Higgins C M 1940 The effect of partial hepatectomy on the action of certain barbiturates and a phenylurea derivative. American Journal of Medical Science 200: 264–268

Sear J W 1983 General kinetic and dynamic principles and their application to continuous infusion anaesthesia. Anaesthesia 39: 10–25

Sharpless S K 1970 Hypnotics and sedatives. In: Goodman L S, Gilman S (eds) The pharmacological basis of therapeutics, 4th edn. Macmillan, New York. ch 9

Shideman F E, Kelly A R, Adams B J 1947 The role of the liver in the detoxication of thiopental (Pentothal) and two other thiobarbiturates. Journal of Pharmacology and Experimental Therapeutics 91: 331–339

Shideman F E, Kelly A R, Adams B J 1948 Blood levels of thiopental (Pentothal) following repeated administration to the dog. Federation Proceedings 7:255

Shideman F E, Kelly A R, Lee L E, Lowell V F, Adams B J 1949 The role of the liver in the detoxication of thiopental (Pentothal) in man. Anesthesiology 10: 421–428

Stanski D R, Greenblatt D J, Lowenstein E 1978 Kinetics of intravenous and intramuscular morphine. Clinical Pharmacology and Therapeutics 24: 52–59

Stoeckel H, Hengstmann J H, Schuttler J 1979 Pharmacokinetics of fentanyl as a possible explanation for recurrence of respiratory depression. British Journal of Anaesthesia 51: 741–745

Toner W, Howard P J, McGowan W A W, Dundee J W 1980 Another look at acute tolerance to thiopentone. British Journal of Anaesthesia 52: 1005–1008

Walker J M, Wynn Parry C B 1949 Effects of hepatectomy on action of certain anaesthetics in rats. British Journal of Pharmacology 4: 93–97

Wilkinson G R, Shand D G 1975 A physiological approach to hepatic drug clearance. Clinical Pharmacology and Therapeutics 18: 377–390

Woods M A, Stanski D R, Curtis J, Rosen M, Shnider S M 1982 The role of the fetal liver in the distribution of thiopental from mother to fetus. Anesthesiology 57:A390

ADDITIONAL READING

Berkowitz B A, Nagi S H, Yang J C, Hempstead B S, Spector S 1975 The disposition of morphine in surgical patients. Clinical Pharmacology and Therapeutics 17: 629–635

Boobis A R, Lewis P 1982 Drugs in pregnancy: altered pharmacokinetics. British Journal of Hospital Medicine 28: 566–573

Chamberlain G V P, Wilkinson A W 1979 Placental transfer. Pitman, London

Curry S H 1980 Drug disposition and pharmacokinetics, 3rd edn. Blackwell, Oxford

Hull C J 1979 Pharmacokinetics and pharmacodynamics. British Journal of Anaesthesia 51: 579–594

Mather L E, Tucker G T, Pflug A E, Lindop M J, Wilkerson C 1975 Meperidine kinetics in man. Clinical Pharmacology and Therapeutics 17: 21–30

Norman J 1979 Drug-receptor reactions. British Journal of Anaesthesia 51: 595–601

Rowland M, Tozer T N 1980 Clinical pharmacokinetics: concepts and applications. Lea & Febiger, Philadelphia.

Stanski D R, Greenblatt D J, Lowenstein E 1978 Kinetics of intravenous and intramuscular morphine. Clinical Pharmacology and Therapeutics 24: 52–59

Tucker G T 1979 Drug metabolism. British Journal of Anaesthesia 51: 613–616

5

Barbiturates: chemistry and drugs

Clinical grouping

The classical grouping of the barbiturates is based on the expected duration of action of normal therapeutic doses in animals and embraces both drugs given by mouth and those injected intravenously. Many textbooks have distinguished three to four groups as follows:

Long	Oral (or intramuscular) preparations used mostly as sedatives
Medium and short	Usually employed as oral (or intramuscular) sedatives, but can be given intravenously
Ultra-short	Drugs normally given by intravenous injection for induction of anaesthesia

This terminology is illogical and should be abandoned. The intravenous barbiturate anaesthetics are not ultra-short acting, their clinical effect is related to dose and, even after apparent return of consciousness, mental clouding persists for some time. Failure to appreciate this has led to unfortunate accidents. Even the so-called short acting compounds can, in suitable doses, cause drowsiness for many hours, and the duration and intensity of action depends partly on the route of administration. A number of workers have doubted whether there is any important difference between the clinical effects of the long and short acting groups. Parsons (1963) found that the hypnotic action of 100 mg doses of phenobarbitone (long acting), butobarbitone (medium acting) and quinalbarbitone (short acting) was indistinguishable, whereas with 200 mg doses quinalbarbitone produces a more profound effect than the other two drugs. At neither dose level was the 'hangover' more marked after phenobarbitone than following the so-called short-acting drugs.

This book is not concerned with the long acting drugs and differences between these will not be discussed. The remainder of the drugs will be grouped as follows:

Short acting (short and medium group)	Oral sedative which can also be given parenterally, but where there is some delay in onset of action after intravenous injection.
Rapidly acting	Intravenous anaesthetics with no delay in onset of action and dose-related duration.

Of all the factors which contributed to the almost universal acceptance of hexobarbitone and thiopentone as intravenous anaesthetics, in preference to pentobarbitone or amylobarbitone, the ability of effective doses to cause sleep in one arm-brain circulation time was undoubtedly the most important. With pentobarbitone and amylobarbitone there is invariably a delay of 20 to 30 s and this makes their incremental use difficult and even dangerous. Where abnormal effects from a barbiturate can be anticipated — an example is hypotension in poor-risk patients — the slow injection of small doses is desirable, but this can only be done safely with 'rapidly-acting' drugs. The 'rapidly-acting' drugs can be given also by mouth as hypnotics but this is not of immediate clinical importance.

There is a fairly clear relationship between this suggested clinical classification and the chemical structure of the drugs and this will be discussed.

CHEMISTRY

The terminology of the barbiturates varies

between the USA and Britain, the USA using the ending '*al*' and Britain '*one*'. This leads to some confusion as there are several drugs which have been available commercially only in one or other country and therefore are known only by one suffix so that they may not conform to the accepted terminology.

The drugs used in clinical practice are the water-soluble sodium salts prepared by the interactions of urea and malonic (propanedioc) acid.

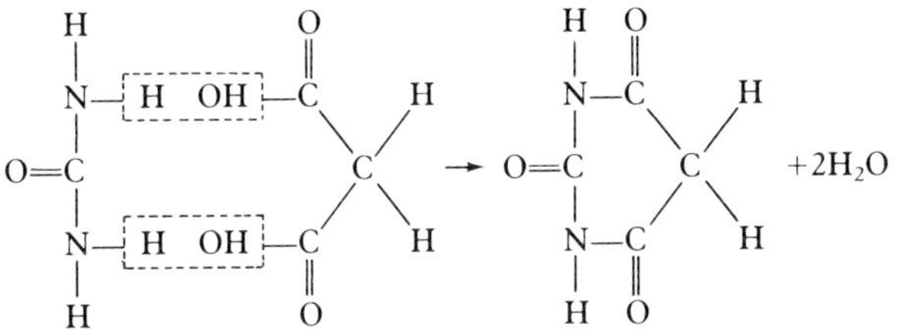

$+2H_2O$

Urea and malonic acid → barbituric acid and water

Although it is more correct to regard barbituric acid as a pyrimidine derivative it is usually depicted as the cyclical ureide of malonic acid in either the keto or enol form, with four common sites of substitution as shown in Figure 5.1. The acidity is due to the hydrogen ion which migrates from the nitrogen in the '1' position. In aqueous solution it dissociates into hydrogen ion and barbiturate ion. The sodium (in position '3') salts are water-soluble and can be administered parenterally.

Barbituric acid is inert as a hypnotic but substitution of the 5-hydrogens by organic radicals endows the resultant drugs with the ability to depress consciousness. Such radicals may be aliphatic, aromatic or heterocyclic. The term 'barbiturate' is used here to embrace the drugs used as induction agents; this is not strictly correct for many of these are in fact thiobarbiturates (prepared by using thiourea rather than urea).

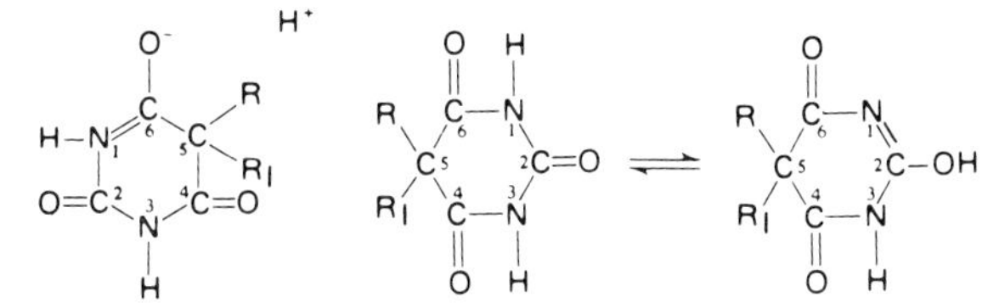

Pyrimidine derivative — Keto form — Enol form

Cyclical ureide of malonic acid

Fig. 5.1: Differing forms of representation of barbituric acid.

The synthesis of the barbiturates is described in Appendix 1, while Appendix 3 describes the methods of detection and estimation of concentrations in biological fluids.

Structure–activity relationship

Many possible side chains can be used in the '5' and '5' positions, but these are mainly concerned with potency and have less effect on the basic action of the drugs than changes in the '1' and '2' positions (Table 5.1). A sulphur atom in position '2' invariably results in a rapidly acting drug. The introduction of a methyl (CH_3) group in position '1' (Fig. 5.1) usually results in a more rapid onset of action, but also produces a very high incidence of dose-related excitatory phenomena, such as tremor, hypertonus and spontaneous involuntary muscle movements.

Oxybarbiturates, except those with a methyl radical in the '1' position, have a limited use in clinical anaesthesia because of the delay in onset of sleep from effective doses. They are sometimes used to produce light sleep during operations under local analgesia or in psychiatric practice. Their main use, however, is as hypnotics or sedatives, usually given by mouth and occasionally by intramuscular injection, especially as preanaesthetic medication. Some methylated barbiturates (methyl barbiturates) undergo rapid demethylation in the body to form active long-lasting compounds and these are unsuitable for anaesthetic practice.

The number of derivatives which can be formed from the parent substances by substitution in the 5 position is virtually limitless. Both hydrogen ions must be replaced by alkyl (straight saturated or unsaturated, branched or cyclical) or aryl (aromatic, e.g. phenol) groups in order to confer hypnotic properties on the barbiturate. Within certain limits an increase in the length of side chain is accompanied by enhancement of narcotic potency and shortening of duration of action. This has attributed to the resulting increase in molecular weight, but that cannot be the sole answer since one of the side chains at the 5 position must be kept relatively simple. A marked dissimilarity is often found between the two side chains of effective drugs (Fig. 5.2). Compounds

Table 5.1 Relationship of chemical grouping to clinical action of barbiturates.

Group	*Substituents* position 1	*Substituents* position 2	*Group characteristics when given intravenously*
(Oxy)barbiturates	H	O	Delay in onset of action, degree depending on 5 and 5′ side chains. Useful as basal hypnotics. Prolonged action
Methylated barbiturates	CH_3	O	Rapidly acting, usually with rapid recovery. High incidence of excitatory phenomena
Thiobarbiturates	H	S	Rapidly acting, usually smooth onset of sleep and fairly prompt recovery
Methylated thiobarbiturates	CH_3	S	Rapid onset of action and very rapid recovery but with so high an incidence of excitatory phenomena as to preclude use in clinical practice

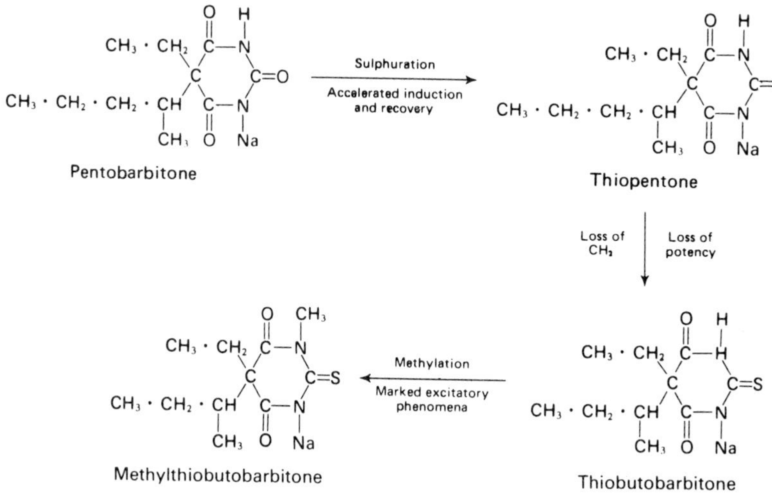

Pentobarbitone

Sulphuration → Accelerated induction and recovery

Thiopentone

Loss of CH_3 ↓ Loss of potency

Thiobutobarbitone

Methylation → Marked excitatory phenomena

Methylthiobutobarbitone

Fig. 5.2 Chemical relationship between 4 compounds and the effects produced by various structural alterations (Dundee & Barron, 1962)

with two simple similar side chains have low hypnotic potency and prolonged action. Double bonds on alkyl substitution groups produce compounds that are more vulnerable to tissue oxidation and therefore are shorter-acting.

As long ago as 1925 Dox stated that the '5' and '5″ side chains must contain not less than four and not more than eight carbon atoms. This applies to all compounds in current use, with the exception of methohexitone which has a total of nine carbons in the two side chains. There is a loss of hypnotic potency if the side chains are too long and convulsant and other toxic properties might appear. Halogenation of the alkyl substitute groups also increases the potency and intensity of action of the barbiturates. Bromine is the only halogen in clinical use for this purpose.

Alterations in the '5' side chains will produce a comparable change in the action of the drugs in each of the four groups in Table 5.1 (Dundee & Barron, 1962). A compilation of data from currently available or abandoned hypnotics and anaesthetic drugs (Table 5.2) illustrates this clearly, the relative potency of each pair of oxy- and thiobarbiturate varying with the '5' and '5″ side chains (Dundee, 1974). Thioethamyl, the sulphur derivative of amylobarbitone, was studied under the trade name of Venesetic by Cullen & Rovenstine (1938) and, apart from having half the potency of thiopentone, was found to be a satisfactory rapidly acting induction agent.

Thus, the net effect of substitutions at four possible sites can be predicted with a reasonable degree of certainty. This is illustrated in Figure 5.2 which shows a barbiturate (pentobarbitone) with a slow onset of action when injected intra-

Table 5.2 Side chains and relative potency of four oxybarbiturates and their equivalent thiobarbiturates

Position on barbiturate molecule 5	5′	2			*Relative potency*	
$CH_3—CH_2—$	$CH_3—CH_2—CH_2—CH—$ | CH_3	O	Pentobarbitone	(Nembutal)	1.0	
		S	THIOPENTONE	(Pentothal)		1.0
$CH_2═CH—CH_2—$	$CH_3—CH_2—CH_2—CH$ | CH_3	O	Quinalbarbitone	(Seconal)	1.1	
		S	THIAMYLAL	(Surital)		1.1
$CH_3—CH_2—$	$CH_3—CH—CH_2—CH_2—$ | CH_3	O	Amylobarbitone	(Amytal)	0.5	
		S	THIOETHAMYL	(Venesetic)		0.5
$CH_3—CH_2—$	$CH_3—CH_2—CH—$ | CH_3	O	Butobarbitone	(Soneryl)	0.7	
		S	THIOBUTOBARBITONE	(Inactin)		0.7

from Dundee (1974)

venously and its rapidly acting thio-analogue (thiopentone). Removal of one CH_2 linkage produces the less potent thiobutobarbitone (Inactin) which has an action similar to thiopentone with no higher incidence of side effects (Dundee & Riding, 1960). Methylation of thiobutobarbitone resulted in a most unsatisfactory drug, methylthiobutobarbitone (B 137), which was abandoned because of the excessively high incidence of excitatory phenomena (Dundee et al, 1960).

Individual drugs*

The intravenous barbiturates of clinical importance and some historical drugs, together with their commonly used proprietary names, are listed in Table 5.3. (The historical drugs, although shown here for convenience, are discussed in Chapter 17). There is much similarity in the side chains of the thiobarbiturates in this table and, as expected, there is no marked difference in the actions of the different compounds. The two methylated barbiturates possess the group characteristics produced by the addition of the methyl radical as mentioned above.

Methohexitone is a racemic mixture of alpa-d and alpha-l isomers (that is, the optically active isomers are present in such proportions as to render the mixture optically inactive). It has been found by Gibson and colleagues (1955) that the beta-isomer produced excessive motor activity. The most desirable configuration proved to be alpha-dl which is available in the commercial compounds Brietal and Brevital Sodium.

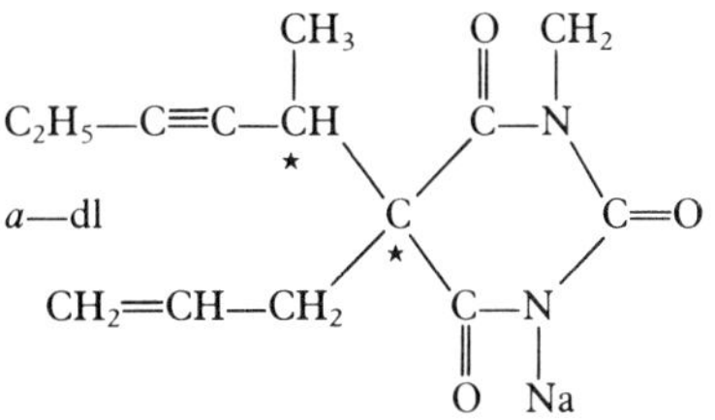

```
                 CH3     O  CH2
                 |       ‖  |
C2H5—C≡C—CH      C—N
                 *  \   /     \
a—dl              C          C=O
                /  *\       /
CH2=CH—CH2      C—N
                         ‖   |
                         O  Na
```

* Denotes centres of asymmetry

The original compound (22451) which was first submitted to clinical trial contained both alpha and beta isomers and produced an undesirably high incidence of muscle movements. This was replaced by compound 25398 which is of the alpha-dl configuration and since its introduction one has been aware of fewer excitatory side effects as purer preparations have become available.

* Using the International Union of Pure and Applied Chemistry nomenclature we have:
Thiopentone sodium:
4, 6 (1H, 5H)-Pyrimedinedione, 5-ethyldihydro -5-(1 methylbutyl)-2-thioxo-monosodium salt
Methohexitone sodium:
2, 4, 6 (1H, 3H, 5H)-Pyrimidinetrione, 1-methyl-5-(1-methyl-2-pentynyl)-5-(2-propenyl)-monosodium salt
Hexobarbitone sodium:
2, 4, 6 (1H, 3H, 5H)-Pyrimidinetrione, 5-(1-cyclohexen-1-yl)-1, 5-dimethyl-monosodium salt
The widely accepted barbiturate terminology is preferred to the above and is used throughout this book.

Table 5.3 Formulae of some intravenous barbiturates

Cyclic ureide of malonic acid	Pyrimidine derivative
R_1, R on C_5; C_6(=O)—N_1(H); C_4(=O)—N_3(Na); $_2C$=2	O^- Na^+ on C; N^1; ^5C with R, R_1; 2=C_2; $_4C$=O; ^3N—H

Preparation	*1*	*2*	*5 R*	*5′ R_1*
Hexobarbitone (Evipan, Evipal, Cyclonal, Hexanol)	CH_3	O	CH_3—	—C(=CH—CH_2)—CH_2—CH_2—CH_2 (ring: CH—CH_2, CH_2, CH_2—CH_2)
Thiopentone* (Pentothal, Intraval, Nesdonal, Trapanal)	H	S	CH_2—CH_2—	—CH—CH_2—CH_2—CH_3 | CH_3
Thiobutobarbitone (Inactin)	H	S	CH_3—CH_2—	—CH—CH_2—CH_3 | CH_3
Thialbarbitone (Kemithal, Kemithene)	H	S	CH_2=CH—CH_2—	—C(=CH—CH_2)—CH_2—CH_2—CH_2 (ring: CH—CH_2, CH_2, CH_2—CH_2)
Thiamylal (Surital, Thioseconal)	H	S	CH_2=CH—CH_2—	—CH—CH_2—CH_2—CH_3 | CH_3
Buthalitone (Baytinal, Transithal, Ulbreval)	H	S	CH_2=CH—CH_2—	—CH_2—CH(CH_3)(CH_2)
Methohexitone (Brietal, Brevital)	CH_3	O	CH_2=CH—CH_2-	—CH—C≡C—C_2H_5 | CH_3
Methitural (Neraval, Thiogenal)	H	S	CH_3—S—CH_2—CH_2—	—CH— CH_2—CH_2—CH_3 | CH_2
Enibomal (Narcodorm, Narkotal, Eunarcon)	CH_3	O	(CH_3)(CH_3)CH—	—CH_2—CBr—CH_2

Hexobarbitone	sodium 1-methyl-5-methyl-5′-cyclohexenyl-2-barbiturate
Thiopentone	sodium 5-ethyl-5′-(1-methylbutyl)-2-thiobarbiturate
Thiobutobarbitone	sodium 5-ethyl-5′-(1-methylprohyl)-2-thiobarbiturate
Thialbarbitone	sodium 5-allyl-5′-cyclohexenyl-2-thiobarbiturate
Thiamylal	sodium 5-allyl-5′-(1-methylbutyl)-2-thiobarbiturate
Buthalitone	sodium 5-allyl-5′-isobutyl-2-thiobarbiturate
Methohexitone	sodium 1-methyl-5-allyl-5′-(1-methyl-2-pentynyl)-2-barbiturate
Methitural	sodium 5-methyl-thioethyl-5′-(1-methylbutyl)-2-thiobarbiturate
Enibomal	sodium 1-methyl-5-isopropyl-5′ (2-bromallyl)-2-barbiturate

* The formula for thiopentone can be remembered by recalling that the drug was originally known as thionembutal and that the trade name Nembutal (pentobarbitone) was based on the chemical structure—*Na Ethyl Methyl BUTyl* barbiturate; AL is the recognised American suffix for barbiturates—THIOPENTAL

PHYSICAL PROPERTIES AND SOLUTIONS

All drugs are prepared for clinical use as sodium salts and, with the exception of enibomal, are available in powder form to be dissolved in water or saline before use. Although 5% dextrose can be used to make up solutions, this is less desirable than other solvents because the relatively low pH of the solution might interact with the barbiturate and cause precipitation of free acid. Moreover, solutions prepared in dextrose tend to be sticky. The use of lactated Ringer's (Hartmann's) or similar solutions will often result in a haze or precipitate formation within one hour. Adequate mixing is essential to avoid 'layering'.

The sodium salt of thiopentone is a pale yellow hygrospopic powder with a bitter taste and a melting point of 158 to 159°C (compared with 127 to 134°C for thiamylal and 93°C for methohexitone). The drug is readily soluble in water, partly soluble in 96% alcohol, and insoluble in solvent ether and benzene. Commercial preparations of most barbiturates contain a mixture of six parts of anhydrous sodium carbonate and 100 parts (w/w) of the barbiturate. This additive prevents precipitation of the insoluble free acid by atmospheric carbon dioxide. There is a slight difference between thiopentone sodium BP and thiopental sodium USP. The British Pharmacopoeia defines the product on the basis of the combined weight of the barbiturate plus sodium carbonate while the USP defines the product on the basis of the barbiturate component alone. Thus 1 g thiopental contains approximately the same amount of active drug as 1.06 g thiopentone.

Aqueous solutions are strongly alkaline and the pH of 2.5% thiopentone is about 10.5. The solutions are incompatible with acids which include most of the analgesics, the phenothiazine derivatives, adrenaline and noradrenaline and some preparations of tubocurarine chloride. Although the precipitate which forms when thiopentone and suxamethonium are mixed dissolves in excess thiopentone, hydrolysis of the relaxant occurs when the mixture is allowed to stand, with a 50% loss of activity in 90 minutes (Fraser, 1954).

Hexobarbitone, methohexitone and enibomal, being non-sulphur containing, are clear compounds whose solutions are readily distinguishable from the thiobarbiturates.

The iso-osmotic concentratton of an aqueous solution of thiopentone sodium BP is 3.31%, while for thiopental sodium USP it is 3.12%. The corresponding figure for methohexitone is 3.7%. Isotonic determinations with red blood cells showed no effects with concentrations in the range of 2 to 3.4% thiopentone sodium BP. Haemolysis was found when the concentration was below 2% or above 3.4%.

Thiopentone is usually prepared for clinical use in a 2.5% solution and in some centres in North America a 2% solution is popular. Solutions of thiamylal and thiobutobarbitone are similar, but 5 to 10% solutions are required to avoid the otherwise excessive volumes needed for hexobarbitone, but if the 10% concentration is desired an appreciable time must be allowed for the substance to dissolve completely.

Although the manufacturers recommend that methohexitone be prepared as a 1% solution, this strength has little to commend it over the more convenient 2% solution which allows smaller syringes to be used and is less hypotonic.

Because of their high alkalinity, solutions of barbiturates possess a bacteriostatic effect against a wide range of micro-organisms. However, since they contain no added bacteriostatic agent, extreme care in preparation, handling.and storage should be exercised to prevent contamination. Solutions of thiobarbiturates may remain stable at room temperature for up to two weeks after preparation, while methohexitone often can be used for up to six weeks. Solutions will remain clearer for a longer time if stored at 4°C but should never be used if they have become cloudy.

The remarkable stability of properly stored ampoules of thiopentone is demonstrated by the unique study of Nielsen & Spoerel (1959). In 1957 they used ampoules of Pentothal received as samples in 1935; solutions were clear and no difference could be detected from those prepared from fresh powder and anaesthesia was uneventful. This does not mean that powder which has been kept indefinitely should be used. Pentothal sodium (Abbott) carries a five year expiry date and the manufacturers of methohexitone recommend that there should be a two year limit on storage. The material should invariably remain fully potent for at least the stated length of time.

In contrast with these, the preparation of

enibomal known as Narcodorm is available commercially in a 5% solution with a storage life of about three years. This solution also contains 50 mg phenazonum per ml and an unstated amount of glycerine.

BULK SOLUTIONS

It is common practice to use multidose containers for thiopentone and methohexitone. Solutions are normally constituted at the beginning of the working day and discarded at the end of the operating list. This is time saving, particularly when large numbers of patients for short operations are to be anaesthetized.

In some centres the bulk thiopentone is dispensed in syringes (usually containing 20 ml 2% or 2.5% thiopentone or equivalent), which are capped and stored at 4°C until required: they will normally be discarded after 24 hours. Alternatively the containers are left (sometimes without a cap) and syringes filled as required through a sterile cannula. Short-term exposure to air does not appear to do any harm but the drug should be discarded if turbulence or particulate matter are visible: these might be due to precipitation of insoluble thiopentone acid or bacterial contamination. Some packs are available which allow the rapid and sterile preparation of thiopentone solutions and which also facilitate subsequent dispensing of the drug.

With all methods of preparation care should be taken to ensure sterility. Most microbial organisms will not survive in 1% methohexitone but 2% thiopentone seems to be slightly less lethal in this respect (Highsmith et al, 1982). Sterility of the water used as a solvent is also important. Normally this is triple distilled, but alternatively γ-irradiated single distilled water is acceptable (Jacobs & Eisenberg, 1981). The small amount of H_2O_2 in irradiated water is of no clinical significance and does not affect thiopentone.

CURRENT DRUGS

At this time *Thiopentone* is the only intravenous barbiturate which is used worldwide. *Thiamylal* enjoys a limited popularity and apart from being slightly more potent, on a w/w basis, is identical in its action with thiopentone. Since two large 'blind' studies (Tovell et al, 1965; Barron et al, 1966) could not distinguish between the drugs, the potency difference is so small as to be of no clinical significance and hereafter all references to thiobarbiturates will refer to thiopentone, unless specifically stated.

Thiobutobarbitone has a limited use in continental Europe and apart from being 25–30% less potent than thiopentone, the clinical effects of equivalent doses of these drugs are indistinguishable (Dundee & Riding, 1960; Barron et al, 1966).

Methohexitone has a place in shorter operations and outpatient procedures and enjoys a limited use for these purposes in Britain and North America. It will be discussed in subsequent chapters.

The original methyl-barbiturate *Hexobarbitone* is still used outside major centres but is clearly not as satisfactory a drug as methohexitone.

RELATIVE POTENCY

Relative potency can have many different meanings, such as the amount of drug required to produce a desired degree of cerebral depression, the minimal amount required to produce sleep or the dose required to produce a given duration of anaesthesia. The MAC value (minimal alveolar concentration required to obtund movement in response to a surgical stimulus in 50% of patients) is obviously inapplicable to intravenous anaesthetics and blood levels are valueless in potency studies because of the phenomenon of acute tolerance.

Table 5.4 Potency of various intravenous barbiturates relative to thiopentone.

	Relative potency	*Relative dose* (g)
Thiopentone	1.0	1.0
Thiamylal	1.0–1.1	0.9–1.0
Thiobutobarbitone	0.7–0.8	1.2–1.4
Hexobarbitone	0.5–0.6	1.8–2.0
Methohexitone	2.5–3.3	0.3–0.4

In clinical practice the dose of drug required 'to produce anaesthesia' compared with that for thiopentone is usually taken as the relative potency but, except for methohexitone, this has not been studied in any great detail. The most commonly accepted figures are given in Table 5.3. The commonly used value for hexobarbitone (0.5 potency of thiopentone) is possibly an underestimate.

Opinions vary as to the potency of methohexitone relative to thiopentone. When a method which employs a standard operation (and hence a standard duration of sleep) is involved the figures are lower (1.5 to 2.7) than those obtained when the dose required to produce a given depth of narcosis is studied (2.7 to 3.5). The most extensive study is that of Clarke and his associates (1968) who gave varying doses rapidly during a period of forearm reactive hyperaemia half-a-minute following release of a tourniquet which had occluded the arterial circulation for two-and-a-half minutes and noted the time until the patient stopped counting. The scatter of readings is such that one can easily determine the minimal dose with an average onset time of 10 to 10.5 s or that which causes sleep in 11 s in 90% of patients. When these two end-points are employed, the figure for potency of methohexitone relative to thiopentone (3.2 to 3.3) is greater than that obtained by other workers. In practice it is recommended that methohexitone be considered about three times as potent as thiopentone, as was suggested by Stoelting (1957) in the original clinical publication on the drug.

Isomerism

The anaesthetic barbiturates are commonly considered to be structurally non-specific drugs whose action depends primarily on their ability to penetrate the central nervous system rather than on any structural affinity to specific sites of action on target cells in the brain. There is some evidence (Andrews & Mark, 1982) suggesting that this is an oversimplification. Drugs such as thiopentone or pentobarbitone have a chiral centre in the methyl-butyl sidechain and the (−) enantiomer is considerably more potent than the (+) form. There is also a difference in the duration of action of the two forms which cannot be explained on a metabolic basis; the sleep time following the (+) form is shorter while the (−) isomer is destroyed more rapidly. The general distribution of the two forms in the body is similar but one can postulate that the (+) isomer is slightly better absorbed into the brain. With compounds such as methohexitone there are two possible sites of asymmetry which lead to four possible stereoisomers. In practice the use of racemic compounds rather than pure optical isomers may result in a high incidence of excitatory side effects. Good examples of this are the early preparations of methohexitone (Lilly 22451) which were much more excitatory than the currently available alpha-dl form (Lilly 25398).

Steric differences in attachment of stereoisomers of a drug to microsomal enzyme protein frequently result in a discrepancy in rate of biotransformation between enantiomers.

REFERENCES

Andrews P R and Mark L C 1982 Structural specificity of barbiturates or related drugs. Anesthesiology 57: 314–320

Barron D W, Dundee J W, Gilmore W R, Howard P J 1966 Clinical studies of induction agents. XVI: A comparison of thiopentone, buthalitone, hexobarbitone and thiamylal as induction agents. British Journal of Anaesthesia 38: 802–811

Clarke R S J, Dundee J W, Barron D W, McArdle L with technical assistance from Howard P J 1968 Clinical studies of induction agents. XXVI: The relative potencies of thiopentone, methohexitone and propanidid. British Journal of Anaesthesia 40: 593–601

Cullen S C, Rovenstine E A 1938 Sodium thio-ethamyl anesthesia: a preliminary report of observations during its clinical use. Anesthesia and Analgesia 17: 201–205

Dox A W 1925 Barbitursauren und die Pikrinsaureaktion. Zeitzchrist fur physiologische Chemie 150: 118–120

Dundee J W 1974 Molecular structure-activity relationships of barbiturates. In: Halsey M J, Millar R A, Sutton J A (eds) Molecular mechanisms in general anaesthesia. Churchill Livingstone Edinburgh, p 16–31

Dundee J W, Barron D W 1962 The barbiturates. British Journal of Anaesthesia 34: 240–246

Dundee J W, Barron D W, King R 1960 The effect of methylation on ethyl methyl propyl thiobarbiturate. British Journal of Anaesthesia 32: 566–575

Dundee J W, Riding J E 1960 A comparison of Inactin and thiopentone as intravenous anaesthetics. British Journal of Anaesthesia 32: 206–218

Fraser P J 1954 Hydrolysis of succinylcholine salts. British Journal of Pharmacology 9: 429–436

Gibson W R, Swanson E E, Doran W J 1955 Pharmacology

of a short-acting non-sulphur barbituric acid derivative. Proceedings of the Society for Experimental Biological Medicine 89: 292–294

Highsmith A K, Greenhood G P, Allen J R 1982 Growth of nosocomial pathogens in multiple-dose parenteral medication vials. Journal of Clinical Microbiology 15: 1024–1028

Jacobs G P, Eisenberg E 1981 The reconstitution of powders for injection with γ-radiated water. International Journal of Applied Radiation and Isotopes 32: 180–181

Nielsen J S, Spoerel W E 1959 Pentothal sodium: 1935–1957. Anesthesia and Analgesia . . . Current Researches 38: 29–31

Parsons T W 1963 Clinical comparison of barbiturates as hypnotics. British Medical Journal ii: 1035–1037

Stoelting V K 1957 Use of a new intravenous oxygen barbiturate 25398 for intravenous anesthesia. Anesthesia and Analgesia . . . Current Researches 36: 49–51

Tovell R M, Anderson C C, Sadove M S, Artusio J F Jr, Papper E M, Coakley C S, Hudon F, Smith S M, Thomas C J 1955 A comparative clinical and statistical study of thiopental and thiamylal in human anesthesia. Anesthesiology 16: 910–926

6

Barbiturates: pharmacokinetics

Early reports on the use of thiopentone suggested that it was rapidly broken down in the body, hence the term 'ultra-short acting', by which it became known (p. 60). However, isolated clinical reports of prolonged narcosis following its use appeared from time to time, and in 1938 Veal & Reynolds pointed out that the effects of repeated injections of small doses were not comparable with the administration of continuous open drop ether. In the following year in animal experiments, Reynolds (1939) demonstrated that thiopentone had a marked cumulative action, the repeated administration of the same dose resulting in a gradual prolongation of narcosis with each successive injection. These findings have since been confirmed by Wyngaarden et al (1949) and have been shown to apply also to thiamylal and thioethamyl.

To explain the cumulative action of thiopentone and the prolonged narcosis which follows large total doses, Reynolds postulated that normal organs are incapable of destroying more than a certain amount of the drug. He also suggested that thiopentone caused liver dysfunction; the initial dose thereby reduced the ability of this organ to deal with supplementary doses.* Another explanation was that the breakdown of thiopentone might involve the formation of a longer acting barbiturate such as pentobarbitone (Maynert & van Dyke, 1949).

Thus until about 1948 it was believed that the duration of action of thiobarbiturates was determined by the rate of their metabolic transformation. A clearer understanding followed the perfection of techniques for the quantitative determination of these drugs in plasma and tissues. Brooks et al (1948) were the first to show that rapid diffusion of thiopentone to non-nervous tissues occurred and was responsible for the short action of small doses. Many other studies have followed and, owing to the work of Jailer & Goldbaum (1946), Bollman and his colleagues (1950) and Brodie and his co-workers (1950, 1952, 1953) new light has been shed on the distribution and fate of these drugs. Before reviewing the present state of knowledge several points must be clarified.

First, it is important to reiterate that the term 'ultra-short acting' is not a correct description of the duration of action of the thiobarbiturates. Brevity of action is related to redistribution rather than to metabolism and patients regain consciousness with a large amount of undetoxified drug in the body. Secondly, blood and tissue levels are changing continuously and since many factors might be affecting them at the same time, often in different directions, it is not always possible to predict what will happen in any given set of circumstances. Thirdly, there is not a good correlation between the clinical depth of anaesthesia and blood thiopentone levels and it might be difficult to correlate changes in tissue levels with clinical effects.

The three most important drug factors affecting the distribution and fate of barbiturates are *lipoid solubility* (partition coefficient), *protein binding* and the degree of *ionisation*. Table 4.5 shows that there is a good correlation between the pharmacological

* It is interesting to note that methitural, a thiobarbiturate developed about 20 years later, contained a methyl-thioethyl in the side chain which it was hoped would liberate methionine and protect the liver from the toxic effects of the barbiturate (p. 314).

action of five barbiturates and their affinity for a non-polar solvent. In addition to their more rapid onset of action (and brevity of effect), the highly lipoid soluble agents tend to be more rapidly degraded metabolically with minimal renal excretion.

Protein binding

Immediately on injection a large proportion of the barbiturate is rendered pharmacologically inactive by being bound to the non-diffusible constituents of plasma (Goldbaum & Smith, 1954). Thiobarbiturates are bound to a greater extent than their oxygen analogues, the figure for thiopentone being 60–85%. The degree of binding varies with the pH, passing through a maximum of about pH 8.0. With increasing barbiturate concentration the percentage of bound drug diminishes, although the total amount activated by this means increases and at low concentrations practically all the drug is bound to the plasma protein, especially to the albumin. This is well shown in the study by Morgan et al (1981a, b) who found 96.7% binding at a concentration of 0.2 $\mu g\ ml^{-1}$ and 60.4% at 150 $\mu g\ ml^{-1}$ in normal subjects. By contrast over a clinical range of 7–90 $\mu g\ ml^{-1}$ Burch & Stanski (1981a) were unable to demonstrate concentration-dependent binding of thiopentone. Enhancement of the action of thiopentone from this cause, if it occurs at all, would seem to be limited to the immediate effects of very large doses.

There are differences in the reported fractions of bound thiopentone, depending on the method of estimation. In the clinical range (10–50 $\mu g\ ml^{-1}$) Morgan et al (1981a) found 78% binding with ultrafiltration compared with 75% with equilibrium dialysis. The extent of plasma thiopentone binding is unaffected by operations of moderate severity: the potential displacement of thiopentone from the binding sites, due to the elevated free fatty acids which accompany any operation does not appear to occur. However, pretreatment with oral probenecid or intravenous acetylsalicylic acid, drugs which have a high affinity for albumin binding sites, reduces the induction doses of thiopentone, and this could be due to the effect on plasma binding of the barbiturate (McMurray et al, 1984).

The binding of drugs such as the barbiturates to plasma albumin is an unstable bonding readily reversible with changes in concentration. It can be considered as a means of barbiturate transport in the blood stream, somewhat analagous to oxygen transport by haemoglobin except that the oxygen in haemoglobin exists as a chemical compound whereas albumin and barbiturate form a loose structural complex held together by van der Waals and other forces of physical attraction acting at their surfaces. Unbound, undissociated barbiturate molecules of either steric configuration pass blood–brain and other blood tissue barriers at speeds related to their lipid solubilities. It is these solubilities that are the prime determinants of the speed of transit of the barbiturates across the blood–brain barrier. This varies with the overall structure of the molecule and not with the steric configuration. Thus the stereoselective binding to plasma proteins is not a major factor in determining the distribution of these drugs in the brain. Thiopentone enters but is not extensively carried in red cells; their concentration of the drug is about 40% of that found in the plasma. Concentration-dependent localisation in cells does not appear to occur.

Uptake

The effects of l-methylation and 2-sulphuration on the uptake and distribution of barbiturates are important as all clinically used agents fall into one or other of these groups. The main action is on lipoid solubility of un-ionised forms of the drugs. The partition coefficients between lipoid solvent and aqueous buffer at pH 7.4 (C_a value) for thiopentone and thiamylal are 16 and 21 times as high as those of their corresponding barbiturates, pentobarbitone and quinalbarbitone. The difference between the coefficients of hexobarbitone (methylated) and nor-hexobarbitone (non-methylated) is of the same order (Bush et al, 1966). Methylation of pentobarbitone, quinalbarbitone and amylobarbitone produced similar effects of the C_a values (Bush, 1963).

As shown in Chapter 4 the rate at which barbiturates penetrate the central nervous system can be correlated with the lipoid solubility of the un-ionised molecules or the partition coefficient between lipoid solvents and aqueous buffer (Brodie et al, 1960; Bush, 1963; Schanker, 1963). It is known that, paralleling its effect by mouth, there is a marked delay in onset of soporific action following the intravenous injection of barbitone (diethyl barbituric acid); Butler (1950) has demonstrated that this is due to slow penetration of the brain. The onset of action and penetration of the brain is quicker after the more lipoid soluble ethyl-n-hexyl barbiturate.

The onset of hypnotic action following intravenous pentobarbitone is slower than following comparable doses of thiopentone (Fig. 4.4) owing to the differences in partition coefficients of the two drugs shown in Table 4.3 and supported by results of analyses of their rate of passage into the brain (Mark et al, 1958). Thiopentone is largely non-ionic at plasma pH and has a very high partition coefficient, while pentobarbitone is less ionised at pH 7.4 and is much less protein-bound, but its penetration is slower because of the low partition coefficient of the non-ionised form.

Thus, to summarise, the rapid onset of sleep following the intravenous injection of adequate doses of thiopentone, thiamylal, methohexitone and similar drugs is due to their high lipoid solubility and lack of ionisation leading to immediate penetration of the blood-brain barrier (Brodie, 1952; Schanker, 1963).

Barbiturates are weak acids and, at a pH near 1 in the stomach, they are practically non-ionised. Absorption from the stomach will vary with their lipoid solubility. The methylated or thio compounds are very rapidly absorbed by mouth and cause a brief period of intense hypnosis. Bush et al (1966) found that oral administration of about 10 mg kg^{-1} of thiopentone, hexobarbitone or methohexitone produced rapid intense sedation of short duration.

Following a single injection of thiopentone, the high cerebral blood flow results in a rapid increase in brain barbiturate content (Fig. 6.1) and the effects on the electroencephalogram can usually be detected in 8 to 15 s and usually consciousness is lost after one deep inspiration. The temporal relationship of this respiratory effect to the onset of anaesthesia suggests that it is mediated by the chemoreceptors in the carotid body. The brain continues to take up thiopentone for a further 30 to 60 s or so, and thereafter the concentration of the drug in the efferent venous blood slightly exceeds the afferent arterial level; the brain concentration thus falls as the drug is removed from the brain (Fig. 6.1). Thus, the maximum depressant action of thiopentone on the nervous system does not occur until half a minute or so after its initial effect.

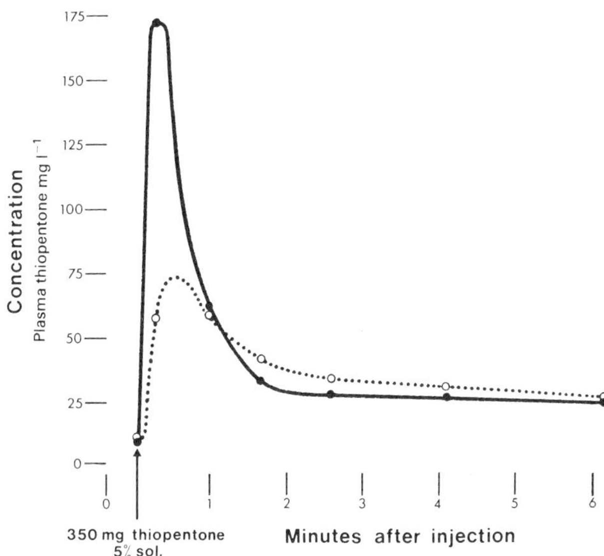

Fig. 6.1 Plasma thiopentone (mg l^{-1}) concentration following 350 mg injected rapidly.
Arterial samples ——, Internal jugular venous samples . . . (Price, 1961).

The immediate uptake of thiopentone by the brain is accompanied by a similar rapid uptake in other important non-nervous tissues such as the liver and kidneys (vital organs) and the plasma level falls quickly. The concentration of drug reaching the brain is thus lowered and, as its brain content falls, anaesthesia lightens. Tissue analysis reveals that the initial peak concentration of drug in the liver exceeds that in the plasma and thereafter they decline at a similar rate. The cerebrospinal fluid concentration reaches a level almost as high as that of the unbound drug in the plasma and thereafter it declines as in other tissues.

Redistribution

With the exception of muscle and fat, the maximum tissue concentration of thiopentone is reached within one minute of a single intravenous injection. It is the rapid redistribution which is responsible for the short action of small doses. Equilibrium with the muscles is not attained until about a quarter of an hour after injection, and thereafter its concentration declines at a rate parallel to the plasma level. Despite the affinity of thiopentone for fat, because of the poor blood supply, uptake of the drug in adipose tissues is relatively slow and maximum deposition only occurs after one and a half to two and a half hours. By this time, the fat level greatly exceeds that of other tissues. In 1963 Mark emphasised that, although maximum deposition of thiopentone in fat does not occur until one hour or so after uptake by muscle has ceased, about one third of the injected dose is located there within 30 min and half of the drug is in fat depots in 90 min. In this respect thiopentone differs from pentobarbitone. Brodie (1952) found the ratio of concentration in fat to plasma three hours after injection in the dog to be 6.2 for thiopentone and only 1.1 for pentobarbitone.

In 1960 Price presented a mathematical analysis of the kinetics of thiopentone distribution (Figure 4.5) and validated his conclusions by direct measurements of drug concentrations in tissues (Price et al, 1960). He demonstrated that following a bolus injection of the drug, the course of anaesthesia depended passively upon a competition between nervous and non-nervous tissues for thiopentone. His concept was that of injection into a central 'pool' of blood with the rapid onset of anaesthesia resulting from the high blood supply and affinity of the central nervous system for thiopentone. Within one minute after injection the blood has given up 90% of the injected dose to the highly perfused tissues, principally the central nervous system, heart and liver. During the subsequent half-hour they were depleted as a result of further redistribution, with about 80% of the thiopentone given up by these highly perfused viscera to other aqueous 'lean' tissues in the body, while the remainder entered fat. The blood supply to fat is so low, relative to other tissues, that it cannot begin to store thiopentone to any significant degree until the central nervous system has lost over 90% of its peak content; his findings here are at variance with those of previous workers in regard to the role played by body fat in concentrating thiopentone and the importance of this in limiting the duration of anaesthesia. He calculated that fat should still contain 55–60% of the injected dose 8 to 10 hours after its administration and with small bolus injections it is hard to conceive that the uptake by fat plays any major part in hastening the removal of sufficient drug from the brain to affect the duration of narcosis in normal subjects.

Figure 6.2 differs from Figure 4.5 in that it allows for early metabolism of thiopentone. This is based on the work of Saidman & Eger (1966) who studied differences between arterial and hepatic venous concentrations. They concluded that although the uptake in muscle still plays a dominant role in the early fall of arterial concentration, this is equalled by the additive effects of metabolism and uptake in fat. In their early studies Brodie and colleagues calculated that 10–15% of thiopentone is broken down per hour.

The positive role of the liver in the metabolism of thiopentone is now recognised (p. 76) since virtually none of the drug is eliminated unchanged in the urine. Stanski & Watkins (1982) have calculated the range of thiopentone hepatic extraction to be in the region of 0.08–0.20 (with a total body clearance of the drug ranging from 1.6 to 4.3 mg kg^{-1} min^{-1}). Burch & Stanski (1981b) quote the extraction ratio as 0.14–0.18, while Morgan et al (1981a, b) found the value to be

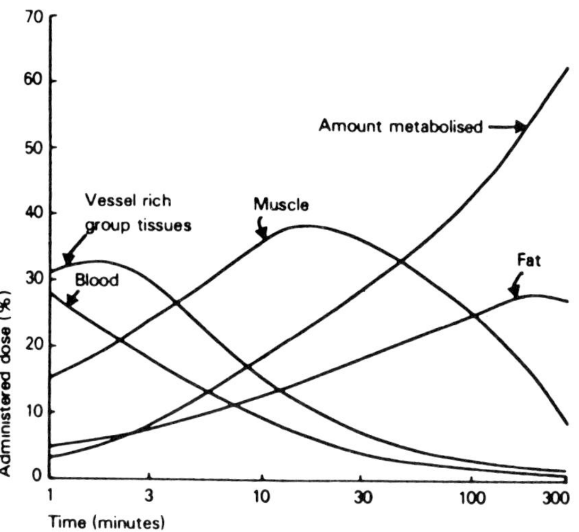

Fig. 6.2 Tissue distribution of thiopentone following intravenous injection according to Saidman (1966).

0.10. These values are lower than the 0.3 ratio used by Saidman in calculating Figure 6.2. The lower values suggest a less important, but not insignificant role of drug metabolism in early recovery from thiopentone. As will be discussed later animal experiments and observations in humans have shown that prolongation of the action of thiopentone in the presence of hepatic dysfunction only occurs after very large doses. The low hepatic extraction shows that thiopentone has capacity-limited binding-sensitive elimination. Thus changes in protein binding and in hepatic enzyme activity will affect the clearance of the drug but this is probably of little clinical significance (Burch & Stanski, 1981c).

Compartmental concept

It is possible to correlate readily the above views with the more modern approach to pharmacokinetics. Figure 6.3 shows the log plasma concentration related to the time after administration of an intravenous bolus of 6.4 mg kg^{-1} of thiopentone (Stanski & Watkins, 1982). In this the individual plasma concentrations correlate well with a tri-exponential equation determined by non-linear regression. Thus, in this patient the distribution of thiopentone showed the characteristics of a three-compartmental model. Comparing this with Figures 4.5 and 6.2 the initial distribution phase would represent uptake into highly perfused tissues, the slow distribution phase uptake by lean tissues (with some contribution by fat) and the elimination phase metabolism of the drug and redistribution to poorly perfused tissues (Fig. 6.4).

Slight differences in methodology including duration of sampling time has resulted in slightly different pharmacokinetic constants by different workers (Table 6.1). The early calculation of 15% metabolism per hour (Brodie et al, 1950) would give an elimination half-life of approximately five hours. This work was carried out on volunteers and in some of the reported studies (Morgan et al, 1981a), where the elimination half-life is at the upper level of the accepted range, the patients were undergoing surgical operations which might have influenced the findings, as occurs in the case of midazolam (Harper et al, 1986).

Table 6.1 summarises the pharmacokinetic data of four studies carried out in normal subjects using clinical doses of thiopentone. This does not include some of the earlier work in which the

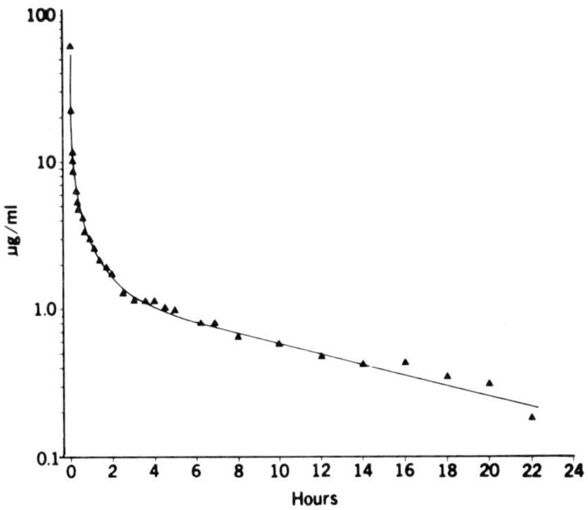

Fig. 6.3 Log plasma concentration v. time data from a patient given 6.4 mg kg^{-1} thiopentone as an intravenous bolus. The solid line represents the triexponential equation determined by nonlinear regression. The triangles represent the measured thiopentone plasma concentrations in plasma (Stanski, 1982).

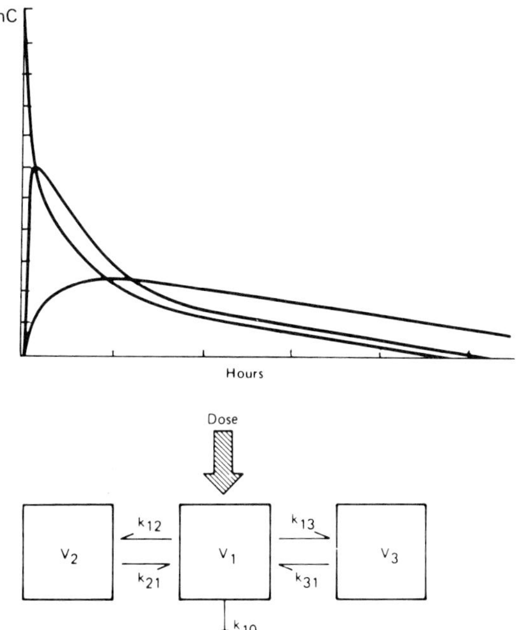

Fig. 6.4 Log-concentrations in all compartments of a three-compartment open model and the corresponding model diagram (Hull, 1984).

Table 6.1 Some pharmacokinetic parameters of thiopentone, methohexitone and pentobarbitone in humans

		Distribution half-life (min) Fast	Slow	*Elimination half-life (h)*	*Clearance (ml kg^{-1} min^{-1})*	Vd_{ss} *(l kg^{-1})*
THIOPENTONE						
Ghoneim and van Hamme	(1978)	2.4	47	5.1–5.7	4.3	1.45
Morgan et al	(1981a)	4.6	38	11.5	1.6	2.50
Hudson et al	(1983)	8.5	63	11.6	3.4	2.50
Pandale et al	(1983)			8.8	3.9	2.30
METHOHEXITONE						
Breimer	(1976)	6.2		1.5	12.1	1.13
Hudson et al	(1983)	5.6	58	3.9	10.9	2.20
PENTOBARBITONE						
Brodie et al	(1953)			17.2		
Smith et al	(1973)	4.0		50.0	0.37	1.94
Ehrenebo	(1974)			22.3	0.48	0.99
Reidenberg et al	(1976)			26.5	0.36	0.82

duration of sampling was short and thus resulted in the calculation of a much longer elimination half-life. Stanski (1981) attributes the longer $t\frac{1}{2}\ \beta$ values to more sensitive methods of assay and longer periods of blood sampling, and these are probably the correct values. Some patients demonstrated 2-compartment pharmacokinetics and thus the values for slow distribution half-life shown here are calculated for smaller numbers of patients than those in the initial fast redistribution. Also included in this table for later discussion are the data from some studies with methohexitone and pentobarbitone.

The influence of sampling site on the kinetics of thiopentone is usually ignored as it is only important for the first 10–15 minutes after administration. Thiopentone concentrations in arterial and venous samples do not differ significantly after 2 min, although there may be considerable variability for up to 9 min (Barratt et al, 1984). Concentrations in arterial plasma are significantly higher than in peripheral venous plasma for at least the first two minutes after administration. Effros et al (1972) have shown that, in dogs, thiopentone is taken up rapidly by the lung and released as the perfusing concentrations decrease. This could occur after slow injection, during which the mixed venous drug concentration should be high and decrease rapidly at the end of the injection. The arterial concentration should then exceed the mixed venous, as the drug leaves the lungs. Variability in time taken for these processes could account for the variability in central venous plasma concentrations.

Prolonged administration and large doses

Attention must also be given to the redistribution of thiopentone following the termination of either a period of intermittent injection or constant infusion. As more of the drug is administered, the concentration in some tissues approaches equilibrium with the thiopentone in blood. Since the central nervous system equilibrates rapidly with blood, and thus ceases to take up the drug, continuous administration will result in an increasing proportion of the total dose administered being located in non-nervous tissues. Thus the body gradually loses its ability to remove the thiopentone from the brain and theoretically there should be a grave risk of overdosage and very prolonged narcosis. According to Price's calculations, after a continuous infusion of one or two hours, the rate at which the central nervous system can be depleted of thiopentone (by means of redistribution to non-nervous tissues) is so slow that recovery of consciousness must depend upon other factors.

Studies in a small number of patients given the very large infusion doses of thiopentone used in cerebral resuscitation have shown a change in elimination from the expected first-order (rate of elimination and elimination half-life constant, irrespective of plasma concentration) to non-linear or Michaelis–Menten elimination, in which the rate of elimination varies with the plasma concentration (Stanski et al, 1980). This results in a decrease in the rate of elimination and an increase in the apparent elimination half life as the plasma concentration increases. With the highest doses (477–600 mg kg^{-1}) the calculated $t\frac{1}{2}\beta$ values were in the range of 16 to 30 hours, compared with the accepted 6–12 hours (Table 6.1) after smaller doses. This is presumably due to progressively increasing saturation of the hepatic enzyme systems that oxidise thiopentone. With doses of this order desulphuration occurs to an appreciable degree and at the end of the infusions plasma pentobarbitone concentrations were approximately 10% of thiopentone levels. Both factors will combine to increase the time until an assessment of neurological status is possible.

Cloyd et al (1979) reported similar findings in two patients given very large doses of thiopentone as treatment for uncontrollable seizures.

Placental transfer

For many years it was believed that the placenta formed an appreciable barrier to the passage of thiopentone to the fetus. This was based on work by Hellman et al (1944) who found minimal amounts of the drug in the newborn infant up to seven minutes after administration to the mother while Cohen and his colleagues (1953) found that the fetal levels never reached those in the mother. Kahn et al (1953) and McKechnie & Converse (1955) have thrown doubts on these views by demonstrating maximum barbiturate concentration in fetal blood within three min of injection and an equal maternal-fetal content of the drug. Crawford et al (1956) have substantiated these latter findings and it seems that the placenta offers no barrier to the passage of barbiturates to the fetus (Morgan et al (1981b). These same workers found an extremely high correlation between umbilical venous and arterial plasma concentrations at delivery ($r = 0.98$; $P < 0.001$) and also between maternal and umbilical venous thiopentone levels at delivery ($r = 0.88$; $P < 0.001$). This is what one would expect from the passage of highly lipoid soluble agents across a barrier like the placenta.

Studies by Flowers & Hill (1958) show that thiamylal and methitural behave in a manner similar to thiopentone, and that equilibrium between the concentration in the maternal circulation, umbilical vein and umbilical artery occurs in about two to three minutes.

pH effect

This picture of the redistribution of the thiopentone in the body might give the impression that it behaves very much like the gaseous and volatile anaesthetics the action of which is controlled by the changing tissue gradients. Thiopentone has a pK value of 7.6, and the degree of ionisation of such a drug can change considerably with physiological variations in blood pH. The effect of such changes can be best understood by regarding thiopentone as being distributed in vitro between two immiscible phases; one (mainly a water phase) consists of blood and parenchymatous tissues, and the other (the organic phase) is fat (Brodie, 1952). The concentration of undissociated acid relative to that which is ionised largely determines the distribution of a weak organic acid, like barbituric acid, between an aqueous buffer and an immiscible organic solvent. The lower the pH, the more drug will be in the organic phase, while at a higher pH the opposite is true. Brodie and his colleagues (1950) found that by decreasing the pH of plasma of dogs to 6.8 by the inhalation of 10% carbon dioxide he reduced the concentration of thiopentone in the plasma by about 40%. On stopping the inhalation, the blood pH returned to near the control level and the plasma level of the drug rose rapidly. However, the brain content would rise with acidosis which would enhance the effect of the drug (Table 4.6). Similar findings have been reported by Rayburn et al (1953) and Waddell & Butler (1957) have shown acidosis to have a similar effect on the distribution of phenobarbitone.

Renal excretion

The degree of ionisation governs the renal excretion of the un-ionised drug which appears in the glomerular filtrate, diffusing back into the circulation through the renal tubules. This will be less if the drug is ionised and with weak organic acids ionisation will be maximal at a high (alkaline) pH. Only a very minimal amount of thiopentone or methohexitone is excreted unchanged in the urine. Alkalinisation of urine will not facilitate excretion.

METABOLISM

Site of metabolic transformation

Evidence from animal studies is conclusive in showing that the liver is the primary site of inactivation of the barbiturates. Cameron & de Saram (1939) and Pratt and colleagues (1932) demonstrated prolongation of pentobarbitone anaesthesia in proportion to the degree of impairment of liver function; the duration of the effect of barbitone, 85% of which is excreted in the kidney, was unaffected (Pratt, 1933). Others have demonstrated the ability of tissue slices and homogenates to break down the drug (Dorfman & Goldbaum, 1947; Shideman et al, 1947). Although Scheifley & Higgins (1940) and Masson & Beland (1945) also observed prolongation of the action of pentobarbitone after partial hepatectomy, this did not apply to thiopentone. The enormous reserve and rapid recovery of function of the liver was not fully realised at first, and later Shideman and his co-workers (1947) demonstrated marked prolongation of the action of thiopentone in rats following subtotal (85–90%) hepatectomy. This was later verified by Walker & Wynn-Parry (1949), who also showed that it applied to thiamylal and thioethamyl. The positive role of the liver was finally proven by Shideman and co-workers (1953), who found that only 27% of the administered dose of thiopentone disappeared within 12 h of administration from the body of rats with partial (70%) hepatectomy, compared with 90% in normal animals. Other workers, using different methods of study, have confirmed the role of the liver in this process (Kelly & Shideman, 1949; Shideman, 1952; Meyers & Peoples, 1954; Rappaport et al, 1956).

The evidence for hepatic detoxication of thiopentone in man was less convincing than in animals. Shideman et al (1949) found a longer sleeping time in patients with abnormal liver function than in normal subjects while Dundee (1952) found that temporary liver damage prolonged the action of large doses of the drug. He also found that smaller doses were required to maintain anaesthesia for 60 min in the presence of severe hepatic dysfunction. Gibson et al (1955) have shown that the liver plays a major role in the detoxication of methohexitone.

Evidence for detoxication of barbiturates by other organs is meagre. In the case of kidney damage, prolongation of sleep might be due to reasons other than metabolism of the drug (Richards et al, 1953; Dundee & Richards, 1954; Dundee & Annis, 1955). However, the inclusion of the kidney in the dog heart-lung preparation accelerated removal of thiopentone from the plasma (Shideman, 1952) although to a lesser extent than with the liver, while bilateral nephrectomy decreased the rate of disappearance of the drug from the body (Shideman et al, 1953). Although tissue incubation studies (Gould & Shideman, 1952; Cooper & Brodie, 1955) demonstrated some breakdown of barbiturate by the kidney, it is much less effective than the liver in this respect. Brain tissue is reported as being capable of metabolising thiopentone, thiamylal and pentobarbitone, while there is some evidence that muscle can inactivate thiopentone (Dorfman & Goldbaum, 1947; Gould & Shideman, 1952; Cooper & Brodie, 1957). Richards (1947) has reported some metabolism of thiopentone by human erythrocyte suspension but plasma is devoid of this property. The anatomical location of the lung is such that it receives substantial exposure to drugs, irrespective of the route of administration. Lung parenchyma contains enzymes which are capable of metabolising drugs, although these enzymes appear to be more selective and less active than the corresponding hepatic enzymes (Stanski & Watkins, 1982). There are no data on the metabolism of barbiturates by this route.

Thiopentone and similar drugs are broken down by non-synthetic (phase 1) reactions (p. 332), mainly oxidation, the resulting polar compound having no hypnotic activity and being inactivated by the kidney. Oxidative metabolism is catalysed by enzyme systems located mainly in the smooth endoplasmic reticulum of liver cells. These contain a unique electron transport system containing a group of pigmented haemoproteins, collectively termed the cytochrome P 450 system, the characteristics of which have been fully described by Stanski & Watkins (1982). Its role in metabolising drugs in humans has been definitely established.

The complex topic of metabolism of the barbiturates is reviewed in Appendix 2, from which it can be seen that in humans only two of the routes are applicable to thiopentone. The main route of metabolism is w-oxidation to the pharmacologically inactive thiopentone carboxylic acid (p. 334)

$$—\underset{\displaystyle CH_3}{\underset{|}{CH}}—CH_2—CH_2—CH_3 \rightarrow \underset{\displaystyle CH_3}{\underset{|}{CH}}—CH_2—CH_2—COOH$$

The role of desulphuration to pentobarbitone is only important following the administration of very large doses and possibly might contribute to delayed recovery in appropriate circumstances.

ENZYME INDUCTION

From studies with various animal species, Quinn et al (1958) have demonstrated an interesting and important correlation between the activity of liver enzyme systems and the duration of hexobarbitone narcosis (Table 6.2). They noted that female rats slept longer than males after hexobarbitone and correlated this finding with enzyme activity; female rats masculinised with testosterone awakened as quickly as male rats, while males feminised with oestradiol slept as long as females.

Acceleration of barbiturate metabolism occurs in animals pretreated with a number of drugs including phenobarbitone, which increase hepatic microsomal enzyme activity and also the synthesis of enzyme protein in the liver (Conney et al, 1960; Conney & Burns, 1962). This enzyme-stimulating response to phenobarbitone can be completely prevented by a preceding injection with ethionine, an aminoacid antagonist which inhibits the synthesis of liver protein. The simultaneous administration of ethionine will also completely block the action of phenobarbitone in enhancing the metabolism of barbiturates. The importance of enzyme induction in the clinical situation is not known, but it might play a part in 'resistance' to intravenous anaesthetics shown by patients who have been receiving large doses of sedative and analgesic drugs, although cross tolerance of the central nervous system to the drug is probably more important. It may be important in non-cirrhotic patients with chronic alcoholism, in whom following a single bolus dose of 3–9 mg kg^{-1} thiopentone, Couderc et al (1984) found clearance of 5.4 ml kg^{-1} min^{-1}, compared with 3.7 in otherwise matched non-alcoholic controls. This supports the finding of Rubin & Leiber (1968) who demonstrated stimulation of hepatic microsomal enzymes in man and rat by ethanol.

In their study Couderc found that $t\frac{1}{2}\beta$ averaged 684 min in the alcoholics, which did not differ significantly from 750 min in their controls.

Table 6.2 Duration of action of 100 mg kg^{-1} hexobarbitone intraperitoneally (except dog, 50 mg kg^{-1} i.v.) in different species related to liver microsomal enzyme activity

Species	*Duration of action (min)*	*Hexobarbitone half-life (min)*	*Enzyme activity* (μg kg^{-1} hr^{-1})
Mouse	12 ± 8	19 ± 8	598 ± 184
Rabbit	49 ± 12	60 ± 11	196 ± 28
Rat	90 ± 15	140 ± 54	134 ± 51
Dog	315 ± 105	260 ± 20	36 ± 30

from Quinn et al (1958)

METHOHEXITONE

Methohexitone is the only drug which has been studied to the same extent as thiopentone (Mark et al, 1960; Brand et al, 1963; Sunshine et al (1966); Breimer, 1976; Whitwam, 1972; 1976).

Table 6.3, based on a study of the two drugs by one group of investigators, leaves no doubt in regard to the shorter elimination half-life and the greater clearance of methohexitone as compared with thiopentone and these changes are reflected in the more rapid recovery from equivalent doses of the oxybarbiturate (Bahar et al, 1982; Carson et al, 1975).

As pointed out previously, minor differences in technique including sampling time result in differences in pharmacokinetic parameters but these are avoided in the definitive study of Hudson et al (1983) who compared the pharmacokinetics of methohexitone and thiopentone. Some of the data

Table 6.3 Pharmacokinetic parameters of thiopentone and methohexitone (mean ± SD)

	Methohexitone	*Thiopentone*
Dose (mg kg^{-1})	2.4 ± 0.4	6.7 0.7
Distribution half-lives (min)		
Rapid	5.6 ± 2.7	8.5 ± 6.1
Slow*	58.3 ± 24.6	62.7 ± 30.4
Elimination half-life (h)	3.9 ± 2.1^{x}	11.6 ± 6.0^{x}
Clearance (ml kg^{-1} min^{-1})	10.9 ± 3.0^{+}	3.4 ± 0.5^{+}
Vc (l kg^{-1})	0.35 ± 0.10	0.38 ± 0.09
Vd_{ss} (l kg^{-1})	2.2 ± 0.7	2.5 ± 0.10

* Slow distribution phase for the three patients given methohexitone and the eight patients given thiopentone exhibiting triexponential kinetics
^{x} $P < 0.005$ $^{+}$ $P < 0.001$
(from Hudson et al, 1983)

from this are included in Table 6.1 but their full findings are reproduced again in Table 6.3. There were 9 patients in each series and the doses of barbiturates were clinically equivalent. For both drugs the volumes of distribution were similar and the value for clearance of methohexitone was similar to that described by Breimer (1976). The hepatic extraction ratio of methohexitone was approximately 0.5, indicating that the liver metabolised about half the amount of methohexitone passing through it during any given passage. This is higher than the comparable figure for thiopentone. The clearance of a drug with such a high hepatic extraction is dependent largely on the magnitude of hepatic blood flow. Although the distribution half-life and VD_{ss} were similar there were major differences between methohexitone and thiopentone disposition. Methohexitone was cleared three times more rapidly than thiopentone, thus the elimination half-life of methohexitone was one-third that of thiopentone. Using complicated pharmacokinetic calculations Burch & Stanski (1981b) have calculated the fraction of thiopentone lost from the central compartment which they could attribute to metabolism. Applying these principles to methohexitone, Hudson et al (1983) estimated that at 30 min the ratio of metabolic loss to total loss is 0.38 for methohexitone and 0.22 for thiopentone, a difference which is statistically highly significant ($P < 0.001$).

The metabolic fate of methohexitone has not been studied to the same extent as that of thiopentone. Less than 1% of the administered dose can be found in bile and urine (Sunshine et al, 1966). The major pathway is w-1-oxidation of the triple bond side chain, resulting in hydroxymethohexitone (Murphy, 1974).

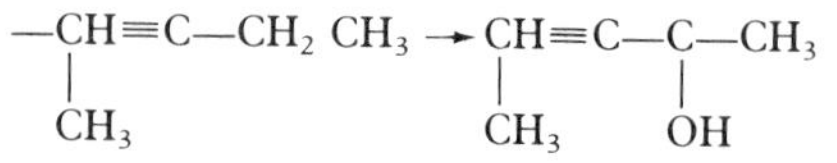

```
—CH≡C—CH2 CH3 → CH≡C—C—CH3
 |                |   |
 CH3              CH3 OH
```

The data for pentobarbitone in Table 6.1 show that it behaves differently from both thiopentone and methohexitone. Here we have a drug with a fairly long elimination half life and a slow clearance. Stanski & Watkins (1982) have illustrated these differences graphically in Figure 6.5.

OTHER BARBITURATES

No other drugs have been studied to the same extent as thiopentone and methohexitone and one is dependent on clinical impressions as to their pharmacokinetic profile. Our experience of thiamylal, thiobutobarbitone and hexobarbitone are as follows:

Thiamylal: appears in all ways to be comparable with thiopentone.

Thiobutobarbitone: apart from being less potent (60–70%) than thiopentone, appears to be comparable in other respects.

Hexobarbitone slightly more than half as potent as thiopentone, with a more prolonged recovery.

FACTORS INFLUENCING PHARMACOKINETICS

Pregnancy

In patients anaesthetised for caesarean section, Morgan et al (1981b) noted a small secondary peak in plasma concentration around the time of delivery, spanning on an average a duration of about 5 min (Fig. 6.6). Otherwise the pharmacokinetics were very similar to those in non-pregnant subjects. This phenomenon was not observed in the previous study (Morgan et al, 1981a) of non-pregnant women undergoing gynaecological operations. Manipulations involving the uterus, removal of the fetus, pressure on maternal blood

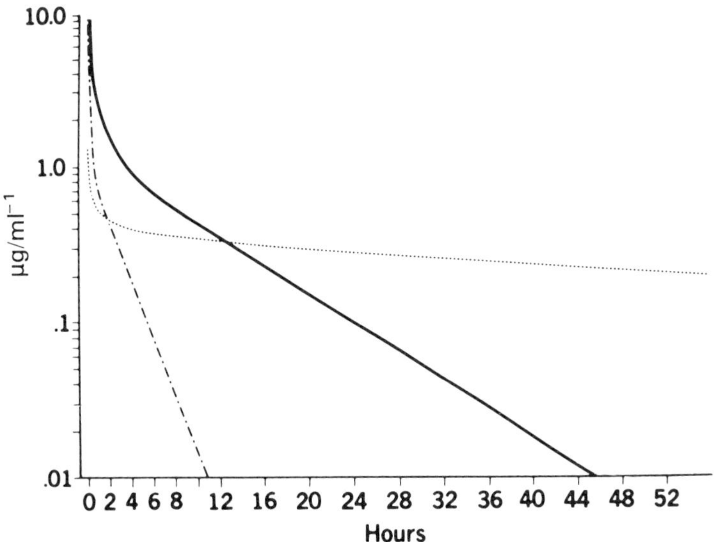

Fig. 6.5 A comparison of the pharmacokinetic profile of thiopentone, methohexitone and pentobarbitone. The plasma decay curves are calculated from the data of Ghoneim and Van Hamme (1978) for thiopentone (——), Breimer (1976) for methohexitone (-.-.-.) and Smith et al (1973) for pentobarbitone (.....) (from Stanski & Watkins, 1982).

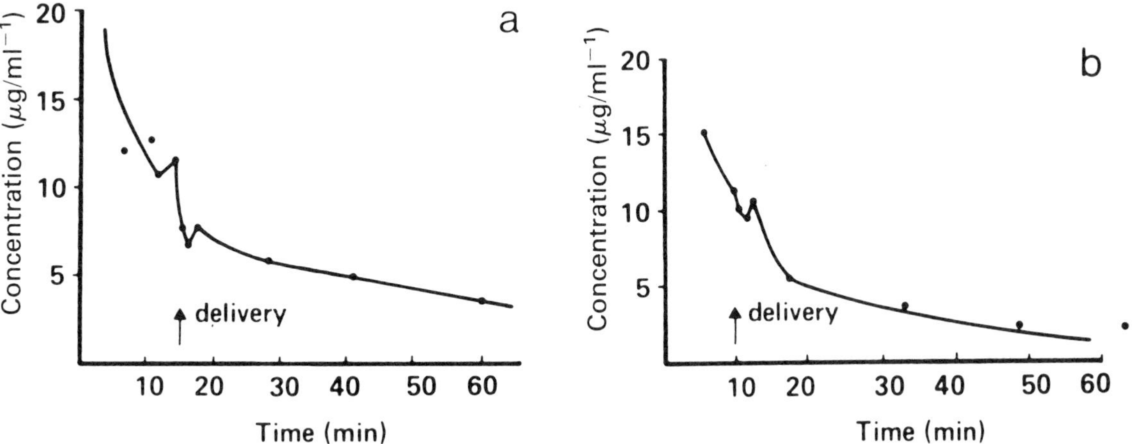

Fig. 6.6 Typical plasma concentration-time profiles of thiopentone in the first hour following drug administration in patients undergoing Caesarean section (Morgan et al, 1981).

vessels and disruption of normal blood flow in the pelvis might have given rise to these peaks. There were a number of other differences in distribution of the drug in the group of pregnant patients, notably the wide variations in elimination half-life. These ranged from 6 to 46 hours (mean 26.1 hours) compared with 10–13 hours (mean 11.5) in the non-pregnant group. The clearance of thiopentone was greater in the pregnant patients and this longer elimination half-life is due to a larger volume of distribution of the drug. The higher V_d in pregnant subjects might be partly due to changes in haemodynamics resulting from the pregnancy and delivery and also to a higher body weight. The trend to a higher clearance of thiopentone, which is a low clearance drug, is most likely due to induction of the hepatic drug metabolising enzymes, particularly near term. This has been shown with a number of drugs and persists for several weeks post-partum.

The widely recognised phenomenon of an alert infant being born to a mother anaesthetised with thiopentone must be capable of explanation on a pharmacokinetic basis, apart from the so-called 'adaptability response' of the infant to birth (Flowers & Hill, 1958). Suggested explanations include a preferential uptake of thiopentone by the fetal liver (Finster et al, 1966; 1972), the higher relative water-content of the brain (Flowers & Hill, 1958) and the fall in carbon dioxide tension at delivery. There is also potentially more rapid redistribution of drug into maternal tissues, causing a rapid reduction in maternal to fetal concentration gradient in addition to the dilution in the fetal circulation. A combination of these factors might prevent thiopentone from achieving sufficiently high concentration in the fetal brain to cause depression of the infant at birth. The studies of Morgan et al (1981b) suggest that the rapid redistribution of thiopentone in the maternal tissues during the period between induction and delivery is the major factor responsible for the discrepancy in the states of consciousness of the mother and neonate at delivery. Venous plasma concentrations of thiopentone in the umbilical cord, which should be similar to those entering the fetal brain, were well below the arterial plasma concentrations required to produce anaesthesia in adults.

On the reverse side of this there are the problems of awareness in the mother which have been reported during caesarean section. The wide inter-subject variation in pharmacokinetics of the drug during pregnancy, including activation of hepatic enzymes (Davis et al, 1973) as well as the inter-subject variation in the placental transfer of thiopentone might be important in relation to awareness following thiopentone during operative obstetrics. Inter-subject variations in plasma proteins could also be a factor.

Renal disease

In chronic renal failure Dundee & Richards (1954) noted that the dose of thiopentone necessary to induce anaesthesia was reduced to about one half. The plasma protein binding of the drug is markedly reduced in patients with chronic renal failure (Ghoneim & Pandya, 1975). This results in an increased free fraction of drug which could explain the need for decreased dosage. Burch & Stanski (1981c) have examined this hypothesis and estimated that the increased free drug concentration in chronic renal failure resulted in a larger total drug clearance because elimination is proportional to the amount of free drug available. Vd_{ss} (ml kg^{-1}) was increased due to the increased free fraction in plasma available for tissue distribution. Since changes in clearance and volume of distribution were equal, the terminal elimination half-life was unaffected. Clearance was estimated as 4.5 mg kg^{-1} min^{-1} compared with 3.2 in normal subjects and elimination half-life was 9.7 h compared with 10.2 h in a corresponding control series. Thus it would seem that the pharmacokinetic changes are due solely to alterations in binding of thiopentone to plasma proteins; clinically it is necessary to reduce the induction dose but recovery should not be prolonged. A slow rate of injection is advised to avoid very high free thiopentone concentrations reaching the central nervous system with consequent toxic effects.

Liver disease

We have already said that it was only with very large doses of thiopentone that early workers on this subject were able to detect a prolongation of action in patients with liver dysfunction. In the clinical dose range Ghoneim & Pandya (1975) found an increase in the free thiopentone fraction and the pharmacokinetic basis of an altered response to thiopentone in patients with hepatic dysfunction is probably similar to that described earlier for chronic renal failure patients.

Hepatic cirrhosis indicates a severe derangement of liver function and in such patients Pandele and colleagues (1983) have demonstrated an increase in free thiopentone fraction similar to that mentioned above. In normal subjects this was 14.5% but was increased significantly to 25.2% in patients with cirrhosis. The intrinsic clearance of the drug was decreased from 28.3 ml kg^{-1} min^{-1} in the control series to 18.2 ml kg^{-1} min^{-1} in those with cirrhosis: this difference was not significant but it does suggest that patients with very severe liver dysfunction might have a decreased capacity to metabolise thiopentone. The risk of a prolonged effect following thiopentone administration is unlikely in patients with cirrhosis provided small doses are given and the other toxic effects of the drug should also be no more marked provided the injections are not given too rapidly.

Obesity

In clinical practice thiopentone is given on an approximate bodyweight basis, but if adhered to in the case of patients with morbid obesity it would result in very large doses being given. Jung and his colleagues (1982) have studied the disposition of the drug in lean and obese patients undergoing operations. The average volume of distribution at the terminal disposition stage of steady state was significantly larger in obese as compared with age-matched lean patients. The clearance of total drug adjusted for body weight was not significantly different between obese and lean patients but total body clearance not so adjusted was significantly larger in the obese than in lean patients. The elimination half-life was significantly longer in the obese (27.8 h) than in lean patients (6.3 h), this difference being primarily due to the larger apparent volume of distribution of thiopentone in the obese. It was not possible to correlate changes in binding with the degree of obesity. Further work is required on this subject but on the basis of present knowledge one can expect a more delayed recovery when a weight-related dose is given to an obese as compared to a lean patient.

Poor risk patients

This ill-defined group includes patients with cardiovascular and other diseases that most affect the pharmacokinetic mechanisms which influence the induction dose of and recovery from thiopentone. The most important factor in all of these is probably the exaggerated pharmacokinetic effect seen in patients with cardiac failure and hypervolaemia. The depressant cardiovascular effect of thiopentone will alter the initial redistribution phase of the drug. Many of these patients will also have alterations in plasma proteins and the effects of this have already been mentioned: here the slow injection of a small dose is important. There might also be acid-base disturbances and, while these have to be marked to alter the amount of free drug, severe acidosis will decrease the plasma concentration of thiopentone due to an increased un-ionised fraction, increase penetration into the brain and enhance its depressant effect. This includes the effect on the vasomotor and respiratory centres as well as those responsible for consciousness.

Age

The induction dose of thiopentone in elderly patients is significantly lower than in the young (Christensen & Andreasen, 1978; Christensen et al, 1981; 1982; Dundee et al, 1982). Christensen and his colleagues however did not find an age difference in the venous and arterial blood concentrations on induction of anaesthesia, comparing patients aged 60–80 with younger ones. Using a three-compartment open model to describe the disappearance of thiopentone from venous blood, they found a significant increase in $t_{\frac{1}{2}}\,\beta$ from 8 to 13 h in the elderly. This however would not explain the lower induction dose, though a significantly decreased early redistribution rate constant ($K_{1.2}$) which is found in the early stage could be responsible. In previous studies Christensen et al (1980) had suggested that the initial redistribution rate-constant rather than the size of Vd_{ss} is the important factor in determining the induction dose of the drug. Cardiac output is a major determinant in this redistribution and in

Table 6.4 Mean 'induction' dose of thiopentone (mg kg^{-1}) using a standard method of administration in males and females. Series are divided into three age groups representing the young and adolescent (under 15 yr), adult (16–64 yr) and the elderly (over 65 yr)

Age (yr)	*Male*	*Female*
–15	3.22	3.06
16–64	3.71	3.49
65+	3.19	2.86

Scatter of dose is omitted for the sake of clarity but there was a highly significant difference ($P < 0.001$) between average adult dose and that required at extremes of age and in each group females required a significantly higher average dose ($P < 0.01$) than males. (from Dundee et al, 1982)

young subjects Christensen et al (1980) have demonstrated a positive relationship between the cardiac output before induction and the dose that was necessary for induction. The depressant effect of thiopentone on cardiac function is well recognised and is normally compensated for by an increase in heart rate so that cardiac output is maintained; however this compensation might be impaired in the elderly in whom the cardiovascular effects of the drug are more marked. This explanation can also apply to other patients classified as poor risk; clinical experience has shown that these people need a lower induction dose than normal, and that the response of their cardiovascular systems to a normal dose is exaggerated.

One definitive study (Sorbo et al, 1984) which examines the pharmacokinetics of thiopentone in 16 healthy children, with an average age of 6 (5 months to 13 years) showed that distribution kinetics did not differ from those of adults (Table 6.5), but the elimination half-life was about one half of the adult value. In addition, clearance of thiopentone was twice as great in infants and children as in adults. The ratio of $t\frac{1}{2}$ β to age did not reach statistical significance, but clearance significantly decreased with age (Fig. 6.7). Plasma binding was similar in adults and children.

The finding of a higher induction dose of thiopentone in children, as compared with adults (Cote et al, 1981; Duncan et al, 1984) is difficult to explain purely on a pharmacokinetic basis (decrease in free drug and increased binding or more rapid early distribution), and may be due to

Table 6.5 Pharmacokinetic data for paediatric (5 months to 13 yrs) and adult patients given 4 mg kg^{-1} thiopentone

Parameter	*Paediatric patients*	*Adult patients*
Distribution $t_{1/2}$ (min)		
Rapid	6.3 ± 6.8	3.7 ± 1.1
Slow	43.0 ± 16.0	61.0 ± 34.0
Elimination $t_{1/2}$ (h)	6.1 ± 3.3*	12.0 ± 6.0
Clearance (ml kg^{-1} min^{-1})	6.6 ± 2.2ˣ	3.1 ± 0.5
Vd_{ss} (1 kg^{-1})	2.1 ± 0.71	2.2 ± 0.11
V_c (1 kg^{-1})	0.4 ± 0.19	0.28 ± 0.11
Free thiopentone (% unbound)	13.2 ± 1.5	13.6 ± 1.3

* $P < 0.0005$ significant difference ˣ $P < 0.001$
Sorbo et al (1984)

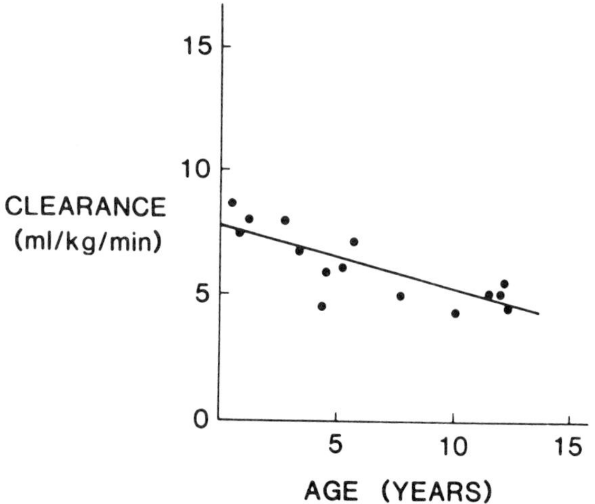

Fig. 6.7 Relationship between age and clearance (ml kg^{-1} min^{-1}) of thiopentone (Sorbo et al, 1984).

decreased sensitivity of the brain to thiopentone as compared with adults.

Sex

Using a standard method to estimate the 'induction' dose of thiopentone Dundee et al (1982) found a significantly lower ($P < 0.001$) dose requirement in women compared with men (Table 6.4). This observation, which confirmed that of Edwards & Ellis (1973), applied irrespective of the age of the patients. With a similar fixed method of administration Christensen & Andreasen (1981) were however unable to demonstrate any difference in induction dose between the sexes but the number of their cases was very small. They did however find a higher venous concentration at the moment of sleep in elderly men (34.3 μg ml^{-1}) as compared with women of the same age group (19.2 μg ml^{-1}). Thus the early distribution differs between men and women and the relatively large apparent initial volume of distribution in women might reflect distribution to more accessible tissues than in men. In practice the sex differences are minimal as compared with the influence of age or pathological factors.

Drugs

Clearly hypnotic and sedative drugs will reduce the induction doses of intravenous agents but this is not due to changes in their pharmacokinetics.

An elevated free thiopentone level can occur if a second drug with affinity to the same binding sites on albumin is given. In vitro studies by Chaplin et al (1973) have shown that acetylsalicylic acid (aspirin), indomethacin, mefenamic acid, phenylbutazone and naproxen can all increase the fraction of free thiopentone but very high concentrations of these drugs are required before significant displacement of binding occurs. In practice many patients on clinical doses of these drugs must have been induced with thiopentone and there are no reports of interactions in the literature. However, it has been shown by McMurray et al (1985) that pretreatment with the equivalent of 1 g acetylsalicylic acid (1.8 g of lysine) did reduce the induction dose of thiopentone to a significant degree. Intravenous acetylsalicylic acid is widely used in continental Europe and these findings could be of clinical significance.

In animal experiments Ylitalo et al (1976) have found that pretreatment with probenecid prolongs both thiopentone and ketamine anaesthesia in mice and rats. Although probenecid has no hypnotic effect, Kaukinen et al (1980) found that the duration of anaesthesia in patients anaesthetized with thiopentone (7 mg kg^{-1}) was prolonged by about 50% by probenecid 0.5–1.0 g compared with a control series. These observations were made in patients premedicated with pethidine but even in the absence of this opiate, probenecid 0.5 g prolonged anaesthesia by 26%. The duration of smaller doses (4 mg kg^{-1} thiopentone) was also markedly prolonged by probenecid. Using a standard method of estimating the 'induction' dose McMurray et al (1984) found that pretreatment with 1 g of probenecid significantly reduced the average 'induction' dose of thiopentone from 5.3 mg kg^{-1} to 4.2 mg kg^{-1} in a constant patient population of healthy young women who received no other anaesthetic premedication. These findings could be explained by the fact that probenecid, which is 80–90% bound to plasma proteins, affects thiopentone binding and results in a higher amount of free drug, thus altering the initial distribution in the body. A greater amount of free drug should lead to a more rapid breakdown and a more rapid recovery and thus might not be the full explanation. It has also been shown to reduce 'induction' time with the highly bound midazolam (Halliday et al, 1984) (see p. 188).

Probenecid is used in clinical practice to delay elimination of penicillin in urine by preventing its active renal tubular excretion. It may be administered just before operation when penicillin is used prophylactically to prevent wound infection. Under these circumstances it is important to know that it can affect both the induction dose of thiopentone and the duration of action of clinical doses.

CLINICAL SIGNIFICANCE OF BARBITURATE PHARMACOKINETICS

The fact that recovery from thiopentone is the result of redistribution of the drug to non-nervous tissues, as well as of detoxication, means that consciousness is regained while a large amount of drug remains in the body. This is of clinical as well as pharmacological interest for a number of reasons.

If a small dose of thiopentone is injected immediately upon recovery from a previous administration a marked cumulative effect is observed for the first 60–90 min (Fig. 6.8); thereafter each dose lasts for approximately the same time. This cumulative effect of large single doses can be detected for up to 24 h in both man and animals (Fig. 6.9) and this could be of clinical significance. In animal experiments Wyngaarden

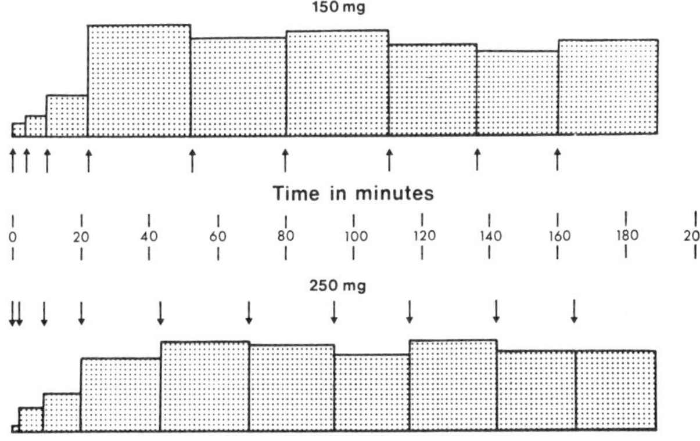

Fig. 6.8 Duration of sleep after repeated doses of thiopentone in fit, unpremedicated adults. Drug injected at arrow when subject opened eyes after previous dose (Dundee, 1955a).

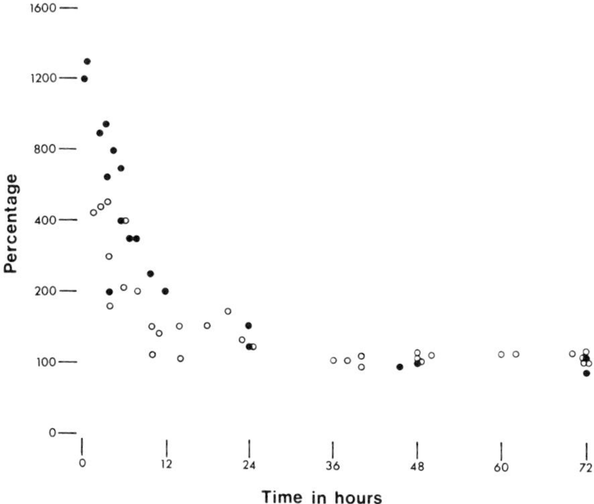

Fig. 6.9 Degree of cumulative action of thiopentone in man (•) and dog (o) when identical doses were given at the time intervals shown. Ordinate expresses the duration of sleep at the second occasion as a percentage of that from the first dose, while abscissa gives time (h) between injections. Doses of thiopentone were 8–10 mg kg^{-1} in man and 15–20 mg kg^{-1} in dogs (Dundee, 1955b).

et al (1949) have demonstrated that thiamylal is less cumulative than thiopentone, while Dundee (1955b) found that a cumulative effect could not be demonstrated in the dog 12 h after thiamylal, as compared with 20–24 h after thiopentone. This difference has not been confirmed in humans.

If anaesthesia is maintained by intermittent injection of a barbiturate — with or without nitrous oxide — supplementary doses required to maintain a constant level of narcosis will become progressively smaller during the first hour of anaesthesia. This sequence will be discussed more fully under Infusion Anaesthesia (Ch. 17). This technique was once employed in obstetrics where Browne (1950) reported very long periods of narcosis following the use of 0.33% solution to control the convulsions of eclampsia; patients received an average dose of 4.9 g over 25 h and recovery of consciousness took 6 to 12 h. Much has been learnt about the pharmacokinetics of thiopentone from this pioneering work.

Because of the dual means of removal of thiopentone and similar drugs from the bloodstream, prolongation of narcosis in the presence of hepatic dysfunction is not a major problem unless very large doses of drug are given or the liver condition is accompanied by malnutrition, dehydration, emaciation, or other complications of terminal malignancy. This is well demonstrated in the studies referred to above in which careful observation and statistical analyses were required to demonstrate any undue sensitivity to the drug in patients with moderately severe liver dysfunction.

Dundee (1955a) has reported seven patients who received repeat anaesthetics within a few hours and the following cases illustrate the sequence of events.

A 27-year old woman was given 850 mg thiopentone intermittently over 10 min for a hysterosalpingogram and was conscious and talking 5 min after the end of the procedure. Twenty-five min later 250 mg thiopentone sufficed for curettage and tubal insufflation lasting 15 min and the patient was deeply unconscious at the end of the procedure.

The sequence of events was similar in a 30-year old woman in whom 500 mg thiopentone was required for the first procedure while 30 min later 250 mg was adequate for the second operation. This patient had no memory of the period between the two events.

A continuous infusion of 9 g thiopentone controlled eclamptic convulsions over 36 h and the patient was fully conscious 24 h later. At this stage a dose of 250 mg re-established a satisfactory level of narcosis for over one hour and following recovery from this a similar effect was produced by 50 mg.

A 60-year old man received 500 mg thiopentone for insertion of a suprapubic catheter and appeared to be fully awake in 10 min. Seven and a half hours later the same procedure was carried out under 300 mg thiopentone and consciousness was not regained for half an hour.

With a large amount of undetoxicated drug in the body on recovery of consciousness the electroencephalographic effects can persist for some time (Brazier et al, 1956) and it is not surprising that there are reports of 'reinduction' of anaesthesia by sedatives and analgesics given in the early postoperative period. The effect of a normal clinical dose of an opiate given for pain relief can be enhanced to the extent of a patient losing consciousness and breathing being depressed. Diazepam also can readily reinduce anaesthesia, even after small doses of barbiturates.

Of greater clinical importance is the enhancement of the action of alcohol after normal adult clinical doses of thiopentone or methohexitone. Doenicke and his colleagues (1966, 1967) clearly showed that EEG changes could be detected for up to 24 h after these barbiturates but not after an equivalent dose of propanidid which is rapidly hydrolysed in the body (Fig. 6.10). Amounts of

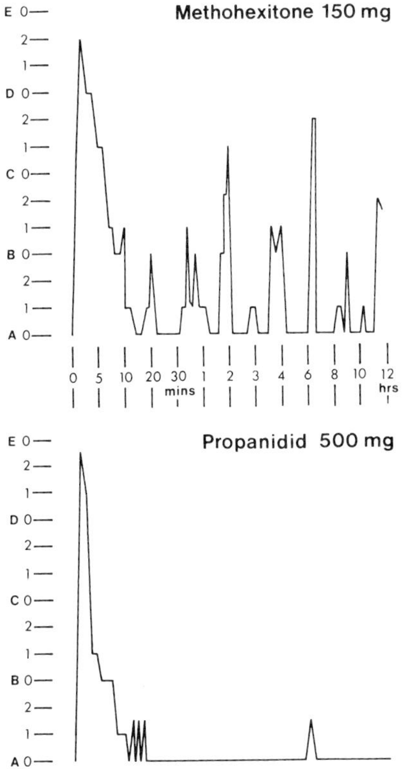

Fig. 6.10 Depth of sleep assessed from the electroencephalographic tracing according to Loomis' classification (varying A; very light sleep, to E; deep sleep), during and after propanidid 500 mg (lower trace) and methohexitone 150 mg (upper trace) (Doenicke et al, 1967).

alcohol that had little effect on the normal subject produced drunkenness when given up to 11 h after the barbiturate. At the time of taking the alcohol, the patients showed little or no evidence of persistence of the hypnotic effect of the anaesthetic. This is quite different from the behaviour of patients after propanidid, which is rapidly hydrolysed in the body and 11 h after which the effect of alcohol did not differ from that in a normal subject.

It is important to appreciate the time taken for normal mental faculties to return following clinical doses of the barbiturates (Osborn et al, 1967). This does not coincide with the apparent return of full consciousness. Hypnotic doses of an oral barbiturate might impair overall driving efficiency for as long as 14 h (Perry & Morgenstern, 1966) while Felsinger et al (1953) have demonstrated significant impairment of visual perception, attention and arithmetic performance for between five and eight and a half hours after the oral administration of 100 mg pentobarbitone. On recovery from sleep 85% of subjects complained of fatigue or grogginess as compared with 50% of those given a placebo. These effects are frequently observed on recovery from intravenous barbiturates and the probability of some degree of mental impairment is such that under no circumstances should patients who have recently received these drugs be allowed to leave for home unaccompanied. This is of major importance in outpatient dental practice. It is not surprising that a committee on Dental Anaesthesia (1967) recommended that following barbiturate anaesthesia, patients be warned not to drive a car and to restrict activities, especially the use of machinery, until the following day. In a detailed study of recovery from clinical doses of methohexitone anaesthesia given for minor 5–10 min procedures, Hutchinson & McNeill (1963) found that although 47 of the 50 patients were awake and talking rationally within five min of the end of the procedure, 23 went back to sleep after their initial waking. The second period of sleep averaged 2.1 (0.5–7.0) h. All patients had amnesia for the time of the first waking. This sequence is well illustrated in Figure 6.10 which shows a return to sleep 2 h after recovering from 150 mg methohexitone. In this instance, sleep or extreme drowsiness lasted for about 4 h.

The following two cases illustrate some of these dangers in routine clinical practice:

> A fit young man was admitted to hospital as a day case for oesophagoscopy which was carried out under thiopentone and a relaxant. It was arranged that a relative should take him home by car on the evening of the operation. Two to three h after return of consciousness the patient seemed quite normal and was told to dress as he would soon be leaving hospital. Without waiting for his escort he set off for home on a complicated journey which he negotiated satisfactorily, getting off at the correct bus stop. He was, however, unable to find his home and was found one h later wandering around in a dazed condition. This occurred about 8 h after the anaesthetic and 4 to 5 h after the return of consciousness. On enquiring later, neither the ward nurse nor one of the bus conductors who knew the patient personally recalled having noticed anything abnormal in his behaviour.

The next report, concerning hexobarbitone, is much more dramatic and resulted in a claim for damages being brought against a dental surgeon (Medicine and the Law, 1949):

A dental surgeon intended to extract seven teeth in a patient for whom nitrous oxide-oxygen was deemed unsuitable. The patient was told that he would be given an intravenous anaesthetic and that he would 'probably be very drowsy for at least one hour after the extractions'. His own doctor administered 500 mg hexobarbitone, the teeth were extracted and the patient was carried to a couch. Nikethamide was given 'to accelerate recovery'. About one quarter of an hour later the dental surgeon went to lunch, instructing the nurse to report to him when the patient began to come round. Within a few minutes the nurse reported that the patient was fingering his shirt collar; returning immediately the surgeon found the patient apparently asleep so he returned to lunch.

Twenty minutes later the nurse, who had kept looking in from time to time, found that the patient had gone. It transpired that he had driven off in his car, and when stopped by traffic lights, had been spoken to by a policeman who, suspecting that something was amiss, kept him in conversation. The constable learned that the patient had just had teeth extracted and offered to drive him home but the offer was refused. On reaching his garage about one mile further on, the patient collided with a wall and a petrol pump; on getting out of the car he collapsed and was helped upstairs. He remained unconscious for a further four to five hours. The dental surgeon's claim for the amount of his fee was met by a counter-claim for damages to the car arising through negligence in that, *inter alia*, the nurse had not prevented the patient from leaving the surgery while still under the influence of the drug.

The case was defended successfully on the grounds that the patient had been warned of possible side effects and he had made an error of judgement in going by car to the operation without arranging for someone else to drive him home. Moreover, it was argued that on the way home the patient had recovered to the extent of making a sound independent judgement of his movements and whether he should accept the constable's offer to drive him home. (This argument is open to debate and it is hard to believe that a patient is in a fit state to make such a decision with so much barbiturate in his body). His decision to drive himself home without the dentist's permission constituted a *novus actus interveniens*, which broke the claim for causation of the damage.

Thiopentone and methohexitone are the only barbiturates from which recovery time has been studied in any detail (Egbert et al, 1959). In studies using a complex performance test (Miles Trainer driving apparatus), Elliott et al (1962) and Green et al (1963) gave 0.88 mg kg^{-1} methohexitone and 2.64 mg kg^{-1} thiopentone to volunteers in a crossover design. Although patients slept slightly longer after methohexitone than following thiopentone, by 35 min 78% of those given methohexitone had recovered compared with 34% after thiopentone. Performance 15 min after drug administration was more variable after thiopentone than after methohexitone. In another experimental study using a Maddox wing to measure extraocular muscular balance Hannington & Kiff (1970) found a slower recovery after 3.6 mg kg^{-1} thiopentone than following 1.2 mg kg^{-1} methohexitone: however, the clinical relevance of these findings is not clear.

There are a large number of clinical studies comparing recovery from these barbiturates. Barry et al (1967) studied 260 urological patients and found a more rapid recovery after methohexitone but the difference was only significant in patients under the age of 60. Psychiatric patients were studied by Burnheim et al (1966) using a battery of tests and they demonstrated a more rapid recovery after methohexitone but not to the extent that they had expected. These two barbiturates have also been used as standard preparations in studying recovery from non-barbiturate agents. Carson et al (1975) and Bahar et al (1982) both noted a more rapid recovery from methohexitone as compared to the equivalent doses of thiopentone.

Some idea of the actual recovery time from these drugs can be gleaned from the work of Vickers (1965). He used four endpoints (pegboard, static ataxia, flicker fusion threshold and reaction time) and the average findings of his study are:

Methohexitone		*Thiopentone*	
mg kg^{-1}	min	mg kg^{-1}	min
1	45–60	2.5	60–75
2	60–90	5.0	135–210

These point to superiority of methohexitone over thiopentone, especially where high doses are used. The clinical observation that recovery occurs quicker after rapid injection is in fact a clinical manifestation of the phenomenon of acute tolerance. It has been observed that within certain limits the higher the initial dose of thiopentone the greater will be the plasma level at recovery (Dundee et al, 1956). This phenomenon will be discussed in Chapter 8.

When given by intermittent injection, methohexitone is less cumulative than thiopentone. When the average requirements of the two drugs (given with nitrous oxide-oxygen for body surface operations lasting at least one hour) are expressed as ratio of total to induction dose, Clarke & Dundee (1966) found that they differed significantly ($P < 0.05$) at 15 and 30 min after induction, and this difference became even more marked ($P < 0.02$) at 45 and 60 min. In studies of liver function Bittrich et al (1963) administered intermittent thiopentone, methohexitone or thiamylal with nitrous oxide-oxygen to comparable groups of patients undergoing body surface operations. Methohexitone was much less cumulative than either thiopentone or thiamylal.

It will be obvious that the main clinical significance of barbiturate pharmacokinetics is based on the fact that recovery is largely due to their translocation in non-nervous tissues, resulting in a cumulative effect on repeated injection, a delay in return of full mental faculties and the ability to enhance the soporific action of drugs given in the early postoperative period. The complexity of their distribution and fate in the body is such that their action may be potentiated not only by sedatives and hypnotics but by a variety of drugs such as antihistamines (Winter, 1948), 2,4-dinitrophenols (Brody & Killam, 1952), glucose (Lamson et al, 1949), as well as compounds which compete for protein binding (Lasser et al, 1963) such as probenecid and acetylsalicylic acid.

The influence of age and operation on the pharmacokinetics of methohexitone have been investigated by Ghoneim et al (1985) and by Harper and his colleagues (1986). Surgery and increase in age did not separately affect the kinetics of the drug. However the elimination half-life was longer in elderly patients than the young unoperated volunteers. All of the subjects studied by Harper and colleagues underwent surgery and these workers did not find any influence of either increasing age or major operations on its pharmacokinetics.

REFERENCES

Bahar M, Dundee J W, O'Neill M P, Briggs L P, Moore J, Merrett J D 1982 Recovery from intravenous anaesthesia: comparison of disoprofol with with thiopentone and methohexitone. Anaesthesia 37: 1171–1175

Barratt R L, Graham G G, Torda T A 1984 Kinetics of thiopentone in relation to the site of sampling. British Journal of Anaesthesia 56: 1385–1391

Barry C T, Lawson R, Davidson D G D 1967 Recovery after methohexitone and thiopentone. Anaesthesia 22: 228–234

Becker K E 1978 Plasma level of thiopental necessary for anesthesia. Anesthesiology 49: 192–196

Bittrich N M, Kane A V'R, Mosher R E 1963 Methohexital and its effect on liver function tests. Anesthesiology 24: 81–90

Bollman J L, Brooks L M, Flock E V, Lundy J S 1950 Tissue distribution with time after single intravenous administration of pentothal sodium. Anesthesiology 11: 1–7

Brand L, Mark L C, Snell M McM, Vrindten P, Dayton P G 1963 Physiologic disposition of methohexital in man. Anesthesiology 24: 331–335

Brazier M A B, Hamlin H, Delgado J M R, Chapman W P 1956 The persistence of electroencephalogram effects of pentothal. Anesthesiology 17: 95–102

Breimer D D 1976 Pharmacokinetics of methohexitone following intravenous infusion in humans. British Journal of Anaesthesia 48: 643–649

Briggs L P, Dundee J W, Bahar M, Clarke R S J 1982 Comparison of the effect of di-isopropyl phenol (ICI 35 868) and thiopentone on response to somatic pain. British Journal of Anaesthesia 54: 307–311

Brodie B B 1952 Physiological disposition and chemical fate of thiobarbiturates in the body. Federation Proceedings 11: 632–639

Brodie B B, Burns J J, Mark L C, Lief P A, Bernstein E, Papper E M 1953 Fate of pentobarbital in man and dog, and method for its estimation in biological material. Journal of Pharmacology and Experimental Therapeutics 109: 26–34

Brodie B B, Kurz H, Schanker L S 1960 The importance of dissociation constant and lipid-solubility in influencing the passage of drugs into the cerebrospinal fluid. Journal of Pharmacology and Experimental Therapeutics 130: 20–25

Brodie B B, Mark L C, Papper E M, Lief P A, Bernstein E, Rovenstine E A 1950 Fate of thiopental in man and method for its estimation in biological material. Journal of Pharmacology and Experimental Therapeutics 98: 85–96

Brody T M, Killam K F 1952 Potentiation of barbiturates in anesthesia by 2,4-dinitrophenol. Journal of Pharmacology and Experimental Therapeutics 106:375

Brooks L M, Bollman J L, Flock E V, Lundy J S 1948 Tissue distribution with time following single intravenous administration of sodium pentothal. American Journal of Physiology 155:429

Browne O 1950 Treatment of eclampsia: preliminary report of present Rotunda treatment of eclampsia by soluble sodium thiopentone and concentrated salt free dextrose solution with particular reference to control of convulsions. Journal of Obstetrics and Gynaecology of the British Empire 57: 573–582

Burch P G, Stanski D R 1981a Thiopental protein binding. Anesthesiology 55:A253

Burch P G, Stanski D R 1981b Metabolism and termination of thiopental effect. Anesthesiology 55:A175

Burch P G, Stanski D R 1981c Fentanyl pharmacokinetics in obese and nonobese patients. Anesthesiology 55:A176

Burnheim R B, Terry P M, Herron J T 1966 Comparative recovery of mental functions after ECT with methohexital and thiopental anesthesia. Medical Journal of Australia 1: 625–627

Bush M T 1963 Sedatives and Hypnotics. 1: Absorption, Fate and Excretion. In: Root W S, Hoffman F G (eds) Physiological pharmacology: a comprehensive treatise, 1st edn. Academic Press, London.

Bush M T, Berry G, Hume A 1966 Ultra-short acting barbiturates as oral hypnotic agents in man. Clinical Pharmacology and Therapeutics 7: 373–378

Butler T C 1950 The rate of penetration of barbituric acid derivatives into the brain. Journal of Pharmacology and Experimental Therapeutics 100: 219–226

Cameron G R, de Saram G S W 1939 The effect of liver damage on the action of some barbiturates. Journal of Pathology and Bacteriology 48: 49–54

Carson I W, Graham J, Dundee J W 1975 Clinical studies of induction agents. XLIII: Recovery from Althesin — a comparative study with thiopentone and methohexitone. British Journal of Anaesthesia 47: 358–364.

Chaplin M D, Roszkowski A P, Richards R K 1973 Displacement of thiopental from plasma proteins by nonsteroidol anti-inflammatory agents. Proceedings of the Society of Experimental Biology and Medicine 143: 667–671

Christensen J H, Andreasen F 1978 Individual variation in response to thiopental. Acta Anaesthesiologica Scandinavica 22: 303–313

Christensen J H, Andreasen F, Jansen J A 1980 Pharmacokinetics of thiopentone in a group of young women and a group of young men. British Journal of Anaesthesia 52: 913–917

Christensen J H, Andreasen F, Janssen J A 1981 Influence of age and sex on the pharmacokinetics of thiopentone. British Journal of Anaesthesia 53: 1189–1195

Christensen J H, Andreasen F, Janssen J A 1982 Pharmacokinetics and pharmacodynamics of thiopentone: a comparison between young and elderly patients. Anaesthesia 37: 398–404

Clarke R S J, Dundee J W 1966 Clinical studies of induction agents. XV: A comparison of the cumulative effects of thiopentone, methohexitone and propanidid. British Journal of Anaesthesia 38: 401–405

Cloyd J C, Wright B D, Pevser D 1979 Pharmacokinetic properties of thiopental in two patients treated for uncontrollable seizures. Epilepsia 20: 313–318

Cohen E N, Paulson W J, Wall J, Elert B 1953 Thiopental curare and nitrous oxide anesthesia for Cesarean section with studies on placental transmission. Surgery, Gynecology and Obstetrics 97: 456–462

Conney A H, Burns J J 1962 Factors influencing drug metabolism. Advances in Pharmacology 1: 31–58

Conney A H G, Davison C, Gastel R, Burns J J 1960 Adaptive increases in drug-metabolising enzymes induced by phenobarbital and other drugs. Journal of Pharmacology and Experimental Therapeutics 130: 1–8

Cooper J R, Brodie B B 1955 Enzymatic oxidation of hexobarbital. Journal of Pharmacology and Experimental Therapeutics 114: 409–417

Cote C J, Goudsouzian N G, Liu L M P, Dedrick D F, Firestone S 1981 Thiopental: a dose-response study in unpremedicated children. Anesthesia and Analgesia 60: 246–247

Couderc E, Ferrier C, Haberer J P, Henzel D, Duvaldestin P 1984 Thiopentone pharmacokinetics in patients with chronic alcoholism. British Journal of Anaesthesia 56: 1393–1397

Crawford J S, Kane P O, Gardiner J E 1956 Some aspects of obstetric anaesthesia. British Journal of Anaesthesia 24: 146–158

Davis M, Simmons C J, Dordoni B, Maxwell J D and Williams R 1973 Induction of hepatic enzymes during normal human pregnancy. British Journal of Obstetrics and Gynaecology, 80, 690–694

Dental Anaesthesia 1967 Report of a Joint Subcommittee of the Standing Medical and Dental Advisory Committees, Ministry of Health. HMSO, London

Doenicke A, Kugler J, Laub M 1967 Evaluation of recovery and 'street fitness' by EEG and psychodiagnostic tests after anaesthesia. Canadian Anaesthetists' Society Journal 14: 567–583

Doenicke A, Kugler J, Schellenberger A, Gurtner T 1966 The use of electro encephalography to measure recovery time after intravenous anaesthesia. British Journal of Anaesthesia 38: 580–590

Dorfman A, Goldbaum L R 1947 Detoxication of barbiturates. Journal of Pharmacology and Experimental Therapeutics 90: 330–337

Duncan B B A, Zaimi F, Newman G B, Jenkins J G, Aveling W 1984 Effect of premedication on the induction dose of thiopentone in children. Anaesthesia 39: 426–428

Dundee J W 1952 Thiopentone narcosis in the presence of hepatic dysfunction. British Journal of Anaesthesia 24: 81–100

Dundee J W 1955a Observations on the dosage and cumulative action of thiopentone. Anaesthesia 10: 139–157

Dundee J W 1955b Cumulative action of four thiobarbiturates: with special reference to thiopentone and thiamylal. Anaesthesia 10: 391–400

Dundee J W, Annis D 1955 Barbiturate narcosis in uraemia. British Journal of Anaesthesia 27: 114–123

Dundee J W, Hassard T H, McGowan W A W, Henshaw J 1982 The 'induction' dose of thiopentone. A method of study and preliminary illustrative results. Anaesthesia 37: 1176–1184

Dundee J W, Price W L, Dripps R D 1956 Acute tolerance to thiopentone in man. British Journal of Anaesthesia 28: 344–352

Dundee J W, Richards R K 1954 Effect of azotemis upon the action of intravenous barbiturate anesthesia. Anesthesiology 15: 333–346

Edwards R, Ellis F R 1973 Clinical significance of thiopentone binding to haemoglobin and plasma protein. British Journal of Anaesthesia 45: 891–893

Effros R M, Corbeil N, Chinard F P 1972 Arterial pH and distribution of barbiturates between pulmonary tissue and blood. Journal of Applied Physiology 33:656

Egbert L D, Oech S R, Echenhoff J E 1959 Comparison of the recovery from methohexital and thiopental anesthesia in man. Surgery, Gynecology and Obstetrics 109: 427–430

Ehrnebo M 1974 Pharmacokinetics and distribution properties of pentobarbital in humans following oral and intravenous administration. Journal of Pharmacy and Science 63: 1114–1118

Elliott C J, Green R, Howells T H, Long A H 1962 Recovery after intravenous barbiturate anaesthesia. Comparative study of recovery from methohexitone and thiopentone. Lancet ii: 68–70

Felsinger J M von, Lasagna L, Beecher H K 1953 The persistence of mental impairment following a hypnotic dose of a barbiturate. Journal of Pharmacology and Experimental Therapeutics 109: 284–291

Finster M, Mark L C, Morishima H O, Moya F, Perel J M, James L S, Dayton P G 1966 Plasma thiopental concentration in the newborn following delivery under thiopental-nitrous oxide anesthesia. American Journal of Obstetrics and Gynecology 95: 621–629

Finster M, Morishima H O, Mark L C, Perel J M, Dayton P G, James L S 1972 Tissue thiopental concentration in the fetus and newborn. Anesthesiology 36: 155–158.

Flowers C E, Hill C 1958 The placental transmission of barbiturates and thiobarbiturates and their pharmacogical action on the mother and infant. American Journal of Obstetrics and Gynecology 78: 730–740

Ghoneim M M, Pandya H 1975 Plasma protein binding of thiopental in patients with impaired renal or hepatic function. Anesthesiology 42: 545–549

Ghoneim M M, Chiang C K, Schoenwald R D, Lilburn J K, Dhanara J 1985 The pharmacokinetics of methohexitone in young and elderly subjects. Acta Anaesthesiologica Scandinavica 29: 480–482

Ghoneim M M, Van Hamme M J 1978 Pharmacokinetics of thiopentone: effects of enflurane and nitrous oxide anesthesia and surgery. British Journal of Anaesthesia 50: 1237–1241.

Gibson W R, Swanson E E, Doran W J 1955 Pharmacology of a short-acting non-sulphur barbituric acid derivative. Proceedings of the Society for Experimental Biology and Medicine 89: 292–294

Goldbaum L R, Smith T K 1954 The interaction of barbiturates with serum albumin and its possible relation to their disposition and pharmacological actions. Journal of Pharmacology and Experimental Therapeutics 111: 197–209

Gould R C, Shideman F E 1952 The in vitro metabolism of thiopental by a fortified cell-free tissue preparation of the rat. Journal of Pharmacology and Experimental Therapeutics 104: 427–439

Green R, Long H A, Elliott C J R, Howells T H 1963 A method of studying recovery after anaesthesia: a critical assessment of recovery following methohexitone and thiopentone using a complex performance task. Anaesthesia 18: 189–200

Halliday N J, Dundee J W, Loughran P G, Harper K W 1984 Age and plasma proteins influence the action of midazolam. Anesthesiology 61:A 357

Hannington-Kiff J G 1970 Measurement of recovery from outpatients general anaesthesia with a simple ocular test. British Medical Journal iii:132

Harper K W, Collier P S, Dundee J W, Elliott P, Halliday N J, Lowry K G 1985 Age and nature of operation influence the pharmacokinetics of midazolam. British Journal of Anaesthesia 57: 866–871

Harper K W, Collier P S, Dundee J W, McClean E 1986 Methohexitone kinetics in surgical patients. Irish Journal of Medical Science 155:332

Hellman L M, Shettles L B, Manahan C P, Eastman N J 1944 Sodium pentothal anesthesia in obstetrics. American Journal of Obstetrics and Gynecology 48: 851–860

Hudson R J, Stanski D R, Burch P G 1983 Pharmacokinetics of methohexital and thiopental in surgical patients. Anesthesiology 59: 215–219

Hull C J 1984 General principles of pharmacokinetics. In: Prys-Roberts C, Hug C C Jr (eds) Pharmacokinetics of anaesthesia. Blackwell, Oxford, p 20

Hutchinson B R, McNeill T D M 1963 Recovery from methohexitone anaesthesia. New Zealand Medical Journal 62: 428–430

Jailer J W, Goldbaum L R 1946 Studies on plasma concentration and tissue distribution of sodium pentothal [sodium ethyl (1-methylbutyl) thiobarbiturate]. Journal of Laboratory and Clinical Medicine 31: 1344–1349

Jung T, Mayersohn M, Perrier D, Calkins J, Saunders R 1982 Thiopental disposition in lean and obese patients undergoing surgery. Anesthesiology 56: 269–274

Kahn J B Jr, Nicholson D B, Assali N S 1953 Placental transmission of a thiobarbiturate in parturient women. Obstetrical and Gynecological Survey 1: 663–667

Kaukinen S, Eerola M, Ylitalo P 1980 Prolongation of thiopentone anaesthesia by probenecid. British Journal of Anaesthesia 52: 603–607

Kelly A R, Shideman F E 1949 Liver as major organ involved in detoxification of thiopental by dog. Federation Proceedings 8:306

Lamson P D, Greig M E, Robbins B H 1949 The potentiating effect of glucose and its metabolic products on barbiturate anesthesia. Science 110: 690–691

Lasser E C, Elizondo-Martel G, Granke R C 1963 Potentiation of pentobarbital anesthesia by competitive protein binding. Anesthesiology 24: 665–671

McKechnie F B, Converse J G 1955 Placental transmission of thiopental. American Journal of Obstetrics and Gynecology 70: 639–644

McMurray T J, Dundee J W, Henshaw J S 1984 The influence of probenecid on the induction dose of thiopentone. British Journal of Clinical Pharmacology 17:224P

McMurray T J, Robinson F P, Dundee J W, Riddell J G, McClean E 1985 A new method for producing constant plasma drug levels — application to methohexitone. British Journal of Anaesthesia, 58:

Mark L C 1963 Thiobarbiturates. In: Papper E M, Kitz R J (eds) Uptake and distribution of anesthetic agents. New York, McGraw-Hill, ch 23

Mark L C, Brand L, Dayton P, Blaber P, Papper E M 1960 Behaviour of methohexital in man. Federation Proceedings 19:274

Mark L C, Burns J J, Brand L, Campomanes C I, Trousof N, Papper E M, Brodie B B 1958 The passage of thiobarbiturates and their oxygen analogs into brain. Journal of Pharmacology and Experimental Therapeutics 123: 70–73

Masson G M C, Beland E 1945 Influence of the liver and the kidney on the duration of anesthesia produced by barbiturates. Anesthesiology 6: 483–491

Maynert E W, van Dyke H B 1949 Metabolism of barbiturates. Pharmacological Reviews 1: 217–242

Medicine and the Law 1949 After effects of intravenous anaesthesia. Lancet i: 285–286

Meyers F H, Peoples D 1954 The positive role of the liver in the rapid metabolism of thiopental. Anesthesiology 15: 146–149

Morgan P J, Blackman G L, Paull J D, Wolff L J 1981a Pharmacokinetics and plasma binding of thiopental. I: Studies in surgical patients. Anesthesiology 54: 468–473

Morgan P J, Blackman G L, Paull J D and Wolff L J 1981b Pharmacokinetics and plasma binding of thiopental. II: Studies in Caesarean section. Anesthesiology 54: 474–480

Murphy P J 1974 Biotransformation of methohexital. International Anesthesiology Clinics 12 (2): 139–143

Osborn A G, Bunker J P, Cooper L M, Frank G S, Hilgard E R 1967 Effects of thiopental sedation on learning and memory. Science 157: 574–576

Pandele G, Chaux F, Salvadori C, Farinotti M, Duvaldestin P 1983 Thiopentone pharmacokinetics in patients with cirrhosis. Anesthesiology 59: 123–126

Perry C J G, Morgenstern A L 1966 Drugs and driving.

Journal of the American Medical Association 195: 376–379
Pratt T W 1933 A comparison of the action of pentobarbital (Nembutal) and sodium barbital in rabbits as related to the detoxicating power of the liver. Journal of Pharmacology and Experimental Therapeutics 48: 285–187
Pratt T W, Vanlandingham H W, Talley E E, Nelson J M, Johnson E O 1932 Studies of the liver function of dogs. American Journal of Physiology 102: 148–152
Price H L 1960 A dynamic concept of the distribution of thiopental in the human body. Anesthesiology 21: 40–45
Price H L 1961 In: Dripps R D, J E Eckenhoff, Vandam L D (eds) Introduction to Anaesthesia, 2nd edn. Saunders, London, p 131
Price H L, Kovnat P J, Safer J N, Conner E H, Price M L 1960 The uptake of thiopental by body tissues and its relation to the duration of narcosis. Clinical Pharmacology and Therapeutics 1: 16–22
Quinn G P, Axelrod J, Brodie B B 1958 Species, Strain and sex differences in metabolism of hexobarbitone, amidopyrine, antipyrine and aniline. Biochemical Pharmacology 1: 152–159
Rappaport A M, Hiraki G Y, Rosenfeld B, Cowan C R, Lang J 1956 Effect of autoperfusion of the liver on detoxication of thiopental sodium. American Journal of Physiology 186: 193–198
Rayburn J C, Whitehead R W, Draper W B 1953 The influence of respiratory acidosis on the plasma levels of thiopental and on the depth of anesthesia. Current Researches in Anesthesia 32: 280–285
Reidenberg M M, Lowenthal D T, Briggs W, Gasparo M 1976 Pentobarbital elimination in patients with poor renal function. Clinical Pharmacology and Therapeutics 150: 118–121
Reynolds C 1939 Dangers of prolonged pentothal sodium anesthesia from pharmacological standpoint. Current Researches in Anaesthesia 18: 270–273
Richards R K 1947 Experiments on the inactivation of Pentothal. Federation Proceedings 6: 188–189
Richards R K, Taylor J D, Kueter K E 1953 Effect of nephrectomy on the duration of sleep following administration of thiopental and hexobarbital. Journal of Pharmacology and Experimental Therapeutics 108: 461–473
Rubin E, Lieber C S 1968 Hepatic microsomal enzymes in man and rat: induction and inhibition by ethanol. Science 162:690
Saidman L J, Eger E I 1966 The effect of thiopental metabolism on duration of anesthesia. Anesthesiology 27: 118–126
Schanker L S 1963 Penetration of drugs into the central nervous system. In: Papper E M, Kitz R J (eds) Uptake and distribution of anesthetic agents. McGraw-Hill, New York, ch 13, p 157–163
Scheifley C H, Higgins C M 1940 The effect of partial hepatectomy on the action of certain barbiturates and a phenylurea derivative. American Journal of Medical Sciences 200: 264–268
Shideman F E 1952 In vitro metabolism of barbiturates. Federation Proceedings 11: 640–646
Shideman F E, Gould T C, Winters W D, Peterson R C, Wilner W K 1953 The distribution and in vivo rate of metabolism of thiopental. Journal of Pharmacology and Experimental Therapeutics 107: 338–378
Shideman F E, Kelly A R, Adams B J 1947 The role of the liver in the detoxication of thiopental (Pentothal) and two other thiobarbiturates. Journal of Pharmacology and Experimental Therapeutics 91: 331–339
Shideman F E, Kelly A R, Lee L E, Lowell V F, Adams B J 1949 The role of the liver in the detoxication of thiopental (Pentothal) in man. Anesthesiology 10: 421–428
Smith R B, Dittert L W, Griffen W O, J T Doluisio 1973 Pharmacokinetics of pentobarbital after intravenous and oral administration. Journal of Pharmacokinetics and Biopharmaceutics 1: 5–16
Sorbo S, Hudson R J, Loomis J C 1984 The pharmacokinetics of thiopentone in pediatric surgical patients. Anesthesiology 61: 666–670
Stanski D R 1981 Pharmacokinetic modelling of thiopental. Anesthesiology 54: 446–448
Stanski D R, Mihm F G, Rosenthal M H, Kalman S M 1980 Pharmacokinetics of high-dose thiopental used in cerebral resuscitation. Anaesthesiology 35: 169–171
Stanski D R, Watkins D W 1982 Drug disposition in anesthesia. Grune & New York, Stratton
Sunshine I, Whitwam J G, Fike W W, Finkle B, LeBeau J 1966 Distribution and excretion of methohexitone in man. A study using gas and thin layer chromatography. British Journal of Anaesthesia 38: 23–28
Veal J R, Reynolds C 1938 Cumulative effects of Pentothal Sodium. Southern Medical Journal (Birmingham, Alabama) 31: 649–650
Vickers M D 1965 Measurement of recovery from anaesthesia. British Journal of Anaesthesia 37: 296–302
Waddell W J, Butler T C 1957 The distribution and excretion of phenobarbital. Journal of Clinical Investigation 36: 1217–1266
Walker J M, Wynn Parry C B 1949 Effects of hepatectomy on action of certain anaesthetics in rats. British Journal of Pharmacology 4: 93–97
Whitwam J G 1972 The pharmacology of brietal sodium (methohexitone sodium) Anaesthesiologie und Wiederbelebung 57: 1–19
Whitwam J G 1976 Methohexitone (editorial). British Journal of Anaesthesia 48: 617–619
Winter C A 1948 Potentiating effect of antihistaminic drugs upon the sedative action of barbiturates. Journal of Pharmacology and Experimental Therapeutics 94: 7–11
Wyngaarden J B, Woods L A, Ridley R, Seevers M H 1949 Anesthetic properties of sodium 5-allyl-5-(1-methyl-butyl)-2-thiobarbiturate (Surital) and certain other thiobarbiturates in dogs. Journal of Pharmacology and Experimental Therapeutics, 95: 322–328
Ylitalo P, Saarnivaara L, Ahtee L 1976 Effect of ketamine anaesthesia on the content of monoamines and their metabolites in the rat brain. Acta Anaesthesiologica Scandinavica 20: 216–220

A. C. McKay MD FFARCS

Barbiturates: mode of action

Much progress has been made in recent years in the understanding of the molecular and neurophysiological mechanisms of anaesthetic action. At molecular level barbiturates have generally been assumed to share an essentially similar mode of action with the volatile and other intravenous anaesthetics. In this area, therefore, little of the literature refers specifically to barbiturates. At the neurophysiological level, by contrast, a great deal of specific data has been accumulated on the actions of barbiturates on individual neurones and on larger CNS structures.

MOLECULAR MECHANISMS

Historically, theories of anaesthesia have been based on the assumption of a common non-specific mechanism of action for all agents. This assumption was based on the observed lack of correlation between chemical structure and the ability to produce anaesthesia, and on the striking correlation between anaesthetic potency and solubility in a non-polar medium. This correlation has been extended to include the barbiturates (Franks & Lieb, 1978) and barbiturate anaesthesia, like that of other agents, is reversible by the application of high pressure (Miller et al, 1973). The critical volume hypothesis (Mullins, 1954), based on earlier observations of this type with inhalational agents, proposed a unitary mechanism, whereby anaesthesia ensues when a critical volume fraction of anaesthetic is achieved in a lipid environment, generally agreed to be a phospholipid membrane. It assumed that this occurred through the physical effect of the expansion on specialised membrane functions.

However, several observations have led to a radical revision of this all-inclusive hypothesis.

Firstly, while membrane expansion and increased fluidity caused by anaesthetics has been demonstrated by some workers (Seeman, 1972; Lawrence & Gill, 1975), others have been unable to show this at clinical concentrations (Franks & Lieb, 1978). Secondly, the critical volume hypothesis predicts that anaesthetic potency should increase with increasing temperature, while in fact the opposite occurs. Thirdly, the relationship between anaesthetic potency and pressure should, according to the hypothesis, be linear and of equal slope for all agents, but this is not the case (Halsey et al, 1978). Interestingly, intravenous agents have the most anomalous behaviour; the potency of methohexitone decreases non-linearly with increasing pressure and reaches a minimum at 58 atm . These workers proposed that, rather than interacting only with a simple bulk solvent, anaesthetics can act at more than one type of molecular site. Some of these molecular sites would have a finite size and therefore be capable of being saturated by anaesthetic molecules or by the effects of pressure. The most likely location of these latter sites is in hydrophobic clefts in the surface of membrane-embedded proteins, and potency-related conformational changes in the haemoglobin molecule might be induced by inhalational agents (Brown & Halsey, 1980).

This explanation is more satisfactory than the simpler critical volume hypothesis, since, by postulating a variety of sites with different characteristics, it enables the obvious clinical and neurophysiological differences among anaesthetics to be accommodated. While some of the sites may be envisaged as comparatively homogenous and non-specific, others, with limited occupancy, more closely resemble specific receptor sites.

It is not unreasonable to suppose that this type of site would be particularly important for larger molecules such as the barbiturates, with their stereo-specificity and marked structure-activity relationships. It is notable that the larger molecules deviate most from the behaviour predicted by the critical volume hypothesis in that not only are they non-linear in their pressure-potency relationships, but also some mixtures of these agents show non-additivity of potency. Althesin–methohexitone mixtures are synergistic (Archer et al, 1977) and methohexitone-nitrous oxide mixtures are non-additive (Wardley-Smith & Halsey, 1981), suggesting that these agents act at different sites: on the other hand, these latter workers found that thiopentone-propanidid mixtures were additive at high pressure. It appears likely, then, that at molecular level barbiturates act, like other anaesthetics, in a hydrophobic environment, but that their mode of action in this environment has more of the characteristics of a classical drug-receptor combination than does that of the smaller volatile anaesthetic molecules.

METABOLIC EFFECTS

In theory there are a number of possible ways in which these molecular changes could affect neuronal function to produce anaesthesia. One such possibility, which has been thoroughly investigated, is by depression of metabolism. Quastel & Wheatley (1932) noted that clinical concentrations of barbiturates caused dose-related inhibition of cerebral oxidation of glucose, lactate and pyruvate but not succinate. Subsequent studies suggest that barbiturates depress mitochondrial respiration by a specific inhibition of electron transfer from NADH to flavoprotein (Cohen, 1973). Krnjevik (1974) has suggested a mechanism whereby anaesthetic interference with mitochondrial function could lead to neurophysiological effects, in that blockade of ATP-dependent mitochondrial uptake of calcium ion would be expected to lead to increased neuronal membrane potassium permeability, and hence reduced membrane excitability. However, it is now generally regarded as unlikely that the metabolic effects of barbiturates, while they might be clinically relevant in certain situations, are involved in producing the anaesthetic effects of the drugs (Cohen, 1973). In most studies, the concentrations of barbiturate required to affect mitochondrial respiration significantly are in excess of those that produce anaesthesia. A more likely mechanism of action would be a direct effect of barbiturates and other anaesthetics on the specialised proteins of the neuronal membrane.

NEUROPHYSIOLOGICAL MECHANISMS

The neurophysiological effects of barbiturates have been widely studied in both vertebrate and invertebrate preparations. Far from pointing to a nonspecific or simple mechanism of barbiturate anaesthesia, the evidence indicates that their effects are highly complex and varied.

Since the work of Larrabee & Posternak (1952) who showed that ether, pentobarbitone and chloroform depressed synaptic transmission through sympathetic ganglia at lower concentrations than those required to block the nerve compound action potential, it has been generally accepted that general anaesthetics exert their clinical effects primarily through modification of synaptic transmission. Although it has been suggested (Seeman, 1972; Krnjevik, 1974) that conduction in fine preterminal axons might be more susceptible than in larger fibres, Richards (1982) compared the action of pentobarbitone on synaptic transmission with that of the sodium channel blocker tetrodotoxin, which has no direct effect on synapses. At concentrations of the two agents which depressed synaptic transmission to the same extent, tetrodotoxin depressed the presynaptic action potential while pentobarbitone did not, suggesting that the action of the barbiturate was entirely on synaptic rather than axonal processes. Barker (1975) showed that the ability of a number of agents, including pentobarbitone, to depress sodium-dependent excitatory synaptic transmission is significantly correlated with hydrophobicity. Since hydrophobicity is strongly correlated with anaesthetic potency in vivo, this finding also supports the view that synaptic effects are of prime importance in the mechanism of general anaesthesia. However, it remains true that the pre-terminal axon is potentially a highly sensitive component in the synaptic chain since a small change in its polarity, such as might be caused by a change in presynaptic inhibition as well as a direct effect of a drug, can profoundly alter the efficacy of synaptic transmission (Eccles, 1973).

In general, the weight of evidence suggests that excitatory synaptic transmission is mainly depressed by barbiturates, while inhibitory synaptic transmission is usually unaffected or enhanced. It is important to determine which component(s) of the synaptic transmission process are affected, and in particular to establish the relative importance of pre-synaptic and post-synaptic effects.

Comparatively few investigators have studied the effects of barbiturates on the release of transmitter at synapses. Matthews & Quilliam (1964) showed that amylobarbitone reduces the quantity of acetylcholine released in response to afferent stimulation of mammalian sympathetic ganglia and neuromuscular junctions. However, other workers (Westmoreland et al, 1971; Procter & Weakly, 1976) have found that barbiturates increase the number of quanta of acetylcholine released in response to afferent stimulation at the vertebrate neuromuscular junction, although overall nueromuscular transmission is depressed, implying that there must be a marked reduction in postsynaptic sensitivity. Weakly (1969) analysed the effects of thiopentone and pentobarbitone on excitatory postsynaptic potentials (EPSPs) in cat spinal cord motor neurones. He showed that the drugs reduced the size of the EPSP caused by stimulation of a Ia afferent nerve fibre, but that the mean amplitude of individual miniature EPSPs was unchanged. He thus concluded that the reduction in evoked EPSP size was due, not to a drug effect on the sensitivity of the postsynaptic membrane, but to a decrease in the number of quanta of transmitter released.

Collins (1980) studied the effects of pentobarbitone on the evoked release of putative neurotransmitters from isolated rat olfactory cortical slices. Release of the presumed excitatory transmitters aspartate and tacrine was depressed by the drug, while that of the inhibitory transmitter gamma-amino butyric acid (GABA) was enhanced (Fig. 7.1).

No unifying theory can as yet explain these different effects of barbiturates on neurotransmitter release at different sites. At present, the most likely explanation for the depressant effects is probably a direct action of the drug on the excitation-secretion coupling process, perhaps through an effect on the influx of calcium into the neurone (Blaustein & Ector, 1975).

There have been many studies of the effects of barbiturates on the postsynaptic neurone, mainly making use of iontophoretic techniques. [For full reviews, see Nicoll (1978) and Richards (1978)]. In the vertebrate nervous system, there is ample evidence that barbiturates depress excitatory postsynaptic responses, at a wide variety of sites, both to acetylcholine and to aminoacid putative transmitters.

In the isolated guineapig olfactory cortex, neuronal discharges, which can be produced by iontophoretically-applied L-glutamate, are depressed by clinical concentrations of pentobarbitone, as well as alphaxalone and several volatile agents (Richards & Smaje, 1976). Galindo (1969) also reported that pentobarbitone decreased neuronal sensitivity to glutamate. Crawford (1970) studied the effects of pentobarbitone, administered both systemically and iontophoretically, on the spontaneous activity and response to applied DL-homocysteic acid and acetylcholine of cat cortical neurones. Both spontaneous activity and sensitivity to these excitatory transmitters were reduced by subclinical doses of the barbiturate. However, Smaje (1976) found that pentobarbitone had no consistent effect on the muscarinic responses of olfactory cortical neurones to acetylcholine.

The effects of barbiturates on postsynaptic inhibitory responses are, however, less consistent. While several workers found that inhibitory responses were unaffected by barbiturates (Galindo, 1969; Crawford, 1970) others have shown enhancement of these responses, especially those mediated by GABA (Nicoll, 1975; Barker & Ransom, 1978). Enhancement of presynaptic inhibition by pentobarbitone was reported by Eccles et al (1963). The available evidence suggests that barbiturate enhancement of GABA-mediated inhibition is due to a direct action of the

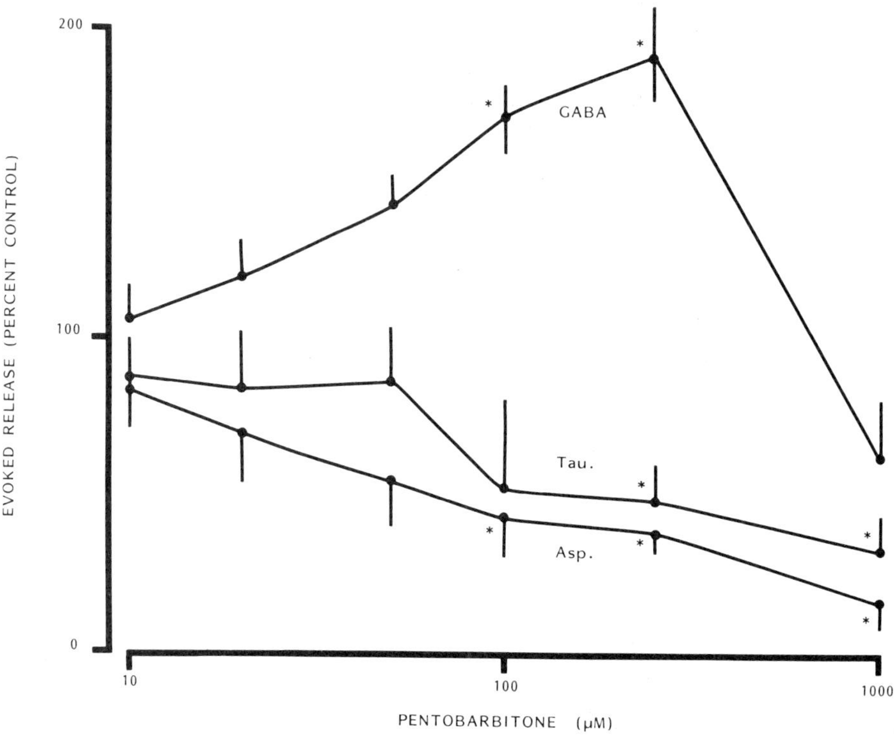

Fig. 7.1 Effect of pentobarbitone on the release of GABA, aspartate (Asp) and taurine (Tau) accompanying supramaximal electrical stimulation of the lateral olfactory tract of rat olfactory cortex slics. From Collins (1980) p. 521.

drugs at the transmitter receptor site, or its associated ion channel, and not an indirect effect such as inhibition of GABA removal.

Studies in invertebrate preparations and at the mammalian neuromuscular junction have enabled the ionic conductance changes that underlie these different effects of barbiturates to be examined (Judge, 1983). Results have tended to confirm that barbiturates depress postsynaptic sensitivity to excitatory transmitters. Barker (1975) showed that pentobarbitone and other anaesthetics in clinical concentrations depressed postsynaptic excitatory responses which depend on changes in sodium conductance, whether the transmitter involved was acetylcholine or glutamate. Pentobarbitone antagonism of the response to acetylcholine was non-competitive. It appears, therefore, that in this situation, the action of the barbiturate might be selective for a particular type of ion channel rather than for a particular receptor. Judge et al (1979) found that clinical concentrations of thiopentone depressed chloride-dependent inhibitory responses to applied acetylcholine and glutamate. This selectivity suggests that the site of action of the drug is at a component of the ion channel control mechanism rather than on its associated receptor.

In the vertebrate neuromuscular junction, Adams (1974) showed that thiopentone increased the rate of decay of miniature endplate currents produced by applied acetylcholine, indicating that the average open time of ion channels was reduced. This effect was more pronounced in previously activated channels ('use dependence') suggesting that the drug gains access to its binding site via the channel mouth. Such electrophysiological evidence of direct interaction of barbiturates with ion channels is in agreement with the current state of opinion on the molecular mechanisms of anaesthesia in that it implies a specific action at a protein site.

The effects of barbiturates on the various pathways and subsystems of the central nervous system (CNS) represent the total effect of these complex and diverse actions of the drugs on many millions of individual neurones. For obvious reasons, pathways subserving the maintenance of consciousness and centripetal transfer of sensory information have been the main objects of study in investigations of barbiturate action.

The spinal cord dorsal horn is known to have an important modulatory role in the onward transfer of sensory information. Monosynaptic spinal reflexes are depressed by barbiturates among other anaesthetics (Somjen & Gill, 1963) as are spontaneous and evoked activity in dorsal horn cells, especially those in laminae IV and V (Wall, 1967; Kitahata et al, 1975). Thus, action at spinal cord level clearly contributes to the overall picture of barbiturate anaesthesia.

In contrast, the classical sensory pathways of the spinal cord and brain stem, which contain only two or three synapses, appear to be relatively resistant to the effects of barbiturates and other anaesthetics, a finding which presumably reflects the high level of efficiency built into their synaptic organisation. However, information also travels cortically in the multisynaptic reticular formation. The demonstration, by Moruzzi & Magoun (1949), that stimulation of the reticular formation causes electroencephalographic (EEG) and behavioural arousal, suggested that the formation might have a role in the production of the anaesthetised state. French et al (1953) showed that pentobarbitone and ether blocked sensory and auditory cortical evoked responses by a direct action on the reticular formation, while Arduini & Arduini (1954) showed that the EEG arousal response to direct reticular stimulation was blocked by pentobarbitone. Abrahamian et al (1963) analysed the effects of thiopentone on the human sensory evoked response. The late component of the response, which is believed to be due to reticular stimulation, was blocked at anaesthetic doses of the drug, while the early, specific component was left intact. Results such as these are strongly suggestive that reticular formation blockade is an essential component of the mechanism of barbiturate action on the brain. King et al (1957) showed that barbiturates depressed transmission through the ventrobasal thalamus, and attributed this to an effect on reticular tone, while Angel (1977) has suggested that functional denervation of the cortex, through increased inhibitory and decreased facilitatory reticular stimulation of the ventrobasal thalamus, might be a general mechanism of anaesthesia. However, observations with other anaesthetics show that there is no simple relationship between the concentration of a drug which produces anaesthesia and that which blocks cortical evoked responses (Clark & Rosner, 1973). In addition, the complex effects of barbiturates and other anaesthetics on synaptic transmission in isolated slices of cortex (see above) provide evidence of the probable importance of direct cortical effects, as well as those on ascending systems, in the mechanism of barbiturate anaesthesia.

REFERENCES

Abrahamian H A, Allison T, Goff W R, Rosner B S 1963 Effects of thiopental on human cerebral evoked responses. Anesthesiology 24: 650–657

Adams P R 1974 The mechanism by which amylobarbitone and thiopentone block the endplate response to nicotinic antagonists. Journal of Physiology 241:41P

Angel A 1977 Modulation of information transmission in the dorsal column-lemniscothalamic pathway by anaesthetic agents. In: Huloz E, Sanchez-Hernandez J A, Vasconcelos G (eds) Anaesthesiology: Proceedings of the VI World Congress of Anaesthesiology. Excerpta-Medica, Amsterdam and Oxford, p 82

Archer E R, Richards C D, White A E 1977 Non-additive anaesthetic effects of alphaxalone and methohexitone. British Journal of Pharmacology 59:508P

Arduini A, Arduini M G 1954 Effect of drugs and metabolic alterations on brain stem arousal mechanism. Journal of Pharmacology and Experimental Therapeutics 110: 76–85

Barker J L 1975 CNS depressants: effects on postsynaptic pharmacology. Brain Research 92: 35–55

Barker J L, Ransom B R 1978 Pentobarbitone pharmacology of mammalian central neurones grown in tissue culture. Journal of Physiology 280: 355–372

Blaustein M P, Ector A C 1975 Barbiturate inhibition of calcium uptake by depolarised nerve terminals in vitro. Molecular Pharmacology 11: 369–378

Brown F F, Halsey M J 1980 Interactions of anesthetics with proteins. In: Fink B R (ed) Molecular mechanisms of anesthesia (Progress in Anesthesiology, vol 2). Raven Press, New York. p 385

Clarke D L, Rosner B S 1973 Neurophysiologic effects of general anaesthetics. I: The electroencephalogram and sensory evoked responses in man. Anesthesiology 38: 564–582

Cohen P J 1973 Effects of anesthetics on mitochondrial function. Anesthesiology 39: 153–164

Collins G G S 1980 Release of endogenous amino acid neurotransmitter candidates from rat olfactory cortex: possible regulatory mechanisms and the effects of pentobarbitone. Brain Research 190: 517–528

Crawford J M 1970 Anesthetic agents and the chemical sensitivity of cortical neurones. Neuropharmacology 9: 31–46

Eccles J C 1973 The understanding of the brain. McGraw-Hill, New York. ch 3

Eccles J C, Schmidt R F, Willis W D 1963 Pharmacological studies on presynaptic inhibition. Journal of Physiology 168: 500–530

Franks N P, Lieb W R 1978 Where do general anaesthetics act? Nature (Lond) 274: 339–374

French J D, Verzeano M, Magoun H W 1953 An extralemniscal sensory system in the brain. Archives of Neurology and Psychiatry 69: 505–518

Galindo A 1969 Effects of procaine, pentobarbital and halothane on synaptic transmission in the central nervous system. Journal of Pharmacology and Experimental Therapeutics 169: 185–195

Halsey M J, Wardley-Smith B, Green C J 1978 Pressure reversal of anaesthesia — a multi-site expansion hypothesis. British Journal of Anaesthesia 50: 1091–1097

Judge S E 1983 Effect of general anaesthetics on synaptic ion channels. British Journal of Anaesthesia 55: 191–200

Judge S E, Norman J, Walker R J 1979 The effects of thiopentone on excitation and inhibition in the central nervous system of *Helix*. Comparative Biochemistry and Physiology 64C:255

King E E, Naquet R, Magoun H W 1957 Alterations in somatic afferent transmission through thalamus by central mechanisms and barbiturates. Journal of Pharmacology and Experimental Therapeutics 119: 48–63

Kitahata L M, Ghazi-Saidi K, Yamashita M, Kosaka Y, Bonikos C, Taub A 1975 The depressant effect of halothane and sodium thiopentone on spontaneous and evoked activity of dorsal horn cells: lamina specificity, time course and dose dependence. Journal of Pharmacology and Experimental Therapeutics 195: 515–521

Krnjevik K 1974 Central actions of general anaesthetics. In: Halsey M J, Millar R A, Sutton J A (eds) Molecular mechanisms in general anaesthesia. Churchill Livingstone, London. p 65–89

Larrabee M G, Posternak J M 1952 Selective actions of general anaesthetics on synapses and axons in mammalian sympathetic ganglia. Journal of Neurophysiology 15: 91–114

Lawrence D K, Gill E W 1975 Structurally specific effects of some steroid anaesthetics on spin-labelled liposomes. Molecular Pharmacology 11: 280–286

Matthews E K, Quilliam J P 1964 Effects of central depressant drugs upon acetylcholine release. British Journal of Pharmacology 22: 415–440

Miller K W, Paton W D M, Smith R A, Smith E B 1973 The pressure reversal of general anaesthesia and the critical volume hypothesis. Molecular Pharmacology 9: 131–143

Moruzzi G, Magoun H W 1949 Brain stem reticular formation and activation of the EEG. Electroencephalography and Clinical Neurophysiology 1: 455–473

Mullins L J 1954 Some physical mechanisms in narcosis. Chemical Reviews 54: 289–323

Nicoll R A 1975 Pentobarbital: action on frog motoneurones. Brain Research 96: 119–123

Nicoll R A 1978 Selective actions of barbiturates on synaptic transmission. In: Lipton M A, DiMascio A, Killam K F (eds) Psychopharmacology: a generation of progress. Raven Press, New York. p 1337

Procter W R, Weakly J N 1976 A comparison of the presynaptic and postsynaptic actions of pentobarbitone and phenobarbitone in the neuromuscular junction of the frog. Journal of Physiology 258: 257–268

Quastel J H, Wheatley A H M 1932 Narcosis and oxidations in the brain. Proceedings of the Royal Society, Series B, Biological Science 112:60

Richards C D 1978 Anesthetics and membranes. International Reviews in Biochemistry 19: 157–220

Richards C D 1982 The actions of pentobarbitone, procaine and tetrodotoxin on synaptic transmission in the olfactory cortex of the guinea pig. British Journal of Pharmacology 75: 639

Richards C D, Smaje J C 1976 Anaesthetics depress the sensitivity of cortical neurones to L-glutamate. British Journal of Pharmacology 58: 347–357

Seeman P 1972 The membrane actions of anesthetics and tranquillizers. Pharmacological Reviews 24: 583–655

Smaje J C 1976 General anaesthetics and the acetylcholine sensitivity of cortical neurones. British Journal of Pharmacology 58: 359–366

Somjen G G, Gill M 1963 The mechanism of the blockade of synaptic transmission in the mammalian spinal cord by diethyl ether and by thiopental. Journal of Pharmacology and Experimental Therapeutics 140: 19–30

Wall P D 1967 The laminar organisation of the dorsal horn and effects of descending inputs. Journal of Physiology 188: 403–424

Wardley-Smith B, Halsey M J 1981 Behaviour of mixtures of anaesthetics at pressure: support for the multi-site expansion hypothesis of anaesthetic action. British Journal of Anaesthesia 53: 187P

Weakly J N 1969 Effect of barbiturates on quantal synaptic transmission in spinal motoneurones. Journal of Physiology 204: 63–77

Westmoreland B F, Ward D, Johns T R 1971 The effect of methohexital at the neuromuscular junction. Brain Research 26: 465–468

8

Barbiturates: pharmacodynamics

CENTRAL NERVOUS SYSTEM

Sleep

The effects of increasing doses of barbiturates on the nervous system are first manifested by a gradual depression of consciousness. Environmental contact and the performance of voluntary movement are progressively impaired; the ability to answer questions is gradually abolished and a state of euphoria often develops before consciousness is lost. Hypersensitivity to touch or pain stimuli might be present just before loss of consciousness and is a constant finding once this has occurred. Concurrently there might also be hyperexcitability of the pharyngeal and laryngeal reflexes. The response evoked by stimuli is at first purposeful, attempting to remove or withdraw from the cause. It later assumes the form of a mass withdrawal reflex which gradually diminishes and is completely abolished in deep anaesthesia.

The eyeball begins to move slightly before consciousness is lost. During the stage of hyperexcitability it might deviate from the midline and gradually become central, remaining so during the deeper planes of anaesthesia. In the absence of stimuli, or large doses of mydriatic drugs, the pupil remains small until paralytic or hypoxic dilatation occurs in deep narcosis. Reflex dilatation might, however, occur immediately after the loss of consciousness, but this response is quickly lost as anaesthesia deepens.

Following an adequate anaesthetic dose of thiopentone (3.5 to 4.5 mg kg^{-1}) injected over 10 to 20 s, consciousness is rapidly lost, although the 'maximum depth' of anaesthesia does not occur until 30 to 60 s later. The loss of consciousness is usually smooth and unaccompanied by spontaneous movement or respiratory upset though all these do occur, particularly with methylated drugs (see p. 107). It is often preceded by one or more deep breaths. Since they occur a few seconds before the first effect of the drug on the electroencephalogram can be detected, it is postulated that they result from chemoreceptor stimulation.

Analgesia

Subnarcotic doses of barbiturates increase sensitivity to somatic pain and this state of antanalgesia, which is associated with a low brain barbiturate concentration, also occurs during recovery from large doses (Dundee 1960; Clutton-Brock, 1961). It applies only to deep pain such as produced by pressure on the tibia, since Robson et al (1965) have demonstrated that small doses of barbiturate actually reduce the ability to appreciate a painful stimulus applied to the skin. 'Hyperalgesia' might be a more appropriate word than 'antanalgesia' to describe the increased appreciation of a painful stimulus which occurs with subanaesthetic doses of the intravenous barbiturates (Keats, 1965). Small doses of thiopentone will also antagonize the analgesia produced by nitrous oxide or pethidine (Dundee, 1960). Increased sensitivity to somatic pain has been demonstrated also after small doses of buthalitone, hexobarbitone and methohexitone, the duration of effect varying with the different drugs (Dundee, 1964).

Clutton-Brock (1961) has postulated that antanalgesia might result from the effect of the barbiturate on some inhibitory system in the brain. Brazier (1954) has shown that an early effect of the barbiturates is to lessen the primary responses to a flash of light, as recorded from the cat's cerebral cortex, and to increase the secondary response. The pathway for this secondary response goes through the reticular formation and at this stage of barbiturate anaesthesia some inhibitory system, probably in the diffuse ascending system, has itself been inhibited. A deeper level of anaesthesia can be reached at which this differential depression is lost. It is believed that the pathways for pain may be made up very largely of relays through the central reticular formation, so it is not unreasonable to expect that this pathway could be facilitated in exactly the same way as the secondary response described above.

ANAESTHESIA

In clinical practice the intravenous administration of barbiturates is usually carried out at such a rate that surgical anaesthesia is reached within one or two minutes and the usual signs and stages of anaesthesia cannot readily be detected. However, it has been shown by Etsten and Himwich (1946), who studied the effects of thiopentone when given slowly in a 1% solution, that the pattern of depression of the central nervous system is similar in many respects to that seen with other anaesthetic agents. They classified the stages of thiopentone narcosis and correlated their observations with depression of different parts of the brain (Fig. 8.1). Their concept of progressive depression of the central nervous system is based on the suggestion first made by Hughlings Jackson in 1884, that the phylogenetically newer and higher functional portions of the brain regulate and control the older and lower areas. When function is depressed in a newer layer, the part immediately below assumes dominant control. (It is appreciated that this concept has been justifiably criticised by Wyke (1960; 1965).)

Because of the route of administration and the lack of analgesic power of these drugs, the signs and stages of barbiturate anaesthesia differ somewhat from those observed with inhalation agents. The irritant action of diethyl ether on the tracheobronchial tree causes stimulation of respiration and this, together with irregularities of rhythm and depth of respiration, is rarely seen

Stage	Anesthesia	Characteristics	Site of depression	Brain
1	Clouding	Euphoria Loss of discrimination	Moderate depression of cortex	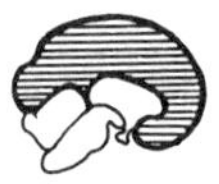
		Impairment of environmental context	Moderate depression of cortex	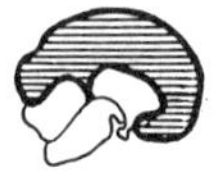
2	Hyper-sensitivity	Loss of consciousness	Predominant control by subcortex	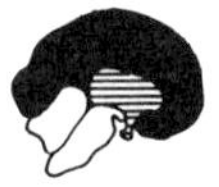
3 Plane 1	Light surgical	Hypoactivity to painful stimulus	Moderate depression of subcortex	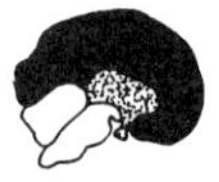
Plane 2	Moderate surgical	Loss of somatic response to pain	Predominant control by midbrain	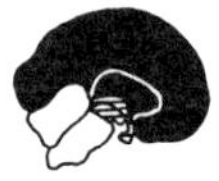
Plane 3	Deep surgical	Loss of visceral response to pain	Moderate depression of midbrain	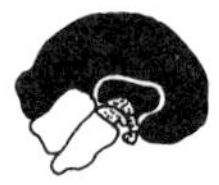
4	Impending failure	Fall in pulse pressure	Moderate depression of pons	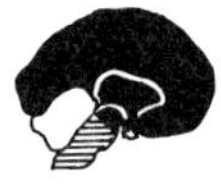

Fig. 8.1 A correlation between the stages of thiopentone anaesthesia and the outstanding clinical signs and their neuro-anatomical allocations (Etsten & Himwich, 1946).

with thiopentone. As with the non-irritant vapours, the degree of respiratory depression is a poor guide to the depth of anaesthesia with the barbiturates in the absence of surgical or other stimuli. Low concentrations of ether and methoxyflurane have a marked analgesic action, in contrast to the hypersensitivity to touch or painful stimuli with thiopentone and a dangerous degree of cerebral depression might be required to abolish this latter completely. Muscular relaxation is also poor with a moderate depth of barbiturate anaesthesia.

With the barbiturates, more than with any other drug used in anaesthesia, the clinical level of anaesthesia is related to the intensity of the surgical stimulus as well as to the degree of cerebral depression. After thiopentone, an undisturbed patient with depressed respiration and abdominal and masseter relaxation, might give a picture of moderately deep surgical anaesthesia, but on application of a surgical stimulus their respiration is stimulated, relaxation lost and there might be reflex movement of a limb. If this patient is given sufficient thiopentone to produce surgical anaesthesia in the presence of strong stimulation, a dangerous degree of respiratory depression might occur when the stimulation ceases. Pretreatment with opioids will reduce the dose of thiopentone required to produce surgical anaesthesia but they also depress respiration and might be long-acting, and a similar state of affairs can be produced at the end of the operation. With the use of nitrous oxide-oxygen to supplement thiopentone it is possible to produce a pattern of anaesthesia somewhat similar to that observed with other drugs without excessive dosage and without causing dangerous and prolonged periods of depression of vital functions.

Dosage and plasma concentrations

In a group of unselected patients one will find a very large scatter of doses of thiopentone required to induce anaesthesia. Even when the technique of administration is standardised the range is still very great — as shown in Figure 8.2, which is based on 2206 consecutive unselected inductions (Dundee et al, 1982). Part of this can be accounted for by the use of different premedicants with their additive or synergistic actions, and the physical condition of the patients. The median dose in this study was 3.5 mg kg^{-1} but most clinicians would place the single bolus induction

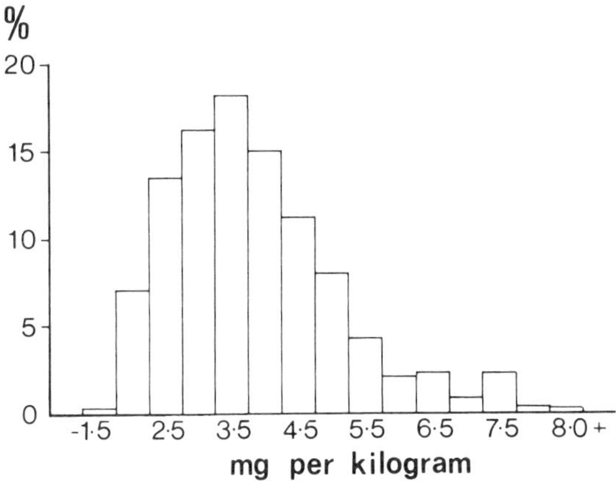

Fig. 8.2 Scatter of induction doses of thiopentone (mg kg^{-1}) in 2006 consecutive unselected inductions.

dose for adults in the region of 4–5 mg kg^{-1}. This might be more than the minimum required to induce loss of consciousness but the margin is essential to allow time for the action of supplementary drugs and for procedures such as tracheal intubation.

In a definitive study, Crankshaw and Allt-Graham (1978) used a cumulative dose-response curve for loss of consciousness to assess the induction dose of thiopentone in premedicated adults. They expressed their findings on the basis of lean tissue mass and found the ED_{50} for thiopentone to be 2.63–2.70 mg kg^{-1}. This might be a helpful figure when comparing the effects of different drugs (as with MAC for inhalational agents) but the clinician is more interested in the ED_{100} which is in the region of 3.5 mg kg^{-1} lean body mass. As pointed out elsewhere (p. 81) the more widely used mg kg^{-1} can easily lead to an overdose in morbidly obese patients.

Reference has already been made to the lower requirements of thiopentone in women and in elderly patients. The situation in respect to young patients is more difficult to define — the data from the under 15 year age group in Table 6.4 were obtained from a wide age range and is of little clinical value. The usual recommended dose in the 5–15 age group is 2–4 mg kg^{-1}, but a planned dose-response study by Cote et al (1981) shows that this should be 5–6 mg kg^{-1}, which is slightly greater than in adults. More recently Duncan et al (1984), using different methodology, have calculated the effective dose of thiopentone in unpremedicated children, aged 1–2 yr, to be 10.5 mg kg^{-1}, although the highest dose used in their study was 8.5 mg kg^{-1}. This is unexpectedly high. An equally important finding was that premedication (trimeprazine, with or without droperidol and methadone, or papaveretum with hyoscine) reduced the ED_{90} to 4–5 mg kg^{-1}.

The increased induction dosage in children cannot fully be explained on a pharmacokinetic basis (p. 82).

In clinical practice a low haemoglobin or a raised plasma urea are the two pathological conditions most likely to reduce the induction dose of thiopentone. Dundee & Hassard (1983) found a positive relationship between the induction dose and haemoglobin levels and an inverse relationship between the induction dose and plasma urea. It is difficult to consider these entities separately but a raised urea had slightly more influence on dosage than a low haemoglobin level. Edwards & Ellis (1973) had previously noted a positive relationship between thiopentone dosage and haemoglobin concentration in a smaller number of subjects.

The clinical impression of lower thiopentone induction requirements in 'cardiac' patients has been confirmed by Christensen et al (1985). Their average control value of 4.7 mg kg^{-1} was reduced to 3.4 mg kg^{-1} in patients on long term therapy with digoxin and a diuretic. However, they could not fully explain their findings on a pharmacokinetic basis and concluded that these were due at least in part to a higher cerebral sensitivity to the drug.

In clinical practice one may precede the administration of thiopentone or methohexitone by a small dose of a short-acting opioid such as fentanyl or alfentanil. This reduces the incidence of excitatory effects with the barbiturates and is particularly helpful in the case of methohexitone, but also markedly reduces the induction dose of these drugs. The combination of a relatively non-toxic opioid with a smaller dose of the barbiturate has much to recommend it in patients with a compromised cardiovascular system. With appropriate doses of fentanyl or alfentanil it is possible to induce anaesthesia with amounts of barbiturates which, if given alone, would not lead to loss of consciousness. The use of the opiates as sole agents or with the neurolept combination is discussed more fully in Chapter 13.

Becker (1978) has shown that the plasma thiopentone level necessary for anaesthesia is in the region of 39 to 42 $\mu g\ ml^{-1}$, with free thiopentone concentration for surgical anaesthesia ranging from 5.9 to 6.3 $\mu g\ ml^{-1}$. The values were obtained in fit surgical patients aged 21–50 yr with no significant history of drug use. It is difficult to get this information following a single dose, as in his study Becker gave an initial dose of 2–2.5 mg kg^{-1} followed by an infusion of 1–1.5 mg $kg^{-1} min^{-1}$. Some of his patients were premedicated with pethidine and he used the loss of corneal reflex and trapezius muscle response as his end point, having previously shown a correlation between these end points and the lack of response of patients to surgical stimuli.

A large number of factors will undoubtedly influence the effective plasma concentration including drug tolerance (acquired and acute), synergism with or potentiation by other drugs as well as the physical condition of the patient. There are no data on the effective plasma thiopentone concentrations in these various situations.

In practice the concomitant use of nitrous oxide is probably the most important factor influencing the dosage of thiopentone and the synergistic action of these two drugs is the basis of current clinical practice. Becker (1978) has put this combination on a sound scientific formulation by demonstrating that 67% nitrous oxide in oxygen reduced effective thiopentone concentrations by 67–71%, with plasma levels averaging 12.6 $\mu g\ ml^{-1}$for unpremedicated patients.

Acute tolerance

Figure 8.3 shows the scatter of venous plasma concentrations at which 201 adults opened their eyes on command after thiopentone. These unselected unpremedicated patients received no volatile or opioid supplements during operation and, even allowing for the imprecision of the end point, there is a very wide range in the plasma concentrations on recovery. Venous, or even arterial blood concentrations might not always reflect the amount of drug in the brain, particularly within the first few minutes after administration. It is recognised that acquired tolerance to one sedative/hypnotic, including alcohol, leads to cross tolerance to others including thiopentone and while this is seen more frequently at induction it can apply to the recovery and might explain part of the scatter in Figure 8.3.

As pointed out previously, recovery from thiopentone occurs when a large amount of the drug remains unchanged in the body, and a cumulative effect is observed after repeated doses (Figs. 6.8, 6.9). Increments necessary to maintain sleep become gradually less as tissue equilibrium is reached, until after two to three hours only small doses are required at long intervals. They not only replace that drug which has been detoxicated but compensate for the increasing tolerance which the

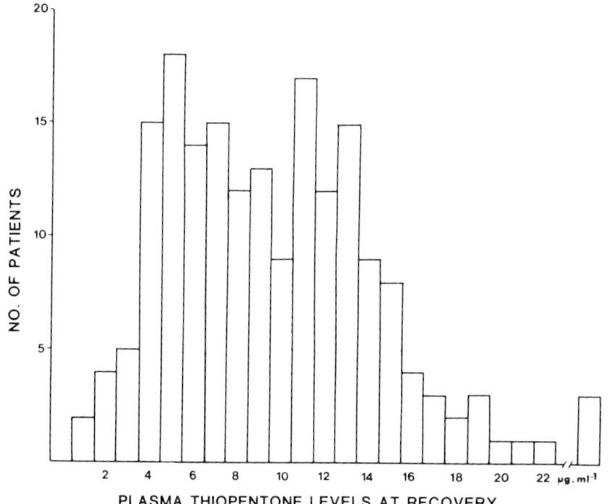

Fig. 8.3 Plasma thiopentone levels on recovery in 201 patients in whom thiopentone was the main anaesthetic agent (Dundee, 1956; Toner et al, 1980).

brain shows to the narcotic effects of thiopentone. As the duration of administration proceeds, the blood drug concentration at which various signs of anaesthesia are elicited increases, and the blood concentration of the drug at recovery becomes higher.

One author (JWD) has conversed lucidly with two subjects who had regained consciousness after a thiopentone infusion but who had venous blood drug concentrations which were much greater than those recorded over an hour previously when both were deeply anaesthetised. A similar phenomenon is reported by Sawada et al (1982) when giving continuous thiamylal to patients with severe head injuries. The total plasma thiamylal concentration required to maintain a burst-suppression pattern in the eeg for up to 10 s increased with time, averaging 20.5 μg ml^{-1} after 15 min administration and increasing to 48.2 after 72 h.

In 1949 Mark et al reported evidence of acute tolerance to thiopentone in humans when a subject was maintained at high plasma concentrations of the drug, the signs of anaesthesia reappeared at higher plasma levels than when he was maintained at low plasma concentrations. As an example one subject was given 3.25 g in 52 minutes and on another occasion 2.0 g in 5 minutes: awakening after the larger dose occurred on plasma level concentrations corresponding to deep anaesthesia in the same subject after the smaller dose (Fig. 8.4). This work, which was later reported in more detail by Brodie et al (1951), was preceded by animal studies by Shideman et al (1948), who noted that with repeat administration of 10 mg kg^{-1} dogs regained their righting reflex with successively higher plasma levels with each additional dose.

In the early 1950s the induction dose of thiopentone in Europe was in the region of 6–8 mg kg^{-1}, though at this time the dose used in most North American centres was half of this. A retrospective survey of total doses used by intermittent injection for body surface operations, in

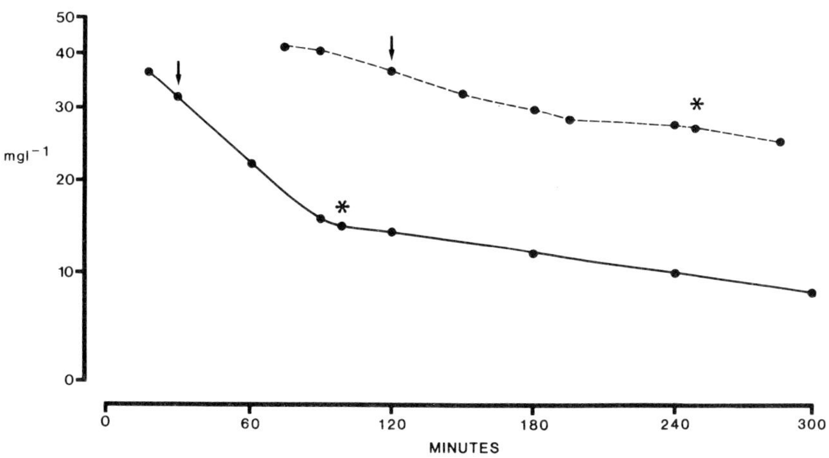

Fig. 8.4 Plasma levels and signs of anaesthesia after two different doses of thiopentone in the same subject (Mark et al, 1949). Upper graph: 1.25 g in 52 min; lower graph: 2.0 g in 5 min (↑ return of consciousness; *orientation).

combination with nitrous oxide-oxygen in one British and one American centre showed the same relationship. Dundee et al (1956) postulated that this might have been due to the initial dose 'setting the sensitivity' for the cerebral response to the drug and hence to dose requirements.

Figure 8.5 shows arterial plasma thiopentone levels at awakening following single intravenous doses of thiopentone ranging from 2 to 14 mg kg^{-1} given to fit unpremedicated subjects. This is the same phenomenon of 'acute tolerance' already referred to. Within certain limits the higher the initial dose of thiopentone the greater will be the increments needed to maintain a constant degree of cerebral depression. It would appear that the greater the peak concentration of the drug attained in the brain, whether at induction or during intermittent administration, the higher will be the blood level at which consciousness is regained (Dundee et al, 1956). This conclusion has been confirmed by Toner et al (1980) in a much larger series of patients, using modern methods of blood analysis. In this study venous blood samples were taken and this might explain the greater scatter of their findings. They also demonstrated a very good relationship between $\log_{10}$ plasma thiopentone concentrations at wakening and time to recovery but the latter was not as long as one would have expected on a purely pharmacokinetic basis.

These findings could explain the failure of Brand and his colleagues (1961) to find a correlation between the blood thiopentone level and the depth of anaesthesia, as recorded on the electroencephalogram and the inability of Kane & Smith (1959) to correlate blood buthalitone levels with the clinical condition of the patient during recovery. In fact, Brand et al explained their findings on the basis of acute tolerance.

The concept of acute tolerance to thiopentone in man has been challenged by Hudson et al (1982; 1983). Using computer-assisted power spectral analysis of the electroencephalograph they were unable to demonstrate a changing relationship between barbiturate blood levels and the 'depth' of anaesthesia following repeated administrations of thiopentone. The depth of anaesthesia was gauged by the spectral edge — the frequency at which 95% of the EEG power is located (Rampil et al, 1980). Using the IC_{50}, the thiopentone serum concentration required to produce 50% of the maximal shift of the spectral edge as a guide to depth of anaesthesia is very different from the end point in a patient responding to a verbal command. The latter will usually occur on a shallow portion of the plasma concentration curve where small errors in identifying the end point will not have a marked effect on the plasma concentration.

More recently Barratt et al (1984) have attempted to explain the findings of Toner et al (1980) and the phenomenon of acute tolerance on a pharmacokinetic basis, related to the site of sampling. They assumed that the brain concentration of thiopentone is closely related to jugular concentration and that patients wake up at a constant brain/jugular concentration. Patients receiving 3.5 to 5.5 mg kg^{-1} thiopentone wake with an average peripheral plasma thiopentone concentration of 7.6 $\mu g\ ml^{-1}$, which would correspond to a jugular concentration of 9.6 $\mu g\ ml^{-1}$, a value which they assumed to be the brain/jugular concentration at awakening. When the thiopentone dose is doubled and the plasma concentration remains proportional to the dose (as with first order kinetics), they calculated that the waking jugular plasma concentration should be reached in about 11 min at which time the predicted peripheral thiopentone concentration would be

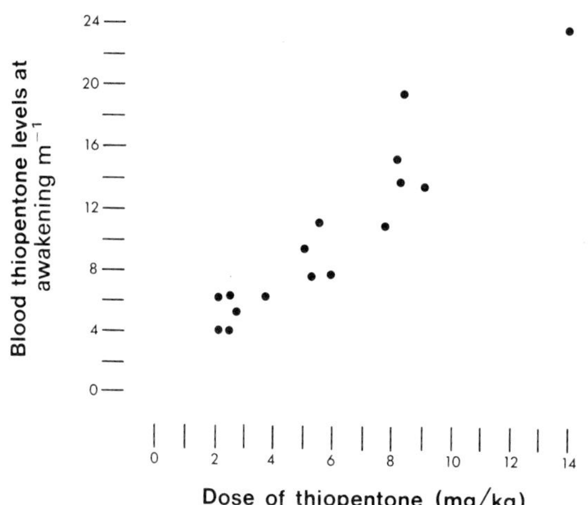

Fig. 8.5 Plasma thiopentone levels at awakening in 15 patients who received single injections of the drug (Dundee et al, 1956).

11.6 $\mu g\ ml^{-1}$: this is close to the actual figure of Toner and his co-workers who found that after 9.5 to 11.5 $\mu g\ ml^{-1}$ on the average patients awakened in 11.3 min with a mean peripheral plasma thiopentone concentration of 13.3 $\mu g\ ml^{-1}$. If the arterial plasma concentration reflects brain concentration at awakening this would be 9.4 $\mu g\ ml^{-1}$ for a 5 mg kg^{-1} dose and 9.1 $\mu g\ ml^{-1}$ for a 10 mg kg^{-1} dose.

This attractive theory does not fully explain the findings of Figure 8.5, and further work is needed for a full understanding of this phenomenon.

Electroencephalographic changes

A number of workers have described the characteristic changes in the electroencephalographic pattern during thiopentone narcosis (Brazier & Finesinger, 1945; Tucci et al, 1949; Kiersey et al, 1951). Some descriptions, such as those of Wyke (1950; 1951; 1957a, b, c; 1958), Brazier (1961; 1963) and Doenicke and his colleagues (1966, 1967), are too detailed for this book; even more detailed are those of Clark & Rosner (1973) and Rosner & Clark (1973), to which readers are referred for further details and an extensive bibliography.

With only minor variations there is general agreement in the pattern of the changes induced by barbiturates and their relation to the depth of anaesthesia. In 1951 they were classified by Kiersey and his colleagues as follows (Fig. 8.6):

1. High amplitude, fast spiky activity of mixed frequencies (10 to 30 cycles/s) with the predominant frequency near 20 Hz. Amplitudes vary greatly; short runs of two, three or more waves with an amplitude of 75 to 80 microvolts are characteristically preceded and followed by similar runs of lower amplitude.
2. Complex pattern of many frequencies differing from the preceding by the presence of predominantly slower wave forms of very irregular contour and random occurrence. There is also much variation in voltage, the larger and predominating waves representing close to 150 microvolts. Superimposed on these slower waves and occupying the intervals between them is a much faster activity, rather spiky in character and irregular in amplitude. The frequency is about 10 Hz and the amplitude is comparable with that seen in the first pattern.
3. Characterised by a progressive suppression of cortical activity, short periods of relative quiescence separating groups or bursts of waves. The bursts are frequently made up of two distinct elements, the first appearing abruptly and consisting of a short series of high voltage waves with a frequency of about 10 Hz and continuing for about one second. The second element follows immediately in the form of two or more slow waves at a frequency of near 2 Hz and tailing off into the next suppression phase. The whole complex occupies a time interval of 2 or more s. In this stage the intervals of quiescence do not exceed 3 s.
4. This differs from the above in that the duration of the periods of cortical inactivity vary from 3 to 10 s.
5. Periods of activity do not appear any more frequently than once every 10 s. There is a reduction in the amplitude of the components which might fall below 25 microvolts.

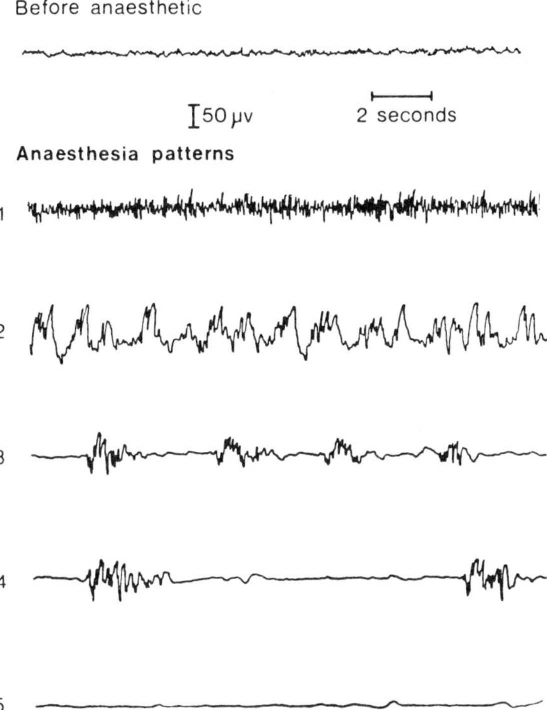

Fig. 8.6 Electroencephalographic changes during thiopentone anaesthesia (Kiersey et al, 1951).

This sequence of events is observed only after cerebral electrical activity attains maturity; the appearances in infants and young children differ in several respects.

During the transition from one pattern to another there is usually a mixture of both patterns. This is especially noticeable in the persistence of fast waves in the second pattern. In fact, an activity of 10 Hz or faster can be followed through into the fifth pattern, where it makes up part of the active elements.

With a rapid injection of an adequate dose of thiopentone the fast spiky pattern 1 might appear within 10 s of injection (Fig. 8.6). Doses of as little as 50 mg given at normal speeds will induce electroencephalographic changes within one minute. Increasing the dosage increases the overall amplitude without altering the frequency during this phase. The patient is still awake and feels drowsy and euphoric. Finesinger et al (1947) and Tucci et al (1949) state that the appearance of the slower waves (2) coincides with the loss of consciousness, although others (Wyke, 1950) report that at this level patients are still only drowsy and will often yawn, but can be readily aroused by gentle stimulation although they will then be slightly confused. Kiersey and his co-workers noted that the exact moment when a person loses contact with the environment depends on the efforts made to retain consciousness. They did not find a consistent relationship to any special electroencephalogram pattern and unconsciousness might sometimes supervene even before the onset of 2.

In pattern 2 at first the lash reflex is present and there is a brisk withdrawal in response to painful stimulation which might produce agitated restlessness. When reflex activity becomes more sluggish, the slower waves predominate and often increase in amplitude. As anaesthesia deepens, the withdrawal reflex is abolished, the corneal reflex disappears and the eyeballs become fixed. There is a slight fall in blood pressure and there might be some respiratory depression. Pupillary reaction to light remains brisk. When this stage is well established, the majority of patients will tolerate a skin incision or a pharyngeal airway.

As the third pattern appears, reduction of respiratory volume becomes most marked. This respiratory depression increases progressively through patterns 4 and 5 and during the latter it might become necessary to aid the respiration. The light reflex remains active throughout all the stages described.

The use of myoneural blocking drugs does not affect these patterns, provided respiratory depression with hypoxia or carbon dioxide retention is avoided.

Recovery from anaesthesia is accompanied by the reverse sequence of events. The patterns characteristic of the deeper planes of anaesthesia are rapidly traversed, but in lighter planes the rate of change diminishes steadily. Even after the patient regains consciousness the alpha activity remains unstable, and for several hours there is more fast beta activity than in the preanaesthetic record. When this is present the subject will

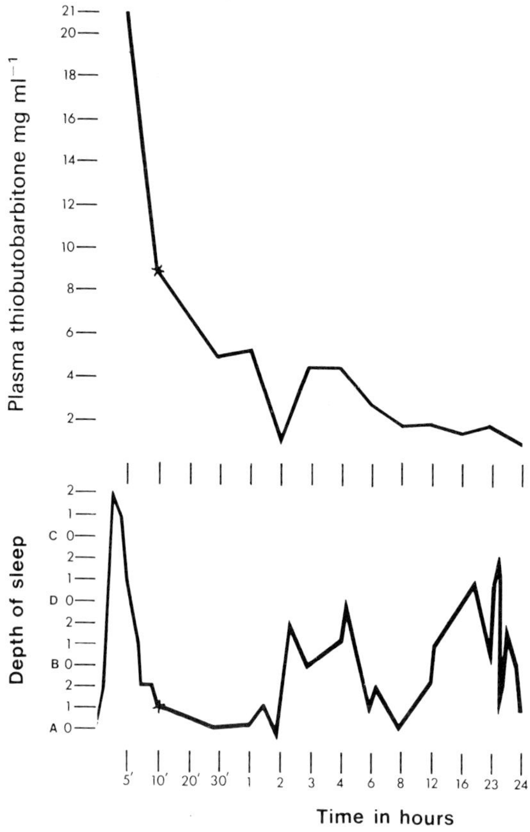

Fig. 7.8 Plasma thiobutobarbitone concentration in $\mu g\ \ell^{-1}$ and depth of sleep expressed as Loomis' classification, following intravenous injection of 500 mg thiobutobarbitone. Patient wakened at X (Doenicke et al, 1967).

readily fall asleep if not in pain; if in pain this period might be associated with agitation.

Doenicke et al (1966) have used the electroencephalographic tracings to study recovery time from intravenous barbiturates. Using a modification of the Loomis classification of depths of sleep (based on eeg patterns) they demonstrated recurring sleep patterns for up to 12 hours after small doses of methohexitone (Fig. 6.10) thiobutobarbitone (Fig. 8.7).

While there is a reasonably consistent correlation between the 'clinical depth' of anaesthesia and the electroencephalographic pattern, this latter is not closely related to plasma barbiturate levels (Kane & Smith, 1959; Brand et al, 1961). In the example shown in Figure 8.7 the plasma level fell rapidly after 500 mg thiobutobarbitone and the patient wakened after 10 min. However, between the second and fifth hours the eeg record showed a return of drowsiness and light sleep. The use of computerised analyses of EEG patterns and the spectral edge as means of assessing the degree of cerebral depression, and hence the 'depth' of anaesthesia, have already been discussed.

Cerebral circulation and intracranial pressure

Cerebral circulation is more dependent on local intrinsic control mechanisms and less influenced by extrinsic humoral and neurogenic factors than other circulatory beds (McDowall, 1971). The effects of barbiturates could be secondary to those on blood pressure since in sudden hypotension cerebral blood flow shows a proportionate acute fall but a small bolus dose of thiopentone can reduce elevated intracranial pressure with minimal effects on perfusion and arterial pressure (Shapiro, 1984). These changes are short lived and also less marked if the blood pressure fall is gradual (Harper, 1965). Herrschaft & Schmidt (1973, 1974) have shown that the effect of methohexitone is shorter than that of thiopentone: after 1 mg kg^{-1} there is a 45% decrease in cerebral blood flow at 30 s, 25% at 5 min and zero at 10 min, whereas the effect of 4 mg kg^{-1} thiopentone (45% reduction) lasted for 10 min. Cunitz et al (1978) have also noted the lesser effect of methohexitone compared with thiopentone.

To maintain blood flow in the presence of a falling blood pressure the cerebral arterioles must relax and so lower cerebrovascular resistence. This autoregulation is lost in certain pathological conditions such as cerebral tumours and infarcts and also if the cerebral vasculature is already widely dilated in response to hypercapnia or hypoxia. Under these circumstances there is a passive pressure-flow relationship in the cerebral circulation (Haggendal, 1965; Harper, 1965) and the results of barbiturate-induced hypotension would be more marked.

Jacobson et al (1963) have pointed out that cerebral venous pressure can also affect cerebral blood flow and changes in this secondary to coughing, straining or breath-holding following induction of anaesthesia can influence the cerebral circulation. The cerebral blood vessels are also very sensitive to changes in carbon dioxide tension and increases in $PaCO_2$ secondary to barbiturate-induced respiratory depression will result in cerebral vasodilation. This occurs particularly in the range of 30–60 mm Hg where Harper (1965) found a 2.5% increase in flow for every 1 mm Hg change in $PaCO_2$.

There is evidence to support the view that reductions in cerebral metabolic activity lead to similar reductions in cerebral blood flow during barbiturate anaesthesia. These cannot be detected with sedative doses of barbiturates, provided changes in arterial blood carbon dioxide tension are taken into account. When barbiturates are given in doses sufficient to produce light general anaesthesia, cerebral blood flow is reduced by approximately one-third while deeper anaesthesia can reduce it by as much as 50%. McDowall (1971) has postulated that this occurs in the following way:

barbiturate anaesthesia
↓
reduced cerebral metabolic activity
↓
reduced cerebral carbon dioxide production
↓
tendency for cerebral tissue carbon dioxide tension to fall

As a result of the reduced cerebral blood flow and accompanying fall in cerebral blood volume, cerebrospinal fluid pressure is reduced by barbiturate anaesthesia. (Ch. 16).

Thiopentone, in normal clinical doses, will reduce the intracranial tension in patients with an acute or chronically elevated intracranial pressure (Shapiro et al, 1973). For this reason intermittent barbiturate administration has been recommended for general anaesthesia in patients with intracranial tumours (Hunter, 1954; 1972; McLeskey et al, 1974). In patients with normal pre-thiopentone pressures the barbiturate produces no significant alteration in intracranial pressure (ICP) even with moderate falls in arterial pressure.

Moss et al (1978) have shown that thiopentone will prevent excessive rises in ICP following tracheal intubation, provided coughing does not occur. This is in contrast with the findings of Burney & Winn (1975) who found dramatic and significant rises in ICP in response to laryngoscopy and intubation. They used suxamethonium, not the tubocurarine used by Moss and his colleagues but, perhaps more important, they gave a larger dose of thiopentone. The role of the relaxant was stressed by McLeskey et al (1974) who reported marked rises in two patients who had tracheal intubation under thiopentone and suxamethonium. The importance of an adequate dose of thiopentone has been further emphasised by the work of Unni and his colleagues (1984) who even recommend the use of a second dose of 1.5 mg kg^{-1} given over 30 seconds in combination with topical analgesia to the larynx immediately before intubation. Although the second dose might cause a significant reduction in arterial pressure this remains within the autoregulatory limits and they have found that, in clinical practice, this technique produces minimal increases in intracranial pressure.

Schulte et al (1978) have shown that while, in appropriate doses, thiopentone and etomidate are equally effective in lowering intracranial pressure in patients with an already raised pressure thiopentone also caused a lower perfusion pressure while etomidate had no effect on arterial or cerebral perfusion pressures. Under similar conditions Cunitz et al (1978) demonstrated a shorter effect of methohexitone as compared with thiopentone.

Cerebral metabolism

Brain metabolism and oxygen consumption are reduced after thiopentone proportionate to the degree of cerebral depression, but not necessarily with the clinical depth of anaesthesia (Schmidt et al, 1945; Homburger et al, 1946; Pierce et al, 1962). Although Etsten et al (1946) and Himwich et al (1947) suggested that oxidation was not decreased to the same extent in all parts of the brain at the lighter levels of narcosis, this was not supported by the findings of Wechsler et al (1951).

In an interesting study in dogs, Altenburg et al (1969) were able to correlate the degree of functional and metabolic depression following a single dose of 10 mg kg^{-1} and following an infusion of 45 mg kg^{-1} thiopentone given over two hours. The depressant effect of the small dose was very transient and had passed off in 60 min, the small residual plasma thiopentone concentration (approx 6 $\mu g\ ml^{-1}$) having no obvious effect on cerebral metabolism. However, when the same infusion was started two hours after a single dose, both the degree of functional depression and metabolic depression were significantly less than after the infusion alone, even though the plasma barbiturate level was higher on this occasion. This shows a rapid development of tolerance to the effect of thiopentone on the brain and might offer an explanation for the findings quoted above. The basis for acute tolerance has not been established, but it is somehow related to the peak levels of thiopentone or the duration of exposure to the drug. In the studies of Altenburg and his colleagues the animals receiving the larger dose (injection followed by infusion) and achieving the highest peak concentration showed less depression of metabolism than those given the infusion alone.

Excitatory effects

Spontaneous involuntary muscle movement, tremor and hypertonus occur occasionally following the administration of thiopentone and more frequently following methylated barbiturates or thiobarbiturates. The incidence increases with dosage and with the rate of administration suggesting that it is related to the cerebral concentration of drug (Barron & Dundee, 1967; Barron, 1968). The occurrence of excitatory effects is also related to the analgesic action of the premedication. Dundee (1965a) studied the incidence of a variety of premedicants which had been found to decrease analgesic sensitivity to somatic pain on excitatory effects of equivalent doses of four barbiturates. Antanalgesic drugs such as promethazine and hyoscine increase the incidence of excitatory effects while analgesics such as morphine and pethidine reduce them. The influence of premedicants was more marked with the methylated compounds as are the effects of dosage and rapid injection.

Table 8.1 shows the incidence of excitatory phenomena followinq equivalent doses of thiopentone and methohexitone injected over 20 s. It can be seen that some premedicants are better avoided with methohexitone. However, as mentioned previously, the currently available preparation of this oxybarbiturate causes much fewer excitatory effects than when the drug was first introduced. It is also worth noting that it were these excitatory effects which led to the almost complete abandonment of hexobarbitone as an induction agent.

It is difficult to offer an explanation for the excitatory effects of the barbiturates but they might be in some way related to their lack of analgesic action. The chemical composition of the premedicants could not play any part in the findings shown in Table 8.1 as this occurs with a wide range of drugs. The spontaneous nature of these movements might have been overemphasized as they could be an exaggerated response to minor stimuli such as a needle prick, application of a face mask or inflation of a sphygmomanometer cuff and this is supported by the view that the movements can be very violent if the patient has a full bladder. Their increased frequence of severity with methylated compounds has been conclusively demonstrated (Dundee, 1965b). It has even been suggested that some convulsive activity can be attributed to the CH_3 side chain (Fig. 5.2).

Table 8.1 % incidence of excitatory phenomena (spontaneous involuntary muscle movement, hypertonus or tremor) following equivalent doses of thiopentone and methohexitone given after different premedicants.

Preanaesthetic medication	*Thiopentone 4 mg kg⁻¹*	*Methohexitone 1.6 mg kg⁻¹*
Atropine or nil	4	17
Hyoscine	18	46
Promethazine	25	70
Pethidine	4	7
Pethidine–hyoscine	6	25
Promethazine–hyoscine	46	87

(Dundee, 1979)

Anticonvulsant/convulsant action

Thiopentone is an effective anticonvulsant and its more widespread use in this field is only hampered by other side effects such as hypotension and respiratory depression. However there is controversy as to the safety of methohexitone as an anticonvulsant and some workers have even described it as a convulsant (Rockoff & Goudsouzian, 1981). There have been a few documented cases of convulsive activity occuring in crypto-epileptics with abnormal EEG recordings (Boston & Unkles, 1969; Ryder, 1969; Redish et al, 1958; Galley, 1963; Male & Allen, 1977). It is necessary to distinguish generalised or non focal seizures which are easily controlled by a number of drugs from focal cortical seizures which are more difficult to treat. It would appear that it is in the latter group that the use of methohexitone might result in epileptiform seizures. In fact methohexitone has been used clinically to activate abnormalities in such patients (Pampiglione, 1965; Paul & Harris, 1970) in whom awake recordings were unrewarding and to provoke epileptic responses during temporal lobectomy. Thiopentone has no such effect (Paul & Harris, 1970). Allen & Male (1982) have commented on the route of administration of methohexitone as a factor in its use in epileptics. The case reports by Rockoff & Goudsouzian (1981) refer to the rectal administration of the drug in children where absorption is erratic and often incomplete. While methohexitone is not contraindicated in epileptic patients thiopentone would remain the intravenous induction agent of choice for epileptics. However, in the emergency control of seizures methohexitone has the advantage of being non-irritant when injected extravenously.

CARDIOVASCULAR SYSTEM

The mechanism of transport of intravenous anaesthetics from vein to brain leads to a high concentration suddenly coming into contact with the heart, vasomotor and respiratory centres. Thus, in clinical practice hypotension and respiratory depression occur more frequently during induction of intravenous anaesthesia than with inhalation agents. The factors involved are often complex and have been studied by many workers and before discussing them in detail it is necessary to make some general observations. With the exception of ketamine the cardiovascular effects of intravenous drugs depend on:

1. The rate of administration and total dose given. As expected the rapid administration of a large dose will have more profound effects than a small dose given slowly. Even quite large doses given as an infusion will often cause less effects than a small rapid injection.
2. The condition of the patient, particularly with regard to blood volume, acid base balance and disease of the cardiovascular system including hypertension. These mainly relate to the ability of the patient to compensate for the effects of peripheral vasodilation.
3. Concurrent or previous administration of drugs which themselves will cause vasodilation or reduce compensatory tachycardia.

It would be impracticable to survey all the publications on this topic, particularly the early studies, in detail and this was done in the First Edition of this book.

Thiopentone has well recognised haemodynamic effects. When given as a bolus it causes a reduction in systemic arterial pressure and cardiac output and an increase in systemic vascular resistance (Chamberlain et al, 1977). Its effect on central venous pressure is variable and some workers have found either no change or an increase or a decrease, varying with the circumstances of their study (Elder et al, 1955; Etsten & Li, 1955; Fieldman et al, 1955; Flickinger et al, 1961; Conway & Ellis, 1969). On administration of thiopentone one immediately sees well marked venedilation and measurements of intrathoracic blood volume (Etsten & Li, 1955; Flickinger et al, 1961) suggest that blood has been transferred from the central pool to the periphery resulting in a reduction in venous return (Eckstein et al, 1961) which in turn reduces cardiac output and arterial pressure.

Opinions are more divided on the effect of thiopentone on the heart; there is little evidence of changes in myocardial contractility with concentrations occurring during anaesthesia but animal work, supported by clinical experience, suggests that the heart will be depressed if a sufficiently large dose is given (Woods et al, 1949; Prime & Gray, 1952; Price & Helrich, 1955). In a study designed to separate myocardial and peripheral cardiovascular effects in animals, Chamberlain et al (1977) found that thiopentone produced minimal depression of the heart in normal doses and it was only in much greater concentrations that significant depression was found. They concluded that the cardiovascular effects of intravenous thiopentone are not a direct effect on the heart, but one must qualify this in relation to the state of the myocardium and the dose of drug given. In clinical practice one finds that with repeated administration, blood pressure takes longer to recover with successive doses suggesting that direct myocardial depressant element is playing a more important part in this depressant effect.

Clinically there is little to choose between the effects of thiopentone and methohexitone although there might be slightly less hypotension with equivalent doses of the latter drug. This is probably due to a greater degree of tachycardia with methohexitone (Doenicke et al, 1974). In direct comparative studies Doenicke et al (1973) and McMillan et al (1974) found the depressant effects of the two drugs to be very similar.

Changes in heart rate following intravenous barbiturates can be very variable, depending not only on compensatory haemodynamic changes, but on resting heart rate and premedication. Broadly speaking, their general effect is to increase relatively slow rates and to decrease rapid rates (Johnstone, 1951). Attention has already been drawn to the more marked tachycardia with methohexitone (Lyons & Clarke, 1972): this had previously been noted for hexobarbitone (Stephen et al, 1953) and might be a feature of the methylated compounds.

The normal cardiovascular response to thiopentone can be illustrated from the study of Becker & Tonnesen (1978) who analysed changes in various cardiovascular parameters in 10 healthy subjects in whom anaesthesia was induced with 2–2.5 mg kg^{-1} thiopentone and maintained with an infusion of 1–1.5 mg kg^{-1} min^{-1}. Increasing depth of anaesthesia was indicated by loss of eyelid reflex, corneal reflex and trapezius response. The latter two would correspond to loss of response to surgical stimulation. Arterial blood pressure, (measured by radial artery catheter), ECG, phonocardiogram and carotid pulse signals were monitored throughout and the interval from the onset of the Q-wave of the ECG to the onset of the second heart sound ($Q–S_2$), R–R intervals on the ECG and left ventricular ejection time (LVET) were determined using a Hewlett-Packard digitiser interfaced with a programmable calculator. For each heart beat $Q–S_2$, LVET and pre-ejection period (PEP) were corrected for heart rate. Ten intervals were averaged for each reading.

The plasma concentrations of thiopentone averaged 38 μg ml^{-1} (5.4 free drug) at loss of corneal reflex and 42 (6.1) at loss of trapezius muscle response. The average findings (Table 8.2) show that heart rate increased on induction of anaesthesia and this increase was maintained with deepening of anaesthesia. Systolic blood pressure decreased to a significant degree only when surgical anaesthesia was achieved. Systolic time intervals were in the high–normal range before induction of anaesthesia and decreased to near normal levels. $Q–S_2$ and LVET showed minor increases as did the average PEP. The ratio of PEP to LVET and the reciprocal of PEP^2 both decreased, the former reaching significant levels both at loss of corneal reflex and trapezius response. PEP correlates well with left ventricular dP/dt while PEP/LVET decreases with stroke volume: $1/PEP^2$ correlates with peak ascending aortic blood flow acceleration.

The changes in systolic time intervals (STI) probably represent some decrease in myocardial contractility with thiopentone while the other changes probably correspond to the decrease in stroke volume that has been found with thiopentone infusions by a number of workers (Etsten & Li, 1955; Fieldman et al, 1955). These findings are very similar to those reported by Filner and Karliner (1976) and Conway and Ellis (1969). From their detailed study Becker and Tonnesen (1978) conclude that in healthy patients the plasma levels of thiopentone producing surgical anaesthesia result in minimal cardiac depression as determined by systolic time intervals.

It is interesting to note that Seltzer et al (1980) found the same degree of cardiovascular depression following a bolus of 4 mg kg^{-1} thiopentone as with incremental doses of 50 mg per 15 s to a total of 5.6 mg kg^{-1}. This suggests that 'depth' of anaesthesia and the corresponding plasma concentration are the important factors rather than total dose.

The studies of Wise et al (1969) with methohexitone deserve special mention. They were carried out during operative dentistry and the findings might have been affected by periods of partial respiratory obstruction and hypoxia. Very light sleep was induced with 50 mg methohexitone or less, and maintained for up to two h with incremental doses of 5 to 10 mg as indicated by the patient's response to stimuli, the total dose averaging 460 mg (range 200–825). Although there was a great difference in findings with individual patients, the overall effect was a pronounced decrease in total peripheral resistance, the blood pressure being maintained only by large increases in cardiac output with a marked tachycardia. Their results suggest that one or two doses of methohexitone cause no great physiological upset, but the administration is cumulative and more

Table 8.2 Mean cardiovascular parameters in 10 fit subjects at different clinical depth of thiopentone anaesthesia.

	Heart rate (bpm)	*Blood presssure (mm Hg)*		*Q-S_2 (s)*	*LVET (s)*	*PEP (s)*	*PEP/LVET*	*1/PEP (s)*
		Systolic	*Diastolic*					
Control	80	136	73	0.532	0.416	0.115	0.279	80
Loss of								
eyelid reflex	94*	130	71	0.552	0.427	0.126	0.296	68
corneal reflex	95*	120	72	0.552	0.418	0.134	0.322	59*
trapezius response	100*	117*	68	0.560	0.427	0.134	0.316	58*

* $P < 0.025$ *cf* controls
(modified from Becker & Tonnesen, 1978)

than 200 mg leads to widespread vasodilation and a fall in peripheral resistance.

In summary the available evidence points to minimal effects from therapeutic doses of thiopentone in healthy subjects but there is some reduction in cardiac output with or without a compensatory increase in total systemic vascular resistance. The intravenous barbiturates appear to cause a reduction in the tone of systemic capacitance vessels leading to a pooling of blood in these sites in preference to the capacitance vessels of the lung. This shift of the blood pool reduces left ventricular diastolic filling and stroke volume (Conway & Ellis, 1969).

Arrhythmias

There is no general agreement on the incidence of barbiturate-induced arrhythmias in man. Volpitto & Marangoni (1938) found no significant changes in the electrocardiogram under thiopentone anaesthesia, while Harrison (1949) detected irregularities of the pulse in one-fifth of 500 patients anaesthetised with thiopentone-relaxant. In a later communication (Harrison, 1953) reported a 21% incidence of arrhythmias during the first 20 min of anaesthesia with thialbarbitone as compared with 5.3% after thiopentone; the majority of these were ventricular extrasystoles. Johnstone (1951) also found pulse irregularities during thiopentone to be ventricular ectopic beats. They are associated with hypercapnia and disappear as soon as the carbon dioxide returns to normal. Irregularities after thialbarbitone might also be associated with carbon dioxide retention.

From their extensive studies, MacCannell & Dresel (1964) concluded that many of the arrhythmias attributable to cyclopropane-adrenaline should more properly be termed thiopentone-cyclopropane-adrenaline arrhythmias. However, the role of barbiturate induction agents was not taken into account in the other studies of the interactions of anaesthetic agents and adrenergic drugs in the causation of cardiac dysrhythmias (Katz et al, 1962; Matteo et al, 1962; 1963) and are secondary in importance to the role of hypercarbia (Katz & Epstein, 1968).

Most workers have found a greater degree of tachycardia with methohexitone than with thiopentone. While it is difficult to quantify the extent of this, one forms an impression that it is more common where there are excitatory effects of the barbiturate. In two large series of patients undergoing electroconvulsive therapy following barbiturate-suxamethonium, Pitts et al (1965) and Woodruff et al (1969) found that methohexitone caused fewer electrocardiographic changes than thiopentone. Wyant & McDonald (1980) found only one notable arrhythmia in 297 electroshock patients given methohexitone and suxamethonium: the very low frequency of disturbances in rhythm in these three series could be due to the minor nature of the procedures.

Clinical implications

In routine clinical practice involving the use of an intravenous induction followed by tracheal intubation under the influence of a relaxant the hypotensive action of the barbiturate might be replaced by a temporary increase in arterial pressure associated with the instrumentation. Thiopentone modifies the vasomotor response to positive pressure inflation of the lungs (Price et al, 1952). Too vigorous controlled respiration, like the Valsalva manoeuvre, increases the intrathoracic pressure and there is a temporary fall in blood pressure, from which recovery occurs by a compensatory vasoconstriction. This compensatory mechanism is abolished by the barbiturates and persistent hypotension may result.

Hypovolaemia might only become apparent when the compensatory vasoconstriction is abolished during the induction of anaesthesia. Thus, shock and allied states make patients unduly susceptible to the depressant action of the barbiturates. Patients with a diseased myocardium, post-coronary thrombosis, valvular heart disease or any degree of decompensation are less able to compensate for the peripheral vasodilating action of the barbiturates, and hypotension might result from small doses of any of the drugs. In the presence of a decreased cardiovascular reserve, hypotension leads to decreased venous return which, in turn, causes a further fall in cardiac output and resulting decreased coronary blood flow. This vicious circle can be easily established and have disastrous results. For this reason, intravenous barbiturate anaesthesia is more frequently contraindicated because of its effects on the cardiovascular system than are the inhalational techniques in which depressant effects occur more gradually and can be more rapidly reversed.

A fast rate of injection increases the hypotensive action of the barbiturates and slow administration is particularly important in the poor risk patient discussed above. However, intermittent administration might lead to prolonged hypotension, as the direct myocardial depressant effect of the drugs becomes evident. This also can be dangerous in the type of patient discussed.

Phenothiazines, opiates and other vasodilatory premedicants will also tend to increase the hypotensive action of the barbiturates, although this is probably relatively unimportant in normal patients. The use of tubocurarine or alcuronium immediately before or following the barbiturate might also result in a greater blood pressure fall, but this does not occur with other relaxants. Mixing of barbiturates with analeptics or vasopressors has been advocated to overcome their depressant action on the cardiovascular system but this cannot be recommended.

It is important to realise that lightening of the depth of barbiturate anaesthesia is not necessarily accompanied by a return of the blood pressure to normal. Hypotension can persist for a long time after the return of consciousness and, if this is accompanied by any degree of respiratory depression, the combined effects of a stagnant and anoxic hypoxia might affect adversely the chances of complete recovery. It is worth noting that deep barbiturate anaesthesia will abolish the blood pressure rise in response to endogenous carbon dioxide, as compared with awake subjects or those under light barbiturate–relaxant–nitrous oxide anaesthesia. This is due to their direct action on the respiratory centre (Dripps & Dumke, 1943 and it might lead to respiratory depression not being detected.

As will be discussed later, many workers have pointed out the less depressant effects of etomidate in comparison with thiopentone (Bruckner et al, 1974; Doenicke et al, 1974; Kettler et al, 1974). The neurolept-opiate combination is preferred to thiopentone in hypertensive patients (Prys-Roberts et al, 1971) and the advantages of opioids will be discussed later. Ketamine (p. 135) differs completely in cardiovascular effect from thiopentone, the only common action being a direct depressant effect on the isolated myocardium.

RESPIRATORY SYSTEM

Apart from the transient stimulation produced by very small doses, barbiturates are more potent central depressants of respiration than any other drugs used in modern anaesthesia. The sequence of events following their administration varies with the patient, the premedication (particularly opioid), the dose and the rate of injection. There is generally an increase in the depth of respiration for 30 to 40 seconds after the injection of a moderate dose; this might be followed by momentary apnoea, when the cerebral barbiturate concentration is at its peak, after which respirations will be resumed with a reduction in tidal volume and rate, depending on the dose administered. The depth of narcosis at which apnoea occurs depends to a great extent on the premedication and the intensity of the surgical stimuli at the time. This latter is of particular clinical importance at the end of anaesthesia. Patients might be breathing satisfactorily when leaving the operating room, but when returned to bed, where they are undisturbed, severe respiratory depression might occur.

As with all anaesthetic agents, the sensitivity of the respiratory centre to carbon dioxide is depressed proportionately to the depth of anaesthesia. Patrick & Faulconer (1952) found that 5% carbon dioxide in the inhaled mixture produced on the average a 72% increase in the minute volume during the second and third electroencephalographic levels of thiopentone anaesthesia in humans but only a 41% increase in levels 4 and 6. In deep anaesthesia the action of hypoxia on the carotid sinus plays an important part in the maintenance of respiration (Moyer & Beecher, 1942). Deep anaesthesia reduces the hypoxic ventilatory response (Knill et al, 1978), the degree of depression varying with depth: under light anaesthesia a relatively brisk hypoxic response was present. This shift of control of respiration from carbon dioxide to hypoxia is accompanied by a decrease in the minute volume and by hypoxaemia (Dripps & Dumke, 1943). On this basis preoxygenation should increase the respiratory depression following a barbiturate induction.

In deep thiopentone anaesthesia $PaCO_2$ rises and pH decreases, even though there might be no clinical evidence of hypoxia. As mentioned previously, carbon dioxide retention might be particularly difficult to detect since the blood pressure rise might be reduced by the anaesthetic. With a barbiturate–nitrous oxide–oxygen sequence the use of a mixture containing not less than 25% oxygen is recommended. This will reduce the hypoxic stimulus which is necessary for maintenance of respiration in deep anaesthesia and there will be less chance of respiratory depression remaining undetected.

The respiratory pattern produced by thiopentone is modified markedly by surgical stimuli or by the concomitant use of opioids or synthetic depressant analgesics. An increase in the respiratory volume in response to tactile stimulation persists until a dangerously deep level of thiopentone narcosis is reached. Eckenhoff & Helrich (1958) have shown that respiratory depression is increased and the response to endogenous carbon dioxide is reduced when thiopentone is given following a moderate dose of morphine or pethidine. These effects are less when a similar dose of thiopentone is given alone. Surprisingly they found that a 50% nitrous oxide–oxygen mixture slightly increased the depressant effects of the barbiturate, although not nearly to the extent of the opioids.

Despite some claims to the contrary, methohexitone has probably the same depressant effect on respiration as its equivalent dose of thiopentone (Doenicke et al, 1973).

Fetal respiration is particularly sensitive to the barbiturates. Dreisbach & Snyder (1943) found that a dose of thiopentone, which decreased the ventilation rate of pregnant rabbits by half, reduced the fetal respiratory rate by 85%. This response was not related to hypoxia, since even during the periods of temporary fetal apnoea the oxygen and carbon dioxide content of the umbilical vein blood remain unaltered. It has been observed clinically that poor-risk subjects with impaired cardiovascular or respiratory function are also particularly prone to dangerous degrees of respiratory depression.

Respiratory reflexes

During anaesthesia, stimuli occurring in the respiratory tract or at the site of operation might lead to a variety of reactions in which the laryngeal muscles are involved. Since their introduction there was a definite impression that thiopentone and similar drugs were followed by a higher incidence of laryngospasm, coughing and breath-holding than the inhalational agents, except cyclopropane. This was confirmed by Harrison (1962) who measured the average duration of responses following the exposure of the respiratory tract to a transient non-injurious stimulus (a single puff of cigarette smoke) in lightly anaesthetised patients. It was longest with cyclopropane, followed by thiopentone, diethyl ether, halothane and nitrous oxide–oxygen in decreasing order of duration. These findings are in keeping with those of Adriani & Rovenstine (1943) who studied the effects of different anaesthetics upon bronchi and bronchioles of excised lung tissues. Thiopentone (1:10 000), cyclopropane and hexobarbitone (1:10 000) caused the greatest degree of constriction.

Clinically it seems that the respiratory tract is hypersensitive to stimuli during light thiopentone anaesthesia. The afferent and efferent pathways of the vagal reflexes are not significantly depressed by this drug (Dille & Horita, 1955). Other reflex paths involved in laryngospasm and other respiratory disturbances are very complex and readers are referred to the comprehensive survey of Rex (1970).

In the conscious subject during breath-holding the vocal cords cannot be held closed voluntarily once the urge to breathe becomes strong. So powerful is the influence of the respiratory centre on the laryngeal reflexes that anaesthetists have administered carbon dioxide to prevent coughing or laryngospasm during laryngoscopy and tracheal intubation in light planes of anaesthesia. The variable duration of laryngeal spasm seen with different anaesthetic agents might be due to a dissimilar degree of depression of the respiratory centre. Thus, theoretically, laryngeal spasm and associated effects would be prolonged with an agent which produces depression of the respiratory centre to its normal chemical and afferent nervous stimuli, in a plane of anaesthesia in which there is little depression of the appropriate reflex arc. On the other hand with an agent which does not depress the respiratory centre at light levels of anaesthesia, the increasing $PaCO_2$ would stimulate respiration and cause abduction of the vocal cords and interruption of the reflex response of laryngeal spasm, coughing and breath-holding. It is well known that deep cyclopropane and thiopentone anaesthesia result in marked respiratory depression and that they depress the response of the centre to endogenous carbon dioxide, but this is little altered in light anaesthesia where laryngospasm can also occur (Harrison, 1962). The relationship between these two aspects of the action of drugs in the respiratory system is worthy of further study.

Laryngospasm was a dreaded complication in the early days of intravenous thiopentone, particularly when the drug was given without adequate means of resuscitation. Although very uncommon it is still potentially life-threatening but its dangers have been markedly reduced by the availability of suxamethonium. In the largest ever survey of its frequency — 136 929 patients given 156 064 anaesthetics–Ollson & Hallin (1984) found an incidence of just over 8 in 1000 anaesthetics. Barbiturate induction was not an important factor in perioperative laryngospasm in adults but might be in children under 10 years of age. The highest overall incidence of laryngospasm was found in this latter age group and was associated with bronchial asthma and respiratory tract infection.

Bronchospasm has been reported to occur with most anaesthetics and here again thiopentone and cyclopropane have been particularly incriminated. The heightened sensitivity of the respiratory reflexes might play an important role here. However, the term 'bronchospasm' is often wrongly used, as the inability to inflate the lungs might be due to reflex spasm of the intercostal and other muscles. This could explain the relief produced by relaxants which have no effect on the smooth muscles of the bronchi.

It has been claimed that thiobarbiturates produce more respiratory disturbances than barbiturates (Stoelting et al, 1950; Volpitto, 1951) but this is not true. A number of factors increase the tendency to cough and hiccough, but taking all factors into consideration there is no doubt that methitural, buthalitone and methohexitone are the worst drugs in this respect yet only two of them are thiobarbiturates. Table 5.3 shows no obvious chemical grouping associated with this side effect, although each has one complicated side chain in position 5. However, those who have used methohexitone since its introduction are aware that the currently available drug is followed by less respiratory upset (and muscle movement) than the original compound 25398.

As with excitatory phenomena, the frequency and severity of respiratory disturbance increases with dosage (Barron & Dundee, 1967) and fast injection (Barron, 1968), but are not influenced by opioid premedication. The occurrence of cough or hiccough is less after methohexitone in patients premedicated with atropine or hyoscine. This effect is less marked with thiopentone and thiamylal in subjects given no antisialogogue (Haslett & Dundee, 1968).

INDUCTION CHARACTERISTICS

The induction characteristics of rapidly acting intravenous barbiturates are largely determined by their action on the central nervous, cardiovascular and respiratory systems. Before discussing other actions on the body, the important factors known to influence these induction characteristics are reviewed in Table 8.3. This is fairly self-explanatory and should clarify some aspects of the action of intravenous drugs as seen in routine clinical practice.

LIVER FUNCTION

This term includes a number of conjugating, detoxicating, enzymatic and other actions, many of which are affected by both the nature and duration of the operation, by hypoxia, hypotension, pre- and postoperative medication and by complications during the recovery period. Consequently it is difficult to assess specifically the action of barbiturates alone. Chronic sepsis,

Table 8.3 Summary of some factors known to influence side effects of barbiturates

Factor	*Excitatory phenomena*	*Respiratory upset*	*Hypotension*
Chemistry	CH_3 group increases incidence and severity	No obvious relation	No obvious relation
Premedication	Reduced by analgesics	Reduced by atropine/hyoscine	Increased by opiates/phenothiazines
Dose relation	+ Worst with methylated compounds	+	++ (Related to rate of injection)
Rate of injection	ditto	+	+ (Related to dose administered)

+ Positive relationship ++ Very marked relationship

pulmonary tuberculosis, thyrotoxicosis, intestinal obstruction, advanced carcinoma and burns are all clinical conditions which will cause impairment of hepatic function and which might increase the toxic action of drugs on the liver. These variables have not always been taken into consideration in the early studies on the effect of barbiturates on liver function which are of limited value (Carraway, 1939; Mordinovia, 1948; Pohle, 1948; Fairlie et al, 1951). This also applies to the case of 'Toxic Jaundice following administration of Pentothal' reported by Vaizey in 1938. An anaemic patient was anaesthetised for haemorrhoidectomy with thiopentone alone following opiate premedication, and hypoxia or hypercapuia could not be excluded as contributory factors.

Various 'liver function tests' have been used by different workers, each of which only deals with one particular aspect of hepatic function. These include the ability of the liver to remove substances from the bloodstream (bromsulphthalein retention, hippuric acid excretion, serum bilirubin and urinary urobilinogen), levels of various enzymes (pseudocholinesterase, transaminases, alkaline phosphatase etc), flocculation tests (thymol turbidity etc) and prothrombin time. In most studies a number of tests have been used to investigate different aspects of liver function and minor degrees of dysfunction might be detected. To complicate matters further, liver function might be affected not only directly by drugs but indirectly by alterations in blood flow or oxygen tension or a hypersensitivity reaction. Thus, the interpretation of liver function tests is not always straightforward and their clinical significance might be difficult to assess.

Hepatic blood flow

Liver function can be affected by blood flow: using the bromsulphthalein method Habif et al (1951) found a decrease in the estimated hepatic blood flow with an increase in the hepatic arterio-venous oxygen difference during anaesthesia with thiopentone or cyclopropane. Hepatic blood flow is, to some extent, dependent on the splanchnic blood flow but in the absence of hypotension or hyper/hypocarbia this is little affected by thiopentone or balanced techniques using it as an induction agent (Levy et al, 1961). Hypercarbia increases splanchnic resistance and splanchnic blood flow decreases accordingly. Hyperventilation, which is an integral part of some anaesthetic techniques, and the associated changes in airway pressure will impede flow by about 30% (Cooperman et al, 1968). However, the ensuing hypocapnia will diminish sympathetic activity and splanchnic resistance will be less than at normocapnia with a similar ventilatory pattern and airway pressure (Cooperman, 1972).

Hepatic impairment follows the use of thiopentone in some animals; the smaller the animal, the more marked are the effects (Reynolds et al, 1938; Richards & Appel, 1941). During prolonged thiopentone anaesthesia in dogs Booker (1946) found a progressive decrease in the ability of the liver to remove bromsulphthalein from the blood. Walton et al (1950) found that small doses of thiopentone were mildly toxic to both the normal and damaged liver of the dog which effect could be overcome by adequate ventilation with oxygen. Doses of 20 mg kg^{-1} thiopentone given twice daily to normal dogs for periods of two to three weeks

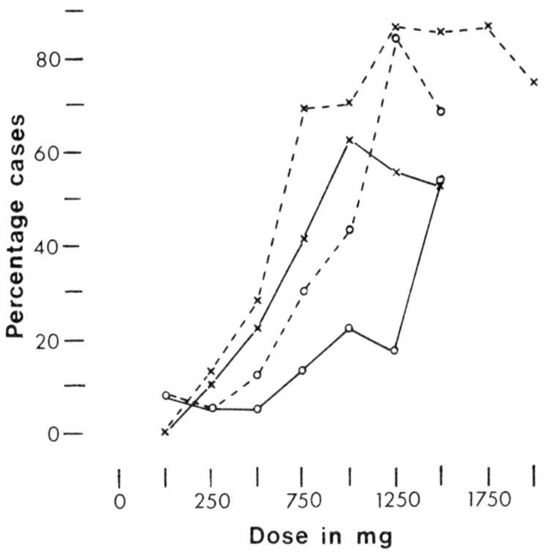

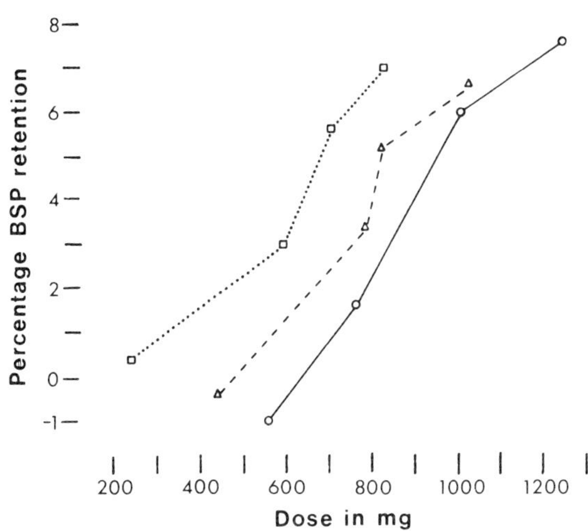

Fig. 8.8 Findings of two studies showing the relationship of dosage of barbiturate to impairment of liver function.
Left: incidence of: definite (————) and possible (---------) liver dysfunction (as detected by abnormal excretion of urobilinogen) with increasing dose of thiopentone; O = patients undergoing minor gynaecological operations; X = abdominal operations. (Dundee, 1955)
Right: correlation of change in bromsulphathalein to dosage of: ———— methohexitone; --------- thiopentone; .... thiamylal. (Bittrich, Kane and Mosher, 1963).

caused a mild depression of hepatic function, as judged by the prothrombin time and serum bilirubin level, with complete return to normal four days after the last injection (Walton et al, 1951). In contradistinction to the effects of small doses, adequate oxygenation did not reduce the toxicity of repeated large doses of thiopentone.

Figure 8.8 shows the results of two early controlled studies which relate the dose of the drug given to the incidence of detected liver dysfunction (Bittrich et al, 1963; Dundee, 1955). In two comparable groups, each of 232 adults receiving thiopentone as an induction (average 400 mg) or main (average 1170 mg) anaesthetic agent, the incidence of excessive postoperative urobilinogen excretion could be related to the dose of the drug given. By excluding intravascular haemolysis as a possible cause of increased urobilinogen output it was shown that detectable liver dysfunction occurred in an appreciable number of patients when the dose of thiopentone exceeded 750 mg. With adequate ventilation the then available muscle relaxants (tubocurarine, gallamine, laudexium) did not increase the hepatic toxicity of thiopentone. Using a battery of tests Bittrich et al (1963) demonstrated a dose-related toxicity for methohexitone, thiopentone and thiamylal. On a weight basis methohexitone was more toxic than thiopentone or thiamylal but in equivalent anaesthetic doses the reverse was the case. An important observation was that in patients with pre-existing liver dysfunction, methohexitone did not increase the depression more than in patients with normal liver function.

The importance of the severity of the operation as a factor in inducing liver dysfunction is shown by the studies of Clarke et al (1965) who studied changes in serum bilirubin, alkaline phosphatase, pseudocholinesterase and glutamic pyruvate transaminase at 3 and 36 hours after operation in two groups of 100 patients each, anaesthetised with nitrous oxide-oxygen and either thiopentone (average dose 315 mg) or propanidid (average dose 573 mg) for minor gynaecological operations. No significant abnormality of liver function was detected in either series. Following the longer surgical procedures in which very large doses of drugs were given (average of 1260 mg thiopentone and 4860 mg propanidid), abnormalities in liver function were detected after both agents. These changes were statistically, but probably not clinically significant.

In a series of studies, which used a common protocol (Dundee et al, 1980; Blunnie et al, 1981;

Kawar et al, 1982), the effect of a number of induction agents was studied under comparable conditions, using a battery of enzyme tests. Patients were either undergoing minor gynaecological or body surface operations and the induction was either given by intermittent administration as main anaesthetic or by infusion, combined with nitrous oxide-oxygen. There was no evidence of hepatic dysfunction using small doses of ketamine, thiopentone, Althesin, etomidate, midazolam or propofol. However infusions caused readily detectable enzyme changes associated with the use of large doses (ketamine 3.7 mg kg^{-1}, thiopentone 13.1 mg kg^{-1}, Althesin 1.6 mg kg^{-1}, etomidate 0.9 mg kg^{-1}): these changes were most marked with Althesin and ketamine. In pooling data from different studies it becomes very apparent that large doses of intravenous anaesthetics cause a greater derangement of liver function than that which occurs using a balanced technique for the same operation. It is not possible to estimate the duration of liver dysfunction but, except after Althesin, the effects were becoming less marked by the 15th postoperative day.

The remarkable resilience of the liver to the hepatotoxic effect of intravenous anaesthetics is illustrated by a case report of the use of continuous methohexitone in a disturbed patient (Dunkin, 1972). By the ninth day he had been given 16.6 g with no evidence of liver dysfunction. On the llth day, after 22.1 g the serum glutamic oxalacetic transaminase had risen to 56 units and by the 15th day (total dose of 33.6 g) to 85 units with serum glutamic pyruvate transaminase of 23 units. Enzymatic evidence of hepatotoxicity had disappeared within five days of the end of the infusion.

There is no suggestion that barbiturates cause a hypersensitivity reaction such as occurs occasionally with halothane (Sherlock, 1971). Intravenous anaesthetics have been repeated so frequently in patients over the past 50 years that a case would almost certainly have been reported by now if sensitisation were common but the possibility of this occurring should not be completely dismissed (Rosenmann et al, 1972). Induced hypersensitivity to barbiturates in other forms is discussed in Chapter 14.

There are two isolated reports of hepatitis following thiopentone. A much quoted early report (Vaizey, 1938) describes the occurrence of jaundice following thiopentone, but this could be explained on grounds other than the anaesthetic. Most recently Hasselstrom & Kristoffersen (1979) described a patient who developed pyrexia and jaundice following repeated anaesthesia, and suggested that thiopentone was the causative factor. This patient had nine anaesthetics and developed jaundice on three occasions when thiopentone was used for induction: halothane was used on only one of these occasions. Although these authors suggest that thiopentone should be considered as a possible factor in 'halothane jaundice' when the drug is used for induction, absence of further reports would not support this view.

RENAL FUNCTION

The effects of anaesthesia and operation on renal haemodynamics and kidney function are complex (Rosen, 1972) and have not been as fully investigated as their action on liver function. Maloney et al (1950) found glomerular filtration to be high in dogs during light thiopentone anaesthesia but depressed during deep narcosis. Their findings concerning effective renal plasma flow were inconclusive. In the studies of Habif et al (1951) the glomerular filtration rate was measured by the inulin clearance and the effective renal plasma flow by the para-aminohippurate (PAH) clearance test. All values fell promptly during induction with thiopentone and there was little further alteration during the subsequent surgical operations. Electrolyte and water reabsorption increased and recovery was almost complete when consciousness was regained. Their results demonstrated a vasoconstrictor response in both the kidney and liver with all forms of anaesthesia, associated with a fall in filtration, urine concentration, excretion of electrolytes and urinary output.

De Wardener (1955) emphasises that, except when there is little or no renal blood flow, urinary output bears little relationship to the amount of blood flowing through the kidney. The rate of urine flow is dependent mainly on the concentration of circulating antidiuretic hormone, which in turn depends on the activity of the supraoptico-hypophyseal system. Nearly all anaesthetic agents stimulate this system and the amount of urine passed during anaesthesia is therefore minimal (0.1 to 0.5 ml min^{-1}), irrespective of any changes occurring in the renal circulation. Some of the action of barbiturates might be secondary to the effect of these drugs on the cardiovascular system, the renal circulation being very sensitive to the blood pressure changes which are liable to occur with the thiobarbiturates.

Silvette (1941) found that thiopentone inhibited the diuretic response to hypotonic sodium chloride and xanthine derivatives in rats. It had no effect on the efficacy of a mercurial diuretic. The administration of thiopentone after posterior pituitary extract did not abolish the antidiuretic effect of the latter, but if the two drugs were given together no antidiuresis occurred.

The temporary oliguria during uncomplicated thiopentone anaesthesia has no effect on blood urea levels. However, if it is accompanied by hyperventilation and gaseous alkalosis with constriction of renal vessels, small rises can occur during prolonged anaesthesia.

No histological evidence of kidney damage has been reported after the use of thiobarbiturates.

REPRODUCTIVE SYSTEM

In therapeutic dosage barbiturates neither depress nor increase the tone of the gravid uterus. Uterine muscle tone is depressed to a variable degree in deep anaesthesia with all agents and there is some inhibition of contractions in light anaesthesia with chloroform and diethyl ether. Muscle relaxants have little effect on the uterine musculature.

Walker & Stout (1952) studied the effect of various anaesthetics on Fallopian tube motility and found thiopentone to have no effect, but there was an increase in the amplitude of contractions when it was combined with curare. Thiopentone, likewise, had no effect on utero-tubal spasm, which was reduced by diethyl ether, chloroform, trichloroethylene and probably nitrous oxide. Morphine, on the other hand, caused increased spasticity.

MUSCLES AND MYONEURAL JUNCTION

Gross and Cullen (1943) observed that thiopentone decreased the contraction of the gastrocnemius muscle, elicited by the intra-arterial injection of acetylcholine or by electrical stimulation of the nerve in the dog. This depression was not abolished by sectioning the nerve to the muscle. This suggests that thiopentone has some curariform action that is much less marked than with diethyl ether and that occurs only when very large doses are used. Blood concentrations of diethyl ether in the region of 100 to 120 mg ml^{-1} reduced the action potentials of the muscles as much as tubocurarine, while clinical doses of thiopentone and cyclopropane had only a very small effect (Comroe et al, 1947). Secher (1951a–d) using the phrenic nerve–diaphragm preparation of the rat, found that barbiturates, but not thiobarbiturates, produced a depression of myoneural transmission.

Barbiturates cause a prolongation of the contraction time of muscles (Sirnes, 1954; Quilliam, 1955). This can explain why Kraatz & Gluckman (1954) demonstrated an increase in muscle contraction after thiopentone and thiamylal, a finding confirmed by Sirnes (1954). Substances which prolong the contraction time augment the twitch response (Brown & von Euler, 1938).

With larger doses of drugs the direct stimulant action on muscles is masked by the simultaneous depression of myoneural transmission, the latter being detected with doses of thiopentone and thialbarbitone not exceeding those used for the production of surgical anaesthesia in the animals (Sirnes, 1954). A synergistic effect was noted between thiopentone and tubocurarine chloride. As a result of these studies, Sirnes has suggested that part of the respiratory depression which occurs in barbiturate overdose is due to the peripheral action of the drugs. However, Sirnes compared the effects of direct and indirect stimulation of the muscles alternately on the same preparation. Since the motor end-plate was intact one cannot be certain that the results of direct stimulation did not also include effects resulting from impulses arising at the myoneural junction.

The curariform effect of doses of barbiturates used in anaesthesia is not very obvious compared

Table 8.4 Respiratory depressant effects of 50 mg suxamethonium given immediately after induction in four large groups of patients

Induction agents	*Barbiturates*	*Althesin*	*Eugenols*	*Ketamine*
Average duration (s)				
Apnoea	196.10	211.9	326.11	328.13
Respiratory depression	321.11	311.10	459.31	451.18

(Clarke et al, 1964; 1967; Bovill et al, 1971; Carson et al, 1973

to that of diethyl ether but it might explain the ease with which tracheal intubation may be carried out following thiopentone in myasthenic subjects. No marked potentiation of tubocurarine chloride by thiopentone has been reported to date and the two drugs have been combined in anaesthesia with complete safety.

There is no evidence to suggest that the intravenous barbiturates influence the intensity or duration of action of the non-depolarising relaxants in clinical practice — it would be impossible to obtain such data as patients have first to be anaesthetised with some agent before administration of the relaxant. Table 8.4 shows that the duration of action of suxamethonium is shorter following a barbiturate than in patients induced with propanidid or ketamine. This is in keeping with the absence of anticholinesterase activity after a single dose of a barbiturate.

Thiopentone has a protective effect against the pain and stiffness caused by a single dose of suxamethonium chloride (Craig, 1964). This protection is of short duration, having nearly disappeared after five minutes and is probably related to the direct action of barbiturates on muscle. Others (Manani et al, 1981) although noting a reduction in fasciculations with thiopentone did not confirm its effect on post-suxamethonium myalgia.

BLOOD

Because of the high alkalinity of solutions, thiobarbiturates cause in-vitro haemolysis, visible to the naked eye, when added to blood to a final concentration of as low as 1:1000. Using the method for detecting intravascular haemolysis based on the presence of carbonic anhydrase in the urine, Dundee (1955) detected evidence of haemolysis in 20% of cases when large (mean 1170 mg) doses were used as the main anaesthetic and in 15% when it was used only for induction of anaesthesia (average dose 440 mg). The incidence of haemolysis however seems to be related to the nature and duration of the operation rather than to the dose of thiopentone. In all cases the degree of haemolysis was so slight that the absorption spectrum for haemoglobin could not be detected. There are no reported cases of haematuria after barbiturates, and there is no evidence to suggest that the degree of intravascular haemolysis referred to above is of clinical significance.

Suggestions that barbiturates tend to cause haemodilution are based on animal experiments with amylobarbitone or pentobarbitone, but some studies have included thiopentone. Haemodilution is due to dilation of the spleen, which is maximal 20 min after induction of anaesthesia with thiopentone in dogs (Hausner et al, 1938). There is no evidence to suggest that this is important in humans, although Magora et al (1974) found a slight decrease in haematocrit after thiopentone. These workers found no change in blood viscosity or fibrinogen concentration with this agent.

Leucocyte histamine release due to thiopentone might play a part in hypersensitivity reactions (Hirshman et al, 1982). This is considered in Chapter 14.

METABOLISM

A mild hyperglycaemia has been observed by Hrubetz & Blackberg (1938) in animals during thiopentone anaesthesia. Richards & Appel (1941), Booker (1946) and Booker and his co-workers (1949; 1952) have verified this in dogs and studied the effects of thiopentone on carbohydrate metabolism. In animals on a normal diet the liver glycogen was found to be progressively depleted during long anaesthesia. The administration of glucose before the induction of anaesthesia produced hyperglycaemia and glycosuria. Even animals with livers depleted of carbohydrate by starvation before the induction of anaesthesia were unable to convert glucose to glycogen and remained hyperglycaemic. The intermediate metabolism of carbohydrates is also depressed during prolonged thiopentone anaesthesia, as shown by a rise in the blood lactic acid content. All these changes could be mitigated by the use of small doses of insulin, if given along with or immediately following the administration of thiopentone. Disturbances in the intermediate metabolism of proteins also occur. Amino acids given intravenously lead to an increase in the blood level which remains high during anaesthesia, in contradistinction to the normal response of a rise during the first hour, returning to normal by the second hour.

An interesting observation was that animals on a high carbohydrate diet, and given insulin during anaesthesia, required more thiopentone to maintain a constant level of narcosis than animals on a normal diet. Animals on a high protein diet, on a high carbohydrate diet and on normal diet with insulin given before and during anaesthesia follow in the above order as regards the thiopentone requirements during anaesthesia.

Slight hyperglycaemia occurs during thiopentone narcosis in man but is of no clinical importance and its effects are much less than those of diethyl ether or chloroform. Indeed, ether glycaemia is inhibited by induction with thiopentone (Bass et al, 1953). Patients under thiopentone–nitrous oxide–oxygen behave in a similar manner to those receiving thiopentone alone. This also applies to thiopentone–nitrous oxide–tubocurarine, but with this technique the hyperglycaemia is minimised by the use of an opioid during anaesthesia, suggesting that the lack of analgesia during operation might predispose to the rise in blood sugar. Further confirmation for this view comes from the work of Clarke (1968) who found no rise in blood sugar when a single dose of thiopentone is given in the absence of an operation and more recent studies by Hall et al (1978) and Blunnie et al (1983) showing that the hyperglycaemic response to stress is obtunded by analgesics. However avoidance of hypercapnia is important since Dundee & Todd (1958) found the rise in blood sugar with thiopentone to be greater after opioid premedication, thus implicating respiratory depression as a contributory factor.

Stern et al (1945) have reported that glucose tolerance is decreased by thiopentone. They administered 1.5 g of 50% glucose intravenously to three subjects who had been anaesthetised for 45 to 60 min and found a greater rise in blood sugar than when the same amount of glucose was administered in the conscious state. Their findings suggest a similarity in behaviour, with respect to glycogenesis, in man and in dog under thiopentone anaesthesia. These observations are open to criticism, in that the three patients were admitted to hospital with acute alcoholism and their livers might not have been normal.

Further evidence of impairment by thiopentone of the ability of the body to handle dextrose comes from the studies carried out by Dundee (1956b) in six healthy subjects. Blood sugar was estimated on three occasions in each person: a) during thiopentone anaesthesia in the fasting state; b) after 50 g glucose without anaesthesia, and c) during thiopentone anaesthesia induced after oral administration of 50 g glucose. A typical finding is shown in Figure 8.9, the dose of thiopentone being 1.3 g administered over an hour and a half on both occasions. These results were in agreement with those of Booker et al in dogs, and these workers suggested that this is a manifestation of the hepatotoxic action of thiopentone and cite it in support of the detoxication of the drug in the liver.

In a clinical situation Goldsmith & Holmes (1957) found that a slightly greater degree of hyperglycaemia results from intravenous dextrose given to the same patients in the conscious state. Dundee & Todd (1958) confirmed these findings but showed that the additional hyperglycaemia induced by the thiopentone was of no clinical significance (Fig. 8.9).

In interpreting studies on blood sugar changes one must remember that hyperglycaemia, and a rise in plasma cortisol, is part of the endocrine and metabolic response to surgery (Hall, 1985), and might be unrelated to changes in carbohydrate

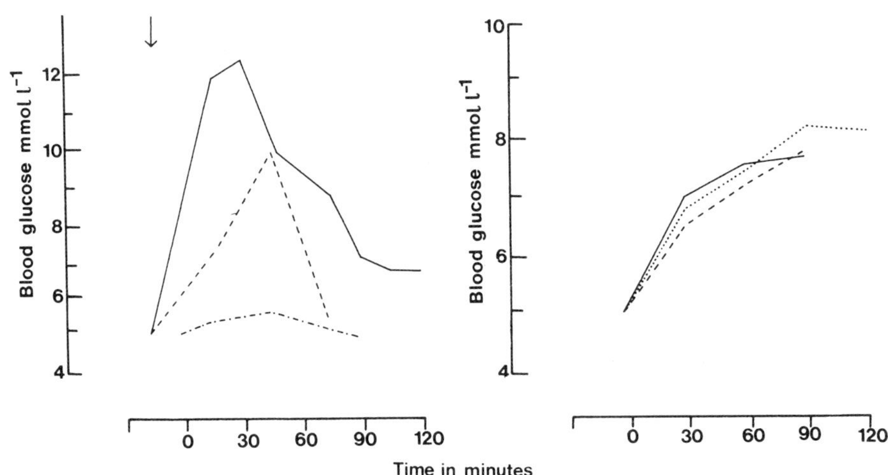

Fig. 8.9 Experimental and clinical data on the effect of thiopentone on glucose tolerance.

Left: normal subjects (no surgery)

-.-.-.-.- Thiopentone anaesthesia, 1.3 g given over 90 minutes

--------- Glucose tolerance curve (no anaesthesia)

——— Glucose tolerance curve under thiopentone (same dose as above)

↓ 50 g glucose given by mouth

(All observations were made on one subject)

(Dundee, 1956b)

Right: average data from groups of 14 to 18 patients infused with 5% dextrose at the rate of 100 ml per hour

--------- No anaesthesia (no surgery)

——— Thiopentone (approx12 mg kg^{-1})—N_2O–O_2 (body surface surgery)

. . . . Thiopentone (approx 8 mg kg^{-1})—N_2O–O_2–tubocurarine (abdominal surgery)

(Dundee and Todd, 1958)

metabolism (Hall, 1985). This response can be modified by afferent neuronal block (epidural or spinal) or by the administration of large doses of potent opioids.

INTESTINAL TRACT

In the dog, Gruber & Gruber (1941) found that 20 mg kg^{-1} thiopentone and 40 mg kg^{-1} thioethamyl might cause complete cessation of action of the pylorus and stomach. A temporary increase in tone was followed by a depression of activity lasting during the period of deep anaesthesia. In some animals an increase in general tonus was again observed during recovery.

Golden & Mann (1943) have studied the effect of various drugs on the tone and motility of the small intestine of the dog, using loops of jejunum and ileum exteriorised in continuity and enclosed in bipedicled tubes of skin. The slow injection of small doses of thiopentone had no effect on intestinal motility but with rapid injection there was a marked loss of tone and cessation of movement persisting for about half the duration of the sleep. When food was given immediately after recovery from thiopentone the normal pattern of peristalsis recurred, irrespective of the dose or rate of administration of thiopentone.

The slow injection of thiopentone, followed by a 50% nitrous oxide-oxygen mixture, did not affect intestinal motility. However, when diethyl ether followed thiopentone, bowel tone was decreased and motility ceased, similar to the effects observed with diethyl ether alone. Golden & Mann also showed the deleterious effects of cyanosis and hypoxia during anaesthesia on smooth muscle tone. In clinical practice the preoperative administration of opioids and atropine appears to be the most important factor influencing the activity of the small intestine.

LOCAL EFFECTS

Clinically used concentrations of barbiturates are

highly alkaline and might also be hypertonic. Pain is not a feature of the intravenous injection of the thiobarbiturates, but does occur frequently with methohexitone (Taylor & Stoelting, 1960). It follows the course of the vein and is more common when small vessels are used. Although reports of its incidence vary (Coleman & Green, 1960; Meagher, 1964; Thornton, 1970), Rowlands (1969) who worked in a small town, found that patients commented on it adversely after leaving hospital and noted that the addition of 1 mg ml^{-1} lignocaine to 1% methohexitone (i.e. 0.5 g methohexitone dissolved in 45 ml water, to which 5 ml 1% lignocaine is added) will almost completely abolish this complication. Precipitation does not occur with this mixture.

Venous thrombosis is uncommon following the injection of intravenous barbiturates. The accumulated data from several large studies (O'Donnell et al, 1969; Carson et al, 1972; Clarke et al, 1972) placed the incidence at between 3 and 4% with thiopentone and slightly higher with methohexitone. In the most extensive comparative study (O'Donnell et al, 1969) it was noticed that 2.5% thiopentone and 1% methohexitone were followed by a lesser incidence of venous damage than the 5 and 2% solutions respectively. These two barbiturates cause less venous damage than etomidate.

Subcutaneous injection results in local tissue irritation, the extent of damage depending on the concentration of the drug and the total amount injected. Patients with a poor peripheral circulation or with sparseness of subcutaneous tissues are more susceptible to the irritant effects; the clinical effects can vary from temporary slight tenderness at the site of injection to extensive tissue necrosis. It would seem that the extravenous injection of methohexitone is followed by fewer sequelae than when a thiobarbiturate is extravasated (Recant, 1960). This could, however, be due to the greater dilution of the oxybarbiturate.

Intramuscular injection

Both thiopentone and methohexitone can be given by deep intramucular injection without any major sequelae. Keown and his colleagues (1957) have recommended intramuscular thiopentone as premedication for cardiac catheterization, and Dhruva (1960) found it useful in paediatric anaesthesia. Miller & Stoelting (1963) have used intramuscular methohexitone in children with no abscesses or sloughs at the site of administration. After 6.6 mg kg^{-1} patients usually lost consciousness within 10 min; thus an accidental extravenous injection should be followed by a smaller than usual intravenous dose.

Intra-arterial injection

This can result in serious damage to the blood supply of the affected limb, with permanent sequelae and is of such importance that it will be discussed in detail. It has been estimated to occur in between 1:3500 and 1:56 000 administrations (Macintosh & Heyworth, 1943; Cohen, 1948; Dundee, 1956a) but the incidence is now much lower than this (Davies, 1979). It is impossible to get a true estimate of its frequency, since there might be few or no untoward effects in many patients and so may remain undetected (Stone & Donnelly, 1961).

The clinical picture varies with the drug used, the dose and the concentration of the solution and with the blood vessels entered. The classical response is one of immediate onset of agonising pain shooting down the forearm and into the hands and fingers, with movement of the arm in an attempt to remove the offending needle and syringe. It has been described by patients as 'like boiling water poured over my hand', 'the hand feeling like a flaming bush' or 'like ice-cold water running down my arms and freezing on the tips of my fingers as icicles, which dropped off after a minute or two'. The severity is such that it cannot be simulated by any other event during induction.

After the intra-arterial injection of a small volume of dilute thiopentone the pain in the arm might subside after a few minutes, but with larger amounts it can persist for several hours. Patients in whom anaesthesia is continued with another agent might still complain of the pain on return of consciousness. A rarer occurrence is for the pain to disappear shortly after the injection and return later. This sequence might be repeated several times and is presumably due to intermittent attacks of vascular spasm. Unfortunately, in an occasional patient no pain might follow the intra-arterial injection of those concentrations of thiopentone which can result in severe damage to a limb (Medico-Legal, 1951).

The intense arterial constriction after injection is manifest by an immediate disappearance of the radial pulse and blanching of the limb. Because of the increased time taken for the anaesthetic to reach the central nervous system, the onset of unconsciousness will be slightly delayed. Severe vasomotor collapse can occur, and the resulting hypotension might be taken as the explanation for the inability to palpate the peripheral pulse. Where the arterial blood flow to the forearm is rapidly restored, blanching of the limb will be followed by reactive hyperaemia. Oedema of the limb occurs quickly where the muscles have been invaded by thiopentone, and mottled patches and echymoses indicate skin involvement.

Where spasm of digital or main vessels persists or where immediate thrombosis occurs, the blanching is followed by increasing cyanosis of the affected part, which becomes a dark purple colour and is followed by gangrene. Cohen (1948) has observed that fingers which developed gangrene did not show oedema while fingers which recovered did. The absence of oedema indicates that the circulation in these fingers has been completely arrested and that the major digital vessels are thrombosed. Extensive oedema of the muscles usually results in flexion of the fingers. It is believed that muscles cannot stand complete ischaemia for more than six hours, and failure of the oedema to subside within this time usually means that the chances of saving the limb are small.

Since the main nerves of the forearm receive their blood supply from the radial and ulnar arteries, interference with the flow in the latter might lead to loss of sensation. The interosseous branch of the ulnar artery is particularly important, as it supplies the median nerve, but where there is a high division of the brachial artery this branch is usually given off by the radial. Consequently it will not be affected unless there had been retrograde spread of the drug.

Thrombosis can develop insidiously and complete occlusion with obliteration of the pulse has been recorded as long as 10 days after the first aggregation of platelets over the damaged site. The thrombosis usually extends proximally as far as the origin of the major collateral vessel above the site of the arterial puncture.

The distal forearm and fingers are affected according to the distribution of the affected vessel. Shunting the drug into the skin might result in discolouration or even sloughing. In muscles it will cause gross oedema, and thrombosis of a major vessel will result in ischaemia and death of the muscle. Gangrene of the fingers results from complete blockage of their blood supply, but it is not unusual to find only the distal portions involved. Cohen (1948) suggests that this is due to intense spasm of the arteriovenous anastomosis followed by clotting in the venous loop. Ischaemia of nerves might result from impairment of their blood supply due either to thrombosis or to pressure from oedema of the surrounding muscles.

The sequelae of an intra-arterial injection can vary from transient pain to gangrene of the forearm. A number of theories have been advanced to explain the events which occur and more than one factor might be involved in many cases. Burn & Hobbs (1959) and Burn (1960) have shown that the intra-arterial injection of thiopentone releases noradrenaline from the vessel walls and this is a possible cause of the vascular spasm that follows the mishap. However, Kinmonth & Shepherd (1959) have shown that the spasm is transitory and alone could not account for the permanent damage. An intense chemical endarteritis develops which rapidly destroys the endothelial and subendothelial tissues and on occasions even the muscle layer itself (Cohen, 1948). This injury is immediate and requires but momentary contact between the drugs and the vessel wall. The initial local response in the tissues adjacent to the damage is oedema which develops shortly after destruction of the intima. It does not encroach upon the lumen of the larger vessels but it assumes increasing importance in smaller arteries and arterioles where blood flow might be greatly reduced or even arrested. Stasis and intimal damage favour thrombosis which has been

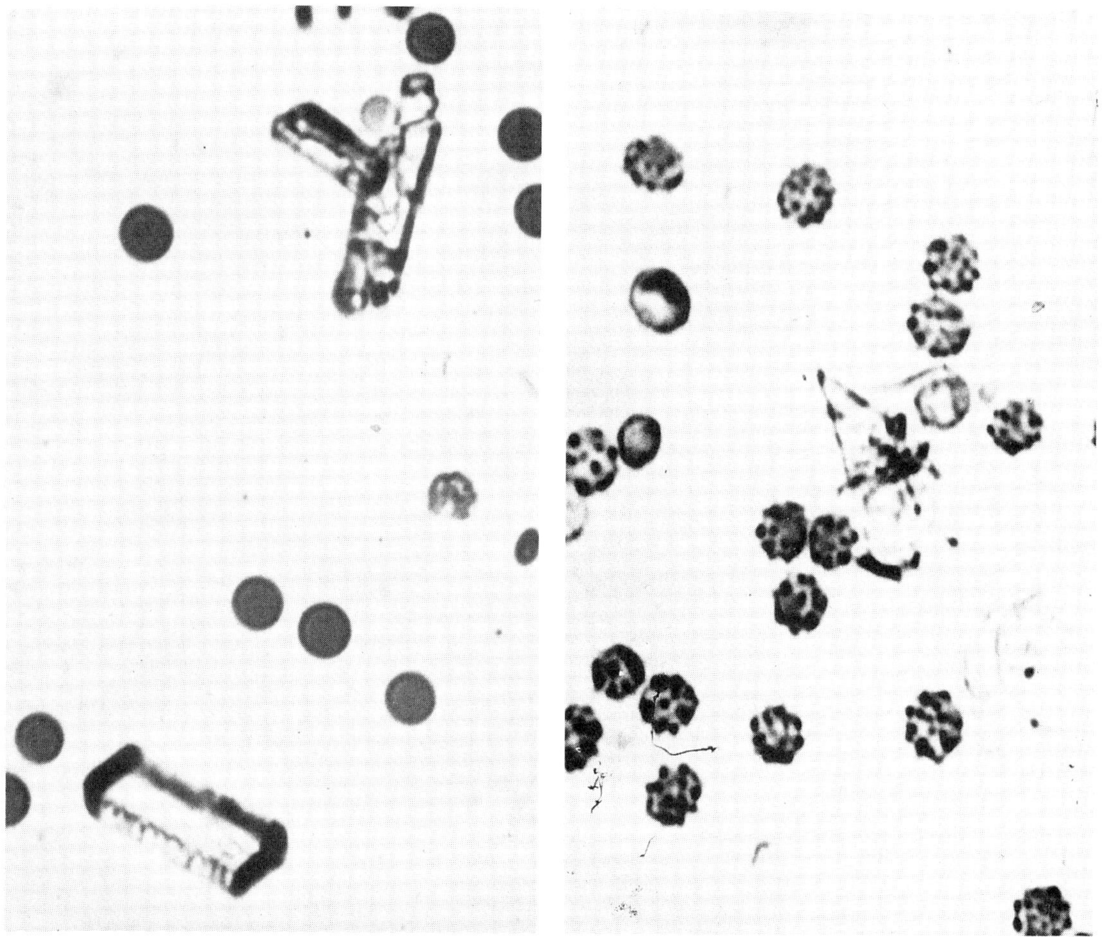

Fig. 8.10 Microphotographs showing size of acid crystals of methohexitone (left) and thiopentone (right) relative to blood cells (Brown et al, 1968).

found in the experimental studies of Kinmonth and Shepherd (1959).

Waters (1966) showed that crystals of insoluble thiopentone acid form in the blood stream after injection and suggested that these are swept along the arterial path and so might block small vessels. This could produce mechanical blockage and bring about the release of noradrenaline and muscular spasm. Waters's evidence of crystal formation was indisputable, but Brown et al (1968) extended the study to show that red blood cell haemolysis and platelet aggregations also occurred and these effects are accentuated by acid crystals. Figure 8.10 is a photomicrograph showing the size and shape of the acid crystals of thiopentone and methohexitone relative to blood cells; these crystals were obtained with the barbiturate concentrations expected after intra-arterial injection, assuming a normal forearm blood flow of 0.5 to 1.0 ml s^{-1} and an injection rate of 1 ml s^{-1}. Release of adenosine triphosphate from damaged red blood cells or platelets and an area of endothelial damage at the puncture site are sufficient reasons for the initiation of thrombosis.

Brown et al (1968) found that although oxybarbiturates might be less likely to form crystals than thiobarbiturates, dilution is the main factor in preventing crystal formation and maximum safety can best be achieved by the use of dilute solutions. Methohexitone is safer in this respect since it need never be used in concentrations exceeding 2% but the absence of a sulphur atom might be the additional safety factor. Crystal formation occurs in veins but is unimportant because of the ever increasing diameter of the vessels and subsequent resolution of the crystals.

Anatomical anomalies (Ch. 2) and the absence of arterial pulsation will increase the risk of accidental arterial injection, but the concentration of solution is a more important factor in clinical practice. Table 8.5, a survey of the sequelae in 65 intra-arterial administrations of thiopentone, confirms this view. There is no comparable report of serious sequelae following the 2.5% solution, although Taff (1982) mentions two anecdotal reports of gangrene.

Table 8.5 A survey of cases showing the sequelae of intra-arterial thiopentone related to the strength of solution used.

		Sequelae				
% Solution	*n*	*Nature*	*Permanent*		*Nil*	
			n	*%*	*n*	*%*
10	11	Amputation required	5	45	2	18
		Gangrene of fingers	3	28		
		Skin slough	1	9		
5	16	Amputation required	3	19	11	69
		Skin slough	1	6		
		Area of hypoaesthesia	1	6		
2.5–5.0	5				5	100
2.5 or less	33	Slight hypoaesthesia	1	3	32	97

(from Dundee & Wyant, 1974; Taffe, 1982; Dundee, 1983).

Extradural thiopentone

There have been four case reports of the inadvertent extradural administration of thiopentone (Forestner & Raj, 1975; Brownridge, 1984; Cay, 1984). All were with 2.0–2.5% solutios, and volumes up to 20 ml were injected. One patient, during a caudal injection, complained of burning pain in the buttocks and legs. When the mistake was realised, saline was injected and there were no permanent sequelae. In another case the injection of 15 ml of 2% thiopentone into the epidural space produced only slight discomfort. When the mistake was realised a mixture of 0.5% bupivacaine and 1.5% lignocaine was injected into the epidural catheter and attempts made at lavage through a lower catheter. The block had resolved completely in two hours and the patient expressed no discomfort, numbness or paraesthesia.

This combination of local analgesics was used in a further patient who had been given 10 ml of 2.5% thiopentone into the epidural space via the sacral hiatus. The injection was slightly painful but the pain was relieved by the local anaesthetic. This patient complained of pain in the anus for four hours after induction but apart from transient urinary retention there were no permanent sequelae. In one patient inadvertently given 20 ml of 2.5% thiopentone extradurally for caesarean section the baby required 3 min of assisted ventilation and had a low Apgar score at birth and at 24 h postoperatively. No neurological changes were detected in the mother.

The treatment in these patients varied from attempting to dilute the thiopentone and attempting to precipitate it with an acid local anaesthetic — a mixture of 20 ml 0.5% bupivacaine and 20 ml 1% lignocaine has a pH of 6.5 and when mixed with 10 ml of 2.5% thiopentone at a pH of 8.2 the mixture forms a precipitate of thiopentone crystals (Cay, 1984). Bupivacaine 0.5% has a pH of 5.8 and perhaps this should be the drug to inject into the epidural space after such an accident. This lowers pH and gives pain relief but it does precipitate thiopentone in the extradural space. If a catheter is still in situ it would seem that dilution of the thiopentone with isotonic saline might be a another possible treatment.

MISCELLANEOUS

Intraocular pressure

Given alone thiopentone will lower intraocular pressure (Joshi & Bruce, 1975). If the administration is followed by suxamethonium it will return the intraocular pressure to normal but if two minutes elapse between thiopentone and suxamethonium intraocular pressure will rise slightly above preanaesthetic levels. More important than either of these drug effects is the significant rise in intraocular pressure which occurs with tracheal intubation.

Histamine release

Using a highly sensitive and specific method for the determination of histamine in human plasma, Lorenz et al (1972) demonstrated that following clinical doses of thiopentone the level of histamine in plasma increased significantly to about 350% of normal. This had dropped to within almost normal limits within 10 min. The injection of saline does not produce this effect. Stimulation of gastric secretions has also been demonstrated after thiopentone accompanied by a fall in basophils suggesting that the histamine in plasma is in a free pharmacologically active form. This observation is of no clinical significance in normal subjects. To date, marked rises in histamine in cases of thiopentone anaphylaxis have not been reported.

Skin rashes

A transient urticarial rash often follows the use of barbiturates. It involves the upper chest and sometimes extends to the neck and face. This occurs with all the drugs and is probably a true allergic response. Occasionally the erythema might progress to vescicles as reported with phenobarbitone. Another type of rash is blotchy, rather than uniform, and is referred to as 'cutis mormorata'.

Delayed reactions

Delayed reactions to thiopentone have been reported by Lemere et al (1952) in 32 out of 1037 patients given an average of 15 administrations of thiopentone as an adjuvant to the treatment of chronic alcoholism. The most common was general malaise with aching, weakness and fever up to 43°C (109°F). This reaction came on from 1 to 24 h after thiopentone and lasted from one to five days unless treated. It sometimes appeared after the first treatment, but usually manifested itself with increasing severity after several treatments has been given. Generalised skin rashes, joint pains and in one case a monoarticular arthritis were also observed. The prompt response of these reactions to ACTH suggests that they might be allergic in nature, but infection from syringes or needles has not been excluded. They have not been observed when amylobarbitone has been substituted for thiopentone.

The fact that delayed reactions after thiopentone have only been reported once in the literature does not necessarily mean that their incidence is very low. After operation other more likely causes are sought to explain the occurrence of pyrexia and other reactions. This also applies when the drug is used with electroconvulsive therapy.

Plasma electrolytes

In animal experiments, Stevenson (1960) found no change in plasma calcium or magnesium concentrations, but a slight fall in potassium after thiopentone. This latter was shown by List (1967) to apply in humans. List, and a number of subsequent workers (Bali et al, 1975a, b; Chestnutt et al, 1985), also found that thiopentone reduced the rise of serum potassium after suxamethonium as compared with patients given halothane. Haw (1972) found that thiopentone had a greater protective action in this respect than methohexitone.

Nausea and vomiting

It is generally agreed that intravenous barbiturates are followed by less sickness than inhalational anaesthetics and that induction with one of these agents reduces emetic sequelae.

The relative emetic effects of different induction agents have been examined in a number of studies which show little difference in the incidence after thiopentone and methohexitone, but both barbiturates were followed by less sickness than either propanidid or ketamine, but more than Althesin (Clarke et al, 1971).

ACUTE SENSITIVITY STATES

Much of what has been said about the action of barbiturates on the body refers to the response of reasonably fit patients. However, even in such patients there is a great variation in response to 'normal doses' of intravenous barbiturates. Certain pathological states and/or drugs engender in patients an acute sensitivity to the barbiturates.

Patients might exhibit an acute anaphylactoid reaction to these induction agents and this is of sufficient importance as to merit separate consideration in Chapter 14.

Elderly patients are, on the whole, more susceptible to the intravenous barbiturates but this might not wholly be due to age *per se*. These people are likely to have some impairment of cerebral, cardiovascular, respiratory or hepatic function, including a slow circulation time. In contrast to the elderly, young children are relatively resistant to these drugs and proportionately larger doses are required for anaesthesia.

Smaller doses are required to induce sleep in patients with renal and liver dysfunction, because of decreased binding in conjunction with low plasma protein levels. A similar sensitivity is exhibited by patients whose level of consciousness is already depressed by drugs or who have some degree of brain damage; the duration of sleep might also be prolonged in these patients.

Synergistic drugs are not limited to barbiturates and other sedatives but include the opiates and certain phenothiazines and benzodiazepines. By the same token, acquired tolerance to any of these drugs will induce cross tolerance to the barbiturates.

Factors which influence the redistribution of drugs will also make patients more sensitive to their cerebral effects. These include uraemia (Dundee & Richards, 1954) and peripheral circulatory failure. The action of thiopentone is also prolonged in severe anaemia (Dundee, 1952a) where plasma binding might be reduced and cerebral cells rendered more susceptible to depressants by prolonged hypoxia (Peterson et al, 1950).

In clinical practice Csogor & Kerek (1970) have shown that 0.1 mg kg^{-1} of 40% sulphafurazole solution significantly reduced the dose of thiopentone required to induce sleep and anaesthesia; this is in agreement with previous animal experiments (Csogor & Papp, 1969). It might be due to interference with the binding of thiopentone to albumin, a factor which might contribute to the potentiating effect of meprobamate in barbiturate narcosis (Di Maggio & Ciacere, 1969). There are no reports of overaction of barbiturates in patients given sulphafurazole, either by tablets or syrup for respiratory or urinary infection or dysentry or as eye drops for infection or trachoma, but this possibility must be borne in mind. The reduction of the induction dose of thiopentone in patients pretreated with soluble aspirin or probenecid has already been discussed. This also applies to the parenteral opiates fentanyl and alfentanil.

Animal experiments suggest that abnormal sensitivity might also occur in patients on disulfiram therapy, or after infusion of hypertonic dextrose, but the clinical importance of these phenomena is not known.

Conditions which render the cardiovascular system unduly susceptible to the barbiturates have already been discussed. The hypotensive effect is greater in the upright or sitting position and these postural effects apply to all types of patients. Asthmatics and the so-called 'vagotonic' subjects are more likely than normal patients to get bronchospasm, laryngospasm, cough or hiccup after the barbiturates, but these effects can be minimized by the slow injection of small doses. Respiratory depression will be greater after opiate premedication and is more likely to occur in patients suffering from dystrophia myotonica (Dundee, 1952b; Hewer, 1957; Lodge, 1958) and myasthenia gravis. The abnormal response of a myotonic patient is probably not specific to barbiturates as they can be unduly sensitive to any central respiratory depressant (Kaufman, 1960).

One might suspect the safety of the barbiturates in patients with varying haemoglobinopathies, e.g. the risk of haemolysis in patients with sickle-cell states. This, however, is not mentioned by Gilbertson (1965) or by Gilbertson & Boulton (1967) in extensive surveys of anaesthetic problems in West African patients with sickle-cell anaemia, haemoglobin SC disease and sickle-cell trait. Avoidance of hypoxia, acidosis, stasis and cooling seems to be more important than the choice of anaesthetic.

Porphyria

Porphyria is an inborn error of metabolism associated with disturbances in porphyrin metabolism and the excretion of porphyrin in the urine. It is characterised by symptoms chiefly associated with the skin and the nervous and alimentary systems. Porphyrins are pigments that possess a basic structure of four pyrrole rings linked by methane bridges. They are found in chlorophyll, haemoglobin and some of the cytochrome and peroxidase systems. They are formed from the percursors, Δ-aminolevulinic acid (ALA) and porphobilinogen. In the liver, ALA synthetase catalyses the rate limiting reaction for haeme production, i.e. the formation of ALA from succinate and glycine within the mitochondria. It therefore controls the rate of synthesis of haeme and porphyrin. ALA synthetase is increased in some types of porphyria.

Exacerbation of acute porphyria in patients who are normally asymptomatic might be precipitated by drugs, hormones and liver disease. Among the drugs which can induce clinical and biochemical manifestations of acute porphyria are the barbiturates, some anticonvulsants, oestrogens, contraceptives and alcohol. For this reason, thiopentone and other intravenous anaesthetics of this group are contraindicated in porphyria. Some of the drugs that precipitate attacks of acute intermittent porphyria increase hepatic ALA synthetase activity, thus compounding the biochemical upset.

Not every type of porphyria is adversely affected by the barbiturates (Leading Article, 1985) but the outcome of administering these drugs to susceptible patients can be so serious that thiopentone should not be given to any of them. Reports of cases are analysed in Appendix 5. In these, 125 attacks of porphyria occurred in 116 patients of whom 65 developed paralysis and 17 died; thiopentone was given 92 times followed by paralysis in 36 (39%) and death in 11 (12%). Eales (1966) found that thiopentone anaesthesia featured in nearly 30% of patients experiencing acute porphyric attacks, half of which were of very great severity. Although Dean (1963) has stated that thiopentone always precipitates an attack of acute porphyria, subsequent reports have shown that this is not so. Ward (1965) reports a 6% incidence of serious complications in 36 barbiturate inductions in known porphyrias (type not stated). A more recent survey (Leading Article, 1985) considers that at least 60% of acute attacks are induced by drugs and that about 5% of attacks severe enough to warrant hospitalisation end fatally. One agrees with the views of Eales (1966) that thiopentone is sufficiently frequently followed by catastrophic attacks as to contraindicate its use. Two attacks have been reported after thialbarbitone but none after methohexitone. In view of the sequelae following other oxybarbiturates it is likely that this latter is due to anaesthetists becoming aware of the dangers of giving any barbiturate.

The term porphyria covers a group of diseases and although, as mentioned above, not all of these are adversely affected by the barbiturates the outcome is so serious that the different types are discussed in detail in Appendix 5.

DRUGS OTHER THAN THIOPENTONE

Reference has frequently been made to *methohexitone* (Brevital, Brietal) and Table 8.6 summarises the important differences between it and thiopentone.

Table 8.6 Clinically important difference between thiopentone and methohexitone.

	Thiopentone	*Methohexitone*
Chemistry	Thiobarbiturate	Methyl-(oxy)-barbiturate
Solution	Slight yellow colouration	Colourless
Usual concentration w/v	2.0–2.5%	1%
Extravenous effects	Concentration related	Less serious than with thiopentone
Relative potency	1	2.5–3.0
Induction	Usually smooth	Frequent excitatory effects*
CVS	Moderate hypotension	Slightly less hypotension, tachcardia
Respiration	Transient apnoea	Frequent cough and hiccough*
Recovery	Smooth	Smooth, more rapid than with thiopentone

* Both reduced by slow injection, excitatory effects by opioid pretreatment and respiratory complications by atropine or hyoscine.

Apart from possibly being slightly more potent, *thiamylal* (Surital) is indistinguishable from thiopentone, as shown by two large comparative studies (Barron et al, 1966; Tovell et al, 1955). Likewise, apart from being about two-thirds as potent, *thiobutobarbitone* (Inactin; Inaktin) is likewise indistinguishable from thiopentone (Dundee & Riding, 1960).

Hexobarbitone, the original Evipan (Evipal, Cyclonal) still has a limited use. It is slightly more than half as potent as thiopentone and is used in a 5 or 10% solution. The latter may be difficult to dissolve fully. Being a barbiturate, it is a clear solution and having a methyl side chain (Table 5.3) it causes an incidence of excitatory effects similar to methohexitone, although the clinical impression is of coarser movements which last longer. Again, unsubstantiated by scientific data is the impression that recovery is more prolonged after hexobarbitone than following equivalent doses of thiopentone.

REFERENCES

Adriani J, Rovenstine E A 1943 The effect of anaesthetic drugs upon bronchi and bronchioles of excized lung tissue. Anesthesiology 4: 253–262

Allen E M, Male C G 1982 Methohexital is not contraindicated in epileptics. Anesthesiology 56: 240–241

Altenburg B M, Michenfelder J D, Theye R A 1969 Acute tolerance to thiopental in canine cerebral oxygen consumption studies. Anesthesiology 31: 443–448

Bali I M, Dundee J W, Assaf R A E 1975a Immediae changes in plasma potassium, sodium and chloride concentrations induced by suxamethonium. British Journal of Anaesthesia 47: 393–397

Bali I M, Dundee J W, Doggart J R 1975b The source of increased plasma potassium following succinylcholine. Anesthesia and Analgesia . . .Current Researches 54: 680–686

Barratt R L, Graham G G, Torda T A 1984 Kinetics of thiopentone in relation to the site of sampling. British Journal of Anaesthesia 56: 1385–1391

Barron D W 1968 Effect of rate of injection on incidence of side effects with thiopental and methohexital. Anesthesia and Analgesia . . . Current Researches 47: 174–176

Barron D W, Dundee J W 1967 Clinical studies of induction agents. XVII: Relation between dosage and side effects of intravenous barbiturates. British Journal of Anaesthesia 39: 24–30

Barron D W, Dundee J W, Gilmore W R, Howard P J 1966 Clinical studies of induction agents. XVI: A comparison of thiopentone, buthalitone, hexobarbitone and thiamylal as induction agents. British Journal of Anaesthesia 38: 802–811

Bass W P, Watts D T, Chase H F 1953 Ether hyperglycemia as influenced by premedication and pentothal induction. Anesthesiology 14: 18–22

Becker K E. 1978 Plasma levels of thiopental necessary for anesthesia. Anesthesiology 49: 192–196

Becker K E, Tonnesen A S 1978 Cardiovascular effects of plasma levels of thiopental necessary for anesthesia. Anesthesiology 49: 197–200

Bittrich N M, Kane A V'R, Mosher R W 1963 Methohexital and its effect on liver function tests. Anesthesiology 24: 81–90

Blunnie W P, McIlroy P D A, Merrett J D, Dundee J W 1983 Cardiovascular and biochemical evidence of stress during major surgery associated with different techniques of anaesthesia. British Journal of Anaesthesia 55: 611–618

Blunnie W P, Zacharias M, Dundee J W, Doggart J R, Moore J, McIlroy P D A 1981 Liver enzyme studies with continuous intravenous anaesthesia. Anaesthesia 36: 152–156

Booker W M 1946 Observations on carbohydrate metabolism during prolonged pentothal anaesthesia in dogs. 1: The blood sugar and liver glycogen. Anesthesiology 7: 405–415

Booker W M, French D M, Molano P A 1949 Further observations on the effect of prolonged thiopental (Pentothal) anesthesia on metabolism of carbohydrates and proteins in dogs. Journal of Pharmacology 96: 145–150

Booker W M, Maloney A H, Tureman J R, Ratcliff C 1952 Some metabolic factors influencing the course of thiopental anesthesia in dogs. American Journal of Physiology 170: 168–172

Boston V, Unkles R 1969 Methohexitone and epilepsy. British Dental Journal 126:394

Bovill J G, Coppel D L, Dundee J W, Moore J 1971 Current status of ketamine anaesthesia. Lancet i: 1285–1288

Brand L, Mazzia V D B, van Poznak A, Burns J J, Mark L C 1961 Lack of correlation between encephalographic effects and plasma concentrations of thiopentone. British Journal of Anaesthesia 33: 92–96

Brazier M A B 1954 Brain mechanisms and consciousness. Oxford: Blackwell

Brazier M A B 1961 Some effects of anaesthesia on the brain. British Journal of Anaesthesia 33: 194–204

Brazier M A B 1963 Electrophysiological effects of barbiturates on the brain. In: Root W S and Hofmann F G (eds) Physiological pharmacology, vol 1, Academic Press, New York, p 219

Brazier M A B, Finesinger J E 1945 Action of barbiturates on cerebral cortex: electroencephalographic studies. Archives of Neurology and Psychiatry 53: 51–58

Brodie B B, Mark L C, Lief P A, Bernstein E, Papper E M 1951 Acute tolerance to thiopental. Journal of Pharmacology and Experimental Therapeutics 102:215

Brown G L,, von Euler U S 1938 The after effects of a tetanus on mammalian muscle. Journal of Physiology 93: 39–60

Brown S S, Lyons S M, Dundee J W 1968 Intra-arterial barbiturates: a study of some factors leading to intravascular thrombosis. British Journal of Anaesthsia 40: 13–19

Brownridge P 1984 More on epidural thiopentone. Anaesthesia and Intensive Care 12: 270–271

Bruckner J B, Gethmann J W, Patschke D, Tarnow J, Weymar A 1974 Untersuchungen zur Wirkung von Etomidate auf den Kreislauf des Menschen. Anaesthesist 23: 322–330

Burn J H 1960 Why thiopentone injected into an artery may cause gangrene. British Medical Journal ii: 414–416

Burn J H, Hobbs R 1959 Mechanism of arterial spasm following intra-arterial injection of thiopentone. Lancet i: 1112–1115

Burney R G, Winn R 1975 Increased cerebrospinal fluid pressure during laryngoscopy and intubation for induction of anaesthesia. Anesthesia and Analgesia 54: 687–690

Carraway B M 1939 Pentothal sodium with nasal oxygen: a report of 3810 consecutive cases. Current Researches in Anesthesia and Analgesia 18: 259–269

Carson I W, Alexander J P, Hewitt J C, Dundee J W 1972 Clinical studies of induction agents. XLI: Venous sequelae following the use of the steroid anaesthetic agent, Althesin. British Journal of Anaesthesia 44: 1311–1313

Carson I W, Clarke, R S J, Dundee J W 1973 Interaction of suxamethonium with intravenous induction agents. British Journal of Pharmacology 47:679P

Cay D L 1984 Accidental epidural thiopentone. Anaesthesia and Intensive Care 12: 61–63

Chamberlain J H, Sede R G F L, Chung D C W 1977 Effect of thiopentone on myocardial function. British Journal of Anaesthesia 49: 865–870

Chestnutt W N, Lowry K G, Dundee J W, Pandit S K, Mirakhur R K 1985 Failure of two benzodiazepines to prevent suxamethonium-induced muscle pain. Anaesthesia 40: 263–269

Christensen J H, Andreasen F, Jansen J A 1985 Increased thiopental sensitivity in cardiac patients. Acta Anaesthesiologica Scandinavica 29: 702–705

Clark D L, Rosner B S 1973 Neurophysiologic effects of general anesthetics: I: The electroencephalogram and sensory evoked responses in man. Anesthesiology 38: 564–582

Clarke R S J 1968 Clinical studies of induction agents. XXIV: The influence of anaesthesia with thiopentone and propanidid on the blood sugar level. British Journal of Anaesthesia 40: 46–52

Clarke R S J, Dundee J W, Carson I W, Arora M, McCaughey W 1972 Clinical studies of induction agents. XL: Althesin with various premedicants. British Journal of Anaesthesia 44: 845–848

Clarke R S J, Dundee J W, Daw R H 1964 Clinical studies of induction agents. XI: The influence of some intravenous anaesthetics on the respiratory effects and sequelae of suxamethonium. British Journal of Anaesthesia 36: 307–311

Clarke R S J, Dundee J W, Hamilton R C 1967 Interactions between induction agents and muscle relaxants. Anaesthesia 22: 235–248

Clarke R S J, Kirwan M J, Dundee J W, Neill D W, Mitchell E S 1965 Clinical studies of induction agents. XIII: Liver function after propanidid and thiopentone anaesthesia. British Journal of Anaesthesia 37: 415–421

Clarke R S J, Montgomery S J, Dundee J W, Bovill J G 1971 Clinical studies of induction agents. XXXIX: CT 1341, a new steroid anaesthetic. British Journal of Anaesthesia 43: 947–952

Clutton-Brock J 1961 Pain and the barbiturates. Anaesthesia 16: 80–99

Cohen S M 1948 Accidental intra-arterial injection of drugs. Lancet 2: 361–371 and 409–416

Coleman J, Green R A 1960 Methohexital: a short acting barbiturate. Anaesthesia 15: 411–423

Comroe J H Jr, Dripps R D, Botelho S Y, Metz H 1947 The curare-like action of ether upon human neuromuscular transmission. Federation Proceedings 6:318

Conway C M, Ellis D B 1969 The haemodynamic effects of short acting barbiturates. British Journal of Anaesthesia 41: 534–542

Cooperman L H 1972 Effects of anaesthetics on the splanchnic circulation. British Journal of Anaesthesia 44: 967–970

Cooperman L H, Warden J C, Prize H L 1968 Splanchnic circulation during nitrous oxide-oxygen anesthesia and hypocarbia in man. Anesthesiology 29: 254–258

Cote C J, Goudsouzian N G, Liu L M P, Dedrick D F, Firestone S 1981 Thiopental: a dose-response study in unpremedicated children. Anesthesia and Analgesia 60: 246–247

Cote C J, Goudsouzian N G, Liu L M, Dedrick P F, Rosow C W 1981 The dose response to intravenous thiopental for induction of general anaesthesia in unpremedicated children. Anesthesiology 55: 703–705

Craig H J L 1964 The protective effect of thiopentone against muscular pain and stiffness which follows the use of suxamethonium chloride. British Journal of Anaesthesia 36: 612–619

Crankshaw D P, Allt-graham J 1978 ED_{50} values for thiopentone, methohexital, propanidid and alfathesin: a clinical experiment. Anaesthesia and Intensive Care 6: 36–43

Csogor S I, Kerek S F 1970 Enhancement of thiopentone anaesthesia by sulpha-furazole. British Journal of Anaesthesia 42: 988–990

Csogor S I, Papp J 1969 Competition between diffusible drugs for the binding sites of plasma proteins. Sixth meeting of the Federation of European Biochemical Society. Madrid. Abstracts of Communications, p 115

Cunitz G, Danhauser I, Wickbold 1978 Comparative investigations on the influence of etomidate, thiopentone and methohexitone on the intracranial pressure of patients. Anaesthesist 27: 64–70

Davies D D 1979 Local complications of thiopentone injection. A further report. British Journal of Anaesthesia 51: 1147–1149

Dean G 1963 The Porphyrias. Pitman, London

de Wardener H E 1955 Renal circulation during anaesthesia and surgery. Anaesthesia 10: 18–33

Dhruva A J 1960 Intramuscular use of pentothal sodium as an aid to pediatric anesthesia. Anesthesia and Analgesia, Current Researches 39: 236–239

Dille J M, Horita A 1955 Actions of thiopental on laryngeal reflex. Federation Proceedings 14:333

Di Maggio G, Ciacere G 1969 The influence of meprobamate on binding of pentothal by plasma proteins. Fourth International Congress on Pharmacology Basel. Abstracts of Communications, p. 449

Doenicke A, Gabanyi D, Lemce H, Schurk-Bulich M 1974 Kreislaufverhalten und Myocardfunktion nach drei kurzwirkenden i.v. Hypnotica Etomidate, Propanidid, Methohexital. Anaesthesist 23: 108–115

Doenicke A, Kugler J, Laub M 1967 Evaluation of recovery and 'street fitness' by EEG and psychodiagnostic tests after anaesthesia. Canadian Anaesthetists' Society Journal, 14: 567–583

Doenicke A, Kugler J, Schellenberger A, Gurtner T 1966 Recovery time after intravenous anaesthesia measured by electroencephalography. British Journal of Anaesthesia 38: 580–590

Doenicke A, Wagner E, Beetz K H 1973 Blutgasanalysen (arteriell) nach drei kurzwirkenden i.v. Hypnotika (Propanidid, Etomidate and Methohexital). Anaesthesist 22: 353–356

Dreisbach R, Snyder F F 1943 The effect on the fetus of pentobarbitone sodium and pentothal sodium. Journal of Pharmacology and Experimental Therapeutics 79: 250–258

Dripps R D, Dumke P R 1943 The effects of narcotics on the balance between central and chemoreceptor control of respiration. Journal of Pharmacology and Experimental Therapeutics 77: 290–300

Duncan B B A, Zaimi F, Newman G B, Jenkins J G, Aveling W 1984 Effect of premedication on the induction dose of thiopentone in children. Anaesthesia 39: 426–428

Dundee J W 1952a The use of thiopentone in anaemic patients. Journal of the Irish Medical Association 31: 351–356

Dundee J W 1952b Thiopentone in dystrophic myotonia. Anesthesia and Analgesia, Current Researches 31: 257–262

Dundee J W 1955 Thiopental as a factor in the production of liver dysfunction. British Journal of Anaesthesia 27: 14–23

Dundee J W 1956a Thiopentone and other Thiobarbiturates. Livingstone, Edinburgh.

Dundee J W 1956b Effect of thiopentone on blood sugar and glucose tolerance. British Journal of Pharmacology 11: 458–461

Dundee J W 1960 Alterations in response to somatic pain. II: The effect of thiopentone and pentobarbitone. British Journal of Anaesthesia 32: 407–414

Dundee J W 1964 Alterations in response to somatic pain associated with anaesthesia. XVI: Methohexitone. British Journal of Anaesthesia 36: 798–800

Dundee J W 1965a Some effects of premedication in the induction characteristics of intravenous anaesthetics. Anaesthesia 20: 299–314

Dundee J W 1965b The Anesthetist and Analgesia. In: Eckenhoff J E (ed) Science and practice in anesthesia. Lipincott, Philadelphia, p 28–34

Dundee J W (1979) Current topics in anaesthesia. 1: Intravenous anaesthetic agents. Arnold, London

Dundee J W 1983 Intra-arterial thiopental. Anesthesiology 59: 154–155

Dundee J W, Fee J P H, Moore J, McIlroy P D A, Wilson D B 1980 Changes in serum enzyme levels following ketamine infusions. Anaesthesia 35: 12–16

Dundee J W, Hassard T H 1983 The influence of haemoglobin and plasma urea levels on the induction dose of thiopentone. Anaesthesia 38: 26–28

Dundee J W, Hassard T H, McGowan W A W, Henshaw J 1982 The 'induction' dose of thiopentone. A method of study and preliminary illustrative results. Anaesthesia 37: 1176–1184

Dundee J W, Price H L, Dripps R D 1956 Acute tolerance to thiopentone in man. British Journal of Anaesthesia 28: 344–352

Dundee J W, Richards R K 1954 Effect of azotemia upon the action of intravenous barbiturate anesthesia. Anesthesiology 15: 333–346

Dundee J W, Riding J E 1960 A comparison of Inactin and thiopentone as intravenous anaesthetics. British Journal of Anaesthesia 32: 206–218

Dundee J W, Todd U 1958 Clinical signifiance of the effects of thiopentone and adjuvant drugs on blood sugar and glucose tolerance. British Journal of Anaesthesia 30: 77–82

Dundee J W, Wyant G M 1974 Intravenous Anaesthesia. Churchill Livingstone, Edinburgh and London

Dunkin L J 1972 Methohexitone in the management of a disturbed patient. British Medical Journal 44: 971–974

Eales L 1966 Porphyria and thiopentone. Anesthesiology 27: 703–704

Eckenhoff J E, Helrich M 1958 Study of narcotics and sedatives for use in preanaesthetic medication. Journal of the American Medical Association 167: 415–422

Eckstein J W, Hamilton W K, McCammond J M 1961 The effect of thiopentalon peripheral venous tone. Anesthesiology 22: 525–528

Edwards R, Ellis F R 1973 Clinical significance of thiopentone binding to haemoglobin and plasma protein. British Journal of Anaesthesia 45: 891–893

Elder J D, Nagano S M, Eastwood D W, Harnagel D 1955 Circulatory changes associated with thiopental anesthesia in man. Anesthesiology 16: 394–400

Etsten B, Himwich H E 1946 Signs and stages of pentothal anesthesia: physiologic basis. Anesthesiology 7: 536–548

Etsten B, Li T 1955 Hemodynamic changes during thiopental anesthesia in humans: cardiac output, stroke volume, total peripheral resistance and intrathoracic blood volume. Journal of Clinical Investigation 34: 500–510

Etsten B, York G E, Himwich H E 1946 Pattern of metabolic depression induced with pentothal sodium. Archives of Neurology and Psychiatry 56: 171–183

Fairlie C, Barso T P, French A B, Jones C M, Beecher H K 1951 Metabolic effects of anaesthesia in man. IV: A comparison of the effects of certain anesthetic agents on the normal liver. New England Journal of Medicine 244: 615–622

Fieldman E J, Ridley R W, Wood E H 1955 Hemodynamic studies during thiopental sodium and nitrous oxide anesthesia in humans. Anesthesiology 16: 473–489

Filner B E, Karliner J S 1976 Alterations of normal left ventricular performance by general anesthesia. Anesthesiology 45: 610–621

Finesinger J E, Brazier M A B, Tucci J H, Miles H H W 1947 Study of levels of consciousness based on electroencephalographic data in pentothal anesthesia. Transactions of the American Neurological Association 72: 183–185

Flickinger H, Fraimow W, Cathcart R T, Nealon T F 1961 Effect of thiopental induction on cardiac output in man. Anesthesia and Analgesia. . .Current Researches 40: 693–700

Forestner J E, Raj P P 1975 Inadvertent epidural injection of thiopental: a case report. Anesthesia and Analgesia . . . Current Researches 55: 406–407

Galley A H 1963 Methohexitone (discussion). Proceedings of the Royal Society of Medicine 56: 377–378

Gilbertson A 1965 Anaesthesia in West African patients with sickle-cell anaemia, haemoglobin S C disease and sick-cell train. British Journal of Anaesthesia 37: 614–622

Gilbertson A A, Boulton T B 1967 Anaesthesia in difficult situations. VI: the influence of disease on preoperative preparation and choice of anaesthetic. Anaesthesia 22: 607–630

Golden R F, Mann F C 1943 The effects of drugs used in anesthesiology on the tone and motility of the small intestine: an experimental study. Anesthesiology 4: 577–595

Goldsmith M W, Holmes F 1957 Thiopentone and carbohydrate metabolism. Anaesthesia 12: 321–325
Gross E C, Cullen S C 1943 The effects of anesthetic agents on muscular contraction. Journal of Pharmacology and Experimental Therapeutics 78: 358–365
Gruber C M, Gruber C M Jr 1941 Effect of barbituric and thiobarbituric acid derivatives on pyloric sphincter and stomach in unanesthetised dogs. Journal of Pharmacology and Experimental Therapeutics 72: 176–183
Habif D V, Papper E M, Fitzpatric H F, Lawrence P, Smyth C McC, Bradley S E 1951 The renal and hepatic blood flow, glomerular filtration rate and urinary output of electrolytes during cyclopropane, ether and thiopental anesthesia, operation and the immediate postoperative period. Surgery 30: 241–255
Haggendal E 1965 Blood flow autoregulation on the cerebral grey matter with comments on its mechanism. Acta Neurologica Scandinavica, Suppl 14, 104–120
Hall G M 1985 The anaesthetic modification of the endocrine-metabolic response to surgery. Annals of the Royal College of Surgeons of England. 61: 25–29
Hall G M, Young C, Holdcroft A, Alaghband Zadeh J 1978 Substrate mobilisation during surgery: a comparison between halothane and fentanyl anaesthesia. Anaesthesia 33: 924–930
Harper A M 1965 Physiology of cerebral blood flow. British Journal of Anaesthesia 37: 225–235
Harrison G 1949 The pulse during anaesthesia with pentothal and curare. Anaesthesia 4: 181–187
Harrison G 1953 Arrhythmia during kemithal anaesthesia. British Journal of Anaesthesia 25: 204–211
Harrison G A 1962 The influence of different anaesthetic agents on the response to respiratory tract irritation. British Journal of Anaesthesia 34: 804–811
Haslett W H K, Dundee J W 1968 Clinical studies of induction agents XXIII: Reduction of respiratory complications by scopolamine and atropine. Anesthesia and Analgesia. . .Current Researches 47: 174–176
Hasselstrom L, Kristoffersen M B 1979 Hepatitis following thiopentone A case report. British Journal of Anaesthesia 51: 801–804
Hausner E, Essex H E, Mann F C 1938 Roentgenologic observations of spleen of dog under ether, sodium amytal, pentobarbital sodium and pentothal. American Journal of Physiology 121: 387–391
Haw M E 1972 Variation in serum potassium during electroconvulsive therapy in patients anaesthetised with thiopentone and methohexitone. British Journal of Anaesthesia 44: 707–711
Herrschaft H, Schmidt H 1973 Behaviour of global and original cerebral blood flow under propanidid, ketamine and sodium thiopentone. Anaesthesist 22: 486–495
Herrschaft, H, Schmidt H 1974 The effect of methohexitone sodium on global and regional blood flow in man. Anaesthesist 23: 340–344
Hewer C L 1957 Thiopentone in dystrophic myotonia. British Journal of Anaesthesia 29:180
Himwich W A, Homburger E, Maresca R, Himwich H E 1947 Brain metabolism in man: unanesthetised and in pentothal narcosis. American Journal in Psychiatry 103: 689–696
Hirshman C A, Peters J, Cartwright-Lee I 1982 Leucocyte histamine release to thiopental. Anesthesiology 56: 64–67
Homburger E, Himwich W A, Etsten B, York G, Maresca R, Himwich H E 1946 Effect of pentothal anesthesia on canine cerebral cortex. American Journal of Physiology 147: 343–345
Hrubetz M C, Blackberg S N 1938 Influence of nembutal, pentothal, seconal, amytal, pentobarbital and chloroform on blood sugar concentration and carbohydrate mobilisation. American Journal of Physiology 122: 759–764
Hudson R J, Stanski D R, Burch P A 1982 Comparative pharmacokinetics of methohexital and thiopental. Anesthesiology 57:A240
Hudson R J, Stanski D R, Saidman L J, Meathe E 1983 A model for studying depth of anesthesia and acute tolerance to thiopental. Anesthesiology 59: 301–308
Hunter A R 1954 Die schmerz-betaubung bei intrakraniellen operationen. Anaesthesist 3:65
Hunter A R 1972 Thiopentone supplemented anaesthesia for neurosurgery. British Journal of Anaesthesia 44: 506–510
Jacobson I, Harper A M, McDowall D G 1963 Relationship between venous pressure and cortical blood flow. Nature (London) 200:173
Johnstone M 1951 Pulse irregularities during thiopentone anaesthesia. Anaesthesia 6: 138–143
Joshi C, Bruce B L 1975 Thiopental and succinylcholine action on intraocular pressure. Anesthesia and Analgesia 54: 471–475
Kane P O, Smith S E 1959 Thiopentone and buthalitone: the relationship between depth of anaesthesia, plasma concentration and plasma protein binding. British Journal of Pharmacology and Chemotherapy 14: 261–264
Katz R L, Epstein R A 1968 The interaction of anesthetic agents and adrenergic drugs to produce cardiac arrhythmias. Anesthesiology 29: 763–784
Katz R L, Matteo R S, Papper E M 1962 The injection of epinephrine during general anesthesia with halogenated hydrocarbons and cyclopropane in man. 2: Halothane. Anesthesiology 23: 597–600
Kaufman L 1960 Anaesthesia in dystrophic myotonia. Proceedings of the Royal Society of Medicine 53: 183–188
Kawar P, Briggs L P, Bahar M, McIlroy P D A, Dundee J W, Merrett J D, Nesbitt G S 1982 Liver enzyme studies with disoprofol (ICI 35868) and midazolam. Anaesthesia 37: 305–308
Keats A S 1965 Pain, analgesia and anti-analgesia. Anesthesiology 26: 1–2
Keown J K, Fisher S M, Downing D F, Hitchcock P 1957 Cardiac catheterization in infants and children. Anesthesiology 18: 270–274
Kettler D, Sonntag H, Donath U, Regensburger D, Schenk H D 1974 Hamodynamik, Myokardmechanik, Sauerstoffbedarf und Sauerstoffversorgung des menschlichen Herzens unter Narkoseeinleitung mit Etomidate. Anaesthesist 23: 116–121
Kiersey D K, Bickford R G, Faulconer A 1951 EEG patterns produced by thiopental sodium during surgical operations: description and classification. British Journal of Anaesthesia 23: 141–152
Kinmonth J B, Shepherd R C 1959 Accidental injection of thiopentone into arteries. British Medical Journal ii: 914–918
Knill R L, Bright S, Manninen P 1978 Hypoxic ventilatory responses during thiopentone sedation in man. Canadian Anaesthetists' Society Journal 25: 366–372
Kraatz C P, Gluckman M I 1954 The actions of barbiturates on the contractions of voluntary muscle. Journal of Pharmacology and Experimental Therapeutics 111: 120–129

Leading Article 1985 Latent acute hepatic porphyria. Lancet i: 197–198
Lemere F, Berard W, O'Halloran P 1952 Thiopentone (pentothal) reactions and their treatment with ACTH. Anesthesiology 13: 86–88
Levy M L, Palazzi H M, Nardi G L, Bunker J P 1961 Hepatic blood flow variations during surgical anesthesia in man, measured by radioactive colloid. Surgery, Gynecology and Obstetrics 112: 289–294
List W F 1975 Digitalis-thiopentone effects on myocardial function. Anaesthesia 30: 624–629
List W F 1967 Serum potassium changes during induction of anesthesia. British Journal of Anaesthesia 39: 480–484
Lodge A B 1958 Thiopentone sensitivity and dystrophia myotonica. British Medical Journal i: 1043–1044
Lorenz W, Doenicke A, Meyer R, Reimann H J, Kusche J, Barth H, Geesing M, Hutzel M, Weissenbacher B 1972 Histamine release in man by propanidid and thiopentone: pharmacological effects and clinical consequences. British Journal of Anaesthesia 44: 355–369
Lyons S M, Clarke R S J 1972 A comparison of different drugs for anaesthesia in cardiac surgical patients. British Journal of Anaesthesia 44: 575–583
MacCannell K L, Dresel P E 1964 Potentiation of thiopental by cyclopropane-adrenaline cardiac arrhythmias. Canadian Journal of Physiology and Pharmacology 42: 627–639
McDowall D G 1971 The cerebral circulation. In: Gray T C, Nunn J F (eds) General anaesthesia, 3rd edn. vol 1, Butterworth, London, ch 18, p 272–290
Macintosh R R, Heyworth P S A 1943 Intra-arterial injection of pentothal. Lancet ii:571
McLeskey C H, Cullen B F, Kennedy R D, Galindo A 1974 Control of cerebral perfusion pressure during induction of anaesthesia in high-risk neurosurgical patients. Anesthesia and Analgesia 53: 985–992
McMillan J C, Brown D M, Smith G, Vance J P 1974 The effect of methohexitone on myocardial blood flow and oxygen consumption in the dog. British Journal of Anaesthesia 46: 729–732
Magora F, London M, Eimerl D, Aronson H B 1974 Blood viscosity during anaesthesia with halothane, cyclopropane, thiopentone and ketamine. British Journal of Anaesthesia 46: 343–347
Male C G, Allen E M 1977 Methohexitone induced convulsions in epileptics. Anaesthesia and Intensive Care 5: 226–230
Maloney A H, Booker W M, Tureman J R, Ratliff C M 1950 Studies on renal function during various stages of anaesthesia produced by thiopental in dogs. Federation Proceedings 9:299
Manani G, Valenti S, Segatto A, Angel A, Meroni M, Giron G P 1981 The influence of thiopentone and Alfathesin on succinylcholine-induced fasciculations and myalgias. Canadian Anaesthetists' Society Journal 28: 253–257
Mark L C, Papper E M, Brodie B B, Rovenstine E A 1949 Quantitative pharmacologic studies with Pentothal. New York State Journal of Medicine 49:1546
Matteo R.S, Katz R L, Papper E M 1962 The injection of epinephrine during general anesthesia with halogenated hydrocarbons and cyclopropane in man. 1: Trichloroethylene. Anesthesiology 23: 360–364
Matteo R S, Katz R L, Papper E M 1963 The injection of epinephrine during general anesthesia with halogenated hydrocarbons and cyclopropane in man. Anesthesiology 24: 327–330
Meagher R P 1964 Methohexital in conjunction with regional anaesthesia. Anesthesia and Analgesia, Current Researches 43: 679–686
Medico-Legal 1951 Finding of negligence against anaesthetist. British Medical Journal i:707
Miller J R, Stoelting V K 1963 A preliminary communication of the sleep-producing effect of intramuscular methohexitone sodium in the pediatric patient. British Journal of Anaesthesia 35: 48–50
Mordinovia N P 1948 Influence of Pentothal Anaesthesia on liver function. Kirurgiya 1:707
Moss E, Powell D, Gibson R M, McDowall D G 1978 Effects of tracheal intubation on intracranial pressure following induction of anaesthesia with thiopentone or Althesin in patients undergoing neurosurgery. British Journal of Anaesthesia 50: 353–360
Moyer C A, Beecher H K 1942 Effects of barbiturate anaesthesia (evipal and pentothal sodium) upon integration of respiratory control mechanism: a study directed toward improvement of methods for preclinical evaluation of anaesthetic agents. Journal of Clinical Investigation 21: 429–445
O'Donnell J F, Hewitt J C, Dundee J W 1969 Clinical studies of induction agents. XXVIII: A further comparison of venous complications following thiopentone, methohexitone nd propanidid. British Journal of Anaesthesia 41: 681–683
Olsson G L, Hallen B 1984 Laryngospasm during anaesthesia. A computer-aided incidence study in 136 929 patients. Acta Anaesthesiologica Scandinavica 28: 567–575
Pampiglione E 1965 A very shorting barbiturate, methohexital : the treatment in the detection of cortical lesions. Electroencephalography and Clinical Neurophysiology 19:314.
Patrick R T, Faulconer A J 1952 Respiratory studies during anesthesia with ether and with pentothal sodium. Anesthesiology 13: 252–274
Paul R, Harris R 1970 A comparison of methohexitone and thiopentone in electrocortography. Journal of Neurology, Neurosurgery and Psychiatry 33: 100–104
Peterson R C, Shideman F E, Johnson L B 1950 Prolongation of thiopental anaesthesia by anoxia. Federation Proceedings 9:307
Pierce E C Jr, Lambertsen C J, Deutsch S, Chase P E, Linde H W, Dripps R D, Price H L 1962 Cerebral circulation and metabolism during thiopental anaesthesia and hyperventilation in man. Journal of Clinical Investigation 41: 1664–1671
Pitts F N, Desmaris G M, Stewart W, Schaberg K. 1965 Induction of anaesthesia with methohexital and thiopental in electroconvulsive therapy. The effect of the electrocardiogram and clinical observations in 500 consecutive treatments with each agent. New England Journal of Medicine 273:353
Pohle F J 1948 Anesthesia and liver function. Wisconsin Medical Journal 47: 476–479
Price H L, Conner E H, Elder J D, Dripps R D 1952 Effect of sodium thiopental on circulatory response to positive pressure inflation of lung. Journal of Applied Physiology 4: 629–635
Price H L, Helrich M 1955 The effect of cyclopropane, diethyl ether, nitrous oxide, thiopental and hydrogen in concentration on the myocardial function of the dog heart-lung preparation. Journal of Pharmacology and Experimental Therapeutics 115: 119–205

Prime F J, Gray T C 1952 Effect of certain anaesthetic and relaxant agents on circulatory dynamics. British Journal of Anaesthesia 24: 101–136

Prys-Roberts C, Greene L T, Meloche R, Foex P 1971 Studies of anaesthesia in relation to hypertension. II: Haemodynamic consequences of induction and endotracheal intubation. British Journal of Anaesthesia 43: 531–547

Quilliam J P 1955 The action of thiopentone sodium on skeletal muscle. British Journal of Pharmacology 10: 141–146

Rampil I J, Sasse F J, Smith N T, Hoff B H, Flemming D C 1980 Spectral edge frequency — a new correlate of anesthetic depth. Anesthesiology 53:S12.

Recant B S 1960 Methohexitone sodium. Oral Surgery 13:1330

Redish C H, Vore R E, Chernish S M, Gruber C M 1958 A comparison of thiopental sodium, methitural sodium and methohexital sodium in oral surgery patients. Oral Surgery 11: 603–606

Rex M A E 1970 A review of the structural and functional basis of laryngospasm and a discussion of the nerve pathways involved in the reflex and its clinical significance in man and animals. British Journal of Anaesthesia 42: 891–899

Reynolds C, Schenken J R, Veal J R 1938 Pathological findings in mice after pentothal narcosis. Current Researches in Anesthesia and Analgesia 17: 357–359

Richards R K, Appel M 1941 The barbiturates and the liver. Current Researches in Anesthesia and Analgesia 20: 64–77

Robson J G, Davenport H T, Sugiyama R 1965 Differentiation of two types of pain by anesthetics. Anesthesiology 26: 31–36

Rockoff M A, Goudsouzian N G 1981 Seizures induced by methohexital. Anesthesiology 54: 333–335

Rosen S M 1972 Effects of anaesthesia and surgery on renal haemodynamics. British Journal of Anaesthesia 44: 252–258

Rosenmann E, Dishon T, Durst A, Boss J H 1972 Kidney and liver damage following anaesthesia with ether and pentobarbitone. British Journal of Anaesthesia 44: 465–468

Rosner B S, Clark D L 1973 Neurophysiologic effects of general anesthetics: II: Sequential regional actions in the brain. Anesthesiology 39: 59–81

Rowlands D E 1969 Pain after methohexitone. Anaesthesia 24:289

Ryder W 1969 Methohexitone and epilepsy. British Dental Journal 126:343

Sawada Y, Sugimoto H, Kobayashi H, Ohashi N, Yoshioka T, Sugimoto T 1982 Acute tolerance to high dose barbiturate treatment in patients with severe head injuries. Anesthesiology 56: 53–54

Schmidt C F, Kety S S, Pennes H H 1945 The gaseous metabolism of the brain of the monkey. American Journal of Physiology 143: 33–51

Schulte am Esch J, Pfeifer G, Thiemig G 1978 Effects of etomidate and thiopentone on the previously elevated intracranial pressure. Anaesthesist 27: 71–75

Secher O 1951a Pilot investigation into the peripheral action of anaesthetics. Acta pharmacologica et toxicologica 7: 82, 103, 231–242

Secher I 1951b The peripheral action of ether estimated on isolated nerve–muscle preparation. II: Synergism of ether and curarizing substances. Acta Pharmacologica et Toxicologica 7: 83–93

Secher O 1951c The peripheral action of ether estimated on isolated nerve–muscle preparation. III: Antagonistic and synergistic actions of ether and neostigmine. Acta Pharmacologica et Toxicologica 7: 103–118

Secher O 1951d The peripheral action of ether estimated on isolated nerve–muscle preparation. IV: Measurements of action potentials in nerve. Acta Pharmacologica et Toxicologica 7: 119–131

Seltzer J L, Gerson J I, Allen F B 1980 Comparison of the cardiovascular effects of bolus v. incremental administration of thiopentone. British Journal of Anaesthesia 52: 527–530

Shapiro H M 1984 Brain resuscitation: the chicken should come before the egg. Anesthesiology 60: 85–87.

Shapiro H M, Heilindo A, Wyte S R, Harris A B 1973 Rapid intraoperative reduction of intracranial pressure with thiopentone. British Journal of Anaesthesia 45: 1057–1062

Sherlock S 1971 Progress Report: Halothane hepatitis. Gut 12:324

Shideman F E, Kelly A R, Adams B J 1948 Blood levels of thiopental (Pentothal) following repeated administration to the dog. Federation Proceedings 7:255

Silvette H 1941 Effect of pentothal-sodium on urine output under various experimental conditions. Journal of Pharmacology and Experimental Therapeutics 72:37

Sirnes T B 1954 Some effects of barbituric acid derivatives on function of mammalian skeletal muscles. Acta Pharmacologica et Toxicologica 10: Suppl 1–170

Stephen C R, Martin R, Nowill W K 1953 Cardiovascular reactions of surital pentothal or evipal combined with muscle relaxants for rapid anaesthesia induction. Current Researches in Anesthesia and Analgesia 32: 361–369

Stern M, Papper E M, Bueding E, Rovenstine E A 1945 Effects of anesthesia and glucose tolerance in man. Journal of Pharmacology and Experimental Therapeutics 84: 157–159

Stevenson D E 1960 Changes caused by anaesthesia in the blood electrolytes of the dog. British Journal of Anaesthesia 32: 353–363

Stoelting V K, Graf J P, Rash G W 1950 Intravenous propyl-methyl-carbinyl allyl barbituric acid for hypnosis during nitrous oxide anaesthesia. Current Researches in Anesthesia and Analgesia 26: 61–67

Stone H H, Donnelly C C 1961 The accidental intra-arterial injection of thiopental. Anesthesiology 22: 995–1006

Taff R H 1982 Intra-arterial thiopental. Anesthesiology 57:543

Taylor C, Stoelting V K 1960 Methohexital sodium. A new ultrashort acting barbiturate. Anesthesiology 21: 29–34

Thornton J A 1970 Methohexitone and its application in dental anaesthesia. British Journal of Anaesthesia 42: 255–261

Toner W, Howard P J, McGowan W A W, Dundee J W 1980 Another look at acute tolerance to thiopentone. British Journal of Anaesthesia 52: 1005–1008

Tovell R M, Anderson C C, Sadove M S, Artusio J F Jr, Papper E M, Coakley C S, Hudon F, Smith S M, Thomas G J 1955 A comparative clinical and statistical study of thiopental and thiamylal in human anesthesia. Anesthesiology 16: 910–926

Tucci J H, Brazier M A B, Miles H H W, Finesinger J E 1949 A study of pentothal sodium anesthesia and a critical investigation of the use of succinate as an antidote. Anesthesiology 10: 25–39

Unni V K N, Johnston R A, Young H S A, McBride R J

1984 Prevention of intracranial hypertension during laryngoscopy and endotracheal intubation: use of a second dose of thiopentone. British Journal of Anaesthesia 56: 1219–1223

Vaizey J M 1938 Toxic jaundice following administration of pentothal. British Journal of Anaesthesia 15: 55–59

Volpitto P J 1951 Experience with ultra short acting intravenous barbiturate combined with decamethonium bromode for endotracheal intubation. Anesthesiology 12: 648–655

Volpitto P P, Marangoni B A 1938 Electrocardiographic studies during anaesthesia with intravenous barbiturates. Journal of Laboratory and Clinical Medicine 23: 575–581

Walker A H C, Stout R J 1952 Effects of anaesthesia upon fallopian tubal mobility. Journal of Obstetrics and Gynaecology of the British Empire 59: 1–24

Walton C H, Saldamando J, Egner W M 1951 The effect of intravenous pentothal sodium with or without inhalation of oxygen on liver function. Anesthesiology 12: 67–72

Walton C H, Uhl J W, Egner W M, Livingstone H M 1950 Use of thiopental sodium intravenously in the presence of hepatic damage. Archives of Surgery 60: 986–994

Ward R J 1965 Porphyria and its relation to anesthesia. Anesthesiology 26: 212–215

Waters D J 1966 Intra-arterial thiopentone (a physico-chemical phenomenon). Anaesthesia 21: 346–356

Wechsler R L, Dripps R D, Kety S S 1951 Blood flow and oxygen consumption of the human brain during anesthesia produced by thiopental. Anesthesiology 12: 308–314

Wise C C, Robinson J S, Heath M J, Tomlin P J 1969 Physiological responses to intermittent methohexitone for conservative dentistry. British Medical Journal ii: 540–543

Woodruff R A Jr, Pitts F N Jr, Craig A. 1969 Electrotherapy : the effect of barbiturate anesthesia, succinylcholine and preoxygenation on EEG. Diseases of the Nervous System 30:180

Woods L A, Wyngaarden J B, Rennick B, Seevers M H 1949 Cardiovascular toxicity of thiobarbiturates: comparison of thiopental and 5-allyl-5 (1 methyl)-2-thiobarbiturate (surital) in dogs. Journal of Pharmacology and Experimental Therapeutics 95: 328-335

Wyant G M, MacDonald W B 1980 The role of atropine in electroconvulsive therapy. Anaesthesia and Intensive Care 8: 445–450

Wyke B D 1950 Electrical activity of the human brain during artificial sleep. I. Journal of Neurology, Neurosurgery and Psychiatry 13: 288–295

Wyke B D 1951 Electrical activity of the human braind during artificial sleep II. Journal of Neurology, Neurosurgery and Psychiatry 14:137

Wyke B D 1957a Electrographic monitoring of anaesthesia. Neuropharmacological aspects, with particular reference to barbiturate narcosis. Anaesthesia 12: 157–173

Wyke B D 1957b Electrographic monitoring of anaesthesia: Clinical and experimental studies of cerebral function during barbiturate narcosis. Anaesthesia 12: 259–275

Wyke B D 1957c Electrographic monitoring of anaesthesia: a method for experimental and clinical study of reversal of barbiturate narcosis. Anaesthesia 12: 373–387

Wyke B D 1958 Electrographic monitoring of anaesthesia. The application of electroencephalography to surgical anaesthesia. British Medical Bulletin 14:58

Wyke B D 1960 Principles of general neurophysiology relating to anaesthesia and surgery. Butterworth, London

Wyke B D 1965 Neurological principles in anaesthesia. In: Evans F T and Gray T C (eds) General Anaesthesia, 2nd edn. Butterworth, London, ch 5, p 157–299

Ketamine

Ketamine produces a condition known as dissociative anaesthesia which is quite different from conventional anaesthesia. It is characterised by catalepsy, light sedation, amnesia and marked analgesia. This state has been described as 'a dissociation of the limbic from the thalamo-neocortical systems' (Corssen et al, 1968).

The first drugs to be used in dissociative anaesthesia belonged to the phenyl cyclohexylamine group. They were phencyclidine, cyclohexamine and ketamine. The first two are no longer used in clinical practice and this chapter is devoted to the actions of ketamine and its isomers.

The non-barbiturate anaesthetic, known as Ketalar and Ketaject is dl 2-(0-chlorophenyl)-2-(methylamino) cyclohexanone hydrochloride. It is chemically related to phencyclidine (CI-395, Sernyl, Sernylan) and cyclohexamine (CI-400).

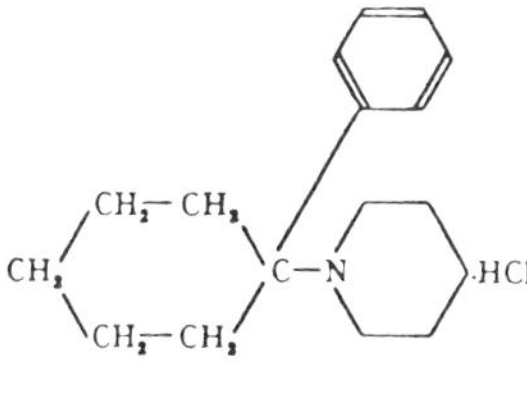

Phencyclidine (CI-395)

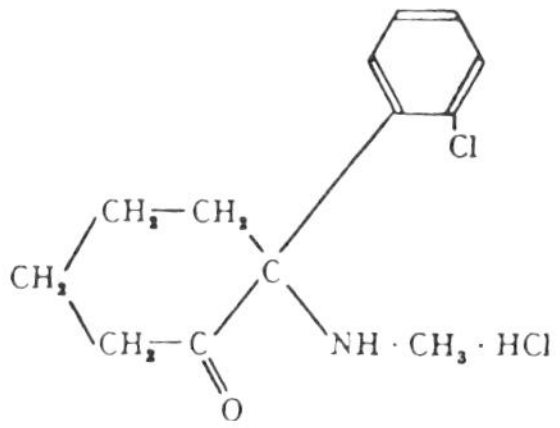

Ketamine (CI-581)

This shows its similarity to phencyclidine which has a cyclohexane ring compared with a cyclohexanone in ketamine. Each contains a phenyl ring, which in the case of ketamine has a chlorine atom. Both have a basic nitrogen attached to the cyclohexane or cyclohexanone ring at the same carbon atom to which the 0-chlorophenyl or phenyl group is attached. The base is a secondary in ketamine whereas in phencyclidine the piperidine ring results in a tertiary base.

Its synthesis is:

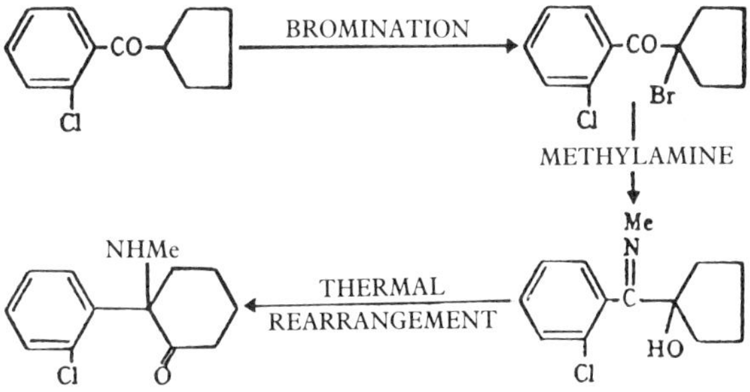

The ketone is brominated to give bromoketone; treatment of this with methylamine yields the imino alcohol which, when heated above its melting point, undergoes a rearrangement leading to the formation of ketamine.

It is an acidic solution (pH 3.5–5.5) available in 10, 50 and 100 mg ml^{-1} strengths and is suitable for intravenous or intramuscular injection. It contains 1 : 10 000 benzethonium chloride as a preservative but this is not included in the dilute solutions marketed in Britain. The 10 mg ml^{-1} solution has been made isotonic with sodium chloride.

A method for estimating ketamine levels in body fluids has been described by Dill et al (1971) based on the fluorimetric assay described by Glazko, Dill and Fransway (1962).

PHARMACOKINETICS

Because of its high lipid solubility the pattern of distribution of ketamine in the body is similar to that of the rapidly acting barbiturates, with short duration of anaesthesia due to both rapid breakdown and redistribution to peripheral tissues

(Wieber et al, 1975). Peak plasma levels occur within one minute of intravenous injection (Cohen et al, 1973; White et al, 1976) and within 5 min of intramuscular injection. Initially it is distributed to highly perfused tissues, including the brain, then to less well perfused organs. Ketamine relies to some extent on biliary excretion and significant prolongation of sleeping time and increase in its plasma concentration is seen after ligation of the common bile duct in rats (Ireland and Livingston, 1980).

The tissue concentrations follow the pattern of a two-compartment open model system (Clements and Nimmo, 1981; Wieber et al, 1975; Zsigmond and Domino, 1980). The initial distribution time ($t\frac{1}{2}\alpha$) is around 10 minutes while the elimination half life is in the region of 2–3 hours following single dose administration, although after continuous infusion Idvall and his co-workers (1979) found it to average 79 min in 31 patients. It is difficult to explain this discrepancy except on the possible grounds that these workers were careful in distinguishing between ketamine and its two main metabolites which accumulated in considerable amounts.

Ketamine is metabolized extensively by liver enzymes and Figure 9.1 shows the suggested pathways (Adams et al, 1981). N-desmethylation via cytochrome P 450 is a major metabolite pathway forming nor-ketamine which can then be hydroxylated at one or more positions in the cyclohexanone ring to form hydroxy-nor-ketamine compounds; these in time can be conjugated to the more water-soluble glycuronide derivatives. Ketamine can also undergo ring hydroxylation (without preceding N-demethylation) but quantitatively this pathway appears to be of minor importance. The resulting compound, which results from high temperatures, might occur as an artifact during gas chromatography.

Less than 4% of ketamine can be recovered from the urine as either unchanged drug or norketamine and only 16% as hydroxylated derivatives. Faecal excretion accounts for less than 5% of injected ketamine.

The main metabolite of ketamine, like that of diazepam, has hypnotic properties, and norketamine is about one third to one fifth as potent as ketamine as an anaesthetic (White et al 1975). This might explain the prolonged residual drowsiness sometimes seen after return of consciousness. More interesting is the suggestion by White et al (1982) that the other metabolites might contribute to the cardiovascular or central nervous system effects of ketamine — the time-pattern could well explain the unpleasant pyschological sequelae which will be discussed later. Alternatively these authors suggest that other metabolites could be devoid of such effect while retaining therapeutically useful analgesic and anaesthetic properties.

As with the barbiturates, at the termination of

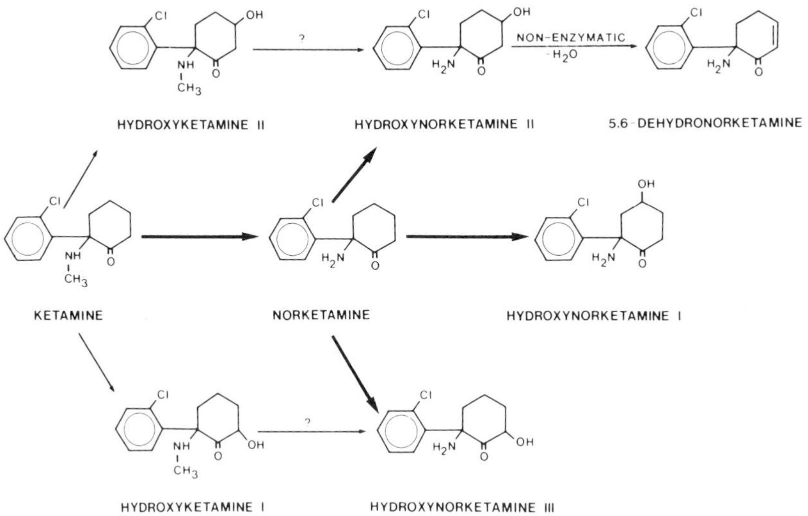

HYDROXYKETAMINE II

HYDROXYNORKETAMINE II

NON-ENZYMATIC
$-H_2O$

5.6 DEHYDRONORKETAMINE

KETAMINE

NORKETAMINE

HYDROXYNORKETAMINE I

HYDROXYKETAMINE I

HYDROXYNORKETAMINE III

Fig. 9.1 Biotransformation of ketamine (White et al, 1982).

ketamine anaesthesia the body will contain a large amount of unchanged drug and this might have significance with regard to a cumulative effect and drug interactions. White and colleagues (1976) have shown that halothane slows distribution of ketamine in the body and inhibits its hepatic metabolism, thus prolonging its clinical action. As expected, ketamine causes a dose-dependent decrease in halothane requirements and even in subhypnotic doses it affected halothane MAC (White et al 1975), an action which might be related to its analgesic action rather than to any effect on metabolism. The elimination half-life of ketamine is prolonged by adjuvants used in anesthesia, particularly diazepam and quinalbarbitone (White, et al 1975; Domino et al, 1984) thus prolonging recovery.

Zsigmond & Domino (1980) reported that an induction dose of diazepam decreased the clearance rate of ketamine — presumably via its effects on liver metabolism. During the relevant period of anaethesia Domino et al (1984) found that pretreatment with diazepam resulted in higher ketamine levels, increased AUC and significantly decreased Cl than ketamine alone, but there was no alteration in the levels of metabolite. Since recovery occurred at the same plasma level (1070–1080 ng ml^{-1}) diazepam prolonged the period of anaesthesia. These studies were done with intermittent ketamine and part of the effect may have been due to alteration in its uptake from tissues. It is not clear whether the non-metabolic effect or analgesia is responsible for the effect of nitrous oxide in reducing the dosage of ketamine required for surgical anaesthesia, described by Wessels et al (1973), but the latter seems a likely explanation.

The gradual resistance which often builds up to repeated administrations of ketamine could be explained by its effect on hepatic drug metabolizing enzymes by a process of self-induction. Marietta et al (1977b) suggest that by increasing the levels of P 450, NADPH reduction and metabolism of type I substance, ketamine behaves like the well established enzyme-inducing drug, pentobarbitone. The significance of this in radiotherapy for small children (Cronin et al, 1972; Bennett and Bullimore, 1973) or burn dressings (Demling, Ellerbee and Jarrett, 1978) has been reported.

PHARMACOLOGY

The pharmacology of ketamine was reported by Chen (1965) and by McCarthy and associates (1965) who described it as being a compound with a cataleptic, analgesic and anaesthetic action but without hypnotic properties. Chen (1969) later defined catalepsy as 'a characteristic akinetic state with a loss of orthostatic reflexes but without impairment of consciousness in which the extremities appear to be paralysed by motor and sensory failure'. The early clinical pharmacological studies of Domino and colleagues (1965) from Ann Arbor, Michigan, led to the drug being used in anaesthesia. It was classed as a 'rapid acting non-barbiturate general anaesthetic' but Corssen and Domino (1966) used the term 'dissociative anaesthesia' characterised by complete analgesia with only superficial sleep (Corssen, 1969). This term has also been used by European workers (Langrehr, 1969).

In early animal studies McCarthy and his colleagues (1965) compared the therapeutic index of ketamine with that for phencyclidine and two barbiturates, using anaesthetic threshold dose (ATD), dose which produces undesirable effects (UED) and minimal lethal dose (MLD). Their findings of a high safety margin with ketamine in rhesus monkeys produced much of the impetus for its continued investigation. It also has a high therapeutic ratio as far as undesirable side effects in monkeys are concerned, but this does not generally apply in humans.

	UED/ATD	MLD/ATD
Phencyclidine	8	26
Ketamine	15	16
Pentobarbitone	3	3.5
Thiamylal	6	6.5

Cardiovascular effects

In contrast to almost all other anaesthetic induction agents, ketamine tends to maintain the integrity of the cardiovascular system under most clinical circumstances by causing a dose-related rise in the rate/pressure product without significant changes in the stroke index (Tweed et al 1972; Idvall et al, 1979). Tokics and coworkers

(1983) have found a relationship between oxygen uptake and cardiac output similar to that seen with some other general anaesthetic techniques. They have not been able to establish a relationship between plasma catecholamine concentrations and central haemodynamics. However, significant cardiovascular depression can ensue when ketamine is used with halothane or enflurane (Bidwai et al, 1975, Stanley, 1973) or in critically ill patients or those who have been subjected to acute trauma (Waxman et al 1980).

In the absence of depressant premedication the rise in systolic pressure in adults receiving clinical doses of ketamine is in the region of 20 to 40 mmHg, with a slightly lower rise in diastolic pressure. In the majority of patients the blood pressure rises steadily over the three to five minutes following injection and then declines to normal limits over the next 10 to 20 minutes. There is often a slight delay in the rise in diastolic pressure which may still be rising when the systolic has begun to drop. In most studies the peak rises occurred between the second and fourth minute after injection as seen in the typical pressure and heart rate graph shown in Figure 9.2. However, it must be remembered that this is a highly individual reaction and on occasions the pressure may be alarmingly high (Corssen and Domino, 1966). The heart rate almost invariably increases following intravenous ketamine in man.

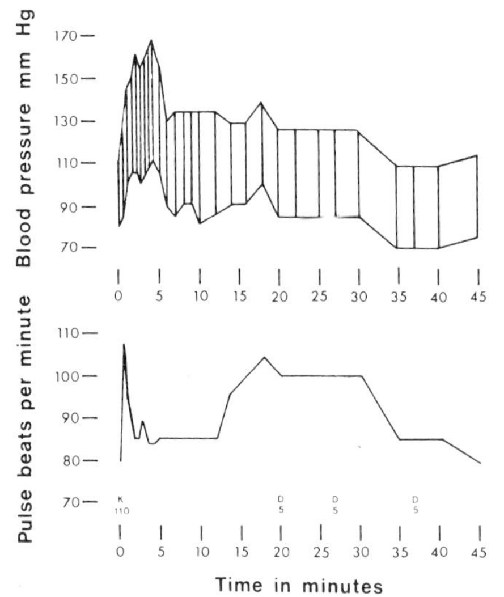

Fig. 9.2 Typical blood pressure and heart rate changes during and after ketamine anaesthesia K110, D5 = diazepam 5 mg.

The cardiovascular stimulating effects of ketamine are almost certainly due to primary direct stimulation of the central nervous system (Chodoff, 1972; Wong and Jenkins, 1974) rather than because of sympathetic activity with enhanced noradrenaline release as originally believed and secondary depression of baroreceptor reflex activity (Dowdy and Kaya, 1968). It has further been shown that ketamine is a direct myocardial depressant (Traber et al 1968; Schwartz and Horwitz, 1975) in the absence of autonomic control and thus the apparent paradoxical response in critically ill patients is likely due to an inability of ketamine and its sympathomimetic effect to counterbalance the direct myocardial depression and vasodilation, a primary effect of the substance on smooth muscle removed from normal autonomic influence (Diaz et al, 1976; Liao et al 1979). Whether ketamine sensitizes the myocardium to adrenaline or whether it might indeed have an antiarrhythmic effect (Hamilton and Bryson, 1974; Koehntop et al, 1977; Idvall et al, 1979; Dowdy and Kaya, 1968; Ivankovitch et al, 1974; 1975) is still controversial. Circumstances do arise where it is desired to block the cardiovascular stimulation from ketamine. This can be achieved with thiopentone (Dobson, 1978), diazepam (Zsigmond et al, 1974; Jackson, et al, 1978; Kumar et al, 1978), or flunitrazepam (Tarnow and Hess, 1979; Tarnow et al, 1979) while lorazepam is ineffective. On the other hand pressure rises when ketamine is given with pancuronium are greater than when tubocurarine or alcuronium are used (Dundee, 1971). This is in keeping with the cardiovascular stimulant action of pancuronium (Kelman and Kennedy, 1970). Tachycardia is also significantly greater with ketamine–pancuronium than when ketamine is given alone or in combination with alcuronium or tubocurarine.

Bovill and Dundee (1972) attempted to control the cardiostimulatory effect of ketamine in man by the prior intravenous administration of droperidol 5 mg, propranolol 5 mg or atropine 2 mg. The latter two produce beta adrenergic and vagal block

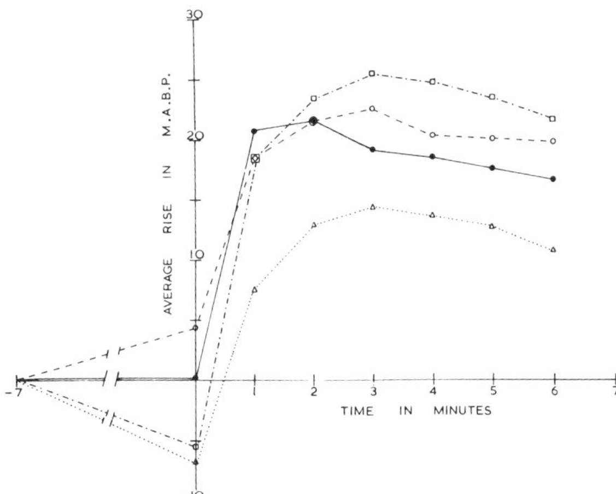

Fig. 9.3 Effects of the prior intravenous administrations of three supplements on the average rise in mean arterial blood pressure caused by ketamine 2.0 mg kg^{-1}.
• control; △ droperidol 5 mg; ○ atropine 2 mg
□ propanolol 5 mg. (Bovill & Dundee 1972).

respectively while the former has a mild α adrenergic blocking action. Figure 9.3 shows that hypertension was reduced to some extent by droperidol, but not by either propranolol or atropine. It would seem that any effect of these drugs on the cardiovascular response to ketamine is due to their action on resting blood pressure and heart rate rather than being a specific effect on the cardiovascular response to ketamine. Sadove et al, (1971a, b) have also shown that droperidol is ineffective in reducing the hypertensive action of ketamine to a significant degree.

Cardiac arrhythmias are very uncommon following ketamine and, in fact, a number of workers have shown that it has an anti-arrhythmic action (Dowdy and Kaya, 1968; Goldberg et al 1970).

Unni and Bovill (1972) found an increase in forearm blood flow during ketamine anaesthesia in unpremedicated subjects, the rise becoming significant after the second minute. The net effect on vascular resistance was a fall which became significant only at the fourth minute of ketamine anaesthesia. These changes were less marked when ketamine was given during nitrous oxide anaesthesia. The combination of cardiac acceleration, increased cardiac output, rise in blood pressure and increased circulating noradrenaline are normally accompanied by vasoconstriction. To explain the discrepancy of vasodilation with ketamine, Unni and Bovill (1972) have suggested the occurrence of an active cholinergic vasodilation as described by Blair et al (1959) during emotional stress; all the patients in their series had emergence delirium, although it is not known whether they had unpleasant dreams during the actual anaesthetic period.

Tweed et al (1972) have studied the circulatory responses to ketamine anaesthesia (2 mg kg^{-1} intravenously) in patients undergoing diagnostic heart catheterization and coronary angiography. There was no difference in response between patients found to have cardiac disease and those with normal hearts. In agreement with other workers, they found that the drug had both cardiac and peripheral effects, causing an increase in blood pressure, cardiac index (29 per cent) and heart rate (33 per cent) and pulmonary arterial pressure (44 per cent) with a constant stroke volume index. In paced patients, a 26 per cent increase in cardiac index occurred with a corresponding increase in stroke volume index, thus indicating that ketamine enhances myocardial contractility. This is accompanied by a rise in oxygen consumption and on this basis these authors advise against the use of ketamine in patients with severe coronary disease.

Hypertensive response

A number of factors are known to influence the blood pressure rise when ketamine is given under clinical conditions.

Dosage

With doses in excess of 1 mg kg^{-1} there is very little variation in the hypertensive action of ketamine which has even been noted with subhypnotic doses (Domino et al 1965; Knox et al, 1970).

Rate of injection

It has been suggested that the rise will be less with slower injection rates, but this is not borne out in

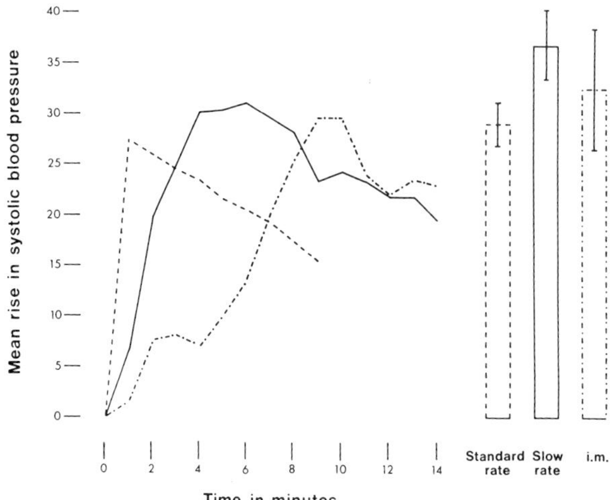

Fig. 9.4 Average rise in systolic blood pressure (mmHg) after ketamine. Columns on right show mean peak rise.

Figure 9.4 which is taken from data of Bovill et al, (1971a). Here a dose of 2 mg kg^{-1} was injected over 20 seconds or at 20 mg min^{-1} and the peak rise is significantly greater at the slow rate as compared with the standard rate of injection. This difference may have resulted from slight agitation during the slower onset of sleep. Podlesch and Zindler (1967) have also noted that injection rate does not influence the hypertensive action of ketamine.

Route of administration

Figure 9.4 also shows that in adults an intramuscular dose of 8 mg kg^{-1} was followed by a similar pressure rise as 2 mg kg^{-1} intravenously. Here the pressure rise did not occur until four to six minutes after injection, reaching its peak in 8 to 10 minutes. This effect lasts longer than that following intravenous injection. In contrast to the effects shown in Figure 9.4, Iwatsuki *et al.* (1967) found a highly significant difference between the hypertensive response to 2 mg kg^{-1} intravenously and that caused by 10 mg kg^{-1} intramuscularly. This difference may be explained by the preponderance of adults in the intravenous series and of children in those given the ketamine by the intramuscular route.

Premedication

On theoretical grounds one might expect premedication with the phenothiazines and butyrophenones to reduce the hypertensive action of ketamine, but there is no support for this view. The only controlled study is that of Bovill et al (1971b) whose findings of average peak pressure rises after 2 mg kg^{-1} ketamine are shown below. Each group contained 50 to 100 patients.

	Atropine	*Opioid*	*Opioid hyoscine*	*Droperidol combinations*
Systolic	33 ± 2.3	25 ± 1.8	23 ± 1.5	29 ± 1.9
Diastolic	24 ± 1.4	21 ± 1.3	14 ± 1.2	23 ± 1.2
Mean	27 ± 1.7	22 ± 1.3	17 ± 1.2	25 ± 1.2

Opioid (Morphine 10 mg, papaveretum 20 mg or pethidine 50–100 mg) and opioid-hyoscine premedication was most effective in minimizing the pressure rise. Hyoscine alone, pentobarbitone, promethazine and diazepam have no effect on the pressure rise (Dundee et al, 1970; Sadove et al, 1971a).

Age

There is no clear relationship between the age of the patient and the hypertensive response to ketamine.

Initial pressure

Contrary to one early opinion (Gjessing, 1968), the detailed study of Knox et al (1970) showed that the initial blood pressure did not affect the degree of hypertension produced by ketamine.

Relatively little is known of the effect of ketamine on the pulmonary circulation in humans. Ketamine causes marked elevation of pulmonary pressure and right ventricular stroke work due to increase in pulmonary vascular resistance (Gooding et al 1977; Tarnow et al, 1979). Gooding and colleagues have shown that there is a 40 per cent increase in pulmonary vascular resistance in individuals free of cardiovascular disease, while Tarnow and co-workers (1979) have shown that ketamine raises pulmonary artery pressure in patients undergoing aorto-coronary bypass operations. Following artificially induced endotoxin injury to the lung in sheep, subsequent administration of ketamine tended to decrease pulmonary arterial pressure and lung lymph flow with simultaneous increase in systemic blood pressure, thus raising the possibility that ketamine might be protective in the face of sepsis (Bodai et al, 1983); Wong and Jenkins (1975) also showed that systemic blood pressure increased significantly in both haemorrhagic and septic experimental shock.

Central nervous system

The effects of ketamine on the central nervous system are intimately related to the profound analgesia it induces and to its propensity of producing dreams and emergence hallucinations. Sparks et al (1973, 1975) have shown that ketamine blocks afferent signals associated with some component of pain perception in the spinoreticular tracts without impairing spinothalamic conduction. Depression of nocipective cells in the medial medullary reticular formation and of the medial thalamic nuclei have been demonstrated by Ohtani et al (1979) and by Massopust et al (1972), respectively. Thus the analgesic effect of ketamine would appear to be largely related to the blockage of the affective–emotional rather than the somatic components of pain perception. Some evidence has been advanced that ketamine binds to opiate receptors (Vincent et al, 1978; Finck and Ngai, 1979; Smith et al 1980), an observation which however was not corroborated by Fratta et al (1980). The analgesia produced by ketamine extends well into the postanaesthetic period (Bjarnesen and Corssen, 1967) and can be produced also by subanaesthetic doses (Bovill and Dundee, 1971; Sadove et al, 1971c; Slogoff et al, 1974). The work of Sadove et al (1971b) suggests that 'subdissociative' doses of approximately 0.4 mg kg^{-1} might be of use in clinical analgesia.

Failure to obtain anaesthesia altogether can occur once in a while and in the opinion of Janis and Wright (1972) can be associated with the absence of appropriate cerebral development. Indeed, he believes that intact cortical function is necessary for the production of analgesia. He supports this contention by citing two cases and we have come across at least one more (Wyant, 1971). This observation is of considerable practical importance since such patients may well come to anaesthesia for neurological investigation. On the other hand Rajanna (1983) has experienced failure to obtain anaesthesia with ketamine even in the presence of a normal central nervous system.

Tremors and spontaneous involuntary muscle movements are not uncommon during induction with ketamine, which is often accompanied by hypertonus. This might involve the jaw muscles to such an extent that the airway becomes obstructed and cyanosis occurs. In contrast to the barbiturates the incidence of excitatory phenomena does not appear to be greatly influenced by premedication. However, on occasions purposeless and tonic-clonic movements of the extremities may occur during the course of anaesthesia. They might be taken erroneously to indicate a light plane of anaesthesia and the need for additive doses, and unless this possibility is recognised one can readily give an overdose.

Ketamine is excitory to the thalamus and limbic system where it provokes a seizure pattern limited to these particular structures but not extending to the cerebral cortex (Kayama and Iwama, 1972; Ferrer-Allado et al, 1973; Corrsen et al 1974). Hence ketamine has been used with impunity in patients with seizure disorders (Sybert and Kyff, 1983). Even anticonvulsant properties have been attributed to the drug (Fisher, 1974; Reder et al 1980).

Although ketamine has been described as a rapid-acting general anaesthetic, the rate of onset is much slower than after the barbiturates. Figure 9.5 shows a comparison of times until patients stopped counting when varying doses of ketamine were injected during the period of reactive hyperaemia which follows arterial occlusion. They are compared with average figures obtained for methohexitone. In contrast to the barbiturates, it is often difficult to get a clear end-point indicative of onset of sleep, particularly after slow injection as patients appear to gaze sightlessly into space and may not close their eyes for several minutes. The eyelash, corneal and laryngeal reflexes remain unimpaired and there is usually increased muscle tone accompanied by grimacing or involuntary muscle movement but there is no response to auditory stimuli. The usual adult induction dose is 2 mg kg^{-1} but Knox et al (1970) found that

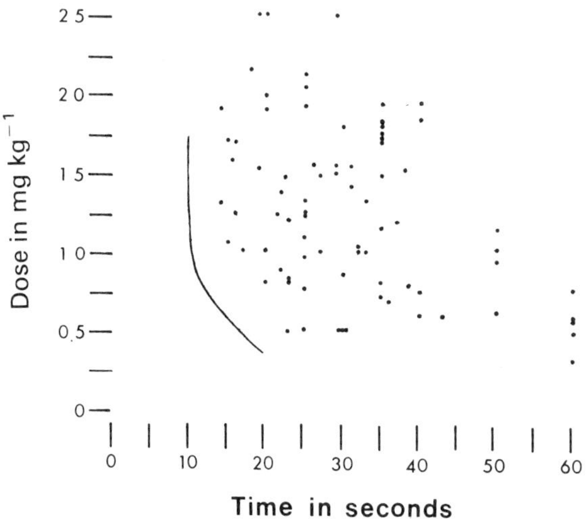

Fig. 9.5 Plotting points: time to onset of anaesthetic action of varying doses of ketamine, judged by time from end of rapid injection until patients stops counting compared with average time (solid line) for methohexitone. (Bovill et al 1971).

most patients will fall asleep with doses as low as 1 to 1.5 mg kg^{-1}.

With intramuscular injections the induction doses are 5 to 10 mg kg^{-1} and consciousness usually is lost in two to four minutes, but the onset may be delayed for six to eight minutes.

Amnesia

In the absence of depressant premedication, Pandit et al (1971) found a negligible incidence of preoperative retrograde amnesia after ketamine. However, memory of events occurring one hour after apparent recovery is often impaired, amnesia increasing with the total dose of ketamine given. A much higher incidence was found when the ketamine was given after heavy premedication, but it was no greater than that encountered when methohexitone is given after the same premedicants.

Electroencephalographic changes

In anaesthetic doses in man, ketamine depresses the alpha rhythm and produces fairly continuous theta waves and rarely delta wave bursts (Domino et al 1965; Virtue et al, 1967). A typical tracing for an eight year old boy is shown in Figure 9.6.

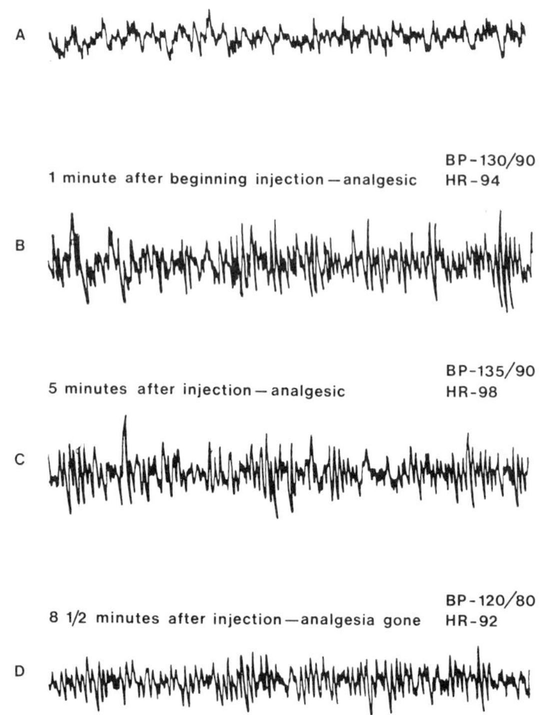

Fig. 9.6 EEG tracing from an eight-year-old boy given ketamine 2.2 mg kg^{-1} over a 30 s period at A. (Corssen et al 1969).

This onset of theta activity coincides with the loss of consciousness, but some theta wave activity persists into the recovery period, even after analgesia has passed off. Ketamine also causes depression of late portions of the auditory evoked response. Detailed studies of the electroencephalogram show a functional dissociation between the thalamo-neocortical and limbic systems, the former being depressed before there is a significant obtunding of the reticular activating and the limbic systems (Corssen et al 1968). The site of action of minimal anaesthetic doses of ketamine thus appears to be on the non-specific thalamo-neocortical system. Miyasaka and Domino (1968) consider that this system seems to be a primary factor in producing the hypersynchronous delta wave burst pattern in the electroencephalogram.

Cerebral blood flow, metabolism and intracranial pressure

In contrast to the action of the barbiturates,

ketamine increases both cerebral blood flow (CBF) and oxygen consumption ($CMRO_2$). In dogs anaesthetized with nitrous oxide-halothane and paralysed with suxamethonium Dawson et al (1971) found that 2 mg kg^{-1} ketamine increased CBF by 80% and $CMRO_2$ by 16%. CBF returned to normal in 30 min and $CMRO_2$ in 20 min. Cerebrospinal fluid pressure changes closely followed changes in CBF. These rises occurred with repeated doses of ketamine. In their study the rise in mean arterial blood pressure was not very marked, presumably due to the concomitant use of halothane. The effects of ketamine on CBF, $CMRO_2$ and cerebrospinal fluid pressure were blocked by the prior injection of thiopentone. These findings are at variance with those of a previous study by Kreuscher & Grote (1967) but the increase in cerebral blood flow has been confirmed by Takeshita et al (1972) who believe that this may account for the concomitant rise in intracranial pressure.

The rise in cerebrospinal fluid pressure after ketamine has been confirmed in its clinical use for pneumoencephalography (Tjaden et al, 1969) and proved advantageous on occasions, although Evans et al (1971) point out that it may be dangerous in certain circumstances, particularly in patients with intracranial pathology where it is more marked (Gibbs, 1972; Shapiro et al, 1972). Sari et al (1972) have shown that the the rise in blood flow, cerebrospinal fluid pressure and intracranial pressure can be abolished by hypocarbia. This latter view is supported by the findings of Pfenninger et al (1984) who found no rise in intracranial pressure with either 0.5 or 2.0 mg kg^{-1} ketamine in animals who were either haemodynamically stable or in haemorrhagic shock, a finding they contribute to the fact that carbon dioxide tension did not rise because of controlled ventilation.

Recovery

Consciousness returns in about 10 to 15 minutes after the normal therapeutic dose of 2 mg kg^{-1} ketamine but, like the onset of anaesthesia, it is difficult to determine the exact moment when this occurs. Muscle tone reverts to normal first, after which there may be a period when the patient seems 'distant' and unaware of his surroundings. The final apparent return of full contact with the environment may be sudden and the time varies from a few minutes to over one hour after first evidence of awakening. Diplopia and other visual disturbances are frequently present on return of consciousness and can be both persistent and distressing. Some patients have thought they were blind at this stage and this was the cause of severe emergence delirium, particularly when accompanied by difficulty in speaking. The variability of psychic reactions which occur during recovery from ketamine will be discussed later in a fuller survey of emergence complications.

Because of the pattern of awakening, it is not possible to study the relationship between dosage and duration of action as with other anaesthetics. Its pharmacokinetics have not been studied although there is a small amount of information available on its cumulative action. Ten subjects had a period of coma lasting from three to eight minutes after 1 mg kg^{-1} which was repeated immediately on recovery and lasted for five to 12 minutes on the second occasion (Domino et al 1965).

Emergence sequelae

There is great discrepancy in reports of the incidence, severity and significance of the sequelae which occur on emergence from ketamine. The psychological manifestations vary in severity from pleasant dreamlike states, a floating feeling, vivid imagery to halucinations and emergence delirium. These may be accompanied by irrational behaviour and may or may not be remembered.

There are three related aspects of this problem which will be discussed together, (*a*) emergence reactions, (*b*) dreams and hallucinations and (*c*) longer term psychotomimetic effects.

It is difficult to improve on the description of emergence sequelae which is given by Domino et al (1965) in the first detailed report of the use of ketamine in man: 'During the recovery period the subjects showed considerable variation in psychic reaction. Some were completely orientated in time and space and showed no significant changes. Others showed marked alteration in mood and affect, some becoming apprehensive and aggressive and others markedly withdrawn. Almost all subjects felt entirely numb, and in extreme instances stated that they had no arms or legs or that they were dead . . . Other reactions noted included feelings of estrangement or isolation, negativism, hostility, apathy, drowsiness, inebriation, hypnogenic states and repetitive motor behaviour.'

Studies of cerebral glucose utilization in animals by Nelson et al (1980) and Crosby et al (1980) have shown that ketamine depresses the medial geniculate nucleus and inferior colliculus, visual and acoustic relay nuclei respectively. This suggests that the psychomimetic emergence phenomena might by due to altered perception or interpretation of visual and auditory stimuli, reinforced by the general analgesia which under the circumstances might well be responsible for the 'out-of-body and floating' experiences so frequently described by patients.

Because of the number of factors which can influence emergence disturbances it is difficult to get reliable figures as to their incidence when other agents were not used. The following figures, taken from the study of Knox et al (1970), only apply to the use of ketamine as the main anaesthetic in women undergoing minor gynaecological operations lasting for 5 to 10 minutes. The percentage incidence of emergence delirium or excitement and visual disturbance was:

	<2 mg kg^{-1}	2–3 mg kg^{-1}	3+ mg kg^{-1}
Severity			
Mild	13	27	9
Severe	19	12	27
Requiring medication	4	6	24
Visual disturbances:			
Nystagmus	4	8	20
Focusing problems	10	6	8
Diplopia	0	6	8
Colours	4	12	8

This shows a relationship in severity of symptoms (as judged by the need for medication) with dosage. This is a much higher incidence than the 2.8 per cent incidence of 'confusion, with or without vocalisation, excitement or irrational behaviour' recorded by Albin and Dresner (1969) in over 12 000 unselected administrations. They may occur if patients are aroused early in the recovery phase (Pannacciulli et al 1966; Corssen et al, 1969b) but this is not a universal finding. Bovill et al (1971c) found that the incidence of disturbing emergence upset is much less after body surface operations (duration 30 to 40 minutes) and even less after abdominal operations which took from 60 to 80 minutes although the duration of anaesthesia *per se* is not an important factor. They also state that it is less common in men than women and that the incidence is reduced markedly by opioid, opioid-hyoscine or opioid-droperidol premedication, but not by diazepam. The intravenous administration of droperidol 5 mg, either immediately before or during recovery, will almost abolish emergence upset after ketamine. When it does occur, it can often be controlled by talking to the patient or, if this is ineffective, a small intravenous dose of 2.5 to 5.0 mg diazepam will exert a rapid calming effect. Larger doses of diazepam may reinduce anaesthesia and cause respiratory depression. A small dose of thiopentone will promptly terminate a severe reaction. Few patients have any memory of emergence delirium, particularly if diazepam is given, and it is more distressing to the attendants than to the patient.

In contrast, dreams can be very upsetting to the patient. These have been described in the literature, as dreams, hallucinations, psychological responses or altered affect. Perhaps the most interesting term is 'sensory and perceptual misinterpretation' (Garfield et al, 1970; 1972). Again we quote from the original description of Domino et al (1965). 'At times some of the subjects had vivid dreamlike experiences or frank hallucinations. Some of these involved the recall of television programmes or motion pictures seen a few days before, or they were at home with their relatives or even in outer space. Some of these phenomena were so real that the subject could not be certain they had not actually occurred.' Corssen and Domino (1966) described the unpleasant type of experience in two patients 'both middle aged, who showed signs of schizophenia during awakening. Both experienced travelling in outer space and thought they had died and were travelling to hell. In one, the episode lasted only a few minutes; in the other restlessness and agitation during the dreaming stage extended to 40 minutes.'

Thus, some patients have severe motor upset during waking with or without dreams, but others only have dreams with no obvious emergence upset. The significance of visual disturbances as a contributory factor to the latter is not clear. Again there is a conflict of evidence as to the incidence and severity of dreams and the following figures are taken from the study already quoted (Knox et al, 1970):

	<2 mg kg^{-1}	2–3 mg kg^{-1}	3+ mg kg^{-1}
Dreams: %			
Pleasant	19	13	18
Unpleasant	23	33	38

This is undoubtedly a worrying aspect of ketamine anaesthesia, and the above incidence unacceptably high. It should be remembered that these data were obtained from unpremedicated women undergoing minor operations. However, the use of 'heavier' premedication is less effective in preventing dreams than in reducing emergence upset. In similar patients (receiving a fixed dose of 2 mg kg^{-1} ketamine) the percentage incidence of dreams, related to premedication was:

	Pleasant	*Unpleasant*
Atropine	22	40
Hyoscine	15	50
Opioid	14	26
Opioid-hyoscine	16	7
Non opioid hypnotic	16	36
Droperidol-opioid	12	23

Neither was the incidence markedly reduced after body surface operations, but unpleasant dreams were uncommon in patients after abdominal operations. In common with emergence delirium, Bovill et al (1971c) found dreams — particularly unpleasant ones — occurred less frequently in men than in women. Other workers (Galloon, 1971; Hervey and Hustead, 1972) have also found an unacceptably high incidence of unpleasant sequelae following minor operations in women.

It is interesting to note that the authors have had experiences with two patients who, following D & C operations under ketamine-nitrous oxide-oxygen anaesthesia, required admission to the psychiatric service. In retrospect both patients had a psychiatric history and the relapse must be assumed to have been triggered by the administration of ketamine.

Premedication with 5 mg diazepam and 5 mg droperidol will reduce both emergence delirium and dreams to acceptable limits, but these complications are not abolished completely (Bovill et al, 1971b). Johnstone (1972) claims that oral premedication with nitrazepam 10 mg and droperidol 20 mg will prevent ketamine dreams, but his studies were carried out in patients undergoing major operations. This mixture also reduces the catatonia frequently seen with ketamine.

A 5 to 10 mg dose of diazepam given intravenously near the end of anaesthesia is very effective in reducing dreams after ketamine, irrespective of whether the patient has had any sedative premedication (Coppel et al 1973). The beneficial effects are less marked after very short procedures but in these cases the combination of 10 mg chlorpromazine given before induction and 5 mg diazepam given at the end of anaesthesia gives good results (Ergbuth et al, 1972). Droperidol is ineffective in this respect. Lorazepam 2–4 mg has been reported to be even more useful than diazepam in this respect (Dundee & Lilburn, 1977; Lilburn et al, 1978; Dundee et al, 1979) and more recently midazolam 0.07 mg kg^{-1} when compared to diazepam 0.12 mg kg^{-1} has been found to reduce the incidence of dreams after ketamine from 29% to 7% in women undergoing short gynaecological procedures (Cartwright & Pingel, 1984). The administration of a small dose of thiopentone (150 mg) at the end of minor operations in patients anaesthetized with ketamine (2 mg kg^{-1}) reduced the incidence and severity of emergence reactions and in this dose thiopentone did not produce respiratory depression (Magbagbedola & Thomas, 1974).

When ketamine is used as an analgesic with nitrous oxide–oxygen following thiopentone induction, sequelae are rare and only consist of slight confusion in 4–5% of patients (Liang & Liang, 1975). If subhypnotic doses of ketamine are given as analgesics for minor procedures without other cerebral depressants unpleasant reactions do occur occasionally but are often minor. Contrary to expectations such sequelae do occur occasionally when the drug is used in less sophisticated surroundings. In a Symposium on its use in small doses 'beyond major centres' there was the occasional report of mild hallucinations in the postoperative period but these occurred no more frequently than after nitrous oxide-oxygen (Boulton, 1985).

Garfield et al (1970; 1972) have looked at the possibility of reducing the patients' tendency to emergence sequelae by detailed preoperative briefing. Apart from establishing that the sequelae were due to the drug the results of a detailed preoperative description as to what to find were disappointing and of no clinical significance.

None of the sequelae in the patients studied by Garfield and colleagues could be classed as hallucinations: rather they were described as illusions, i.e. a misinterpretation of a real external sensory experience. In contrast Collier (1972), from a study of 131 adults receiving ketamine, concluded that the emergence phenomena could be closely related to those described with published experiments in acute sensory deprivation of the Shurley and Hebb types — feelings of depersonalization, sensation of strangeness and even splitting of the body image. One subject described it as a combination of the effects experienced with marihuana and LSD. This may explain why Sklar et al (1981) have shown that psychological techniques can prevent adverse reactions to ketamine and increase its acceptance.

It is of some importance to note that both emergence delirium and dreaming were virtually absent following the administration of ketamine in obstetrics (Moore et al, 1971). This cannot be explained entirely by the other drugs given during labour. Perhaps the altered psychological state of the mother with her new baby may be all-important.

Albin et al (1970) and Albin and Dresner (1971) reported a complex psychological assessment of patients who had ketamine, and of a comparable series anaesthetised with other agents. Using the revised Janis stress scale and the Katz adjustment scale scored for psychopathology clusters and for the arbitrary hallucinogenic symptom complex, they concluded that ketamine does not result in long-term impairment of personality functioning, even after repeated exposures.

Corssen et al (1971) used the MMPI (Minnesota multiphasic personality inventory) to detect prolonged or even permanent, psychic alterations in man. They used three groups of patients having thiopentone, ketamine or no anaesthesia. Unfortunately there was a high drop-out of subjects on their six months' evaluation, but the findings record no adverse effects from the ketamine.

Wilson et al (1969) have evolved the 'ketamine acceptance test' based on the answers to five questions relating to memory of the operation, dreams, recovery and other unpleasant sequelae. This has been useful in showing improved acceptance of the drug on repeated administration, but it has not been used to compare its acceptance to that of other agents, or to study factors which might influence the patients' impression of the anaesthetic.

In contrast to these, Knox et al (1970) and Bovill et al (1971b) adopted the simple manœuvre of visiting patients (all women) 24 hours after minor operations and asking them if they would like the same anaesthetic on another occasion should this be required. The most notable observation was that 83 per cent of patients anaesthetized with methohexitone would like the same anaesthetic again, as compared with only a 29 per cent incidence of patients who would like a second ketamine anaesthetic. Premedication with hyoscine and an opiate or with combinations containing droperidol increased this acceptance rate to over 60 per cent, as did intravenous diazepam given near the end of the operation. In keeping with what has already been discussed, patient acceptance was highest in those undergoing major operations. These findings convincingly condemn the use of ketamine for minor operations in women.

It is probable that neither emergence upset nor unpleasant dreams occur in very young children after ketamine (Ginsberg and Gerber, 1968, 1969; Spoerel and Kandel, 1971). It is difficult to determine the incidence of hallucinations in small children, but Roberts (1967) did not detect any personality disturbance with multiple anaesthetics. Only one of his 20 patients showed any suggestion of possible psychotomimetic effects. However, on close questioning of children of school age Langrehr and Kluge (1969) found that 50 per cent were able to report on the experience of a dissociative dream that they could remember, but none objected to a possible repetition of this form of anaesthesia. MacLennan (1982) has found that hallucinations can occur in small children but none were distressed by the experience. Based on their experience with both adults and children Spoerel and Kandel (1971) are hesitant to recommend the use of ketamine in school-age children.

In an appraisal of the use of ketamine in the aged, Lorhan and Lippmann (1971) did not mention emergence upset or other undesirable sequelae. Although their incidence and severity is greatly reduced in geriatric patients, they are not completely eliminated.

Wilson et al (1969) have correlated certain physiological and psychological effects of ketamine in children undergoing repeat anaesthetics. About one in 20 of the children reacted unfavourably to the repeated administration of the drug, but its 'acceptance' by the remainder improved with successive anaesthetics. None had problems with auditory or visual hallucinations.

In burned adults subjected to daily administrations it noted that disturbing emergence sequelae following the first administration are less after the second and do not occur at all thereafter. Reference has already been made to ketamine causing induction of the enzyme which is responsible for its own metabolism and perhaps one particular breakdown product may have a psychotomimetic action and metabolism to this compound could be reduced by repeat administration. Domino et al (1984) have looked at a similar explanation to explain the reduction of sequelae by the prior administration of diazepam. This benzodiazepine reduces ketamine clearance to a significant degree but there is no evidence that this may have psychomimetic metabolites. Alternatively they suggest that diazepam may enhance gamma-aminobutyric acid-mediated transmission which may be altered by ketamine. It is more likely that diazepam reduces delirium by use of its sedative and/or amnesic properties. This latter would fit in with the protective effect of thiopentone.

Any suggestion that the sequelae are not due to ketamine itself are dispelled by the work of Moretti et al (1984): in a double blind comparison in female volunteers 2.5 mg kg^{-1} ketamine caused a significantly greater incidence of 'abnormalities of mental status' than 5.0 mg kg^{-1} thiopentone. The changes were short-lived and not evident on the following day and there were no long-term sequelae.

Emetic sequelae

When given as a main anaesthetic with minor operations, ketamine is followed by a slightly higher incidence of nausea and vomiting than when similar cases were anaesthetised with a barbiturate. This difference is not obvious when it was used for major operations. When ketamine is given repeatedly anorexia, nausea or vomiting are not severe and the majority of patients can take liquids by mouth shortly after regaining consciousness.

Respiratory effects

Respiratory depression is minimal and transient after clinical doses of ketamine when given in the absence of depressant premedication (Corssen and Domino 1966, Virtue et al, 1967; Coppel and Dundee, 1972) and some workers have even found evidence of respiratory stimulation (Wilson et al 1968; Kelly et al, 1971). The peak depressant effect occurs about two minutes after intravenous injection. Significant respiratory depression with reduction of p_aO_2 occurs only after the rapid single-dose injection of 2 mg kg^{-1} in spontaneously breathing patients on room air (Zsigmond et al, 1976). Respiratory depression and even apnoea have also been noted when ketamine is given after opioid premedication (Podlesch and Zindler, 1967), especially after rapid injection or when it is given intramuscularly to small children. There is a slight increase in respiratory rate in most patients.

As mentioned previously, cough, hiccup or laryngospasm occur very rarely after ketamine, but are more frequent in children than in adults (Brown et al 1970). In animals, El-Hawary et al (1972) found that it dilated the bronchial tree and effectively antagonised the bronchoconstrictive effect of histamine, acetylcholine and 5-hydroxytryptamine (5HT) on both the trachea and bronchi. Ketamine has proved to be a most satisfactory agent for the asthmatic (Corssen et al, 1972). In one patient reported by Betts and Parkin

(1971) the wheezing disappeared when the patient became unconscious and reappeared each time a light level of anaesthesia was reached.

Salivary and tracheo-bronchial secretions are enhanced by the administration of ketamine and prophylactic administration of a drying agent is recommended, particularly in children.

Laryngeal reflexes are not markedly depressed with normal adult doses, but the extent to which the protective reflexes remain intact is not as great as was originally thought (Taylor and Towey, 1971). A report of studies where 20 ml of a radio-opaque contrast medium were injected over the back of the tongue one minute after loss of consciousness shows a low incidence of inhalation of dye after 1 mg kg^{-1} ketamine. There is less frequent protection with 2 mg kg^{-1} and the lungs invariably contained the contrast when any premedication was given prior to the ketamine (Carson et al, 1973). Actual aspiration pneumonitis after ketamine has been reported by Penrose (1972). Taylor et al (1972) also demonstrated the importance of dosage and found a greater depression of reflexes as the duration of anaesthesia continued. It is interesting to note that Yeung and Lin (1972) found active laryngeal reflexes after an intramuscular injection of 4 mg kg^{-1} ketamine in children, with no aspiration of radio-opaque medium placed in the pharynx although half the patients developed laryngospasm. Both the age of the subjects and the relatively small dose of drug may have been significant factors in this situation.

Miscellaneous effects

Long term use

Since many of its properties make ketamine a useful drug in repeated burn dressings (Bjarnesen and Corssen, 1967; Wilson et al 1967; Corssen and Oget, 1971), the studies of Bree et al (1967) with repeated administration in monkeys are important. They found no marked pathological changes in vital organs, although the duration of anaesthesia decreased as the number of anaesthetics increased, suggesting the development of tolerance to ketamine. In this context it is also important to record that Wilson et al (1971) found no evidence of immunosuppression from ketamine.

Muscle tone and relaxation

The effect of ketamine on neuromuscular transmission has not been studied but, as pointed out previously, sleep is usually accompanied by an increase in muscle tone. Corssen et al (1968) record two cases which suggest that it has some anti-epileptic properties, but there is no evidence to show whether this is a central or peripheral action. Animal studies by McCarthy et al (1965) had previously demonstrated some anticonvulsant activity, although it was ineffective against strychnine-induced seizures (Chen et al 1966).

The only study directly related to the action of ketamine on the myoneural junction is that of Bovill et al (1971c), who showed that the average duration of apnoea and respiratory depression from 50 mg suxamethonium was significantly greater when it was given after ketamine than after either thiopentone or methohexitone.

Organ toxicity

Domino et al (1965) and Corssen and Domino (1966) state that ketamine has no adverse effects on hepatic or renal function. Bovill et al (1971c) gave data based on six tests of liver function carried out before and six and 24 hours after 2 mg kg^{-1} ketamine, given for minor operations and detected no evidence of hepatic toxicity.

Others

Corssen and Hoy (1967) and Corssen et al (1968) found slightly increased intraocular pressure following the intravenous administration of ketamine. Yoshikawi and Murai (1971) observed a transient increase after the intramuscular injection of 5 mg kg^{-1} which they attributed to a possible imbalance in the tone of the extraocular muscles. Although Rubli (1971) also found a slight rise, he commented on the relative stability of intraocular pressure under ketamine anaesthesia in children.

Uterine tone does not appear to be depressed with clinical doses of ketamine (Langrehr et al, 1970; Moore et al, 1971); in fact the tendency is towards increased tone (Galloon, 1972). This same author (1973) has also shown that ketamine increases the pressure in the pregnant uterus for 5 to 15 min after injection and during this same period also tends to increase the intensity and frequency of contractions although Nishijima (1972) and Rodrigues & Barreto (1971) reported a decrease in tone. Marx et al (1979) investigated the effects of ketamine in doses ranging from 5 to 100 mg using internal tocography of the uterus immediately following full-term delivery. They concluded that 100 mg or less has no unphysiological effect on the pregnant uterus at term under normal conditions. However during situations in which an increased uterine activity may be harmful such as tetanic contraction, abruptio placenta or cord prolapse the dose of ketamine should not exceed 25 mg. Idvall and coworkers (1982) have established that ketamine increases the basal tone and intensity of contractions of the non-pregnant uterus and that these effects coincide with the phase of haemodynamic stimulation and peak plasma ketamine levels. Moore and his colleagues (1971) found some evidence of increased muscle tone in infants when ketamine was given to the mothers. In clinical practice low Apgar scores (Moore et al, 1971; Little et al, 1972) can be avoided and patient acceptance has been reported as good if low-dose ketamine is used (Chodoff & Stella, 1966; Akamatsu et al, 1974).

Ketamine causes a slight rise in blood sugar but this effect is quite variable. It reaches its peak about 10 to 15 min after injection and has passed off within 2 h. It does not exacerbate the metabolic response to surgical trauma (Lacoumenta et al, 1984).

An erythematous rash is seen in about one-fifth of the patients given ketamine, but this is transient and of no particular significance.

Salivation may be profuse after either route of administration of ketamine and this can cause problems in unatropinised children.

According to Grant and associates (1981) who have tested it in volunteers gastric emptying time is not delayed by intramuscular ketamine.

In common with other intravenous agents (List, 1967) ketamine causes a slight fall in serum potassium levels. When followed by suxamethonium, the rise in potassium is less than in patients induced with thiopentone (Gal and Malit, 1972). Ketamine also appeared to reduce the incidence and severity of fasciculations produced by the relaxant.

KETAMINE ISOMERS

Ketamine enantiomers have been tested in animals (Marietta et al, 1977a; Ryder et al, 1978 and Meliska et al, 1980) and have been subjected to clinical studies by White and associates (1980a and b). Both quantitative and qualitative differences have been demonstrated between the isomers on one hand and the racemic compound on the other. It has been shown that there are unique pharmacodynamic and pharmacokinetic differences between these three substances. While no differences in duration of anaesthesia could be demonstrated for equipotent doses, there was however a definite difference in potency, the ratio being 3.4:1 for the (+) ketamine as compared to (−) ketamine. (+) ketamine seems to produce more effective anaesthesia than either the racemic or (−) ketamine preparation with significantly more psychic emergence reactions and agitated behaviour than with either of the other two preparations. Postoperative pain was more prominent with the racemic and (−) ketamine than with the (+) ketamine variety, while the instance of dreaming was identical for the three groups. In a more general sense patients found the (+) ketamine more acceptable than either of the other two. Since the plasma decay curves and the patterns of appearance in excretion of the ketamine metabolites are parallel in all three groups, the difference can only be explained as being due to pharmacodynamic factors.

Despite the apparent superiority of (+) ketamine over the other two preparations the substance is not in commercial use.

CLINICAL APPLICATIONS

It is clear from what has been said that ketamine is one of the most interesting intravenous anaesthetics to have been introduced into clinical practice. It has properties both desirable and undesirable that are unique in the realm of pharmacology, and it is perhaps because of these that some fifteen years after its introduction into anaesthesia its exact role is still undecided and even controversial.

There can be little doubt that because of the excellent tissue tolerance, its consequent suitability for intramuscular administration, and profound analgesia obtained, it is a most desirable agent in instances when there is difficulty finding a suitable vein or where venipuncture is poorly tolerated. This goes particularly for young children and patients with extensive burns. Its use in these circumstances is not necessarily limited to induction of anaesthesia, but ketamine has also been found to be a very suitable single anaesthetic for minor diagnostic procedures, such as examination under anaesthesia, probing of tear ducts, certain neurological investigations in the absence of intracranial hypertension, paediatric dentistry (Sobczak, 1975) and radiotherapy (Amberg and Gordon, 1976). It has also been used in cardiac catheterization and in this connection Morray et al. (1984) have shown that haemodynamic changes with this method are small and that there is no change in clinical status nor is the information obtained influenced by the anaesthesia. Even the oral route has been found effective in children (Hain, 1983; Morgan and Dutkiewicz, 1983) while Maltby and Watkins (1983) have found the rectal route as acceptable as the intramuscular one for repeat anaesthesia in children. However, this should be seen in the light of the observation of Idvall et al (1983) of the low bioavailability of ketamine when given rectally, compensated for by extension of the analgesia into the recovery period. Grant and associates (1984) have demonstrated delayed and incomplete absorption after oral administration and attribute the efficacy of this route to elevated levels of nor-ketamine. While these paediatric indications are well-established and documented, its use nevertheless is not as widespread as it might be. It has also become clear that tolerance can develop after repeated use of ketamine (Stevens & Hain, 1981; Byer & Gould, 1981) and that limits its usefulness for burn dressings and radiotherapy where multiple sessions are often needed. The possible mechanism to explain this phenomenon has been discussed. Chatterjee & Syed (1983) have suggested ketamine for the operation of pyloromyotomy in infants, an indication which is categorically rejected by Bush (1984) and Battersby and associates (1984).

It has been used for operations on the great vessels in infants with congenital cardiac anomalies and for ophthalmological operations in children (ApIvor, 1973). Here one must be aware of potential rises in intraocular pressure and avoid its use when this would cause problems.

Adults

As far as the non-paediatric patient population is concerned the situation is less clear. It has been recommended to break severe bronchospasm (Fisher, 1977; Rajanna et al, 1982) and is considered by some to be the induction agent of choice in asthmatics (Corssen et al, 1972). Repeated burn dressings is one of the least disputed indications for this drug and it can be rightly extended to include other kinds of painful dressing changes. Ketamine has at one time or other been recommended as the ideal anaesthetic for almost any surgical operation in any age group, but many of these reports have been isolated and few, if any, have been universally accepted. It has been used in conjunction with nitrous oxide and tubocurarine for abdominal and thoracic operations in adults (Vaughan & Stephen, 1974; Houlton et al, 1978) and as a continuous infusion for one-lung anaesthesia (Weinreich et al, 1980); however, Rees & Gaines (1984) did not consider this technique to afford an advantage over enflurane anaesthesia.

In obstetrics and gynaecology ketamine has been used for colposcopy (McKenzie & Tantisira, 1973), abdominal tubal ligation (Azar & Ozomek, 1973) and Caesarean Section (Meer et al, 1973; Peltz & Sinclair, 1973; Downing et al, 1976; Dich-Nielsen & Holasek, 1982), vaginal delivery (Akamatsu et al, 1974; Janeczko et al, 1974; Galloon, 1976) and manual removal of the placenta (Roopnarinesingh & Kalipersadsingh, 1974). There is even a case on record (Bancroft & Lauria, 1983) in which ketamine was used successfully for induction of anaesthesia in an achondroplastic dwarf suffering from acute intermittent porphyria who needed a Caesarean Section.

It has been particularly recommended as the anaesthetic of choice in poor-risk patients (Nettles et al, 1973; Pedersen et al, 1982) such as fixation of fractured neck of femur in geriatrics (Stefanson et al, 1982), for those in hypovolaemic shock (Chasapakis et al, 1973; Bond & Davies, 1974) and in patients with liver damage (Schaps & Hauenschild, 1977). Its use has even been described in one case of hepatic artery ligation in a patient with carcinoid syndrome (Eisenkraft et al, 1981) but here they recommend that it be combined with diazepam to modify catecholamine release.

Despite its proven propensity to cause convulsions, ketamine has nevertheless been recommended and found useful in the control of convulsions (Corssen et al, 1974; Fisher, 1974; Sybert & Kyff, 1983). Ketamine has been used with advantage in paralysis agitans (Hetherington & Rosenblatt, 1980) and has been found safe in patients suffering from acute intermittent porphyria (Rizk et al, 1977), as well as individuals requiring multiple operations for epidermolysis bullosa (LoVerme & Oropollo, 1977). Single patient experience has been reported of successful tracheal intubation under ketamine alone in a patient with Treacher-Collins syndrome (MacLennan & Robertson, 1981), for induction of anaesthesia for an emergency procedure in a patient in Addisonian crisis (Smith & Byrne, 1981), in one with Shy-Drager syndrome (Saarnivaara et al, 1983) and in the patient with a previous history of malignant hyperthermia (Zsigmond, 1971).

As an intravenous infusion in combination with diazepam, ketamine has been found to be a useful anaesthetic in a case of pemphygus vulgaris (Vatashsky & Aronson, 1982). Ketamine has even been administered for the treatment of hiccough (Shanta, 1973).

Ketamine has been administered by continuous intravenous drip (Jastak & Goretta, 1973; El-Naggar et al, 1977; Lilburn et al, 1978) and as a low-dose intravenous infusion to provide amnesia, analgesia and sedation for non-stimulating superficial interventions (Slogoff et al, 1974) and for postoperative analgesia (Nimmo & Clements, 1981). In combination with diazepam, ketamine has been found to be an acceptable and useful adjunct to regional anaesthetic techniques (Beekhuis & Kahn, 1978; Rothe & Schorer, 1980) and Korttila & Levanen (1978) found no more side effects after diazepam-ketamine than in an unpremedicated control group. On the whole it would appear that the combination of intravenous ketamine and diazepam is gaining in popularity.

Of more than passing interest is the observation of Gale (1972) that penile turgescence yields to ketamine and this observation has been confirmed by Ravindran et al (1982). To explain this observation it has been postulated that the dissociative properties of ketamine might block subconscious central responses to peripheral penile stimulation. On the other hand Benzon et al (1983) have failed to confirm the effectiveness of ketamine in the condition. Another unconfirmed finding is reversal of the effect of ketamine by physostigmine (Balmer & Wyte, 1977). This is both unpredictable and transient.

This is indeed a formidable list of uses for ketamine, yet it lacks consistency. Almost everything has been tried at one time or another, but the real indications for this anaesthetic remain elusive. Yet the fact that the drug has survived for a good number of years testifies to its usefulness, at least under some circumstances and in the practice of some anaesthetists.

The situation can be clarified by consideration of the very comprehensive list of indications and contraindications (Table 9.1) proposed by White et al (1982). This table includes outpatient gynaecological and orthopaedic procedures: in some countries these would take less time than the onset of action of ketamine, so that these indications have to be considered in the light of local surgical practice. To these one would add a consideration of its use 'beyond the major centres' and in some emergency or difficult situations.

Elsewhere

A more recent, and as yet imperfectly evaluated, use of ketamine is in subanaesthetic doses 'beyond major centres'. Its use in 'Third World situations' was reported in detail at the 8th World Congress of Anaesthesiologists in Manila (Boulton, 1985) and reference has already been made to the low incidence of psychotic sequelae. In this situation it is used entirely without nitrous oxide, although most patients are given a small dose of atropine. Initial doses are in the region of 0.4–0.5 mg kg^{-1}

with supplements as required. It is difficult to get a suitable endpoint to indicate that patients are ready for operation — nystagmus is unreliable and there are even some patients who will continue to talk after they are sufficiently analgesic to allow minor procedures to be carried out. One must not expect the 'cardavaric' stillness of the patient under full general anaesthesia and certainly surgeons will not have the degree of muscle relaxation provided either by inhalation agents, myoneural blocking drugs or subarachnoid block.

Table 9.1 Clinical uses of ketamine and contraindications to its use

I. Indications for ketamine anaesthesia or analgesia:
- A. Aged and poor-risk patients:
  1. shock or cardiovascular instability
  2. severe dehydration
  3. respiratory failure or bronchospasm
  4. severe anaemia
  5. major thoracoabdominal procedures
  6. cardiac tamponade and constrictive pericarditis
- B. Obstetrical patients:
  1. rapid induction of general anaesthesia
     a) severe hypovolaemia
     b) acute haemorrhage
     c) acute bronchospasm
  2. low-dose for analgesia
     a) supplement regional technique
     b) transient analgesia at the time of delivery or during postpartum period
- C. Adjunct to local and regional anaesthetic techniques:
  1. low-dose for sedation and analgesia during performance of nerve block procedure
  2. supplemental analgesia for inadequate block
- D. Outpatient surgery:
  1. Paediatric anaesthesia
     a) brief diagnostic and therapeutic procedures (e.g. cardiac cath; endoscopy; oral surgery; head and neck surgery; orthopaedic surgery; ophthalmology; radiotherapy)
     b) induction of anaesthesia (e.g. intramuscular or rectal route)
  2. Adult anaesthesia
     a) brief surgical procedures (e.g. gynaecological, head and neck, orthopaedic, urologic)
     b) supplement local and regional techniques
     c) diagnostic and therapeutic procedures (e.g. endoscopy)
- E. Patients with reactive airway disease:
  1. asthmatics with acute bronchospasm
  2. chronic obstructive pulmonary disease with bronchospasm
- F. Patients with thermal injuries:
  1. debridement and skin grafting
  2. dressing changes
- G. Postoperative analgesia:
  1. recovery room
  2. intensive care units

II. Contraindications to the use of ketamine
- A. Cardiovascular disease:
  1. poorly controlled hypertension
  2. intracranial, thoracic or abdominal aneurysms
  3. unstable angina or recent myocardial infarction
  4. right or left heart failure
- B. Central nervous system disorders:
  1. cerebral trauma
  2. intracerebral mass or haemorrhage
- C. Open-globe injury to eye or increased intraocular pressure*
- D. Thyrotoxic states*
- E. Otolaryngologic procedures involving pharynx, larynx or trachea*
- F. Psychiatric disorders (e.g. schizophrenia) or history of adverse reaction to ketamine or one of its congeners*

* indicates a *relative* contraindication to the use of ketamine (White et al, 1982)

Preoperative briefing might minimize the feeling of dissociation and floating in space which sometimes occurs either during operation or in the postoperative period and which might be attributed to the state of analgesia and consequent detachment from their surroundings. Nausea and vomiting has not been a problem in these patients and although conditions are not what one would expect with modern techniques, nevertheless under these circumstances the drug can fill a vacuum where others are not available and furthermore it can, under these circumstances, be administered by the same person who is carrying out the operation or by any available technical assistance.

Difficult situations

The drug has already proved its worth in emergency situations (Rust et al, 1978). Its intrathecal use in war surgery has been investigated by Bion (1984) and while the absence of hypotension and respiratory depression were advantageous, its central effects and short duration of action would appear to limit its use in this field.

Ketamine is invaluable in some difficult situations. Limitation of supplies of anaesthetics might cause problems because of isolation due to geographical distance and inaccessibility or man-made restrictions such as occur during wars or in civil disasters due to logistic difficulties particularly those relating to air transport. Other conditions are the cost of drugs and apparatus and climatic and topographic factors. Ketamine is nonflammable and portable, and requires minimal apparatus. Its administration is not affected by climate or topography, except that additional oxygen will be required at high altitude. Solutions have a shelf life of up to four years at maximum potency provided that they are kept away from light and at an ambient temperature below 30°C; storage in a cool place, or even a refrigerator, is therefore an advantage, and the question of turnover has to be considered if the drug is stored in emergency mobilisation or disaster stores.

Oral and rectal use

Ketamine has been used as a sole agent for analgesia by the oral route in small children to provide analgesia for burn dressing and similar procedures (Morgan & Dutkiwicz, 1983; Hain, 1983); the technique might have a place but further evaluation is required. Ketamine has also been employed as a basal rectal anaesthetic after diazepam premedication for minor operations in children (Saint-Maurice et al, 1979).

REFERENCES

Adams J D, Baillie T A, Trevor A J, Castagnoli N Jr 1981 Studies on the biotransformation of ketamine — identification of metabolites produced in vitro from rat liver microsomal preparations. Biomedical Mass Spectrometry 8: 527–538

Akamatsu T J, Bonica J J, Rehmet R, Eng M, Ueland K 1974 Experiences with the use of ketamine for parturition: I. Primary anesthetic for vaginal delivery. Anesthesia and Analgesia, Current Researches 53: 284–287

Albin M S, Dresner A J 1969 Emergence reactions associated with the administration of ketamine hydrochloride (Ketalar, Parke Davis). Paper read before the International Symposium on L'anesthesie vigile et subvigile, Ostend, Belgium, April 17–20, 1969

Albin M S, Dresner A J 1971 Personality functioning after Ketalar and other anesthetic agents. Ketalar (ketamine hydrochloride-PD & CO), P 137. Parke, Davis & Co Ltd, Montreal

Albin M, Dresner J, Paolino A, Sweet R, Virtue M D, Miller G 1970 Long term personality evaluation in patients subjected to ketamine hydrochloride and other anesthetic agents. Pharmacology: Abstracts of Scientific Papers, pp 166–167. American Society of Anesthesiologists: Annual Meeting 1970

Amberg H L, Gordon G 1976 Low-dose ketamine for pediatric radiotherapy: a case report. Anesthesia and Analgesia, Current Researches 55: 92–94

ApIvor D 1973 Ketamine in Paediatric Ophthalmological surgery. An evaluation of its efficacy and post-operative effects. Anaesthesia 28: 501–508

Azar I, Ozomek E 1973 The use of ketamine for abdominal tubal ligation. Anesthesia and Analgesia, Current Researches 52: 39–42

Balmer H G R, Wyte S R 1977 Antagonism to ketamine by physostigmine. British Journal of Anaesthesia 49:510P

Bancroft G H, Lauria J I (1983) Ketamine induction for cesarean section in a patient with acute intermittent porphyria and achondroplastic dwarfism. Anesthesiology 59: 143–144

Battersby E F, Facer E, Glover W J, Hatch D J, James I, Mackersie A, Sumner E 1984 Ketamine anaesthesia for pyloromyotomy. Anaesthesia 39:381

Beekhuis G J, Kahn D L 1978 Anesthesia for facial cosmetic surgery. Low dosage ketamine-diazepam anesthesia. Laryngoscope 88: 1709–1712

Bennett J A, Bullimore J A 1973 The use of ketamine hydrochloride anaesthesia for radiotherapy in young children. British Journal of Anaesthesia 45: 197–201

Benzon H T, Leventhal J R, Ovassapian A 1983 Ketamine treatment of penile erection in the operating room (letter). Anesthesia and Analgesia, Current Researches 62: 457–458

Betts E K & Parkin C E 1971 Use of ketamine in an asthmatic child: a case report. Anesthesia and Analgisia, Current Researches 50: 420–421

Bidwai A V, Stanley T H, Graves C L, Kawamura R, Sentker C R 1975 The effect of ketamine on cardiovascular dynamics during halothane and enflurane anesthesia. Anesthesia and Analgesia, Current Researches 54: 588–592

Bion J F 1984 Intrathecal ketamine for war surgery. A preliminary study under field conditions. Anaesthesia 39: 1023–1028

Bjarnsen W, Corssen G 1967 CI-581: a new non-barbiturate short acting anesthetic for surgery in burns. Michigan Medicine 66:177

Blair D A, Glover W E, Greenfield A D M, Roddie I E 1959 Excitation of cholinergic vasodilator nerves to human skeletal muscles during emotional stress. Journal of Physiology 148:633

Bodai B I, Harms B A, Nottingham P B, Zaiss C, Demling R H 1983 The effect of ketamine on endotoxin-induced lung injury. Anesthesia and Analgesia, Current Researches 62: 398–403

Bond A C, Davies C K 1974 Ketamine and pancuronium for the shocked patient. Anaesthesia 29: 59–62

Boulton T B (ed) 1985 Anaesthesia beyond the major medical centre. Current techniques with ketamine. Blackwell, Oxford

Bovill J G, Clarke R S J, Davis E A, Dundee J W 1971a Some cardiovascular effects of ketamine. British Journal of Pharmacology 41:411p

Bovill J G, Clarke R S J, Dundee J W, Pandit S K, Moore J 1971b Clinical studies of induction agents. XXXVIII: Effect of premedicants and supplements on ketamine anaesthesia. British Journal of Anaesthesia, 43: 600–608

Bovill J G, Coppel D L, Dundee J W, Moore J 1971c Current status of ketamine anaesthesia. Lancet i: 1285–1288

Bovill J G, Dundee J W 1971 Alterations in response to somatic pain associated with anaesthesia. XX: Ketamine. British Journal of Anaesthesia 43: 496–499
Bovill J G, Dundee J W 1972 Attempts to control the cardiostimulatory effect of ketamine in man. Anaesthesia 27: 309–312
Bree M M, Feller I, Corssen G 1967 Safety and tolerance of repeated anesthesia with CI-581 (ketamine) in monkeys. Anesthesia and Analgesia, Current Researches 46: 596–600
Brown T C K, Cole W H J, Murray G H 1970 Ketamine: a new anaesthetic agent. Australian and New Zealand Journal of Surgery 39: 305–310
Bush G H 1984 Ketamine anaesthesia for pyloromyotomy. Anaesthesia 39:381
Byer D E, Gould A B Jr 1981 Development of tolerance to ketamine in an infant undergoing repeated anesthesia. Anesthesiology 54: 255–256
Carson I W, Moore J, Balmer J P, Dundee J W, McNabb G 1973 Laryngeal competence with ketamine and other drugs. Anesthesiology 38: 128–133
Cartwright P D, Pingel S M 1984 Midazolam and diazepam in ketamine anaesthesia. Anaesthesia 39: 439–442
Chasapakis G, Kekis N, Sakkalis C, Kolios D 1973 Use of ketamine and pancuronium for anesthesia for patients in hemorrhagic shock. Anesthesia and Analgesia, Current Researches 52: 282–287
Chatterjee S C, Syed A 1983 Ketamine and infants. Anaesthesia 38:1007
Chen G 1965 Evaluation of phencyclidine-type cataleptic activity. Archives internationales de pharmacodynamie et de therapie 157: 193–201
Chen G 1969 Pharmacology of ketamine. Anaesthesist 18:24
Chen G, Ensor C R, Bohner B 1966 The neuropharmacology of 2-(O-chlorophenyl)-2-methylaminocyclohexanone hydrochloride. Journal of Pharmacology and Experimental Therapeutics 152: 332–339
Chodoff P 1972 Evidence of central adrenergic action of ketamine: report of a case. Anesthesia and Analgesia, Current Researches 51: 247–250
Chodoff P, Stella J C 1966 Use of CI-581, a phenylcyclidine derivative for obstetric anesthesia. Anesthesia and Analgesia, Current Researches 45: 527–530
Clements J A, Nimmo W S 1981 Pharmacokinetics and analgesiac effect of ketamine in man. British Journal of Anaesthesia 53: 27–30
Cohen M L, Chan S L, Way W L, Trevor A J 1973 Distribution in the brain and metabolism of ketamine in the rat after intravenous administration. Anesthesiology 39: 370–376
Collier B B 1972 Ketamine and the conscious mind. Anaesthesia 27: 120–134
Coppel D L, Bovill J G, Dundee J W 1973 The taming of ketamine. Anaesthesia 28: 293–296
Coppel D L, Dundee J W 1972 Ketamine anaesthesia for cardiac catheterisation. Anaesthesia 27: 25–31
Corssen G 1969 Allgemeine klinische Erfahrungen mit Ketamine bei mehr als 1500 Fallen. Der Anaesthesist 18:25
Corssen G, Domino E F 1966 Dissociative anesthesia; further pharmacologic studies and first clinical experience with the phencyclidine derivative CI-581. Anesthesia and Analgesia, Current Researches 45:29
Corssen G, Domino E F, Bree R L 1969 Electroencephalographic effects of ketamine anesthesia in children. Anesthesia and Analgesia, Current Researches 48: 141–147
Corssen G, Hayward J R, Gunter J W, Groves E H 1969b A new parenteral anesthesia for oral surgery. Journal of Oral Surgery 27: 627–632
Corssen G, Gutierrez J, Reves J G, Huber F C Jr 1972 Ketamine in anesthetic management of asthmatic patients. Anesthesia and Analgesia, Current Researches 51: 588–596
Corssen G, Hoy J W 1967 A new parenteral anesthetic CI-581: its effect on intraocular pressure. Pediatric Opthalmology 4: 20–23
Corssen G, Little S, Tavakoli M 1974 Ketamine and epilepsy. Anesthesia and Analgesia, Current Researches 53: 319–335
Corssen G, Miyasaka M, Domino E F 1968 Changing concepts in pain control during surgery: dissociative anesthesia with CI-581: a progress report. Anesthesia and Analgesia, Current Researches 47: 746–759
Corssen G, Oget S 1971 Dissociative anesthesia for the severely burned child. Anesthesia and Analgesia, Current Researches 50: 95–102
Corssen G, Oget S, Reed P C 1971 Computerised evaluation of psychic effects of ketamine. Anesthesia and Analgesia, Current Researches 50: 397–401
Cronin M M, Bousfield J D, Hewitt E B, McLellan I, Boulton T B 1972 Ketamine anaesthesia for radiotherapy in small children. Anaesthesia 27: 135–142
Crosby G, Tannenbaum S, Sokoloff A 1980 Ketamine alters regional glucose utilization in rat brain. Anesthesiology 53:S6
Dawson B, Michenfelder J D, Theye R A 1971 Effects of ketamine on canine cerebral blood flow and metabolism: modification by prior administration of thiopental. Anesthesia and Analgesia, Current Researches 50: 443–447
Demling R H, Ellerbee S, Jarrett F 1978 Ketamine anesthesia for tangential excision of burn eschar: a burn unit procedure. Journal of Trauma 18: 269–270
Diaz F A, Bianco A, Bello N, Beer N, Velarde H, Izquierdo J P, Jaen R 1976 Effects of ketamine on canine cardiovascular function. British Journal of Anaesthesia 48: 941–946
Dich-Nielsen J, Holasek J 1982 Ketamine as induction agent for caesarian section. Acta Anaesthesiologica Scandinavica 26: 139–142
Dill W A, Chucot L, Chang T, Glazko A J 1971 Determination of ketamine in blood plasma. Anesthesiology 34: 73–76
Dobson M B 1978 Anaesthesia with ketamine and thiopentone for short surgical procedures. Anaesthesia 33: 268–270
Domino E F, Chodoff P, Corssen G 1965 Pharmacologic effects of CI-581, a new dissociative anesthetic in man. Clinical Pharmacology and Therapeutics 6: 279–290
Domino E F, Domino F E, Smith R E, Domino L E, Goulet J R, Domino K E, Zsigmond E K 1984 Ketamine kinetics in unpremedicated and diazepam-premedicated subjects. Clinical Pharmacology and Therapeutics 36: 645–653
Dowdy E G, Kaya K 1968 Studies of the mechanism of cardiovascular responses to CI-581. Anesthesiology 29: 931–943
Downing J W, Mahomedy M C, Jeal D E, Allen P J 1976 Anaesthesia for caesarian section with ketamine. Anaesthesia 31: 883–892
Dundee J W 1971 Ketamine. Proceedings of the Royal Society of Medicine 64: 39–40
Dundee J W, Bovill J, Knox J W D, Clarke R S J, Black

G W, Love S H S, Moore J, Elliott J, Pandit S K, Copple D L 1970 Ketamine: a preliminary report on its use as an induction agent. Lancet i: 1370–1371
Dundee J W, Lilburn J K 1977 Ketamine–lorazepam: attenuation of the psychic sequelae of ketamine by lorazepam. Anaesthesia 37: 312–314
Dundee J W, McGowan A W, Lilburn J K, McKay A C, Hegarty J E 1979 Comparison of the actions of diazepam and lorazepam. British Journal of Anaesthesia 51: 439–445
Eisenkraft J B, Dimich I, Miller R 1981 Ketamine–diazepam anaesthesia in a patient with carcinoid syndrome. Anaesthesia 36: 881–885
El-Hawary M B, Mossad B, Abd El-Wahed S, Tolba H M 1972 Effect of ketamine hydrochloride on the tracheobronchial tree. Middle East Journal of Anaesthesia 3: 455–450
El-Naggar M, Letcher J, Middleton E, Levine H 1977 Administration of ketamine or Innovar by the microdrip technic: a double blind study. Anesthesia and Analgesia 56: 279–282
Erbguth P H, Reiman B, Klein R L 1972 The influence of chlorpromazine, diazepam and droperidol on emergence from ketamine. Anesthesia and Analgesia, Current Researches 51: 693–700
Evans J, Rosen M, Weeks R D, Wise C 1971 Ketamine in neurosurgical procedures. Letter to Editor. Lancet i: 40–41
Ferrer-Allado T, Brechner V L, Dymond A, Cozen H, Crandall P 1973 Ketamine-induced electroconvulsive phenomena in the human limbic and thamalic region. Anesthesiology 38: 333–334
Finck A D, Ngai S H 1979 A possible mechanism of ketamine-induced analgesia. Anesthesiology 51:S34
Fisher M McD 1974 Use of ketamine hydrochloride in the treatment of convulsions. Anaesthesia Intensive Care 2: 266–268
Fisher M McD 1977 Ketamine hydrochloride in severe bronchospasm. Anaesthesia 32: 771–772
Fratta W, Casu M, Balestrieri A, Loviselli A, Biggio G, Gessa G L 1980 Failure of ketamine to interact with opiate receptors. European Journal of Pharmacology 61: 389–391
Gal T J, Malit L A 1972 The influence of ketamine induction on potassium changes and fasciculations following suxamethonium. British Journal of Anaesthesia 44: 1077–1080
Gale A S 1972 Ketamine prevention of penile turgescence. Journal of American Medical Association 219:1629
Galloon S 1971 Ketamine for dilation and curettage. Canadian Anaesthetists' Society Journal 18: 600–613
Galloon S 1972 Measurement of pressure changes on the pregnant uterus following ketamine HCl and other anaesthetics. Proceedings of the fifth World Congress of Anaesthesiologists, Kyoto, September 19–23, 1972, pp 92–93
Galloon S 1973 Ketamine and the pregnant uterus. Canadian Anaesthetists' Society Journal 20: 141–145
Galloon S 1976 Ketamine for obstetrical delivery. Anesthesiology 44: 522–524
Garfield J M, Garfield F B, Stone J G, Hopkins D 1970 The effect of varying preoperative information on psychological responses to ketamine and halothane anesthesia. Abstracts of Scientific Papers. American Society of Anesthesiologists, Annual Meeting 1970, pp 164–165
Garfield J M, Garfield F B, Stone J G, Hopkins D, Johns L A 1972 Comparison of psychologic responses of ketamine and thiopental–nitrous oxide–halothane anesthesia. Anesthesiology 36: 329–338
Gibbs J M 1972 The effect of intravenous ketamine on cerebrospinal fluid pressure. British Journal of Anaesthesia 44: 1298–1302
Ginsberg H, Gerber J A 1968 CI-581: a clinical report on 100 patients. South African Medical Journal 42: 1177–1179
Ginsberg H, Gerber J A 1969 Ketamine hydrochloride: a clinical investigation in 60 children. South African Medical Journal 43: 627–628
Gjessing J 1968 Ketamine (CI-581) in clinical anaesthesia. Acta Anaesthesiologica Scandinavica 12: 15–21
Glazko A J, Dill W A, Fransway R L 1962 Determination of diphenhydramine blood levels using a new fluorescent dye-salt procedure generally applicable to basic organic compounds. Federation Proceedings 21:269
Goldberg A H, Keane P W, Phear W P C 1970 Effects of ketamine on contractile performance and excitability of isolated heart muscle. Journal of Pharmacology and Experimental Therapeutics 175: 388–394
Gooding J M, Dimick A R, Tavakoli M 1977 A physiologic analysis of cardiopulmonary responses to ketamine anesthesia in non-cardiac patients. Anesthesia and Analgesia, Current Researches 56: 813–816
Grant I S, Nimmo W S, Clements J A 1981 Lack of effect of ketamine analgesia on gastric emptying in man. British Journal of Anaesthesia 53: 1321–1323
Grant I S, Nimmo W S, Clements J A 1984 Oral ketamine Anaesthesia 39: 66–67
Hain W R 1983 Oral ketamine. Anaesthesia 38: 810–811
Hamilton J T, Bryson J S 1974 The effect of ketamine on transmembrane potentials of Purkinje fibres of the pig heart. British Journal of Anaesthesia 46: 636–642
Hervey W H Hustead R F 1972 Ketamine for dilatation and curettage procedures: patient acceptance. Anesthesia and Analgesia, Current Researches 51: 647–655
Hetherington A, Rosenblatt R M 1980 Ketamine and paralysis agitans. Anesthesiology 52:527
Houlton P J C, Downing J W, Brock-Utne J G 1978 Intravenous ketamine anaesthesia for major abdominal surgery — an assessment of a technique and the influence of ataractic drugs on the psychomimetic effects of ketamine. Anaesthesia Intensive Care 6: 222–225
Idvall J, Ahlgren I, Aronsen K F, Stenberg P 1979 Ketamine infusions: pharmacokinetics and clinical effects. British Journal of Anaesthesia 51: 1167–1173
Idvall J, Holasek J, Stenberg P 1983 Rectal ketamine for induction of anaesthesia in children. Anaesthesia 38: 60–64
Idvall J, Sandahl B, Stenberg P, Ulmsten U 1982 Influence of ketamine on non-pregnant uterus in vivo. Acta Anaesthesiologica Scandinavica 26: 592–595
Ireland S J, Livingston A 1980 Effect of biliary excretion on ketamine anaesthesia in the rat. British Journal of Anaesthesia 52: 23–28
Ivankovich A D, Miletich D J, Reimann C, Albrecht R F, Zahed B 1974 Cardiovascular effects of centrally administered ketamine in goats. Anesthesia and Analgesia, Current Researches 53: 924–933
Ivankovich A D, El-Etr A A, Janeczko G F, Maronic J P 1975 The effects of ketamine and of Innovar(R) anesthesia on digitalis tolerance in dogs. Anesthesia and Analgesia, Current Researches 54: 106–111
Iwatsuki K, Aoba Y, Sato K, Iwatsuki N 1967 Clinical study on CI-581 a phencyclidine derivative. Tohoku Journal of Experimental Medicine 93: 39–48

Jackson A P F, Dhadphale P R, Callaghan M L, Alseri S 1978 Haemodynamic studies during induction of anaesthesia for open-heart surgery using diazepam and ketamine. British Journal of Anaesthesia 50: 375–378
Janeczko G F, El-Etr A A, Younes S 1974 Low-dose ketamine anesthesia for obstetrical delivery. Anesthesia and Analgesia, Current Researches 53: 828–831
Janis K M, Wright W 1972 Failure to produce analgesia with ketamine in two patients with cortical disease. Anesthesiology 36: 405–406
Jastak J T, Gorretta C 1973 Ketamine HCl as a continuous-drip anesthesic for out-patients. Anesthesia and Analgesia, Current Researches 52: 341–344
Johnstone M 1972 The prevention of ketamine dreams. Anaesthesia Intensive Care 1: 70–74
Kayama Y, Iwama K 1972 The EEG evoked potentials and single unit activity during ketamine anesthesia in cats. Anesthesiology 36: 316–328
Kelly R W, Wilson R D, Traber D L, Priano L L 1971 Effect of two new dissociative anesthetic agents, ketamine and CL-1848C, on the respiratory response to carbon dioxide. Anesthesia and Analgesia, Current Researcnes 50: 262–269
Kelman G R, Kennedy B R 1970 Cardiovascular effects of pancuronium in anaesthetised man. British Journal of Pharmacology 40: 567–568
Knox J W D, Bovill J G, Clarke R S J, Dundee J W 1970 Clinical studies of induction agents. XXXVI: Ketamine. British Journal of Anaesthesia 42: 875–885
Koehntop D E, Liao J C, Van Bergen F H 1977 Effects of pharmacologic alterations of adrenergic mechanisms by cocaine, propolene, aminophylline and ketamine on epinephrine-induced arrhythmias during halothane-nitrous oxyde anesthesia. Anesthesiology 46: 83–93
Korttila K, Levanen J 1978 Untoward effect of ketamine combined with diazepam for supplementing conduction anaesthesia in young and middle-aged adults. Acta Anaesthesiologica Scandinavica 22: 640–648
Kreuscher H, Grote J 1967 Die Wirkung des Phencyclindinderivates Ketamine (CI-581) auf die Durch blutung und Sauerstoffaufnahme des Gehirns beim Hund. Anaesthesist 16: 304–308
Kumar S M, Kothary S P, Zsigmund E K 1978 Plasma-free norepinephrine and epinephrine concentrations following diazepam-ketamine induction in patients undergoing cardiac surgery. Acta Anaesthesiologica Scandinavica 22: 593–600
Lacoumenta S, Walsh E S, Waterman A E, Ward I, Paterson J L, Hall G M 1984 Effects of ketamine anaesthesia on the metabolic response to pelvic surgery. British Journal of Anaesthesia 56: 493–497
Langrehr D 1969 Dissoziative Anästhesie durch Ketamine. Actuelle Chirurgie 4: 71–78
Langrehr D, Kluge J 1969 Zur Anwendung von Ketamine in der Kinderanasthesie. Kinderchirurgie 7: 1–8
Langrehr D, Stolp W, Kluge J, Hans A 1970 Ketamine-anesthesia fur Geburtshilflish-gynakologische Eingriffe. Zeitzchrift fur praktische Anasthesie und Wiederbelebung 3: 145–156
Liang H S, Liang H G 1975 Minimizing emergence phenomena; subdissociative dosage of ketamine in balanced surgical anesthesia. Anesthesia and Analgesia, Current Researches 54: 312–316
Liao J C, Koehntop D E, Buckley J J 1979 Dual effect of ketamine on the peripheral vasculature. Anesthesiology. 51:S116
Lilburn J K, Dundee J W, Moore J 1978 Ketamine infusions. Observations on technique, dosage and cardiovascular effects. Anaesthesia 33: 315–321
Lilburn J K, Dundee J W, Nair S G, Fee J P H, Johnston H M L 1978 Ketamine sequelae-evaluation of the ability of various premedicants to attenuate its psychic actions. Anaesthesia 33: 307–311
List W F 1967 Serum potassium changes during induction of anaesthesia. British Journal of Anaesthesia 39: 480–484
Little B, Chang T, Chucot L, Dill W A, Enrile L L, Glazko A J, Jassani M, Kretchmer H, Sweet A Y 1972 Study of ketamine as an obstetric anesthesia agent. American Journal of Obstetrics and Gynecology 113: 247–260
Lorhan P H, Lippmann M 1971 A clinical appraisal of the use of ketamine hydrochloride in the aged. Anesthesia and Analgesia, Current Researches 50: 448–451
LoVerme S R, Oropollo A T 1977 Ketamine anesthesia in dermolytic bullous dermatosis. Anesthesia and Analgesia, Current Researches 56: 398–401
MacLennan F M 1982 Ketamine tolerance and hallucinations in children. Anaesthesia 37: 1214–125
MacLennan F M Robertson G S 1981 Ketamine for induction and intubation in Treacher-Collins syndrome. Anaesthesia 36: 196–198
Magbagberola J A O, Thomas N A 1974 Effect of thiopentone on emergence reactions to ketamine anaesthesia. Canadian Anaesthetists' Society Journal 21: 321–324
Maltby J R, Watkins D M 1983 Repeat ketamine anaesthesia of a child for radiotherapy in the prone position. Canadian Anaesthetists' Society Journal 30: 526–530
Marietta M P, Way W L, Castagnoli N 1977a On the pharmacology of the ketamine enantiomorphys in the rat. Journal of Pharmacology and Experimental Therapeuties 202: 157–165
Marietta M P, Vore M E, Way, W L, Trevor A J 1977b Characterization of ketamine induction of hepatic microsomal drug metabolism. Biochemical Pharmacology 26: 2451–2453
Marx G F, Hwang H S, Chandra P 1979 Postpartum uterine pressures with different doses of ketamine. Anesthesiology 50: 163–166
Massopust L C Jr, Wolin L R, Albin M S 1972 Electrophysiologic and behavioural responses to ketamine hydrochloride in the rhesus monkey. Anesthesia and Analgesia, Current Researches 51: 329–341
McCarthy D A, Chen G, Kaump D H, Ensor C 1965 General anesthetic and other pharmacological properties of 2-(0-chlorophenyl)-2-methylamino cyclohexanone HCl (CI-581). Journal of New Drugs 5: 21–33
McKenzie R, Tantisira B 1973 Culdoscopy: a new use for ketamine. Anesthesia and Analgesia, Current Researches 52: 351–354
Meer F M, Downing J W, Coleman A J 1973 An intravenous method of anaesthesia and caesarian section, part II: ketamine. British Journal of Anaesthesia 45: 191–196
Meliska C J, Greenberg A J, Trevor A J 1980 The effects of ketamine enantiomers on schedule-controlled behavior in the rat. Journal of Pharmacology and Experimental Therapeutics 212: 198–202
Miyasaka M, Domino E F 1968 Neuronal mechanisms of ketamine-induced anesthesia. Journal of Neuropharmacology 7: 557–573
Moore J, McNabb T G, Dundee J W 1971 Preliminary report on ketamine in obstetrics. British Journal of Anaesthesia 43: 779–782

Moretti R J, Hallan S Z, Goodman L I, Meltzer H Y 1984 Comparison of ketamine and thiopental in healthy volunteers: effects on mental status, mood and personality. Anesthesia and Analgesia 63: 1087–1096
Morgan A J, Dutkiewicz T W 1983 Oral ketamine Anaesthesia 38:293
Morray J P, Lynn A M, Stamm S J, Herndon P S, Kawabori I, Stevenson J G 1984 Hemodynamic effects of ketamine in children with congenital heart disease. Anesthesia and Analgesia, Current Researches 63: 859–899
Nelson S R, Howard R B, Cross R S, Samson F 1980 Ketamine induced changes in regional glucose utilization in the rat brain. Anesthesiology 52: 330–334
Nettles D C, Herrin T J, Mullen J G 1973 Ketamine induction in poor-risk patients. Anesthesia and Analgesia, Current Researches 52: 59–64
Nimmo W S, Clements J A 1981 Ketamine on demand for postoperative analgesia (letter). Anaesthesia 36:826
Nishijama M 1972 Ketamine in obstetric anaesthesia, with special reference to placental transfer and its concentration in drug plasma. Acta Obstetrica et Gynecologica Japonica 19: 80–93
Ohtani M, Kikuchi H, Kitahata L M, Taub A, Toyooka H, Hanaoka K, Dohi S 1979 Effects of ketamine on nociceptive cells in the medial medullary reticular formation of the cat. Anesthesiology 51: 414–417
Pandit S K, Dundee J W, Bovill J G 1971 Clinical studies of induction agents. XXXVIII: Amnesic action of ketamine. British Journal of Anaesthesia 43: 362–364
Pannacciulli E, Sordi L, Trazzi R 1966 The hallucinogen CI-581 and its use in anaesthesiology. Giornale italiano delle malattie de torace 20: 61–67
Pedersen T, Engbaek J, Klausen N O, Srensen B, Wiberg-Jrsensen F 1982 Effects of low-dose ketamine and thiopentone on cardiac performance and myocardial oxygen balance in high-risk patients. Acta Anaesthesiologica Scandinavica 26: 235–239
Peltz B, Sinclair D M 1973 Induction agents for caesarian section. A comparison of thiopentone and ketamine. Anaesthesia 28: 37–42
Pfenninger E, Dick W, Grunert A, Lotz P 1984 Tierexperimentelle Untersuchung zum intrakraniellen Druckverhalten unter Ketamineapplikation. Anaesthesist 33: 82–88
Penrose B H 1972 Aspiration pneumonitis following ketamine induction for a general anesthetic. Anesthesia and Analgesia, Current Researches 51:41
Podlesch I, Zindler M 1967 Erste Erfahrungen mit dem Phencyclidinderivat Ketamine (CI-581) einem neuen intravenösen und intramuskularen Narkosemittel. Der Anaesthesist 16: 299–303
Rajanna P 1983 Failure to produce anaesthesia with ketamine (letter). Anaesthesia 38:698
Rajanna P, Reddy J N, Gupta P K 1982 Ketamine for the relief of bronchospasm during anaesthesia (letter). Anaesthesia 37:1215
Ravindran R S, Dryden G E, Somerville G M 1982 Treatment of priapism with ketamine and physostigmine. Anesthesia and Analgesia, Current Researches 61: 705–707
Reder B S, Trapp L D, Trautman K C 1980 Ketamine suppression of chemical induced convulsions in the two-day-old white leghorn cockerel. Anesthesia and Analgesia, Current Researches 59: 406–409
Rees D I, Gaines G Y 1984 One-lung anesthesia — a comparison of pulmonary gas exchange during anesthesia with ketamine or enflurane. Anesthesia and Analgesia, Current Researches 63: 521–525
Rizk S F, Jocobson J H, Silvay G 1977 Ketamine as an induction agent for acute intermittent porphyria. Anesthesiology 46: 305–306
Roberts F W 1967 A new intramuscular anaesthetic for small children. Anaesthesia 22: 23–28
Rodrigues L J, Barreto H E 1971 Influence of ketamine on uterine contractions during labour. Journal Brasiliero de Ginecologia 71: 223–228
Roopnarinesingh R, Kalipersadsingh S 1974 Manual removal of the placenta under ketamine. Anaesthesia 29: 486–488
Rothe K F, Schorer R 1980 Ataranalgesia — an intravenous anesthetic technique; experience with 978 administrations. Acta Anaesthesiologica Belgica 31: 77–89
Rubli E 1971 Tonometry during general anaesthesia, the influence of halothane, cyclopropane and ketamine on normal intraocular pressure in children. Der Anaesthesist 20: 369–375
Rust M, Landauer B, Kolb E 1978 Stellenwert von ketamin in der notfallsituation. Der Anaesthesist 27: 205–212
Ryder S, Way W L, Trevor A J 1978 Comparative pharmacology of the optical isomers of ketamine in mice. European Journal of Pharmacology 49: 15–23
Saarnivaara L, Kautto U M, Teravainen H 1983 Ketamine anaesthesia for a patient with Shy-Dräger syndrome. Acta Anaesthesiologica Scandinavica 27: 123–125
Sadove M S, Hatano S, Redlin T, Thomason R, Arastounejad P, Roman V 1971a Clinical study of droperidol in the prevention of side effects of ketamine anesthesia. A progress report. Anesthesia and Analgesia, Current Researches 50: 526–532
Sadove M S, Hatano S, Zahed B, Redlin T, Arastounejad P, Roman V 1971b Clinical study of droperidol in the prevention of the side effects of ketamine anesthesia; a preliminary report. Anesthesia and Analgesia, Current Researches 50: 388–393
Sadove M S, Shulman M, Hatano S, Fevold N 1971c Analgesic effects of ketamine administered in subdissociative doses. Anesthesia and Analgesia, Current Researches 50: 452–457
Saint-Maurice C, Laguenie G, Couturier C, Goutail-Flaud F 1979 Rectal ketamine in paediatric anaesthesia. British Journal of Anaesthesia 51:573–574
Sari A, Okuda Y, Takeshita H 1972 The effect of ketamine on cerebrospinal fluid therapy. Anesthesia and Analgesia, Current Researches 51: 560–565
Schaps D, Hauenschild E, 1977 Anwendung von Ketamin bei Lebergeschädigten Patienten. Der Anaesthetist 26: 172–175
Schwartz D A, Horwitz L D 1975 Effects of ketamine on left ventricular performance. Journal of Pharmacology and Experimental Therapeutics 194: 410–414
Shanta T R 1973 Ketamine for the treatment of hiccups during and following anesthesia: a preliminary report. Anesthesia and Analgesia, Current Researches 52: 822–824
Shapiro H M, Wyte S R, Harris A B 1972 Ketamine anaesthesia in patients with intracranial pathology. British Journal of Anaesthesia 44: 1200–1204
Sklar G S, Zukin S R, Reilly T A 1981 Adverse reactions to ketamine anaesthesia. Abolition by a psychological technique. Anaesthesia 36: 183–187
Slogoff S, Allen G W, Wessels J V, Cheney D H 1974 Clinical experience with subanesthetic ketamine. Anesthesia and Analgesia, Current Researches 53: 354–358
Smith D J, Westfall D P, Adams J D 1980 Ketamine

interacts with opiate receptors as an agonist. Anesthesiology 53:S5
Smith M G, Byrne A J 1981 An addisonian crisis complicating anaesthesia. Anaesthesia 36: 681–684
Sobczak O M 1975 Use of ketamine in pediatric dentistry. Anesthesia and Analgesia, Current Researches 54: 248–249
Sparks D L, Corssen G, Sides J, Black J, Kholeif A 1973 Ketamine-induced anesthesia: neural mechanism in the rhesus monkey. Anesthesia and Analgesia, Current Researches 52: 288–297
Sparks D L, Corssen G, Aizenman B, Black J 1975 Further studies of the neural mechanisms of ketamine-induced anesthesia in the rhesus monkey. Anesthesia and Analgesia, Current Researches 54: 189–195
Spoerel W E, Kandel P F 1971 CI-581 in anaesthesia for tonsillectomy in children. Canadian Anaesthetists' Society Journal 17: 37–51
Stanley T H 1973 Blood pressure and pulse rate responses to ketamine during general anesthesia. Anesthesiology 39: 648–649
Stefansson T, Wickstrom I, Haljamae H 1982 Hemodynamic ad metabolic effects of ketamine anaesthesia in the geriatric patient. Acta Anaesthesiologica Scandinavica 26: 371–377
Stevens R W, Hain W R 1981 Tolerance to rectal ketamine in paediatric anaesthesia. Anaesthesia 36: 1089–1093
Sybert J W, Kyff J V 1983 Ketamine treatment of status epilepticus. Anesthesiology 58:203
Takeshita H, Okuda Y, Sari A I972 The effects of ketamine anesthesia on cerebral circulation and metabolism in man. Anesthesiology 36:69
Tarnow J, Hess W 1979 Flunitrazepam-Vorbehandlung zur Vermeidung Narkosevaskulärer Nebenwirkungen von Ketamin. Der Anaesthesist 28: 468–473
Tarnow J, Hess W, Schmidt D, Eberlein H J 1979 Narkoseeinleitung bei Patienten mit koronärer Herzkrankheit: Flunitrazepam, diazepam, ketamin, fentanyl. Eine hamodynamische Untersuchung. Der Anaesthesist 28: 9–19
Taylor P A, Towey R M 1971 Depression of laryngeal reflexes during ketamine anaesthesia. British Medical Journal 2: 688–689
Taylor P A, Towey R M, Rappaport A S 1972 Further work on the depression of laryngeal reflexes during ketamine anaesthesia using a standard challenge technique. British Journal of Anaesthesia 44: 1163–1168
Tjaden R J, Ethier R, Gilbert R G B, Straja A 1969 The use of CI-581 (Ketalar) for paediatric pneumoencephalography. Journal of the Canadian Association of Radiologists 20: 155–156
Tokics L, Brismar B, Hedenstierna G, Lundh R 1983 Oxygen uptake and central circulation during ketamine anaesthesia. Acta Anaesthesiologica Scandinavica 27: 318–322
Traber D L, Wilson R D, Priano L L 1968 Differentiation of the cardiovascular effects of CI-581. Anesthesia and Analgesia, Current Researches 47: 769–778
Tweed W A, Minuck M, Mymin D 1972 Circulatory response to ketamine anesthesia. Anesthesiology 37: 613–619
Unni V K N, Bovill J G 1972 Forearm blood flow during ketamine anaesthesia. British Journal of Anaesthesia 44: 698–703
Vatashsky E, Aronson H B 1982 Pemphigus vulgaris; anaesthesia in the traumatised patient. Anaesthesia 37: 1195–1197
Vaughan R W, Stephen C R 1974 Abdominal and thoracic surgery in adults with ketamine, nitrous oxide and d-tubocurarine. Anesthesia and Analgesia, Current Researches 53: 271–280
Vincent J P, Cavey D, Kamenka J M, Geneste P, Lazdunski M 1978 Interaction of phencyclidines with the muscarinic and opiate receptors in the central nervous system. Brain Research 152: 176–182
Virtue R W, Alanis J M, Mari M, Lafargue R T, Vogel J H K, Metcalf D R 1967 An anesthetic agent: 2-orthochlorophenyl, 2-methylamino cyclohexanone HCl (CI-582). Anesthesiology 28: 823–833
Waxman K, ShoemakerW C, Lippmann M I980 Cardiovascular effects of anesthetic induction with ketamine. Anesthesia and Analgesia, Current Researches 59: 355–358
Weinreich A I, Silvay G, Lumb P D 1980 Continuous ketamine infusion for one-lung anaesthesia. Canadian Anaesthetists' Society Journal 27: 485–490
Wessels J V, Allen G W, Slogoff S 1973 The effect of nitrous oxide on ketamine anesthesia. Anesthesiology 39: 382–385
White P F, Ham J, Way W L, Trevor A J 1980a Pharmacology of ketamine isomers in surgical patients. Anesthesiology 52: 231–239
White P F, Ham J, Way W L, Trevor A J 1980b Pharmacology of ketamine isomers in surgical patients. Proceedings of the 7th World Congress of Anaesthesiologists (Ed. Rugheimer E Zindler M), Excerpta Medica, Amsterdam 732–734
White P F, Johnston R R, Pudwill C R 1975 Interaction of ketamine and halothane in rats. Anesthesiology 42: 179–186
White P F, Marietta M D, Pudwill C R, Way W L, Trevor A J 1976 Effects of halothane anesthesia on the biodisposition of ketamine in rats. Journal of Pharmacology and Experimental Therapeutics 196: 545–555
White P F, Way W L, Trevor A J 1982 Ketamine — its pharmacology and therapeutic uses. Anesthesiology 56: 119–136
Wieber J, Gugler R, Hengstmann J H, Dengler H J 1975 Pharmacokinetics of ketamine in man. Der Anaesthesist. 24: 260–263
Wilson R D, Nichols R J, McCoy N R 1967 Dissociative anesthesia with CI-581 in burned children. Anesthesia and Analgesia, Current Researches 46: 719–724
Wilson R D, Priano L L, Traber D L, Sakai H, Daniels J C, Ritzmann S E 1971 An investigation of possible immuno suppression from ketamine and 100 per cent oxygen in normal children. Anesthesia and Analgesia, Current Researches 50: 464–470
Wilson R D, Traber D L, Evans B L 1969 Correlation of psychologic and physiologic observations from children undergoing repeated ketamine anesthesia. Anesthesia and Analgesia, Current Researches 48: 995–1001
Wilson R D, Traber D L, McCoy N R 1968 Cardiopulmonary effects of CI-581 — a new dissociative anesthetic. Southern Medical Journal 61: 692–696
Wong D H W, Jenkins L C 1974 An experimental study of the mechanism of action of ketamine on the central nervous system. Canadian Anaesthetists' Society Journal 21: 57–67
Wong D H W, Jenkins L C 1975 The cardiovascular effects of ketamine in hypotensive states. Canadian Anaesthetists' Society Journal 22: 339–348

Wyant G M 1971 Intramuscular Ketalar (CI-581) in paediatric anaesthesia. Canadian Anaesthetists' Society Journal 18: 72–83
Yeung M L, Lin R S H 1972 Laryngeal reflexes in children under ketamine anaesthesia. British Journal of Anaesthesia 44: 1089–1092
Yoshikawi K, Murai Y 1971 The effect of ketamine on intraocular pressure in children. Anesthesia and Analgesia, Current Researches 50: 199–202
Zsigmond E K 1971 Malignant hyperthermia with subsequent uneventful general anesthesia. Anesthesia and Analgesia, Current Researches 50: 1111–1112
Zsigmond E K, Domino E F 1980 Ketamine — clinical pharmacology, pharmacokinetics, and current clinical uses. Anesthesiology Review 7: 13–33
Zsigmond E K, Kothary S P, Martinez O A, Matsuki A, Kelsch R C 1974 Diazepam for prevention of the rise in plasma catecholamines caused by ketamine. Clinical Pharmacology and Therapeutics 15: 223–224
Zsigmond E K, Matsuki A, Kothary S P, Jallad M 1976 Arterial hypoxemia caused by intravenous ketamine. Anesthesia and Analgesia, Current Researches 55: 311–314

Etomidate

This drug, which bears no chemical resemblance to any others used in anaesthesia, resulted from research in the Belgian laboratories of Janssen Pharmaceuticals at Beerse. It was originally known as R 26490 and is sold under the trade names of Hypnomidate (Janssen) and Amidate (Abbott, USA). It was the finding of a very high therapeutic index in animals (26.4 cf 6.7 for propanidid and 9.5 for methohexitone) that recommended etomidate for study in man (Janssen et al, 1975). It is a pure hypnotic with no analgesic properties.

The chemical name of etomidate is R-(+)-ethyl-1-(1-methyl benzyl)-1H-imidazole-5-carboxylate sulphate. Its structural formula is shown in Figure 10.1; its empirical formula is $C_{14}H_{16}N_2O_2,H_2SO_4$. Only the dextro isomer is active as a hypnotic.

It is a white crystalline powder with a molecular weight of 342.4. The salt is soluble in water, but unstable in aqueous solution. The base is soluble in propylene glycol and ethanol, freely soluble in polyethylene glycol and chloroform, sparingly soluble in acetone and water, and practically insoluble in ether and n-hexane. The pKa of etomidate is 4.24 (Heykants et al, 1975).

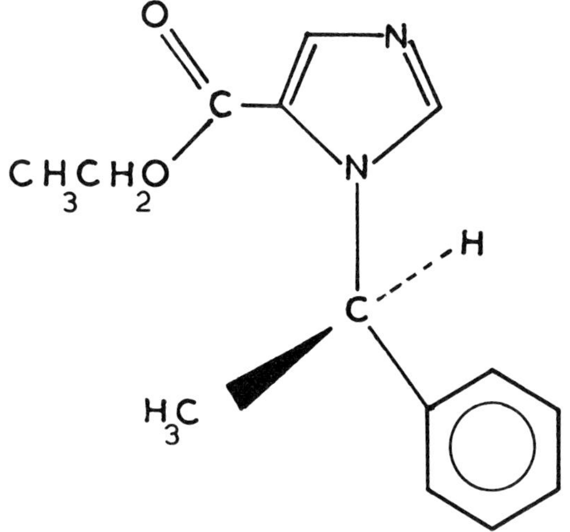

Fig. 10.1 Formula of etomidate.

The aqueous solution has to be freshly prepared. The drug is commercially available as an induction agent in a propylene glycol solvent containing 2 mg ml^{-1} (0.2% solution) and is stable at room temperature for two years. It has also been solubilised in a narrow range (3000 molecular weight) polyethylene glycol solvent, but its use has been suspended since it might be immunologically active and is a possible cause of haemolysis.

Solutions There are two commercially available solutions:

1. Hypnomidate for induction: ampoules containing 20 mg etomidate base in 10 ml solvent (35% propylene glycol v/v in water). pH at 37°C is 4.5–5, osmolarity 550 m.osmol kg^{-1} and viscosity 0.40 Ns m^2. The solution remains stable at room temperature for over two years.
2. Hypnomidate for infusion: a clear colourless liquid of etomidate hydrochloride, equivalent to 125 mg etomidate, base in 1 ml absolute alcohol. When diluted to 1 mg ml^{-1} with normal saline or dextrose, the pH is about 3.5. The volume for infusion will depend on the technique used, but each ampoule should be diluted in at least 50 ml fluid (2–3 μg ml^{-1}) unless a small volumetric syringe pump is used. In preparing solutions one should be aware of a deliberate pharmaceutical overfill of 0.1 ml in each 1 ml ampoule and possible but less important overfill of infusion containers.

Solutions are stable following dilution for up to one week at room temperature.

ONSET OF ACTION AND DOSAGE

In effective doses etomidate is a rapidly acting drug with onset times similar to those of thiopentone (Dundee & Zacharias, 1979) and methohexitone (Kay, 1976). The minimum anaesthetic dose in fit unpremedicated adults is around 0.25 mg kg^{-1} and 0.3 mg kg^{-1} is recommended for clinical use. On a w/w basis etomidate is approximately 12 times more potent than thiopentone and 4–5 times more potent than methohexitone.

The duration of an induction dose of 0.3 mg kg^{-1} is such as to allow for uptake of a volatile agent, or for tracheal intubation with suxamethonium or with a non-depolarising relaxant. Problems of waking may arise because of the slow onset of tubocurarine or pancuronium, but can be obviated by giving the relaxant before the etomidate.

Venous irritation

Pain on injection is a distinct problem with etomidate. The incidence with the three original preparations varied from 10 to 63 per cent with different workers. This occurs in about one quarter of patients given a direct intravenous injection of the propylene glycol preparation (Zacharias et al, 1979) and, as with most drugs, the incidence is higher when small veins are used, particularly on the back of the hand or at the wrist. Dundee & Zacharias (1979) found slow injection to be the major factor influencing the occurrence of pain; presumably the time the drug is in contact with the vein wall is the important factor. Opiate premedication reduces the incidence of injection pain and the common practice of preceding etomidate with fentanyl also minimises the problem. Pain is reduced when the drug is given into a rapidly running infusion (Thomas et al, 1976).

Because of the differing dilutions used by different workers, data on the effects of the alcoholic solution are less easily obtained. It can cause pain when small veins are used but the incidence and severity is much less than with the propylene glycol formulation.

An early study by Kay (1976) showed a low incidence of pain with etomidate in cremophor, but this is of no practical importance. Attempts by the same author to reduce injection pain by combining etomidate with lignocaine were not very successful.

PHARMACOKINETICS

Despite its widespread use, this aspect of the action of etomidate has not been studied in detail and there is some disagreement in findings by different workers. During transport in the blood about 76% of etomidate is bound to plasma proteins. The distribution of the two optical isomers [R (+)] and [S (−)] does not differ substantially in the blood, brain or liver but S(−) has considerably less hypnotic activity, suggesting stereospecificity of the 'receptor' area of the brain.

The first reported pharmacokinetic data of Heykants et al (1973) showed a rapid fall in plasma concentration of unchanged etomidate in a biphasic manner, with an elimination half-life of 75 min. Plasma concentrations of metabolites increase over the first 30 min after administration then decrease with $t\frac{1}{2}B$ of 160 min. Van Hamme et al (1978) followed plasma concentrations following an induction dose of 0.3 mg kg^{-1} etomidate in patients in whom anaesthesia was maintained with 1.5–2% enflurane in nitrous oxide–oxygen. These results are consistent with the drug following a three compartment model distribution, the individual half lives being 2.6, 29 and 275 min respectively. Subsequent studies by Shuttler et al (1980) in patients given 20 mg etomidate, who like those of van Hamme and colleagues also received enflurane, gave plasma levels which were best fitted to a two compartment model with an elimination half life of 68 min. Van Hamme et al (1978) found the apparent volume of distribution to be 4.51 l kg^{-1} and the systemic or plasma clearance rate was 11.7 ml kg^{-1} min^{-1}, the corresponding figures for the Shuttler study being 2.2 l kg^{-1} and 23.8 ml kg^{-1} min^{-1}. The differences between these two studies are not readily accountable (Prys Roberts & Sear, 1984).

More recent work from Shuttler and his colleagues (1982) has shown that, in the presence of a steady state concentration of fentanyl (10 ng ml^{-1}) the clearance of etomidate was reduced from about 1600 to 400 ml min^{-1}, with little alteration of the elimination half-life. However V_1 decreased from 21l to 5l and V_D^B from 160 l to about 40 l. The exact kinetic drug interactions are not known: they might involve saturation of the enzymes responsible for the metabolism of etomidate. If substantiated by subsequent studies, the clinical implications of this opioid-etomidate interaction are important as they suggest prolonged recovery may occur after fentanyletomidate anaesthesia.

Etomidate is metabolised mainly in the liver by ester hydrolysis to pharmacologically inactive metabolites, the main metabolite in man being the corresponding carboxylic acid of etomidate. About three-quarters of the administered dose is excreted in the urine in that form, with only about 2% being excreted unchanged. Clearance is normal in cirrhotic patients but Vd is doubled resulting in a prolonged $t\frac{1}{2}\beta$ (van Beem et al, 1983).

Despite the paucity of data on this aspect of etomidate, it would appear to be a drug suitable for administration by continuous infusion. Etomidate is not cumulative when given by intermittent injection. Rapid changes in plasma (and brain) concentration could be obtained and delayed recovery is unlikely even after large doses.

INDUCTION OF ANAESTHESIA

Etomidate is a reliable induction agent with a variation in range of induction doses similar to thiopentone. The EEG pattern of anaesthesia is similar to that with the barbiturates and propanidid (Doenicke, 1974; Salinas, 1976). However, particularly in young unpremedicated patients, sleep is accompanied by a high incidence of excitatory effects — spontaneous involuntary muscle movement and hypertonus. This can be troublesome if induction is followed by a non-relaxant inhalational sequence, or with intermittent use of etomidate. The frequency and severity of movement is similar to that with equivalent doses of methohexitone (Boralessa & Holdcroft, 1980). There is no connection between the occurrence of pain on venous injection and muscle movements (Kortilla et al, 1981) which appear to be truly central excitatory.

The excitatory effects of etomidate can be reduced markedly by prior administration of an opioid, either as traditional preanaesthetic medication or intravenously 2–3 min before induction (Carlos & Innerairty, 1979; Dundee & Zacharias, 1979). Fentanyl would appear to be the preferred drug for this purpose, but alfentanil would be equally effective. Many clinicians feel that etomidate is clinically only acceptable after such pretreatment. With small doses (50 μg fentanyl or 150 μg alfentanil) it is possible to sustain spontaneous breathing.

Cardiovascular and respiratory effects

Relative lack of cardiovascular toxicity, as compared with thiopentone or Althesin, is one of the outstanding features of etomidate. Janssen and his colleagues (1971) showed this in the first reported animal (rat) studies of this drug and later reported it to have less effect than comparable doses of propanidid or thiopentone (Janssen et al, 1975). In therapeutic doses it has no depressant effect on atrial muscle function or conduction (Xhonneux et al, 1975) and, although doses of 1.25 and 2.5 mg kg^{-1} decreased arterial pressure in the intact dog, it has no effect on dp/dt_{max} in man, or on mean aortic pressure or coronary blood flow (Reneman et al, 1975). Other work on animals has confirmed this lack of direct cardiovascular toxicity (Weymar et al, 1974).

In general, clinical studies have confirmed this low cardiovascular toxicity (Zindler, 1975). In fit patients Bruckner (1976) and Bruckner and colleagues (1974) found that 0.3 mg kg^{-1} produced a slight increase in cardiac index, accompanied by a slight fall in heart rate, a slight fall in arterial pressure (14%) and peripheral resistance (17%); dp/dt_{max} rose (9%) with maximum effects occurring about three minutes after injection. They considered changes to be small in comparison with the effects of other intravenous anaesthetics.

In a comprehensive comparative study, Kettler & Sonntag (1974) investigated coronary blood flow and myocardial oxygen consumption (MVO_2) in healthy patients. Increases in heart rate are in the main responsible for the increases in MVO_2 which were found with propanidid (+82%) ketamine (+78%), Althesin (+63%), thiopentone (+55%) and methohexitone (+44%). In contrast, etomidate did not produce significant changes in MVO_2. Coronary arteriovenous difference was not significantly altered by any of the agents and etomidate alone seemed to have a true but weak coronary vasodilator effect. In another study the same group of workers (Kettler et al, 1974) gave an induction dose of 0.3 mg kg^{-1} etomidate followed by an infusion of 0.12 mg kg^{-1} min^{-1}; they found that coronary blood flow was increased by 19% and coronary resistance decreased 19%, leaving a constant coronary perfusion pressure.

Clinical doses of etomidate reduce peripheral vascular resistance (Kettler & Sonntag, 1974; Hempelmann et al, 1974). This action may be potentiated by other drugs (Dubois-Primo et al, 1976; Kettler et al, 1974; Zacharias et al, 1978). More recent reports which deal mostly with infusions of etomidate (Scorgie, 1983; Lees, 1983; Cohn et al, 1983; Edbrooke et al, 1983) or its use in poor-risk patients (Oduro et al, 1983), confirm this comparative lack of cardiovascular toxicity. However, it is established practice to give etomidate with fentanyl (Lees, 1983) or more recently with alfentanil (Versichelen et al, 1983). This group of opioids has minimal effects on the cardiovascular system and pretreatment with them will reduce the induction dose of etomidate. This might play some part in the reported low cardiovascular toxicity of etomidate, but nevertheless it remains the drug of choice for many anaesthetists in dealing with poor-risk patients.

Etomidate causes a reduction in cerebral blood flow and of intracranial pressure equal to that of thiopentone (Lazarevic et al 1976, Van Aken & Rolly, 1976). It has been used therapeutically for patients with head injuries (Dearden & McDowall, 1985) and also for neurosurgical anaesthesia, but in view of the adverse effects of prolonged infusions on adrenocortical function the justification for this application is in doubt.

Etomidate does not cause cough and hiccough as frequently as methohexitone. These are of short duration and do not interfere with the course of anaesthesia: frequency and severity are reduced by premedication with an opioid or diazepam.

In well-controlled crossover studies in volunteers Choi et al (1985) found that equipotent doses of etomidate (0.3 mg kg^{-1}) and methohexitone (1.5 mg kg^{-1}) cause a similar shift in the CO_2 response curve, indicating a similar depression of the medullary centres that modify the ventilatory drive in response to changing CO_2 tensions. However at any given CO_2 tension ventilation was greater after etomidate than after methohexitone. They interpret this as indicating that etomidate causes a CO_2-independent stimulation of ventilation. It would thus have advantages as an induction agent where maintenance of spontaneous ventilation is desirable. In practice etomidate is so often preceded by a short-acting opioid that it is difficult to comment on its respiratory depressant effects, but one can certainly maintain spontaneous respiration using it as the main agent for prolonged body surface operations in association with nitrous oxide-oxygen.

A most important observation is that the sparing effect of etomidate on both the cardiovascular and respiratory systems also applies to poor-risk patients with demonstrable cardiac and pulmonary disease (Gooding & Corssen, 1975; Gooding et al, 1979; Lindeburg et al, 1982).

Interactions with relaxants

Etomidate is a non-competitive, as well as a competitive, inhibitor of pseudocholinesterase (Calvo et al, 1979; Burr, 1980). In view of the possible interaction between etomidate and suxamethonium Dundee & Zacharias (1979) measured the plasma cholinesterase in 21 patients before and 2, 10 and 60 min after etomidate (without suxamethonium). Butylthiocholine was used as the substrate in the colorimetric method employed. There was a progressive fall in the average cholinesterase level during the study period, the changes being statistically significant at 60 min; however, all changes fell within the known range of error of the test method and are probably of no clinical significance.

The same workers also measured the average duration of respiratory depression (based on clinical observations) and apnoea following 50 mg

Table 10.1 Average duration (± SEM) and range of apnoea and respiratory depression (s) after 50 mg suxamethonium in an unselected group of fit unpremedicated patients.

	Etomidate (0.15%)	*Thiopentone (2.5%)*
APNOEA		
Average and range	178 ± 7 (0–530)	194 ± 17 (0–480)
RESPIRATORY DEPRESSION:		
Average and range	250 ± 9 (90–625)	300 ± 20 (145–630)

suxamethonium. This study was initiated because of the early clinical impression that suxamethonium was less effective when given with etomidate than with thiopentone (Dundee & Zacharias, 1979; Bruckner et al, 1974). The results (Table 10.1) show little difference in the duration of apnoea with the two induction agents but, on the average, respiratory depression lasted significantly longer in those patients induced with thiopentone. It is doubtful if this difference is of great clinical significance. However, there can be some problems when etomidate–suxamethonium is used for bronchoscopy with the apnoeic-ventilation technique or for electroconvulsive therapy.

One should be aware of the possibility of a prolonged action when suxamethonium is given after etomidate in patients with low plasma pseudo-cholinesterase activity (Booij, 1984). Etomidate also potentiates the non-depolarising relaxants (Booij & Crul, 1979).

Histamine release

Unlike other intravenous anaesthetics, etomidate does not release significant amounts of histamine. As supporting evidence for this Doenicke and his colleagues (1973) found a steady basophil count during anaesthesia. However, there are reports of rashes occurring in varying parts of the body, mainly head, neck and upper trunk, following etomidate (Popescu, 1976; Doom & Mundeleer, 1976; Holdcroft et al, 1976). Dundee & Zacharias (1979) found a very low incidence (3 in 1400) of rashes. However, in one series, a woman having repeat administrations of etomidate–suxamethonium for electroconvulsive therapy developed a marked generalized rash each time the drug was given. The propylene glycol formulation was used and the rash occurred immediately on injection before any other drugs had been given. She showed no other evidence of histamine release and had no bronchospasm or hypotension.

Watkins (1983) has made a convincing case for considering etomidate to be an 'immunologically safe' anaesthetic agent. As pointed out in Chapter 14, the possibility of a genuine immune response occurs, on repeated exposure to any drug, in addition to the normal risk of an anaphylactoid response. This risk might be increased by underlying pathology, for example myasthenia gravis or the myasthenic syndrome in cancer of the bronchus. No adverse reaction involving repeated exposure to etomidate has yet been reported.

Watkins (1982) has pointed out that against a background of some 10 000 to 15 000 severe reactions a year to the established hypnotic and neuromuscular drugs in the UK, France and Germany, the absence of sub-clinical histamine release boded well for etomidate. From its introduction in 1978 until 1982 (some 3 000 000 induction doses later) no convincing anaphylactoid reactions to the drug were reported. Watkins et al (1979) investigated five possible reactions, all involving only immediate widespread cutaneous flushing or urticaria, followed in two cases by extensive perioperative vomiting. All patients showed cardiovascular stability and no plasma protein involvement was detected. It was felt that the patients' own underlying pathology could have contributed to the reactions. A few similar cases were reported at the Janssen conference on etomidate infusion held in Beerse in 1980 and this might be typical of 'etomidate reactions'. Watkins concluded that etomidate has a very low incidence of adverse reaction compared with other intravenous hypnotics. Those reactions which are reported appear notably free from severe cardiovascular effects and on this basis he recommends the use of etomidate in high-risk patients such as those who previously have had severe anaphylactoid response.

The situation has become less clear since Sold (1985) drew attention to two case reports in the German literature. Krumholz and colleagues (1984) observed generalised erythema, severe urticaria and hypotension when 4 mg etomidate was given near the end of an anaesthetic in a patient who had already received a number of drugs. The second patient (Sold & Rothhammer, 1985) was given five drugs at induction including 4 mg etomidate and developed a severe tachycardia and hypotension which, on the basis of subsequent skin tests, was likely to be due to etomidate. The latter workers point out that although Doenicke and his co-workers (1973) in an experimental study in human volunteers found no evidence for direct histamine liberation they were able to demonstrate an effect when etomidate was used in conjunction with suxamethonium, alcuronium, pancuronium or lormetazepam (Lorenz & Doenicke, 1978; Doenicke, 1980; Doenicke et al, 1980), i.e. synergistic histamine release. Watkins (1985) admits that Sold & Rothhammer may have reported the first genuine anaphylactic reaction involving etomidate but he considers that, since several million people have been anaesthetized with the drug, the risk is very small and "the combination fentanyl–etomidate–pancuronium must still be the safest option open for the anaesthetist for the induction of anaesthesia".

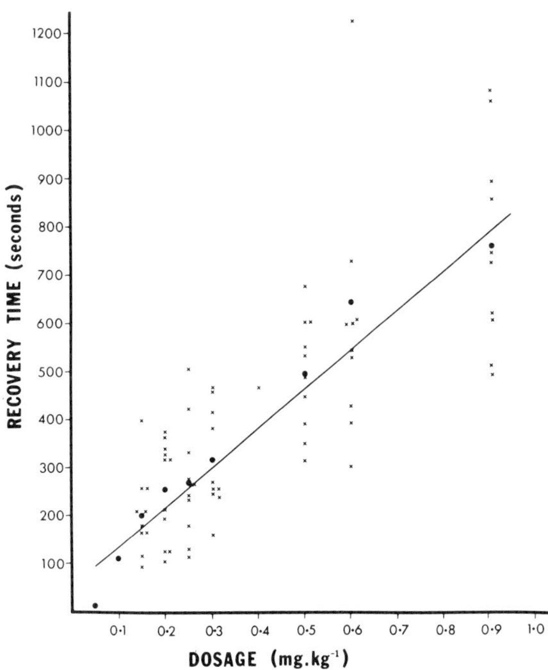

Fig. 10.2 Duration of sleep (time from end of injection until opened his eyes on command) related to the dosage of etomidate. x = individual patients; • = average of groups of 10. (Dundee & Zacharias, 1979).

Liver and kidney function

The effect of etomidate on five liver function tests, namely aspartate aminotransferase, alanine aminotransferase, alkaline phosphatase, gamma glutamyl transpeptidase and plasma cholinesterase has been reported by Dundee & Zacharias (1979). Compared with the preoperative readings no changes were detected on the 3rd–4th and 13th–15th postoperative days in 20 patients given an average of 1.2 mg kg^{-1} etomidate for minor operations lasting about 10–12 min.

The influence of etomidate on renal function has not been studied in detail. Unlike volatile and some other intravenous anaesthetics, it does not decrease renal perfusion (Tarnow et al, 1974).

RECOVERY

Recovery from etomidate is dose-related within the range of 0.1–1.0 mg kg^{-1} (Fig 10.2). In this respect it differs from the barbiturates and resembles propanidid (Clarke & Dundee, 1966). There is a general consensus of opinion that recovery from etomidate is slightly faster than from equivalent doses of methohexitone and markedly shorter than that from thiopentone.

Postoperative emetic effects

There is a distinct impression that when used as the main agent for minor operations (van Oss et al, 1980) or for dental procedures (Boralessa & Holdcroft, 1980) etomidate has a higher incidence of emesis than other induction agents. After minor gynaecological operations in unpremedicated patients under etomidate–nitrous oxide–oxygen anaesthesia, vomiting (with or without nausea) occurred in 26% and nausea alone in 21% of patients during the first six postoperative hours, compared with 14% vomiting and 9% nausea when barbiturates (thiopentone or methohexitone) were used (Dundee & Zacharias, 1979). This is a problem when etomidate is given as an infusion even when combined with an opioid.

Venous sequela

A 2–3 day follow-up has shown a high incidence of venous thrombosis after direct intravenous injection of etomidate. In one study (Zacharias et al, 1978, 1979) this occurred in about 25% of patients with the commercially available preparation. The incidence of this complication was related to the dose of drug injected, increasing from 13% with 0.3 mg kg^{-1} to 37% with doses in excess of 0.9 mg kg^{-1}. In a similar type of study carried out on patients undergoing major operations Olesen et al (1984) found a 24% incidence of thrombophlebitis up to the 14th postoperative day with etomidate, compared with 4% after thiopentone. Although injection pain occurred in 24% of patients after etomidate, there was no correlation between pain on injection and the subsequent thrombophlebitis. Data are not available on the frequency of this complication following infusion of etomidate or the use of the alcoholic solution.

EVALUATION AS AN INDUCTION AGENT

It would be difficult to get a better overall evaluation of etomidate as an induction agent than from the analysis of 4763 anaesthetic records and a controlled comparison of etomidate (325 cases) with thiopentone (311 cases) reported by Schuermans et al (1978). They were from Europe (excluding the United Kingdom) and the United States of America. Premedication was standardised only in the controlled series. They concluded that

> 'etomidate proved to be a safe and effective hypnotic. Sleep was deep and long enough to allow the normal induction and maintenance procedures. Blood pressure and heart rate remained remarkably steady in all groups. The incidence of respiratory depression was higher with thiopental: anesthesiologists' acceptance of etomidate was, however, reduced by the occurrence of venous pain during injection and of associated voluntary muscle movements.'

The authors expressed the hope that these adverse reactions would be largely eliminated by a change in formulation and by giving etomidate shortly after fentanyl. Muscle movement, but not pain, can be eliminated.

INFUSIONS

As pointed out by many workers, the pharmacokinetic profile of etomidate makes it an ideal drug for long-term infusions. This use is recommended for sedation in the intensive care unit to reduce intracranial pressure in patients with head injuries or during and following neurosurgical operations, or as a controllable method of achieving general anaesthesia in combination with an opioid and neuromuscular blocking drugs. However, as will be seen, grave doubts have been cast on its safety for long-term use and for a discussion of etomidate infusion and its use in head injuries the reader is referred to chapter 16.

Adrenocortical function

The safety of long-term use of etomidate was first challenged by Ledingham & Watt (1983) who worked in an intensive care unit in Glasgow. During the years 1981–2 they noted a significant increase in mortality in patients surviving more than five days from the time of injury and whose lungs were mechanically ventilated for respiratory insufficiency. There was no difference in the severity of injury or in the degree of sepsis when they are compared with a lower mortality group who, apart from the sedation, were treated in a similar manner during 1979–80. The more recent group of patients were sedated with etomidate in comparison with morphine and benzodiazepines in the previous group. They suggested that one of the causative mechanisms might be suppression of adrenocortical function by etomidate, possibly by a direct effect on steroid synthesis in the adrenal cortex. This report was much criticised in subsequent correspondence. One comment was by Doenicke (1983) who introduced etomidate into clinical practice. He pointed out that while the control (benzodiazepine) group received up to 60 mg morphine per day the etomidate series has 75–120 mg per day with additional bolus doses of up to 50 mg. High doses of morphine inhibit glucocorticoid synthesis, release prolactin and lengthen the elimination half-life of etomidate — in short the benefits of etomidate could have been negated by the high morphine levels. An outcome of this controversy, which involved a completely new complication of prolonged sedation was a more detailed look at adrenal function during etomidate infusions.

The actual cause of death in the Glasgow patients was usually related to infection, with adrenocortical suppression by etomidate as a possible contributory factor. Steroid replacement might improve the outcome (Newby & Edbrooke, 1983; Fellows et al, 1983; McKee & Finlay, 1983) but not if there has also been failure of adrenocortical hormone response to decreasing serum cortisol concentrations (Logan & McKee, 1984).

Ledingham & Watt's hypothesis was supported by in-vitro animal experiments in which Preziosi and Vacca (1982) and Preziosi (1983) showed that 20 μ mol kg^{-1} d-etomidate inhibited stress and drug induced corticosteroid production in the adrenal gland as well as inhibiting the ACTH-mediated response. Etomidate also appeared to inhibit the rises in prolactin which normally follow surgical or other forms of stress. Some suppression was produced by deep anaesthesia with Althesin, but not with normal doses; neither hydroxydione nor ketamine had such an action. The findings with etomidate were similar to those of another in-vitro study (Lambert et al, 1983), which found etomidate to be an even more potent inhibitor of steroid synthesis than metyrapone, although this study was criticised because of the high drug concentration required to produce this suppression. However, Owen & Spence (1984) have pointed out that all infusion regimes produce plasma concentrations in excess of that required to inhibit corticosteroid production. They also noted that the elimination half-life of etomidate can be substantially increased by high doses of morphine (Doenicke, 1983) and that hepatic clearance is decreased by fentanyl (Shuttler et al, 1980; 1982). These are all factors which could influence its action during infusion in an intensive care situation. An infusion of etomidate might also decrease its own clearance through an effect on hepatic blood flow (van Lambalgen et al, 1982).

Subsequent studies by Sear and his colleagues (1983) confirmed the suppressant effects of etomidate on adrenal function. They compared the response to induction followed by infusion of etomidate to that in similar patients anaesthetised with thiopentone, nitrous oxide and halothane. In response to a similar stimulus plasma cortisol increased significantly with the latter technique, whereas a slight decrease was seen in the etomidate group. Fragen et al (1983) found similar changes in comparing the responses to etomidate and thiopentone. In the etomidate group plasma cortisol concentrations decreased to less than the control concentrations, compared with an increase following thiopentone. In a subsequent publication they (Fragen et al, 1984) reported that in patients who had been given thiopentone both cortisol and aldosterone concentrations were greater than the control level in the second to fourth hours after induction, while with etomidate both levels were below baseline values in the first and second hour after induction and significantly lower than in those who had received thiopentone. Because aldosterone was also suppressed they suggest that etomidate exerts its effect by inhibiting the early stages of steroidogenesis in the adrenal cortex. Similar effects have been demonstrated by Mehta et al (1985) and Wanscher et al, 1985.

The Ledingham & Watt report and subsequent papers led the Committee on Safety of Medicines in the United Kingdom to draw attention to possible hazards with the administration of etomidate (letter 20 June 1983). The licence to promote the use of the drug by infusion was subsequently revoked. In most European countries package inserts have included a warning paragraph, although its use as an infusion is not banned, except in Denmark where the duration of its use is restricted to 12 hours.

Sebel et al (1983) compared plasma cortisol concentrations following induction of anaesthesia with etomidate and with thiopentone. They found no significant differences in the two groups, in both of which cortisol had increased by the end of the operation. A subsequent more detailed study by Wagner & White (1984) comparing induction (bolus) and maintenance (infusion) with thiopentone and etomidate and a third group of patients induced with etomidate and maintained with thiopentone showed no difference in noradrenaline levels between the series, but a very marked decrease in plasma cortisol in those given etomidate. The suppression occurred even when the use of etomidate was limited to induction of anaesthesia. These authors concluded; "Anaesthetists using etomidate should be aware that biochemical adrenocortical suppression may follow even a single induction dose of the drug".

They also point out that adrenal supplementation might be required if patients given etomidate are exposed to an unexpected stress during the operation. These views are compatible with the results of the *in vitro* studies of Kenyon et al (1985).

In a more recent study Wanscher et al (1985) studied the adrenocortical response to a short tetracosactrin (Synacthen) test in patients having major gynaecological operations. Etomidate completely blocked the adrenocortical response to corticotropin stimulation for at least 24 h after operation, but no suppression was found in patients given thiopentone infusion. They conclude that etomidate cannot be recommended for routine induction and maintenance of anaesthesia.

CLINICAL USES OF ETOMIDATE

At the time of writing the use of etomidate is restricted to the induction of anaesthesia. Hence one has to look for circumstances where its sparing effect on the cardiovascular system, in comparison with other induction agents, more than outweighs the disadvantages of injection pain and excitatory effects and the theoretical dangers of adrenocortical suppression. From the patient's viewpoint pain on injection is most important and there is no justification for the administration of this drug into small veins in the back of the hand or at the wrist. Ideally one should inject it into a rapidly running infusion, but this complicates the technique as well as adding additional expense and cannot be justified as routine practice in all patients.

As pointed out previously, pretreatment with fentanyl or preferably alfentanil, makes etomidate an acceptable induction agent, but usually necessitates assisted or controlled ventilation. This would be the technique of choice with this drug and with smaller doses of opioids (particularly alfentanil) it is possible to retain spontaneous breathing. While appreciating the lack of cardiovascular depression one should not forget the stress/strain of the unwanted effects of laryngoscopy and tracheal intubation in such patients and to get maximum benefit large doses of opioids should be given and the etomidate preceded or followed by the appropriate myoneural blocking drug. This technique will have the least deleterious effects on the cardiovascular system, with minimal changes in blood pressure or heart rate.

Uses in porphyria

The uneventful use of etomidate in a known porphyric who had developed acute abdominal pain and lower motor neurone paralysis following injection of a barbiturate suggested that the drug might be safe for induction of anaesthesia in such patients (Famewo, 1985). However, Harrison et al (1985) have carried out experiments on a DDC-primed rat model of latent variegate porphyria which show potential porphyrogenicity of etomidate but not of ketamine when administered as a continuous infusion. Etomidate resulted in a change from control in 5-aminolae-vulimate synthesase (ALAS) activity which increased by 47% with a corroborative 85% increase in corproporphyrin and a 40% increase in photoporphyrin content. This did not occur in untreated rats or with ketamine. On these grounds the drug must be regarded as potentially porphyrogenic when administered as a continuous infusion and in practice it is best avoided in known or suspected porphyrics except where the advantages of its use outweigh the potential danger.

REFERENCES

Booij L H D J 1984 Benzodiazepine and non barbiturate hypnotic drugs. Clinics in Anaesthesia. Intravenous Anesthesiology. Sear J W (ed), vol 2, 65–87

Booij L H D J, Crul J F 1979 The comparative influence of gamma-hydroxy butyric acid, Althesin and etomidate on a neuromuscular blocking potency of pancuronium in man. Acta Anaesthesiologica Belgica 30: 219–223

Boralessa H, Holdcroft A 1980 Methohexitone or etomidate for induction of dental anaesthesia. Canadian Anaesthetists' Society Journal 27: 578–583

Bruckner J B 1976 Etomidate. Abstract 31, Sixth World Congress of Anaesthesiology, Mexico City, April 24–30. Excerpta Medica, Amsterdam.
Bruckner J B, Gethmann J W, Patschke D 1974 Untersuchungen zur Wirkung von Etomidate auf den Kreislauf der menschen. Anaesthesist 23: 322–330
Bruckner J B, Gethmann J W, Patschke D, Tarnow J, Weymar A 1974 Tierexperimentelle Untersuchungen zur Wirkung von Etomidate auf den Kreislauf und die myokardiale Sauerstoffversorgung. Anaesthesist 23:150
Burr R 1980 Die Wirkung von Etomidate auf die aktivitat des menschichen studokolinesterase. Anaesthesist 29: 113–119
Calvo R, Carlos R, Erill S 1979 Etomidate and plasma esterase activity in man and experimental animals. Pharmacology 18: 294–298
Carlos R, Innerarity S 1979 Effect of premedication on etomidate anaesthesia. British Journal of Anaesthesia 51: 1159–1162
Choi S D, Spaulding B C, Gross J B, Apfelbaum J L 1985 Comparison of the ventilatory effects of etomidate and methohexital. Anesthesiology 62: 442–447
Clarke R S J, Dundee J W 1966 Survey of experimental and clinical pharmacology of propanidid. Current Researches in Anesthesia and Analgesia 45: 250–262.
Cohn B F, Rejger V, Hagenouw-Taal J C W, Voormolen J H C 1983 Results of a feasibility trial to achieve total immobilisation of patients in a neurosurgical intensive care unit with etomidate. Anaesthesia 38 Supplement: 47–50
Dearden N M, McDowall D G 1985 Comparison of etomidate and Althesin in the reduction of increased intracranial pressure after head injury. British Journal of Anaesthesia 57: 361–368
Doenicke A 1974 Etomidate, a new intravenous hypnotic. Acta Anaesthesiologica Belgica 25: 307–315
Doenicke A 1980 Pseudo-allergic reactions due to histamine release during intravenous anaesthesia. In: Dukor P, Kallos P, Schlumberger H D, West G B (eds) PAR. Pseudo-allergic reactions. Involvement of drugs and chemicals, vol 1. Karger, Basel. 224–250
Doenicke A 1983 Etomidate. Lancet 2:168
Doenicke A, Lorenz W, Beigl R, Bezecny H, Uhlig G, Kalmar L, Praetorius B, Mann G 1973 Histamine release after intravenous application of short-acting hypnotics. A comparison of etomidate, Althesin CT 1341 and propanidid. British Journal of Anaesthesia 45: 1097–1104
Doenicke A, Lorenz W, Dittman J, Hug P 1980 Histaminfreisetzung nach Diazepam/Lormetazepam in Kombination mit Etomidat. In: Doenicke A, Ott H (eds) Lormetazepam. Springer, Berlin, Heidelberg, New York, pp. 11–15
Doom A, Mundeleer P 1976 Etomidate and tonsillectomy. Proceedings of the Belgian Congress of Anesthesiology II, Brussels, 10–13 September 1975. Acta Anaesthesiologica Belgica 27: 181–186
Dubois-Primo J, Bastenier-Geens J, Genicot C, Rucquoi M 1976 A comparative study of etomidate and methohexital, as induction agents for analgesia anesthesia. Proceedings of the Belgian Congress of Anesthesiology II, Brussels, September 1975. Acta Anaesthesiologica Belgica 27: 187–195
Dundee J W, Zacharias M 1979. Etomidate. In: Dundee J W (ed) Current topics in anaesthesia series. 1: Intravenous anaesthetic agents. Arnold, London, ch 6, p 46–66
Edbrooke D L, Newby T M, Mather S J 1983 Use of etomidate in an intensive care unit. Anaesthesia 38 Supplement: 44–46
Famewo C E 1985 Induction of anaesthesia with etomidate in a patient with acute intermittent porphyria. Canadian Anaesthetists' Society Journal 32: 171–173
Fellows I W, Basto W M D, Byrne A J, Allison S P 1983 Adrenocortical suppression in multiply injured patients: a complication of etomidate treatment. British Medical Journal ii: 1835–1837
Fragen R J, Shanks C A, Molpeni A 1983 Etomidate. Lancet 2:625
Fragen R J, Shanks C A, Molpeni A, Avram M J 1984 Effects of etomidate hormonal responses to surgical stress. Anesthesiology 61: 652–656
Gooding J M, Corssen G 1975 Etomidate: an ultra-short acting non-barbiturate agent for anesthesia induction. Anesthesia and Analgesia. Current Researches 55: 286–289
Gooding J M, Wang J T, Smith R, Beringer J T, Kirby R R 1979 Cardiovascular and pulmonary response following etomidate induction of anaesthesia in patients with demonstrated cardiac disease. Anesthesia and Analgesia 58: 40–41
Harrison P G, Moore M R, Meissner T M 1985 Porphyrinogenicity of etomidate and ketamine as continuous infusions: screening in the DDC-primed rat model. British Journal of Anaesthesia 57: 420–423
Hempelmann G, Hempelmann W, Piepenbrock S, Oster W, Karliczek G 1974 Blood gas analyses and haemodynamic studies on heart surgery patients using etomidate. Anaesthesist 23: 423–429
Heykants J J P, Brugmans J, Doenicke A 1973 Pharmacokinetics of etomidate (R 26490) in human volunteers: plasma levels, metabolism and excretion. Janssen Research Products Information Service, Clinical Research Report R 26490/1.
Heykants J J P, Meuldermans W E G, Michiels L J M, Lewi P J, Janssen P A J 1975 Distribution, metabolism and excretion of etomidate, a short-acting hypnotic drug, in the rat. Comparative study of (R)-(+) and (S)-(−) etomidate. Archives Internationales de Pharmacodynamic et de Therapie 216: 113–129
Holdcroft A, Morgan M, Whitwan J G, Lumley J 1976 Effect of dose and premedication on induction complications with etomidate. British Journal of Anaesthesia 48: 199–204
Janssen P A J, Niemegeers C J E, Marsbook R P H 1975 Etomidate, a potent non-barbiturate hypnotic. Intravenous etomidate in mice, rats, guinea-pigs, rabbits and dogs. Archives Internationales de Pharmacodynamie et de therapie 214: 92–132
Janssen P A J, Niemegeers C J E, Schellekens K H L, Lenaerts F M 1971 Etomidate, R-(+)-ethyl-l-(-methyl-benzyl) imidazole-5-carboxylate (R16659), a potent short-acting and relatively atoxic intravenous hypnotic agent in rats. Arzneimittel-Forschung 21: 1234–1243
Kay B 1976 A clinical assessment of the use of etomidate in children. British Journal of Anaesthesia 48: 207–211
Kenyon C J, McNeil L M, Fraser R 1985 Comparison of the effects of etomidate thiopentone and propofol on cortisol synthesis. British Journal of Anaesthesia 57: 509–511
Kettler D, Sonntag H 1974 Intravenous anesthetics: coronary blood flow and myocardial oxygen consumption (with special reference to Althesine). Acta Anaesthesiologica Belgica 25: 384–399
Kettler D, Sonntag H, Donath U, Regensburger D, Schenk

H D 1974 Haemodynamics, myocardial function, oxygen requirement and oxygen supply of the human heart after the administration of etomidate. Anaesthesist 23: 116–121
Kortilla K, Tammisto T, Aromaa 1981 Comparison of etomidate in combination with fentanyl or diazepam with thiopentone as an induction agent for general anaesthesia. British Journal of Anaesthesia 51: 115–117
Krumholz W, Muller H, Gerlach H, Russ W, Hempelmann G 1984 Ein Fall von anaphylaktoider Reaktion nach Gabe von Etomidat. Anaesthesist 33: 161–162
Lambert A, Mitchell R, Frost J, Ratcliffe J G, Robertson W R 1983 Direct in vitro inhibition of adrenal steroidogenesis by etomidate. Lancet 2:1085
Lazarevic Z D, Rejger V, Popescu D T, Mattigaly R 1976 The influence of hypnomidate on intracranial pressure. Abstract 235, sixth World Congress of Anaesthesiology, Mexico City, April 24–30, Excerpta Medica, Amsterdam.
Ledingham I McK, Watt I 1983 Influence of sedation on mortality in critically ill multiple trauma patients. Lancet 1:1270
Lees N 1983 Experience with etomidate as part of a total intravenous technique. Anaesthesia 38 Supplement: 70–73
Lindeburg T, Spotoff H, Pregard-Sorensen M, Skopsted T 1982 Cardiovascular effects of etomidate used for induction and in combination with fentanylpancuronium for maintenance of anaesthesia in patients with valvular heart disease. Acta Anaesthesiologica Scandinavica 26: 205–208
Logan R W, McKee J I 1984 Etomidate. British Medical Journal 289: 84–85
Lorenz W, Doenicke A 1978 Anaphylactoid reactions and histamine release by intravenous drugs used in surgery and anaesthesia. In: Watkins J, Milford Ward A (eds) Adverse response to intravenous drugs. Academic Press, New York. 83–112
McKee J I, Finlay W E 1983 Cortisol replacement in severely stressed patients. Lancet 1:484
Mehta M P, Dillman J B, Sherman M M, Ghoneim M M, Lemke J H 1985 Etomidate anesthesia inhibits the cortisol response to surgical stress. Acta Anaesthesiologica Scandinavica 29: 486–489
Newby D M, Edbrooke G L 1983 Influence of sedation on mortality in trauma patients. Lancet i:1381
Oduro A, Tomlinson A A, Voice A, Davies G K 1983 The use of etomidate infusions during anaesthesia for cardiopulmonary bypass. Anaesthesia 38 Supplement: 66–69
Olesen A S, Huttel M S, Hole P 1984 Venous sequelae following the injection of etomidate or thiopentone intravenously. British Journal of Anaesthesia 56: 171–173
Owen H, Spence A A 1984 Etomidate: editorial. British Journal of Anaesthesia 56: 55–556
Popescu D T 1976 Clinical study of Althesin and hypnomidate. Proceedings of the Belgian Congress of Anesthesiology II, Brussels, 10–13 September 1975. Acta Anaesthesiologica Belgica 27: 196–207
Preziosi V 1983 Etomidate, sedative and neuroendocrine changes. Lancet 2:276
Preziosi V, Vacca M 1982 Etomidate and the corticotrophic axis. Archives of International Pharmacodynamic and Therapy 256: 308–310
Prys-Roberts C, Sear J W 1984 Non-barbiturate intravenous anaesthetic and continuous infusion anaesthesia. In: Prys-Roberts C, Hug C C (eds) Pharmacokinetics of anaesthesia. Blackwell, London, p. 128–156
Reneman R S, Jageneau A H M, Xhonneux R, Laduron P 1975 The cardiovascular pharmacology of etomidate (R-26490), a new, potent and short-acting intravenous hypnotic agent. In: Arias L, Llaurado M, Nalda M A, Lunn J N (eds) Recent progress in anaesthesiology and resuscitation, Proceedings of the IV European Congress of Anaesthesiology, Madrid 5–11 September 1974 Excerpta Medica, Amsterdam; American Elsevier, New York, p 152–156
Salinas A F 1976 Clinical evaluation of etomidate as an anesthesia-inducing agent. Study of 50 cases. Abstract 191, Sixth World Congress of Anaesthesiology, Mexico City, April 24–30. Excerpta Medica, Amsterdam.
Schuermans V, Dom J, Dony J, Scheijgrond H, Brugman S 1978 Multinational evaluation of etomidate for anesthesia induction: conclusions and consequences. Anaesthesist 27: 52–59
Scorgie B 1983 Etomidate infusion: its use in anaesthesia for general surgery Anaesthesia 38 Supplement: 63–65
Sear J W, Allen M C, Gales M, McQuay H J, Kay N H, McKenzie P J, Moore R A 1983 Suppression by etomidate of normal cortisone response to anaesthesia and surgery. Lancet ii:1028
Sebel P S, Verghese C, Macken H L J 1983 Effect on plasma cortisol concentrations of single induction dose of etomidate or thiopentone. Lancet ii:625
Shuttler J, Lauven P M, Schwilden H, Stoeckel H 1982 Alterations of the pharmacokinetics of etomidate caused by fentanyl. Anaesthesia, Volume of summaries, Sixth European Congress of Anaesthesiology, London, 1982. Abstract 700, p 368
Shuttler J, Wilms M, Lauven P M, Stoeckel H, Koenig A 1980 Pharmakokinetische untersuchungen uber etomidat beim menschen. Anaesthesist 29: 658–661
Sold M J 1985 Etomidate: an 'immunologically safe' anaesthetic agent? Anaesthesia 40: 1014–1015
Sold M J, Rothhammer A 1985 Lebensbedrohliche anaphylaktoide Reaktion nach Etomidat. Anaesthesist 34: 208–210
Tarnow J, Passian Patschke D, Weymar A, Bruckner J B 1974 Nierendurchbultunt unter Etomidate. Anaesthesist 23: 421–422
Thomas B, Meirlaen L, Rolly G, Weyne L 1976 Clinical use of etomidate. Proceedings of the Belgian Congress of Anesthesiology II, Brussels, 10–13 September 1975. Acta Anaesthesiologica Belgica 27: 167–174
van Aken J, Rolly G 1976 Influence of etomidate, a new short-acting anesthetic agent, on cerebral blood flow in man. Proceedings of the Belgian Congress of Anesthesiology II, Brussels, 10–13 September 1975. Acta Anaesthesiologica Belgica 27: 175–180
van Beem H, Manger F W, van Boxtel C, van Bentem N 1983 Etomidate anaesthesia in patients with cirrhosis of the liver: pharmacokinetic data. Anaesthesia 38 supplement: 61–62
van Hamme M J, Ghoneim M M, Ambre J J 1978 Pharmacokinetics of etomidate, a new intravenous anaesthetic. Anesthesiology 49:274
van Lambalgen A A, Bronsveld W, van den Bos G C, Thijs L G, Teule G J J 1982 Cardiovascular and biochemical changes in dogs during etomidate-nitrous oxide anaesthesia. Cardiovascular Research 16:599
van Oss G E C, Rachmat Y, Booij L D H J, Crul J F 1980 Continuous infusion of etomidate as a method for outpatient anaesthesia. Acta Anaesthesiologica Belgica 31: 39–43

Versichelen L, Rolly G, Beerens J 1983 Alfentanil/etomidate anaesthesia for endolaryngeal microsurgery. Anaesthesia 83 supplement: 57–60

Wagner R L, White P F 1984 Etomidate inhibits adrenocortical function in surgical patients. Anesthesiology 61: 647–651

Wanscher M, Tonnesen E, Huttel M, Larsen K 1985 Etomidate infusion and adrenocortical function. A study in elective surgery. Acta anaesthesiologica Scandinavica 29: 483–485

Watkins J 1982 'Hypersensitivity response' to drugs and plasma substitutes used in anaesthesia and surgery. In: Watkins J, Salo M (eds) Trauma, stress and immunity in anaesthesia.and surgery. Butterworths, London, p 254–291

Watkins J 1983 Etomidate: 'immunologically safe' anaesthetic agent. Anaesthesia 38 Supplement: 34–38

Watkins J 1985 Etomidate: an 'immunologically safe' anaesthetic agent? Anaesthesia 40:1015

Watkins J, Thornton J A, Clarke R S J 1979 Adverse reactions to i.v. agents. British Journal of Anaesthesia 51:469

Weymar A, Eigenheer F, Gethmann J W, Reinecke A, Patschke D, Tarnow J, Bruckner J P 1974 Tierexperimentellle Untersuchungen zur Wirkung von Etomidate auf den Kreislauf und die myokardiale Sauerstoffversorgung. Anaesthesist 23:150

Xhonneux R, Carmaliet E, Reneman R S 1975 The electrophysiological effects of etomidate (R 26490), a new, short-acting hypnotic, in various cardiac tissues. In: Arias A, Llaurado R, Nalda M A, Lunn J N (eds) Recent progress in anaesthesiology and resuscitation, Proceedings of the IV European Congress of Anaesthesiology, Madrid 5–11 September 1974, Excerpta Medica, Amsterdam; American Elsevier, New York, p 152–156

Zacharias M, Clarke R S J, Dundee J W, Johnston S B 1978 An evaluation of three preparations of etomidate. British Journal of Anaesthesia 50: 925–929

Zacharias M, Clarke R S J, Dundee J W, Johnston S B 1979 Venous sequelae following etomidate. British Journal of Anaesthesia 51:779

Zacharias M, Dundee J W, Clarke R S J 1978 Evaluation of etomidate. British Journal of Anaesthesia 50: 633–634

Zindler M 1975 In: Arias A, Llaurado R, Nalda M A, Lunn J N (eds) Recent progress in anaesthesiology and resuscitation, Proceedings of the IV European Congress of Anaesthesiology, Madrid 5–11 September 1974. Excerpta Medica, Amsterdam; American Elsevier, New York, p 118–121

11

Propofol

Propofol is a hindered phenol which is chemically dissimilar to any other compounds used in anaesthesia (Fig. 11.1). It is insoluble in water and was originally solubilised in Cremophor EL. The currently available preparation is a 1% w/v aqueous emulsion containing 10% w/v soya bean oil, 1.2% w/v egg phosphatide and 2.25% w/v glycerol (Diprivan). The pH is 6–8.5 and the pKa of the drug in water is 11.

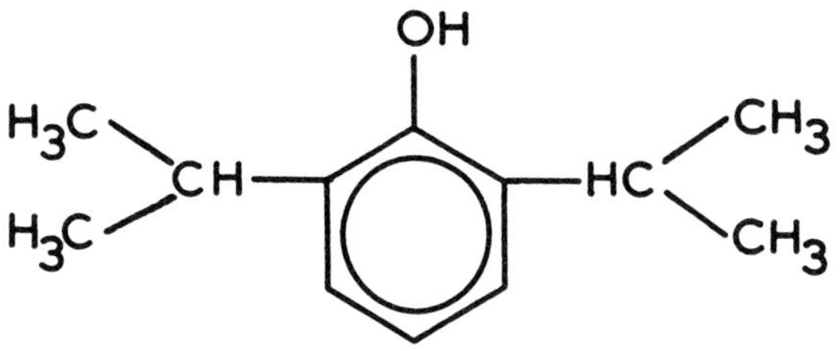

OH

H_3C CH H_3C HC CH_3 CH_3

Fig. 11.1 Formula of propofol.

The emulsion formulation, which contains 10 mg ml^{-1}, is free flowing and is as easy to inject as an aqueous solution. It is made isotonic with glycerol and is sealed under nitrogen. The precautions which apply to intravenous fat emulsions must be taken with propofol, that is it should be stored below 25°C but must not be frozen and the ampoules should be shaken before use. Filters should not be used during administration of the emulsion which should not be mixed before administration with other therapeutic agents or infusion fluids, although it can be administered through a Y-piece close to the injection site into a crystalloid infusion such as isotonic dextrose or normal saline.

PHARMACOLOGY

Animal experiments have shown that in normal doses propofol is ineffective by mouth (Glen et al, 1985) but intravenous propofol rapidly and reliably induces anaesthesia and side effects are comparable with those of other induction agents. However, it has less anticonvulsant and central anticholinergic action than comparable doses of thiopentone. While the emulsion formulation had anaesthetic properties in rats and mice and haemodynamic effects in the mini-pig, similar to those of the previously available cremophor formulation, the administration of the emulsion to dogs caused no untoward effects whereas the cremophor formulation had produced a marked increase in plasma histamine concentration (Glen & Hunter, 1984). Likewise there were no adverse effects following repeat administration of the emulsion preparation to the mini-pig whereas the cremophor formulation had produced anaphylactic responses when a second injection was given one week after an uneventful first exposure (Glen & Hunter, 1984).

In humans propofol is a 'rapidly-acting' induction agent and doses of 2.0 to 2.5 mg kg^{-1} injected at the height of forearm reactive hyperaemia will induce anaesthesia in unpremedicated adults in around 11 s (Robinson et al, 1985). This is similar to the times with equivalent doses of thiopentone.

In contrast to thiopentone (Dundee, 1960) subhypnotic doses of propofol in cremophor do not cause an increase in sensitivity to experimentally induced somatic pain (Briggs et al, 1982). Of more clinical importance are the postoperative findings when the drugs are used as sole agent for minor operations (Fig. 11.2). Thiopentone was

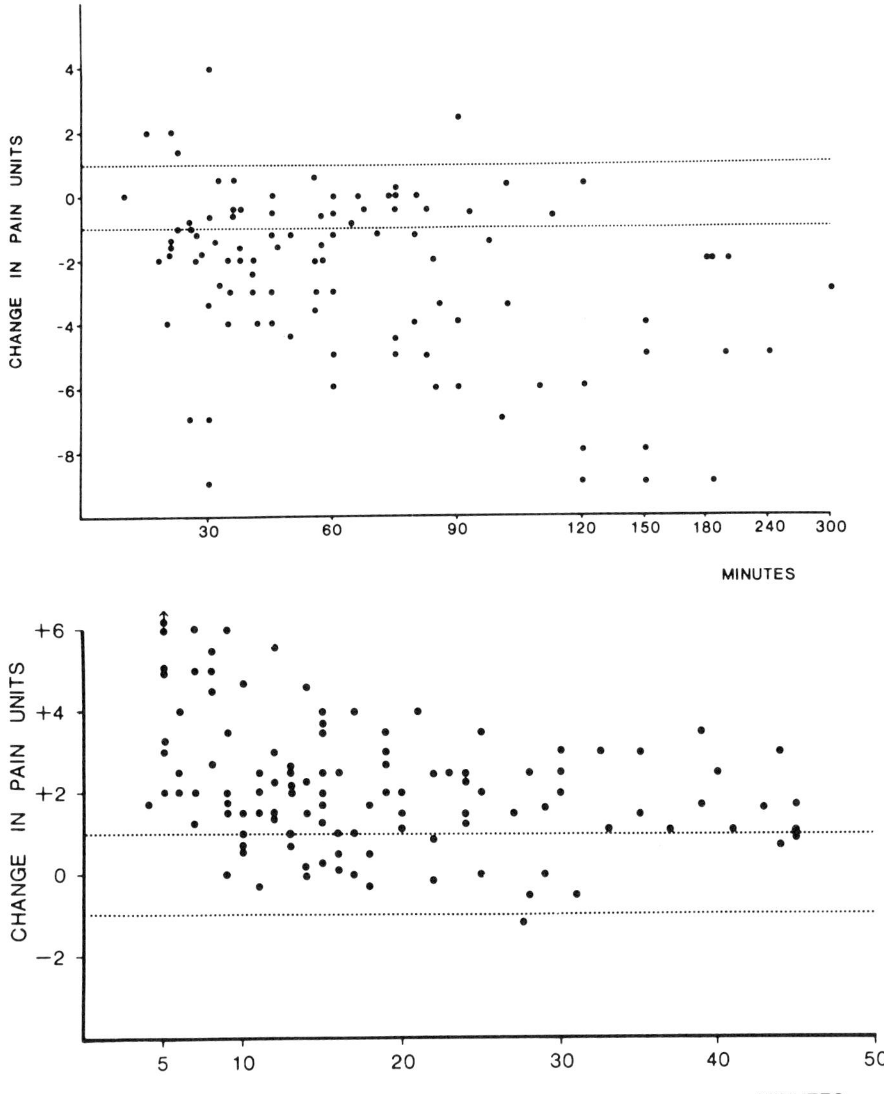

Fig. 11.2 Changes in postoperative pain readings from preoperative controls following large doses of thiopentone (upper) and propofol (lower).
. . . = range of expected normal variations in readings. (Briggs et al, 1982).

consistently followed by hyperalgesia, which lasted for up to 4 hours, while propofol causes a short period of analgesia. Clinical experience confirms the absence of antanalgesia (Briggs & White, 1985; Lees et al, 1985; Grounds et al, 1985).

Dosage

While the induction dose for the cremophor preparation was around 2 mg kg^{-1} for unpremedicated adults (Kay & Rolly, 1977; Briggs et al, 1981) with the emulsion, doses of 2.0 to 2.5 mg kg^{-1} are required (Cummings et al, 1984). More recent reports (Grounds et al, 1985; Plosker et al, 1985; Mouton et al, 1985) have confirmed the higher dose requirement of the emulsion and these and other studies (Fahmy et al, 1985) would therefore place the potency of propofol as 1.6 to 1.8 times that of thiopentone.

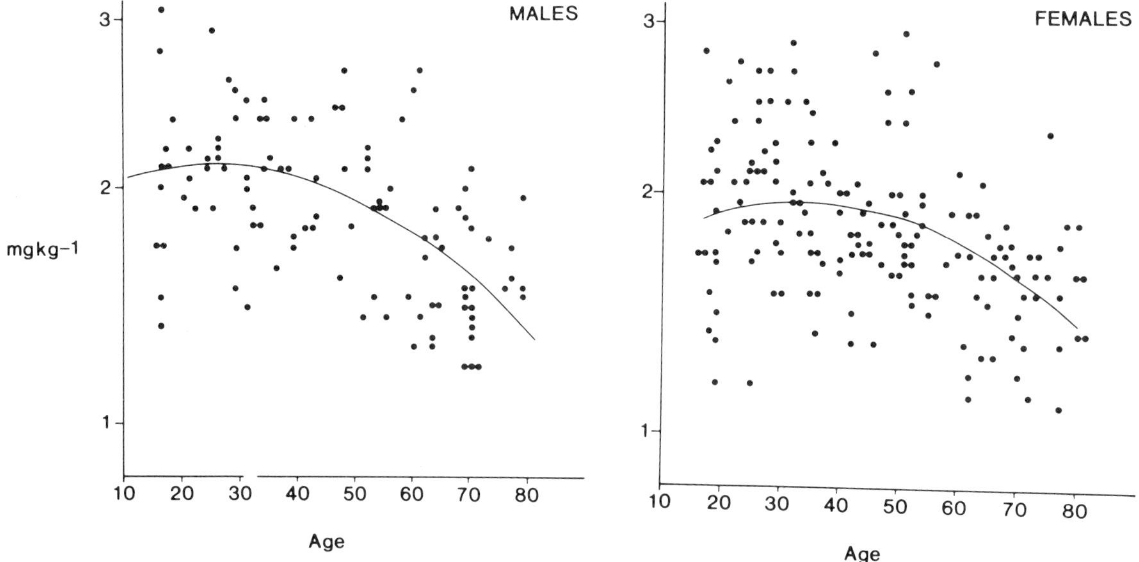

Fig. 11.3 Relationship of age to induction dose of propofol in unpremedicated subjects to whom the drug was administered in a constant manner. (Dundee et al, 1986).

However propofol exhibits a very marked relationship between the age of the subject and the induction dose (Fig. 11.3) and Dundee et al (1986) have shown this using a standard method of administration of the drug (1.25 mg kg^{-1} injected over 20 s followed by 10 mg at 15 s intervals until the eyelash reflex and contact with the patient is lost). The reduction in dosage with increasing age became clinically obvious at 60 yr: the dose for patients under 60 yr averaged 2 mg kg^{-1} while that for patients older than 60 yr was 1.6 mg kg^{-1}. There was some slight, but not significant, difference in the requirements for males and females but both sexes followed the above pattern as regards the influence of age on dose. This is further illustrated by another study by the same workers who gave bolus doses ranging from 1.5 to 3.0 mg kg^{-1} to fit patients under or over 60 yr bracket (Table 11.1). In these unpremedicated patients 2.25 mg kg^{-1} was required for the younger age group whereas in the elderly patients a dose of 1.75 mg kg^{-1} sufficed. It is worth noting the increasing cardiorespiratory depression with dosage in both of these series and also the more marked effect in the elderly patients. This will be discussed later.

The preoperative administration of 100 μg fentanyl with 5 mg droperidol reduced the induc-

Table 11.1 Frequency (%) of adequate induction of anaesthesia, hypotension and apnoea with varying single bolus doses of propofol in two age groups (n = 30, except *n = 20)

Dose (mg kg⁻¹)	*Under 60 yr* Anaesthesia induced	*Under 60 yr* Systolic BP fall (mmHg) 21–40	41+	*Under 60 yr* Apnoea (s) 31–60	61+	*Over 60 yr* Anaesthesia induced	*Over 60 yr* Systolic BP Fall (mmHg) 21–40	41+	*Over 60 yr* Apnoea(s) 31–60	61+
1.25						*100 (30)	35	15	10	15
1.50	53 (13)	20	3	17	3	97 (3)	27	13	23	7
1.75	83 (17)	40	0	30	7	100 (0)	50	13	40	7
2.00	87 (10)	23	0	20	10	97 (0)	40	20	53	20
2.25	97 (0)	50	0	30	13	*100 (0)	35	45	30	25
2.50	100 (3)	33	13	64	13					
2.75	100 (0)	40	3	20	40					
3.00	100 (0)	33	10	23	43					

Figures in brackets indicate rapid lightening anaesthesia (Dundee et al, 1986)

tion dose of propofol to as low as 1.5 mg kg^{-1} (Rolly and Versichelen, 1985; Rolly et al, 1985). McCollum et al (1986) who studied the effect of a number of premedicants, found no effect from diazepam 10 mg or pethidine 50–75 mg, but papavaretum 20 mg with hyoscine 0.4 mg, made 1.75 mg kg^{-1} an effective induction dose in young subjects.

PHARMACOKINETICS

A highly lipophilic drug like propofol would be expected to distribute rapidly but extensively from blood to tissues with a high estimated volume of the central compartment and a very high Vd_{ss} (Cockshott, 1985). Studies with single 2 mg kg^{-1} doses of the cremophor preparation showed a decline in blood levels which could be described by a 2-compartment open model with a mean α-phase half-life of 2.5 min and a mean β-phase half-life of 54 min (Adam et al, 1983). The plasma levels were similar, irrespective of whether the drug was injected as a fast bolus or over 20 to 40 s. Patients opened their eyes at an average of 4.4 min after this dose and by 5.2 min they were able to give date of birth on request. This would suggest that with the intermittent injection technique supplementary doses would be required every 4–5 min.

Two studies indicate that the pharmacokinetics of the emulsion preparation of propofol can be described by a 3-compartment open model (Kay et al, 1985; Briggs et al, 1985). Both groups showed a very rapid initial distribution of the drug from blood and a rapid intermediate phase and a slower final elimination. In the post-distributive phase propofol concentration declined biphasically with a mean $t\frac{1}{2}\beta$ in the range of 35–45 min — thought to reflect metabolic clearance of propofol from the blood. A slower final phase was observed in all patients giving a terminal half-life of 200–300 min: it is likely that this phase represents slower return of propofol to blood from a poorly perfused compartment, probably fat. Both studies confirm the high clearance of the drug indicated by the earlier workers, the rate being in excess of the estimates of hepatic blood flow during anaesthesia, suggesting some possible extrahepatic metabolism of propofol. In patients who did not receive fentanyl or halothane clearance has been estimated as 1.8–1.9 l min^{-1} and the volume of distribution 722 to 755 litres.

Briggs and his colleagues (1985) found that both fentanyl and halothane modified these figures. Fentanyl, but not halothane, significantly reduced the clearance from an average of 1.9 to 1.3 l min^{-1}. This was probably because propofol levels were higher in patients pretreated with fentanyl than in a comparable control group, reflecting a reduced degree of propofol distribution in the former.

A similar pharmacokinetic profile was noted when propofol was administered for induction and maintenance of anaesthesia by repeat bolus doses in patients having subarachnoid anaesthetic blocks. The blood concentration declined rapidly between 2 and 6 min after injection, indicating rapid distribution of propofol from blood into tissues (Knell & McKean, 1985) but the administration of a second dose prevented sampling being continued sufficiently long to provide the complete pharmacokinetic profile.

Secondary peaks have been observed in the blood decay concentrations in many patients following propofol. These occur in venous blood shortly after return of consciousness and might reflect local or systemic changes occurring on recovery, such as drug coming from muscle when exercised or other alterations in regional blood flow; despite the magnitude of these increases they appear to have no clinical or dynamic sequelae.

Most (88%) of the radioactivity detected following administration of labelled propofol can be accounted for in the urine in the form of glucuronides of propofol and the corresponding quinol, with approximately 2% in faeces (Cockshott, 1985; Simons et al, 1985a). The metabolic pathways for elimination of propofol have been investigated in man and animals. The drug is completely and rapidly metabolised to the sulphate and glucuronide conjugates of propofol 2, 6-diisopropyl 1, 4 quinol and other related compounds which are mainly eliminated via the kidneys. The actual proportions of these metabolites varies between species (Simons et al, 1985b, Simons personal communication, 1986).

In vitro binding of propofol has been investigated using equilibrium dialysis techniques. Over the concentration range of 0.1 to 20 μl ml^{-1} the drug was 98% bound to proteins in man; data for animals were similar (Cockshott I D, personal communication).

These pharmacokinetic data suggest that propofol would be a drug which would be very suitable for administration by intermittent injection or better still by infusion. Given with nitrous oxide for body surface operations, following an induction dose of 2.5 mg kg^{-1}, the requirements by 40 min range from 6 to 14 mg kg^{-1} and the median of 11.25 mg kg^{-1} h^{-1} would point to the dose for maintenance of anaesthesia (Robinson, 1985). Gepts et al (1985a, b) found that infusion rates of 9 mg kg^{-1} h^{-1} did not consistently maintain the desired hypnotic effect and they suggested that an analgesic premedication followed by an average of 6 mg kg^{-1} h^{-1} might be a simple and convenient method of achieving good operating conditions.

An interim report by Morcos & Payne (1985) suggests that, in patients undergoing major abdominal operations, the pharmacokinetics of propofol are generally similar in patients with impaired renal function to those in normal patients. Cockshott (1985) has also reported interim results in the study of the effect of liver cirrhosis on the pharmacokinetics of propofol: these indicate that even in patients with a reduced capacity for metabolism by liver the clearance of propofol from blood is similar to that in hepatically normal patients. This confirms the high capacity of the liver to metabolise propofol.

PHARMACODYNAMICS

Pain on injection has been reported since the first studies of propofol (Kay & Rolly, 1977). With the cremophor preparation there was a marked association between the site of injection and pain on injection. Briggs et al (1981) reported a 39% incidence when it was injected into a vein at the back of the hand, compared with 3% when veins at the forearm or anticubital fossa were used. While pain is less with the emulsion, the relationship to the site of injection still applies (Briggs & White, 1985). Venous thrombosis is not a clinical problem with the currently available formulation (Mattila & Koski, 1985).

Cardiovascular effects

Most workers have commented adversely on the cardiovascular effects of propofol and many have considered these to be worse than those of equivalent doses of thiopentone (Prys-Roberts et al, 1983; Youngberg et al, 1985; Mouton et al, 1985; Fahy et al, 1985). The last three workers all noted that the changes in the heart rate were less than with thiopentone and that this, together with decreased systemic vascular resistance, could account for the relatively greater hypotensive effect of the propofol. Fahmy et al (1985) found that propofol caused a greater reduction in systemic vascular resistance than equivalent doses of thiopentone. In an in-depth study, Patrick et al (1985) compared the cardiovascular effects of propofol 1.5 mg kg^{-1} and thiopentone 2 mg kg^{-1} for induction of anaesthesia in patients scheduled for elective coronary artery operations. Anaesthesia with propofol was accompanied by a reduction in arterial pressure which was largely due to a decrease in systemic vascular resistance and while thiopentone resulted in a small decrease in arterial pressure there was a greater increase in arterial pressure following tracheal intubation after the barbiturate. In infusion studies Coates et al (1985) found greater haemodynamic changes with the emulsion, as compared with their previous experience with the Cremophor preparation. Arterial hypotension (30% from baseline) was associated with a moderate decrease (19% from baseline) in cardiac output, but little change in heart rate.

Henriksson et al (1985) and Coates et al (1985) have noted that the greater hypotensive effect of propofol as compared with thiopentone is more marked when the drug is given by intermittent administration even for short procedures. Robinson (1985) who gave large doses up to 16 mg kg^{-1} over a period of 40–60 min found that the maximum fall in blood pressure occurred within the first few minutes of administration of the bolus induction dose; thereafter systolic and diastolic blood pressures remained virtually unchanged for the duration of the procedure. She also found a stable heart rate with intermittent administration of propofol.

As mentioned previously, age not only affects the induction dose of propofol but also the cardiovascular response to the drug (Dundee et al, 1986) (Table 11.1). These studies were carried out on patients in ASA status 1 or 2 who were unlikely to have severe undetected cardiac disease. The findings indicate the need for caution in the administration of propofol in the elderly. The importance of speed of injection is shown when one compares the degree of hypotension in the initial dose-finding study reported by the same workers, where the drug was administered slowly over a period which could have been as long as 60–90 s compared with the effect of a bolus administration (over 20 s). Even in the elderly patients hypotension was not a problem with the slow injection whereas Table 11.1 shows a high incidence with rapid administration. These elderly subjects could probably benefit from preparation with a small dose of fentanyl or alfentanil which should reduce the induction dose and minimise the cardiovascular effects, albeit at the risk of causing respiratory depression. Slow injection in the elderly is probably the most important prophylactic measure in reducing adverse cardiovascular effects of propofol.

In a well controlled comparison of the acute cardiovascular effects of 2.5 mg kg^{-1} propofol and 4 mg kg^{-1} thiopentone in patients without cardiovascular disease Grounds et al (1985) found significant differences between the drugs, which are summarised in Figure 11.4. There was a slight fall from baseline in cardiac output with both drugs, this reaching statistical significance ($P < 0.05$) only at 2 min after propofol and 8 min after thiopentone. Heart rate did not change significantly with either drug, although there was a tendency to tachycardia 2 min after thiopentone. Significant falls in mean arterial blood pressure occurred following both drugs, and it was always lower after propofol, but only significantly so at 4 min ($P < 0.05$). Slight falls in central venous pressure were also observed. The authors considered them to be equipotent doses but the equivalent dose of thiopentone to 2.5 mg kg^{-1} propofol should have been nearer 5 mg kg^{-1}.

As with other intravenous anaesthetics, arrhythmias do not appear to be a feature of propofol in man. Animal experiments by Glen and his colleagues (1985) showed that induction and maintenance by propofol increased the threshold to adrenaline arrhythmias as compared with either propofol–halothane or thiopentone–halothane. The same workers found that propofol does not possess any significant ganglion blocking or beta-adrenoreceptor antagonist properties.

It is interesting to note that despite the known cardiovascular effects a number of workers found the drug to be acceptable for induction of anaesthesia in patients who were receiving beta-adrenoreceptor blocking drugs (Al-Khudhairi et al, 1982) and in those with valvular heart disease (Aun & Major, 1984). Even Grounds et al (1985) who showed that propofol has a greater depressant effect on the cardiovascular system than an equivalent dose of thiopentone, concluded that these changes were clinically acceptable in patients without cardiovascular disease.

Respiration

Most workers have commented on the initial profound reduction in tidal volume following a normal induction dose of propofol, often amounting to a period of apnoea varying from 30 to 60 s. There has been no accompanying cough or hiccough and otherwise anaesthesia was smooth. This is not a problem for the clinical anaesthetist and patients easily tolerate artificial ventilation. However, there might be some difficulty in uptake of volatile agents if respiration is not assisted. There seems to be some degree of tachypnoea which Goodman et al (1985) found usually preceded the reduction in tidal volume and was also apparent on the return of respiration after a period of apnoea.

The intravenous injection of 2.5 mg kg^{-1} propofol had no effect on resting bronchomotor tone in the anaesthetised guinea pig (Glen et al, 1985). In man we have encountered one possible case of mild bronchospasm in over 1000 administrations of propofol, and this could have been due to the concurrent administration of suxamethonium. (The manufacturers report four instances in 4500 patients). One forms a distinct clinical

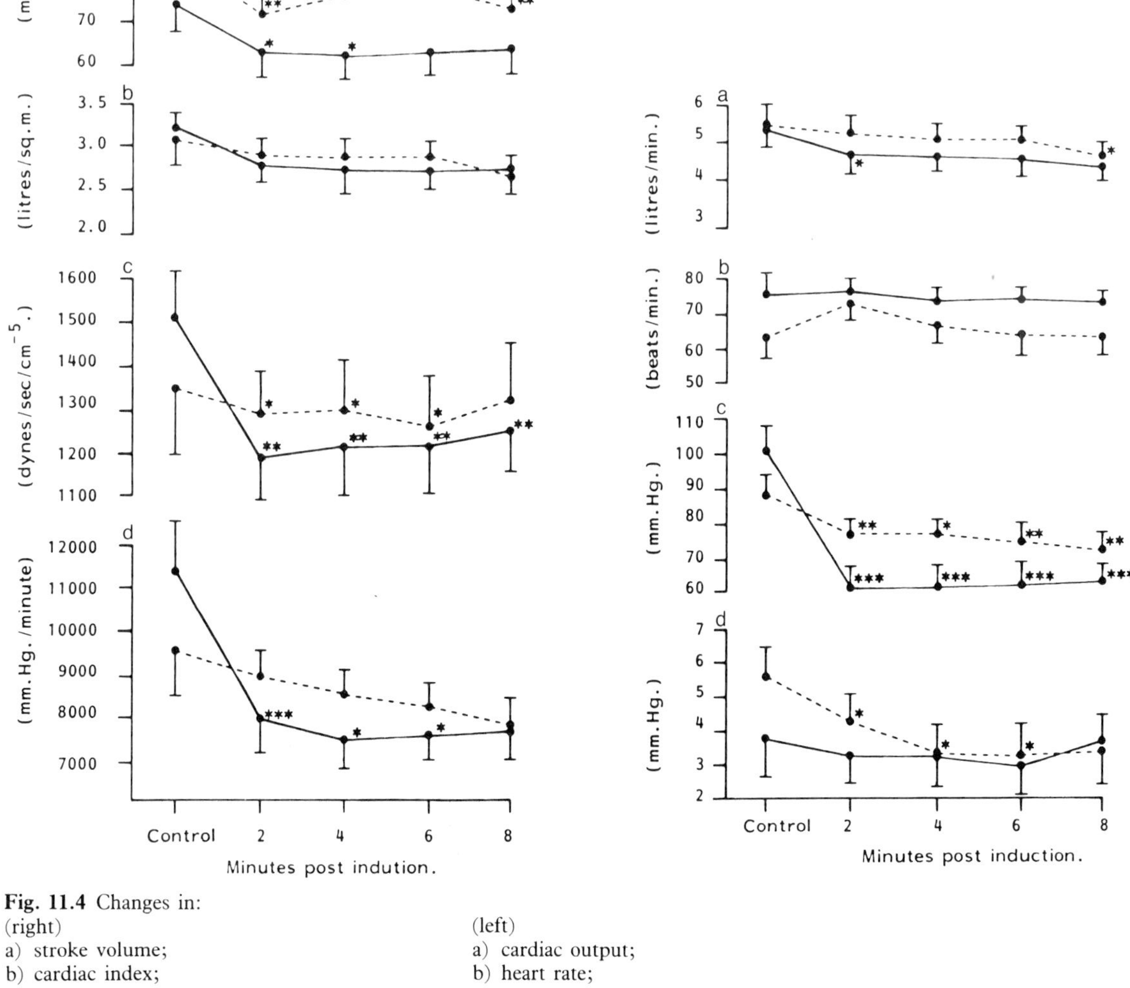

Fig. 11.4 Changes in:

(right)
a) stroke volume;
b) cardiac index;
c) systemic vascular resistances
d) heart rate systolic blood pressure product

(left)
a) cardiac output;
b) heart rate;
c) mean arterial blood pressure
d) central venous pressure

following induction of anaesthesia with propofol 2.5 mg kg^{-1} (●——●) or thiopentone 4.0 mg kg^{-1} (●---●). Points are mean (± SEM). * Significantly different from control (*$P < 0.05$; **$P < 0.01$; ***$P < 0.001$). (Grounds et al, 1985)

impression that, in contrast with thiopentone, propofol depresses laryngeal reflexes, an oropharyngeal airway is tolerated in light anaesthesia and laryngospasm is uncommon after its use. In agreement with this de Grood et al (1985b) found a greater degree of relaxation of the vocal cords after topical lignocaine in patients anaesthetized with propofol as compared with thiopentone.

Adrenocortical function

As will be discussed below, propofol shows promise as a drug for infusion. It is thus important to know whether it will have an effect on steroidogenesis similar to etomidate or whether it can be safely given for prolonged periods. In-vitro studies reported by Robertson et al (1985), Lambert et al (1985) and Kenyon et al (1985) showed that thiopentone, propofol and etomidate all inhibited ACTH-stimulated cortisol secretion in a dose-related manner. Similar inhibition of LH-stimulated testosterone secretion in a dose-related manner was found with thiopentone and propofol but not with etomidate, a finding in keeping with the known inhibitory site of action of the latter drug. The relevance of the findings to the pharmacological action of the drugs is not clear but on the basis of the relationship of inhibition to effective concentrations Robertson and colleagues (1985) suggest that it seems unlikely that either thiopentone or propofol will have any deleterious effect in vivo on adrenal or testicular steroidogenesis while Kenyon et al (1985) conclude that, on the basis of its effects on in-vitro cortisol synthesis 'the clinical use of propofol should not be accompanied by the sort of steroidogenic problems seen with etomidate'.

This view is supported by the animal experiments of Blackburn et al (1985) who found a reduced corticosteroid response to ACTH in rats anaesthetized with etomidate, but not with methohexitone or propofol. On this basis it seemed that the latter two anaesthetics were unlikely to produce adrenocortical hypofunction in a stress situation.

Liver function

There have been two reported studies of the influence of propofol on liver function tests. Kawar et al (1982) gave total doses of the cremophor preparation averaging 3.8 mg kg^{-1}, while Robinson & Patterson (1985) gave similar doses of the emulsion, both with nitrous oxide–oxygen, but without volatile supplements. Each study involved 30 fit women having minor gynaecological operations lasting 4–15 min and tests were carried out preoperatively and on the 2–3rd and 10–15th postoperative days. There were no significant changes in liver enzymes (aspartate transaminase and alanine transaminase) or in serum alkaline phosphatase in either series. There was no incidence of jaundice and on questioning at each post-operative visit, all patients felt generally well with no complaints of side effects. These findings are similar to those with small doses of other induction agents, but one must remember that Blunnie et al (1981) found some derangement of enzyme activity in about 38% of patients having continuous infusions of other agents. Similar studies are needed with continuous infusions of propofol.

Others

In a randomised study in healthy volunteers, Doenicke et al (1985) compared the effects of 2 mg kg^{-1} propofol and 0.05 ml kg^{-1} Althesin on plasma histamine concentration. The only significant rise occurred in the Althesin group and no changes consistent with a propensity to produce anaphylactoid reactions could be seen from measurements of immunoglobulin levels, complement C_3 or plasma histamine concentration in the propofol treated subjects.

The drug has no significant effect on blood coagulation or fibrinolytic activity (Sear et al, 1985). These workers found a significant fall in haematocrit value and haemoglobin concentration following its use, with a slight rise in blood sugar, but their significance is not known (Stark et al, 1985).

Animal studies showed no effect by propofol on gastrointestinal activity, compared with a slight decrease in motility with thiopentone (Glen et al, 1985).

Apart from causing a slight reduction in excretion of sodium ions it does not impair renal function. By contrast thiopentone causes a marked reduction in sodium excretion and a decrease in the elimination of chloride.

Propofol causes a reduction in intraocular pressure similar to that produced by comparable doses of thiopentone (Mirakhur & Shepherd, 1985). These studies were carried out in elderly patients and the authors commented unfavourably on the significant fall in arterial pressure that occurred with propofol.

RECOVERY

There have been several recovery studies with propofol. Bahar et al (1982) compared 2 and 3 mg kg^{-1} propofol (cremophor) with 4 and 6 mg kg^{-1} thiopentone and 1.5 mg kg^{-1} methohexitone. Recovery was faster with methohexitone and slightly slower with thiopentone than with equivalent doses of propofol, although the differences between the latter were small and of neither statistical nor clinical significance. Using reaction times and subjective assessment of coordination Herbert et al (1985) showed a faster return to baseline reaction times after 2.5 mg kg^{-1} propofol (emulsion) as compared with 5 mg kg^{-1} thiopentone, and performance after the latter remained significantly impaired until the morning of the second postoperative day. Grant & Mackenzie (1985) compared recovery from thiopentone and methohexitone used in three different anaesthetic techniques. In all of these propofol was associated with rapid and symptom-free recovery from anaesthesia and in day cases this was more rapid than after methohexitone or thiopentone. Like many other clinicians they comment on the quality of the recovery which is one of the most striking features of this drug.

A number of clinical studies conclude that, when given by intermittent injection for short procedures, recovery from propofol occurs more rapidly than with thiopentone (Henrikksson et al, 1985). In terms of recovery from anaesthesia for minor procedures Noble & Ogg (1985) found no difference between methohexitone (av. 2.8 mg kg^{-1}) and propofol (av. 3.3 mg kg^{-1}). Kay & Healy (1985) found a slightly more rapid recovery after propofol than from methohexitone, with the difference between the two drugs becoming more apparent in the early postoperative period — patients were drowsy for a shorter time, and ate earlier after propofol than after methohexitone.

This is in keeping with the views of Logan et al (1985) who studied recovery after outpatient dental anaesthesia. They found that although recovery was equally rapid after propofol as after methohexitone, propofol appeared to cause less impairment of the motor component of early recovery and of the higher discriminating cerebral functions (critical flicker fusion) 40 min after induction and might be compared to methohexitone for this type of outpatient anaesthesia. Valanne & Korttila (1985) would agree with this view.

There is a very low incidence of postoperative sickness with propofol. McCollum (1986) found a much lower than expected incidence of postoperative vomiting in patients given 'heavy' opioid premedication, suggesting that propofol might have some anti-emetic effect. This needs further evaluation.

INTERACTIONS

No dangerous interactions were found in animals when propofol was administered after daily doses of phenelezine, amitriptyline, or alcohol (Glen et al, 1985). The findings with alcohol, which are summarised in Table 11.2, are surprising when compared with thiopentone. In earlier studies Glen (1980) had found that a single dose of a number of drugs used as preanaesthetic medication (chlorpromazine, diazepam, papaveretum) caused an increase in propofol sleeping time, but the potentiation was less than when the same drugs were given before thiopentone.

No interactions were noted when animals pretreated with the beta-adrenoreceptor antagonists propranolol or atenolol were infused with propofol (Glen et al, 1985). As expected the heart rate remained below the baseline in the propranolol group, who also showed a significant increase in total peripheral resistance after the propofol.

Two clinical studies have shown no interaction between propofol and the neuromuscular blocking drugs, suxamethonium, vecuronium and atracurium (Nightingale et al, 1985; de Grood et al, 1985a). Preliminary studies by Lees et al (1985) suggest some potentiation of vecuronium, but not of atracurium by the emulsion preparation. These contrast with the in-vitro and in-vivo studies

Table 11.2 Effect of oral administration of ethyl alcohol on sleeping and recovery times following anaesthesia with propofol or thiopentone in mice

	Propofol 18 mg kg^{-1}		*Thiopentone 30 mg kg^{-1}*	
Alcohol dose ($g\ kg^{-1}$)	*Sleeping time (min)*	*Recovery of coordination (min)*	*Sleeping time (min)*	*Recovery of coordination (min)*
0	3.6	2.7	2.1	4.9
0.5	2.5	2.1	6.0	6.8
1.0	3.4	2.3	4.8	13.5
1.5	2.4	2.7	4.3	14.9
2.0	6.5	2.6	11.2	14.3

(Glen et al, 1985)

carried out with the cremophor preparation (Fragen et al, 1983; Robertson et al, 1983). In-vitro studies have shown that cremophor potentiates the action of suxamethonium, but antagonizes the action of non-depolarizing neuromuscular blockers, while clinical studies have shown that propofol–cremophor potentiates both atracurium and vecuronium, but does not prolong the duration of action of either drug.

INFUSIONS

While the pharmacokinetic profile suggests that propofol would be a very useful drug for infusion, one must realise that it should not be diluted and that administration must be by a controlled syringe. It is also not recommended that propofol and narcotics be administered from the same syringe, but both can be given simultaneously if injected into a fast-running infusion.

The suitability of propofol emulsion for this purpose has been confirmed by Mackenzie & Grant (1985) who showed its superiority over methohexitone, due to a lower incidence of excitatory effects. After opioid premedication anaesthesia was induced with 2 mg kg^{-1} followed by nitrous oxide-oxygen and an infusion of 0.3 mg kg^{-1} min^{-1}, reduced to 0.2 mg kg^{-1} min^{-1} after 10 min. The infusion was stopped about 10 min after the end of the operation and recovery which was smooth and occurred within 20 min. Their dosage of 12–15 mg kg^{-1} h^{-1} is slightly higher than that used by Robinson (1985) when the propofol was given by intermittent injection, but recovery was similar in the two series.

In view of the great individual variation in requirements of propofol when given by intermittent injection (Wright et al, 1984; Robinson, 1985), one questions the wisdom of using it as sole infusate without analgesic supplementation. When combined with fentanyl de Grood et al (1985a) found 9 mg kg^{-1} h^{-1} to be an adequate dose and recovery times were shorter than those found by Mackenzie & Grant (1985). Lees et al (1985) similarly found that 9 mg kg^{-1} h^{-1}, later reduced to 4.5 mg kg^{-1} h^{-1} and supplemented by fentanyl, provided good anaesthesia. All of these workers have commented that drug requirements decreased as the duration of anaesthesia increased and perhaps an automated variable-rate infusion pump (Ch. 17) might prove to be the answer.

By contrast, two studies (Coates et al, 1985; Uppington et al, 1985) report maintenance of anaesthesia with much smaller doses of propofol (4.5–5.5 μg kg^{-1} h^{-1}). Both workers premedicated their patients with morphine, but this is unlikely to explain the discrepancy: perhaps the patients were older than in the other series and the long delay (not less than 30 min) from induction to incision might have played a part as by that time the tissue depots would be filling and drug requirements decreasing.

Low concentrations of propofol have been used to 'cover' local anaesthesia and have proved very acceptable and controllable (O'Callaghan et al, 1982).

Other clinical aspects

Propofol has not been used sufficiently to comment on any specific clinical indications. It clearly is a reliable induction agent which shows promise as an infusion agent and within the limitations of its safe use which have been outlined above, it will likely find a place in clinical practice.

REFERENCES

Adam H K, Briggs L P, Bahar M, Douglas E J, Dundee J W 1983 Pharmacokinetic evaluation of ICI 35 868 in man. British Journal of Anaesthesia 55: 97–102

Al-Khudhairi D, Gordon G, Morgan M, Whitwam J G 1982 Acute cardiovascular changes following disopropopofol. Effects in heavily premedicated patients with coronary artery disease. Anaesthesia 37: 1007–1010

Aun C, Major E 1984 The cardiorespiratory effects of ICI 35868 in patients with valvular heart disease. Anaesthesia 39: 1096–1100

Bahar M, Dundee J W, O'Neill M P, Briggs L P, Moore J, Merrett J D 1982 Recovery from intravenous anaesthesia: comparison of disoprofol with thiopentone and methohexitone. Anaesthesia 37: 1171–1175

Blackburn T P, Glen J B, Hunter S C, Wood P 1985 Adrenocortical function in rats during anaesthesia with etomidate, methohexitone or propofol. British Journal of Pharmacology 86:497P

Blunnie W P, Zacharias M, Dundee J W, Doggart J R, Moore J, McIlroy P D A 1981 Liver enzyme studies with continuous intravenous anaesthesia. Anaesthesia 36: 152–156

Briggs L P, Clarke R S J, Dundee J W, Moore J, Bahar M, Wright P J 1981 Use of diisopropylphenol as main agent for short procedures. British Journal of Anaesthesia 53: 1197–1202

Briggs L P, Dundee J W, Bahar M, Clarke R S J 1982 Comparison of the effect of diisopropylphenol (ICI 35868) and thiopentone on response to somatic pain. British Journal of Anaesthesia 54: 307–311

Briggs L P, White M 1985 The effects of premedication on anaesthesia with propofol (Diprivan). Postgraduate Medical Journal 61 (Suppl 3): 35–37

Briggs L P, White M, Cockshott I D, Douglas E J 1985 The pharmacokinetics of propofol (Diprivan) in female patients (Abstract). Postgraduate Medical Journal 61 (Suppl 3): 58–59

Coates D P, Prys-Roberts C, Spelina K R, Monk C R, Norley I 1985 Propofol (Diprivan) by intravenous infusion with nitrous oxide: dose requirements and haemodynamic effects. Postgraduate Medical Journal 61 (Suppl 3): 76–79

Cockshott I D 1985 Propofol (Diprivan) pharmacokinetics and metabolism — an overview. Postgraduate Medical Journal 61 (Suppl 3): 45–50

Cockshott I D 1985 Personal communication,

Cummings G C, Dixon J, Kay N H, Windsor J P W, Major E, Morgan M, Sear J W, Spence A A, Stephenson D K 1984 Dose requirements of ICI 35868 (propofol Diprivan) in a new formulation for induction of anaesthesia. Anaesthesia 39: 1168–1171

de Grood P M R M, Ruys A H C, van Egmond J, Booij L H D J, Crul J F 1985a Propofol (Diprivan) emulsion for total intravenous anaesthesia. Postgraduate Medical Journal 61 (Suppl 3): 65–69

de Grood P M R M, van Egmond J, van de Wetering M, van Beem H B, Booij L H D J, Crul J F 1985b Lack of effects of emulsified propofol (Diprivan) on vecuronium pharmacodynamics — preliminary results in man. Postgraduate Medical Journal 61 (Suppl 3): 28–30

Doenicke A, Lorenz W, Stanworth D, Duka Th, Glen J B 1985 Effects of propofol (Diprivan) on histamine release, immunoglobulin levels and activation of complement in healthy volunteers. Postgraduate Medical Journal 61 (Suppl 3): 15–20

Dundee J W 1960 Alterations in response to somatic pain associated with anaesthesia II: The effect of thiopentone and pentobarbitone. British Journal of Anaesthesia 32: 407–414

Dundee J W, Robinson F P, McCollum J S C, Patterson C C 1986 Sensitivity to propofol in the elderly. Anaesthesia 41: 482–485

Fahmy N R, Alkhouli H M, Sunder N, Smith D, Kelley M M 1985 Diprivan: a new intravenous induction agent. A comparison with thiopental. Anesthesiology 63:A363

Fahy L T, van Mourik G A, Utting J E 1985 A comparison of the induction characteristics of thiopentone and propofol (2, 6-di-isopropyl phenol). Anaesthesia 40: 939–944

Fragen R J, Booij L H D J, van der Pol F, Robertson E N, Crul J F 1983 Interaction of diisopropyl phenol (ICI 35868) with suxamethonium, vecuronium and pancuronium in vitro. British Journal of Anaesthesia 55: 433–436

Gepts E, Claeys A M, Camu F 1985a Pharmacokinetics of propofol (Diprivan) administered by continuous intravenous infusion in man. A preliminary report. Postgraduate Medical Journal 61 (Suppl 3): 51–52

Gepts E, Claeys M A, Camu F, Smekens L 1985b Infusion of propofol (Diprivan) as sedative technique for colonoscopies. Postgraduate Medical Journal 61 (Suppl 3): 120–126

Glen J B 1980 Animal studies of the anaesthetic activity of ICI 35868. British Journal of Anaesthesia 52: 731–742

Glen J B, Hunter S C 1984 Pharmacology of an emulsion formulation of ICI 35868. British Journal of Anaesthesia 56: 617–625

Glen J B, Hunter S C, Blackburn T P, Wood P 1985 Interaction studies and other investigations of the pharmacology of propofol (Diprivan). Postgraduate Medical Journal 61 (Suppl 3): 7–14

Goodman N W, Carter J A, Black A M S 1985 Some ventilatory effects of propofol (Diprivan) as a sole anaesthetic agent. Preliminary studies. Postgraduate Medical Journal 61 (Suppl 3): 21–22

Grant I S, Mackenzie N 1985 Recovery following propofol (Diprivan) anaesthesia — a review of three different anaesthetic techniques. Postgraduate Medical Journal 61 (Suppl 3): 133–137

Grounds R M, Morgan M, Lumley J 1985 Some studies on the properties of the intravenous anaesthetic propofol (Diprivan) — a review. Postgraduate Medical Journal 61 (Suppl 3): 90–95

Henriksson B A, Carlsson P, Hallen B, Hagerdal M, Lundberg D, Ponten J 1985 Propofol (Diprivan) versus thiopentone in nitrous oxide/oxygen anaesthesia for short gynaecological procedures (Abstract). Postgraduate Medical Journal 61 (Suppl 3):102

Herbert M, Makin S W, Bourke J B, Hart E A 1985 Recovery of mental abilities following general anaesthesia induced by propofol (Diprivan) or thiopentone. Postgraduate Medical Journal 61 (Suppl 3):132

Kawar P, Briggs L P, Bahar M, McIlroy P D A, Dundee J W, Merrett J D, Nesbitt G S 1982 Liver enzyme studies with disoprofol (ICI 35868) and midazolam. Anaesthesia 37: 305–308

Kay B, Healy T E J 1985 Propofol (Diprivan) for outpatient cystoscopy. Efficacy and recovery compared with Althesin and methohexitone. Postgraduate Medical Journal 61 (Suppl 3): 108–114

Kay B, Rolly G 1977 ICI 35868, a new intravenous induction agent. Acta Anaesthesiologica Belgica 28: 303–316

Kay N H, Uppington J, Sear J W, Douglas E J, Cockshott I D 1985 Pharmacokinetics of propofol (Diprivan) as an induction agent. Postgraduate Medical Journal 61 (Suppl 3): 55–57

Kenyon C J, McNeil L M, Fraser R 1985 Comparison of the effects of etomidate, thiopentone and propofol on cortisol synthesis. British Journal of Anaesthesia 57: 509–511

Knell P J W, McKean J F 1985 An investigation of the pharmacokinetic profile of propofol (Diprivan) after administration for induction and maintenance of anaesthesia by repeat bolus doses in patients having spinal anaesthetic block. Postgraduate Medical Journal 61 (Suppl 3): 60–61

Lambert A, Mitchell R, Roberston W R 1985 Effect of propofol, thiopentone and etomidate on adrenal steroidogenesis in vitro. British Journal of Anaesthesia 57: 505–508

Lees N W, McCulloch M, Mair W B 1985 Propofol (Diprivan) for induction and maintenance of anaesthesia. Postgraduate Medical Journal 61 (Suppl 3): 88–89

Logan M R, Levack I D, Duggan J, Spence A A 1985 Propofol (Diprivan) compared with methohexitone for outpatient dental anaesthesia (Abstract). Postgraduate Medical Journal 61 (Suppl 3):144

McCollum J S C, Dundee J W, Carlisle R J T 1986 Effect of preanaesthetic medication on induction of anaesthesia with propofol. British Journal of Anaesthesia 58: 1330p

Mackenzie N, Grant I S 1985 Propofol (Diprivan) for continuous intravenous anaesthesia. A comparison with methohexitone. Postgraduate Medical Journal 61 (Suppl 3): 70–75

Mattila M A K, Koski E M J 1985 Venous sequelae after intravenous propofol (Diprivan) — a comparison with methohexitone in short anaesthesia. Postgraduate Medical Journal 61 (Suppl. 3): 162–164

Mirakhur R K, Shepherd W F I 1985 Intraocular pressure changes with propofol (Diprivan): comparison with thiopentone. Postgraduate Medical Journal 61 (Suppl 3): 41–44

Morcos W E, Payne J P 1985 The induction of anaesthesia with propofol (Diprivan) compared in normal and renal failure patients. Postgraduate Medical Journal 61 (Suppl 3): 62–63

Mouton S M, Bullington J, Davis L, Fisher K, Ramsey S, Wood M 1985 A comparison of Diprivan and thiopental for the induction of anesthesia. Anesthesiology 63:A364

Nightingale P, Petts N V, Healy T E J, Kay B, McGuinness K 1985 Induction of anaesthesia with propofol (Diprivan) or thiopentone and interactions with suxamethonium, atracurium and vecuronium. Postgraduate Medical Journal 61 (Suppl 3): 31–34

Noble J, Ogg T W 1985 The effect of propofol (Diprivan) and methohexitone on memory after day case anaesthesia. Postgraduate Medical Journal 61 (Suppl 3): 103–104

O'Callaghan A C, Normandale J P, Grundy E M, Lumley J, Morgan M 1982 Continuous intravenous infusion of disopropofol (ICI 35868, Diprivan). Comparison with Althesin to cover surgery under local anaesthesia/analgesia. Anaesthesia 37: 295–300

Patrick M R, Blair I J, Feneck R O, Sebel P S 1985 A comparison of the haemodynamic effects of propofol (Diprivan) and thiopentone in patients with coronary artery disease. Postgraduate Medical Journal 61 (Suppl 3): 23–27

Plosker H, Sampson I, Cohen M, Kaplan J A 1985 A comparison of diprivan and thiamylal sodium for the induction and maintenance of outpatient anaesthesia. Anesthesiology 63:A366

Prys-Roberts C, Davies J R, Calverley R K, Goodman N W 1983 Haemodynamic effects of infusions of diisopropyl phenol (ICO 35868) during nitrous oxide in anaesthesia in man. British Journal of Anaesthesia 55: 105–111

Robertson E N, Fragen R J, Booij L H D J, van Egmond J, Crul J F 1983 Some effects of diisopropyl phenol (ICI 35868) on the pharmacodynamics of atracurium and vecuronium in anaesthetized man. British Journal of Anaesthesia 55: 723–727

Robertson W R, Reader S C J, Davison B, Frost J, Mitchell R, Kayte R, Lambert A 1985 On the biopotency and site of action of drugs affecting endocrine tissues with special reference to the antisteroidogenic effect of anaesthetic agents. Postgraduate Medical Journal 61 (Suppl 3): 145–151

Robinson F P 1985 Propofol ('Diprivan') by intermittent bolus with nitrous oxide in oxygen for body surface operations. Postgraduate Medical Journal 61 (Suppl 3): 116–119

Robinson F P, Dundee J W, Halliday N J 1985 Age affects the induction dose of propofol (Diprivan). Postgraduate Medical Journal 61 (Suppl 3): 157–159

Robinson F P, Patterson C C 1985 Changes in liver function tests after propofol (Diprivan). Postgraduate Medical Journal 61 (Suppl 3): 160–161

Rolly G, Versichelen L 1985 Comparison of propofol and thiopentone for induction of anaesthesia in premedicated patients. Anaesthesia 40: 945–948

Rolly G, Versichelen L, Herregods L 1985 Cumulative experience with propofol (Diprivan) as an agent for the induction and maintenance of anaesthesia. Postgraduate Medical Journal 61 (Suppl 3): 96–100

Sear J W, Uppington J, Kay N H 1985 Haematological and biochemical changes during anaesthesia with propofol (Diprivan). Postgraduate Medical Journal 61 (Suppl 3): 165–168

Simons P J 1986 Personal communication

Simons P J, Cockshott I D, Douglas E J, Gordon E A, Rowland M, Hopkin K 1985 Personal communication in Cockshott (1985)

Simons P J, Cockshott I D, Douglas E J, Gordon E A, Hopkins K, Rowland M 1985b Blood concentrations, metabolism and elimination after a subanaesthetic intravenous dose of ^{14}C-propofol ('Diprivan') to male volunteers. Postgraduate Medical Journal 61 (Suppl 3): 64

Stark R D 1985 Opening remarks. Postgraduate Medical Journal 61 (Suppl 3):1

Stark R D, Binks S M, Dutka V N, O'Connor K M, Arnstein M J A, Glen J B 1985 A review of the safety and tolerance of propofol (Diprivan). Postgraduate Medical Journal 61 (Suppl 3): 152–156

Uppington J, Kay N H, Sear J W 1985 Propofol (Diprivan) as a supplement to nitrous oxide–oxygen for the maintenance of anaesthesia. Postgraduate Medical Journal 61 (Suppl 3): 80–83

Valanne J, Korttila K 1985 Comparison of methohexitone and propofol (Diprivan) for induction of enflurane anaesthesia in outpatients. Postgraduate Medical Journal 61 (Suppl 3): 138–143

Wright P J, Clarke R S J, Dundee J W, Briggs L P, Greenfield A A 1984 Infusion rates for anaesthesia with propofol. British Journal of Anaesthesia 56: 613–616

Youngberg J A, Grogono A W, Sehon C K, White J, Texidor M 1985 Comparative evaluation of diprivan, thiopental and thiamylal for induction of anesthesia. Anesthesiology 63:A365

12

The benzodiazepines

In the last edition of this book the relevant section was headed 'Tranquillisers', but in the intervening years both the clinical usage and knowledge of the benzodiazepines has increased to the extent of justifying a change in title. For the average anaesthetist the words tranquillisers and benzodiazepines are almost synonymous. About thirty benzodiazepines have been used clinically, but most of these are only available in tablet form. The currently available injectable drugs are listed in Table 12.1 but only four of these are used by anaesthetists. The emphasis here will be laid on diazepam and midazolam, with lesser mention of flunitrazepam and lorazepam. An injectable form of flunitrazepam is not available in Britain, while the use of lorazepam is more in the field of preanaesthetic medication than intravenous anaesthesia. The mode of action and pharmacokinetics will be discussed before reviewing the individual drugs used in anaesthesia.

Table 12.1 The injectable benzodiazepines. Chlordiazepoxide and clonazepam have no use in anaesthetic practice

Generic name	*Brand name*
Chlordiazepoxide	Librium
Diazepam	Valium, Diazemuls, Stesolid
Flunitrazepam	Rohypnol
Lorazepam	Ativan
Clonazepam	Rivotril, Clonoptin
Midazolam	Hypnovel, Dormicum, Dobralam

MODE OF ACTION

All benzodiazepines possess the same range of actions on the central nervous system. They act on specific receptor sites throughout the brain and spinal cord, though radioisotopic binding studies have shown these to be most dense in the cerebral cortex, the hippocampus and the cerebellum (Mohler & Okada, 1978). Their effect is produced by the potentiation of certain inhibitory interneurones which utilise the neurotransmitter gamma-amino butyric acid (GABA). Upon release of GABA into the synapse an increase in the flow of Cl^- ions into the target neurone occurs, resulting in hyperpolarisation. The nerve cell is thus made more refractory to any excitatory impulse (Haefely et al, 1975).

The benzodiazepines receptors are situated in these synapses and by enhancing the response to GABA they will tend to inhibit certain pathways in the central nervous system (Fig. 12.1). This has

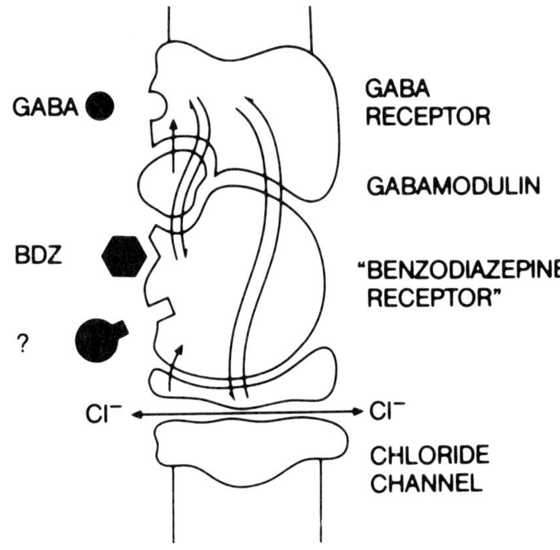

Fig. 12.1 The suggested mode of action of benzodiazepines and their antagonists on their receptors.

been shown to apply to the benzodiazepines used in anaesthesia. In an *in vitro* study, Cheng & Brunner (1981) found that midazolam decreased the re-uptake of GABA in preparations of rat fore-brain synaptosomes. Thus, more GABA was present at the synapse producing greater inhibition of the neurone. Hence, midazolam-induced increase in the flow of chloride ions into certain neurones was demonstrated in rats by Tang et al (1983). This effect also occurred with the benzodiazepine antagonist Ro 15 1788 which indicated it has an agonist action in this respect. With both Ro 15 1788 and midazolam this phenomenon was dose-related.

Similarity of clinical action

There is growing evidence that the benzodiazepines all have a similar pharmacological profile and that their therapeutic use is related more to the pharmaceutical preparation than to any inherent drug differences. The currently available drugs range from those marketed as 'daytime sedatives' to longer-acting drugs which are used as hypnotics. Certain preparations are recommended for control of convulsions and a small number for induction of anaesthesia.

The benzodiazepines cause dose-related cerebral depression, a hypothetical representation of which is shown in Figure 12.2. In increasing doses all of these drugs can cause mild sedation, drowsiness, sleep and even anaesthesia but it is only possible to produce this wide spectrum of actions with a small number which are available both as oral, intravenous and intramuscular preparations. Certain pharmacokinetic differences determine the time of onset of intravenous benzodiazepines but in anaesthetic practice these are less important than their metabolism, particularly their breakdown to hypnotically active metabolites and the duration of action of both the parent compound and the metabolite.

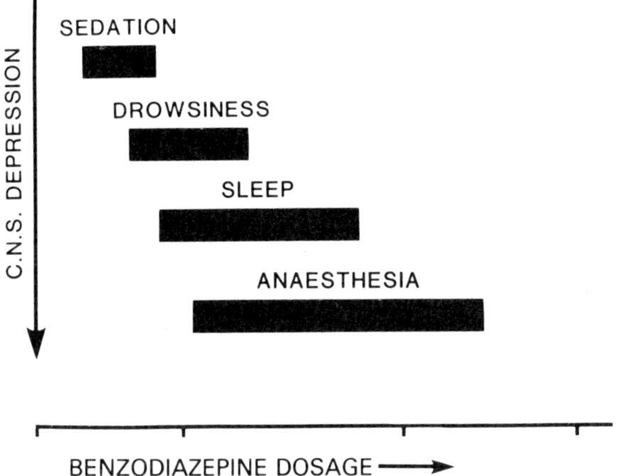

Fig. 12.2 Dose–effect response to an injectable benzodiazepine showing increasing dose requirements and variability in response.

The variability of action of the benzodiazepines is quite different from that of other drugs used in anaesthesia. With increasing cerebral depression there is an increasing variability of dose required to produce the desired therapeutic effect. This difference is more marked in younger patients and is one of the factors limiting their more widespread acceptance as induction agents.

In addition to the actions shown in Figure 12.2 all benzodiazepines have anticonvulsant activity and the injectable ones are useful for this purpose.

CHEMISTRY

As a group the benzodiazepines are insoluble in water and all the commercially available preparations are available in tablet or capsule, and in some cases syrup, form. The chemical structures of the four compounds which are of most interest to anaesthetists are given in Figure 12.3. Midazolam is the newest member of this group and is a water-soluble imidazole benzodiazepine derivative.

Diazepam

Diazepam is 7-chloro-1,3-dihydro-l-methyl-5-phenyl-2H-1,4-benzodiazepin-2-one. It is a colourless crystalline base, insoluble in water with a molecular weight of 285. Diazepam is available both in oral and injectable forms. There are three injectable preparations:

The established preparation (Valium) contains 5 mg ml^{-1} in an aqueous vehicle composed of organic solvents consisting mainly of propylene glycol, ethyl alcohol and sodium benzoate in benzoic acid. This is a slightly viscid solution with

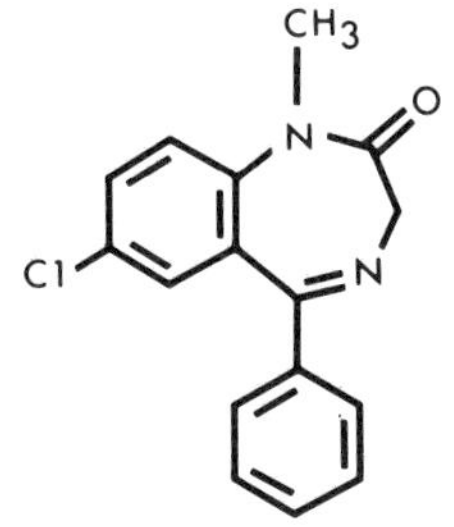

Diazepam 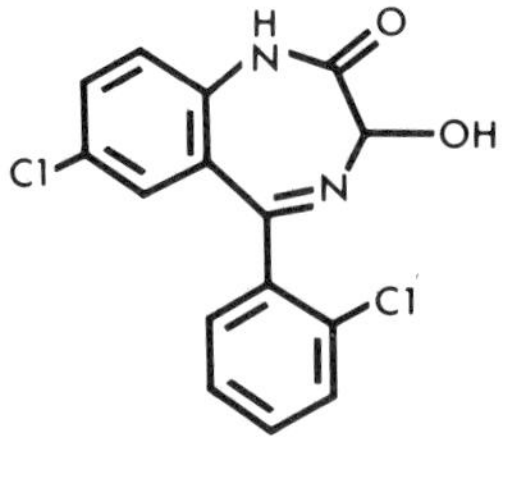 Lorazepam

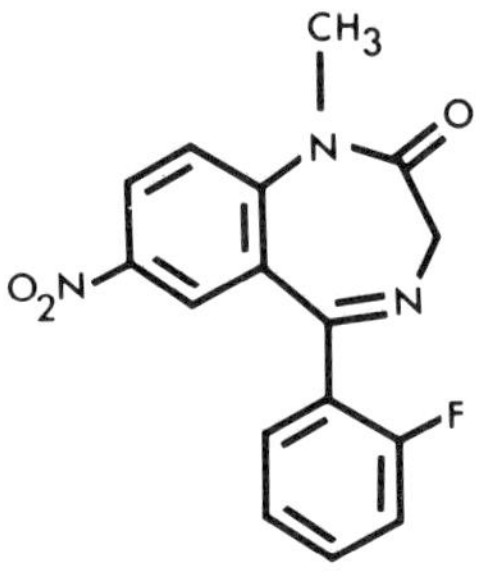

Flunitrazepam 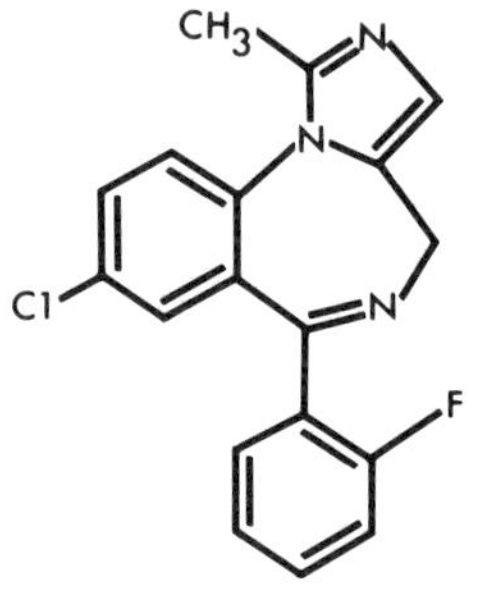 Midazolam

Fig. 12.3 The chemical structures of four injectable benzodiazepines.

a pH in the range 6.4 to 6.9 and it requires a large bore needle for rapid intravenous injection. A similar preparation, Stesolid, is also solubilised in propylene glycol.

An emulsion preparation (Diazemuls) contains 5 mg ml^{-1} in a lipid emulsion made from soya bean oil similar to the fat emulsion used for parenteral nutrition (Intralipid). The solution is easy to inject but the opacity might cause slight difficulty with venepuncture. There was a preparation of diazepam, solubilised in Cremophor EL which is no longer used because of the high incidence of hypersensitivity reactions. This was marketed under the trade name Stesolid which, as mentioned above, is now used for one brand of diazepam BP solubilised with propylene glycol. A micelle preparation of diazepam is undergoing investigation but data are not available at the time of writing.

Diazepam is also available in tablet and capsule form, in suppositories and in a form suitable for rectal administration.

Midazolam

Midazolam [8-chloro-6 (2-fluorophenol)-l-methyl-4H imidazo (1,S-a) (1, 4)] benzodiazepine is an imidazo benzodiazepine derivative. The nitrogen in the imidazole ring, which is attached to positions 1 and 2 in the diazepine ring imparts to the molecule a higher basicity and hence water-solubility, as well as a shorter duration of action than other injectable drugs. It can be prepared as a water-soluble salt with hydrochloric, maleic or lactic acid and is commercially available in a stable aqueous solution as the hydrochloride salt.

Although midazolam is stable in an aqueous solution and is freely water-soluble, its solubility is pH dependent. As shown in Figure 12.4, the ring opens reversibly at pH values below 4, imparting water-solubility. At the pH of plasma the ring closes and the lipid solubility is enhanced, this closing process having a half-life of about 10 minutes. Care should be taken to ensure that midazolam is not mixed with acidic solutions.

Midazolam

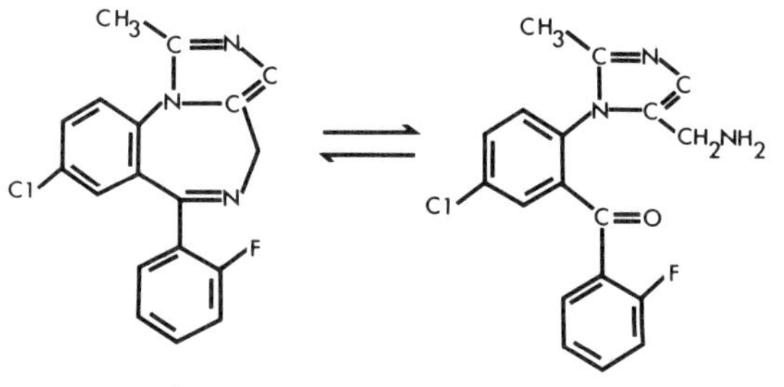

1. 2.

Fig. 12.4 The unique midazolam ring structure.

Flunitrazepam

Flunitrazepam (Rohypnol) is 5(2 fluorophenyl)-1,3 dihydro-7-nitro-1-methyl-2H-1,4-benzodiazepin-1-one. It is marketed widely as a hypnotic and in some countries in an injectable form (1 mg ml^{-1}) for induction of anaesthesia and sedation. Like diazepam the solution is made up in an organic solvent.

Lorazepam

Lorazepam (Ativan) is 7-chloro-5-(0-chlorophenyl)-1,3-dihydro-3 hydroxy-2H-1, 4-benzodiazepam-2-one. This is available in tablet form (differing strengths in different countries) and as a solution (organic solvent) containing 4 mg ml^{-1}.

Mode of presentation

There are two important clinical aspects of the mode of presentation of injectable benzodiazepines. These relate to bioavailability and to the irritant effect of the injectable preparation, i.e. pain on injection and venous thrombosis.

Bioavailability

This only applies to injectable diazepam. Anecdotal reports that the emulsion preparation (Diazemuls) was 'less potent' than Valium, which contains an organic solvent, led Fee et al (1984a) to compare plasma levels following 10 mg of each given intravenously in a randomised crossover study in volunteers. The concentration was consistently 20–30% higher following Valium as compared with Diazemuls. The overall bioavailability, as shown by average $AUC_{24\,h}$, was also very significantly greater ($P < 0.001$) with Valium. (Fig. 12.5)

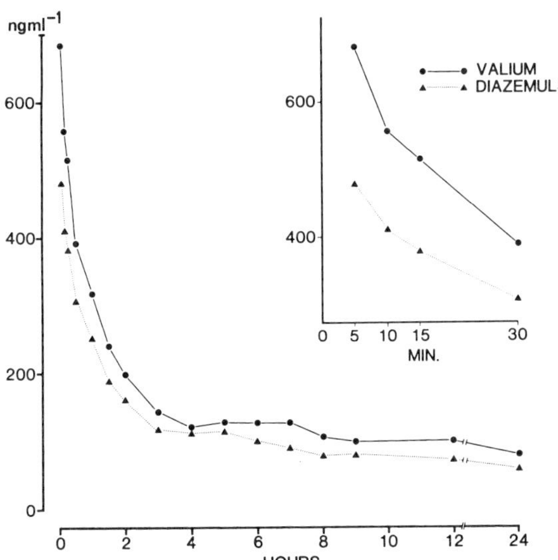

Fig. 12.5 Mean plasma diazepam levels following administration of 10 mg Valium (solid line) and 10 mg Diazemuls (broken line) given intravenously to 8 subjects (From Fee et al, 1984a).

Venous irritation

Pain accompanying direct intravenous injection occurs in about 40% of patients given Valium brand of diazepam, and its use is followed by a similar incidence of venous thrombosis. Many early reports of its use did not mention thrombosis since in many incidences this might not appear until the 7th to 10th day after administration (Hegarty & Dundee, 1977). Both injection pain and venous thrombosis are more likely to occur with the use of small veins in the dorsum of the hand. Valium-induced thromboses occur more commonly in elderly patients, very long sections of veins might be involved and such thromboses might persist for many weeks as painless cord-like structures.

A number of means have been suggested for reduction of these troublesome complications, such as dilution of the drug (even though this results in a cloudy solution of small droplets), injection into a fast-running infusion, or preceding administration by a small dose of intravenous lignocaine. However, the simplest solution is to employ Diazemuls, the introduction of which has virtually eliminated these problems, which are very important to the patient (Kawar & Dundee, 1982).

Venous sequelae have been reported in only 15% of patients given lorazepam 4 mg and in 5% following 1 mg flunitrazepam (Hegarty & Dundee, 1977). Injection pain is uncommon with midazolam, which likewise causes a low incidence of venous sequelae (Kawar & Dundee, 1982). The complication incidence with flunitrazepam and midazolam is similar to that associated with thiopentone and both cause less injection pain than methohexitone although followed by a similar low incidence of thrombosis.

PHARMACOKINETICS

Protein binding

The benzodiazepines are all highly bound to plasma albumin, ranging from 80% in the case of flunitrazepam to 98% with diazepam (Greenblatt et al, 1982). The rank order for binding of other injectable benzodiazepines and for temazepam is

Table 12.2 Rank order of certain properties which influence the pharmacokinetics of the benzodiazepines

Property	*Rank order*
Lipid solubility	MDZ < FNZ < TMZ < LZ < DZ
Plasma protein binding	LZ < FNZ < MDZ < TMZ < DZ
Volume of distribution	LZ < FNZ < MDZ < TMZ < DZ
Elimination half-life	MDZ < TMZ = LZ < FNZ < DZ
Plasma clearance	LZ = FNZ < DZ < TMZ < MDZ

DZ = diazepam, MDZ = midazolam,
LZ = lorazepam, FNZ = flunitrazepam, TMZ = temazepam

shown in Table 12.2. Small changes in protein binding will produce large alterations in concentrations of available free drug and will markedly affect the clinical action of the benzodiazepine. This has been demonstrated to be important in clinical practice in the case of midazolam (Dundee et al, 1984a and b). Patients with liver or renal disease and in states of malnutrition with resulting hypoalbuminaemia, have an enhanced response to benzodiazepines as compared with normal subjects (Reves et al, 1981) and this might be attributable to differences in plasma binding.

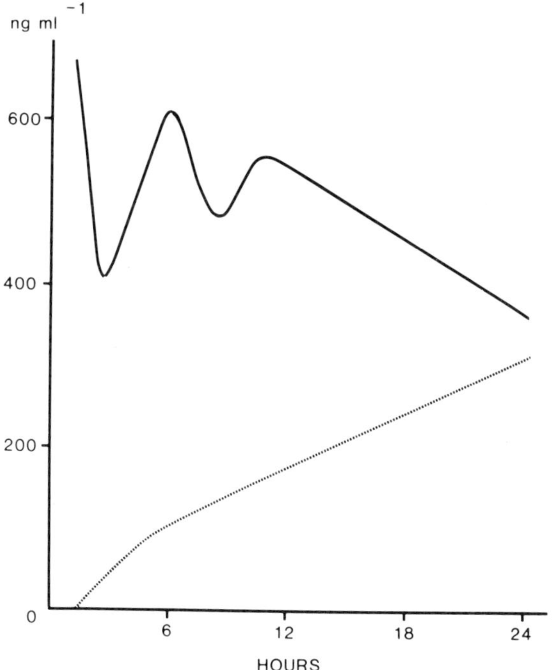

Fig. 12.6 Average plasma levels of diazepam (——) and its metabolite, N-desmethyl diazepam (. . .) up to 24 hours following 1 mg kg^{-1} intravenously. Freehand drawing of average readings in 10 patients: calculated from unpublished data.

Distribution and metabolism

The disappearance of benzodiazepines from the plasma is in the biphasic manner of a two-compartment model, although there is great inter-individual variability in the pharmacokinetics of these drugs. As an example, diazepam has a range of elimination half-lives varying from 20 to 70 hours. However, pharmacokinetic parameters do not vary with the dose of drug given or with repeat administration and as a rule the benzodiazepines follow first order kinetics.

Following intravenous injection there is the usual initial distribution phase to vessel-rich tissues including the central nervous system, kidneys, liver and heart from where it is distributed to muscle and later to body fat. The elimination phase is then dependent on hepatic biotransformation. Some degree of 'enterohepatic recirculation' occurs with diazepam: following biliary excretion of the drug into the gastrointestinal tract, there is reabsorption by the intestinal mucosa which results in a second peak effect as illustrated in Figure 12.6. This usually occurs within about 4 to 6 hours after the initial administration and might be accompanied by a period of re-sedation. The second peak shown in this Figure is often difficult to detect and is probably only of clinical significance when very large doses are given, as was the case with these data. There are alternative theories for the cause of this second peak but these are less important than is the realisation that this is a common occurrence.

The elimination of the benzodiazepines follows one of the patterns shown in Table 12.3. Oxidation occurs in the liver; drugs can be considered to have a low extraction ratio when the hepatic clearance is lower than hepatic blood flow. Available evidence suggests that benzodiazepine oxidation is a 'susceptible' metabolic pathway and it might be impaired in subjects with liver disease and in some elderly patients. Furthermore it is impaired by the administration of drugs which are known to inhibit the activity of microsomal oxidizing enzymes, such as cimetidine, ioniazid

Table 12.3 Classification of benzodiazepines according to their route of metabolism and extraction ratios

Metabolic process	*Low extraction*	*High extraction*
Oxidation	Diazepam Flunitrazepam	Midazolam
Conjugation	Oxazepam Lorazepam Temazepam	
Nitroreduction	Nitrazepam Clonazepam	

(modified from Dundee et al 1984c, Greenblatt 1982, 1983)
Some commonly used benzodiazepines which are not used in intravenous anaesthesia have been included to put the topic into perspective.

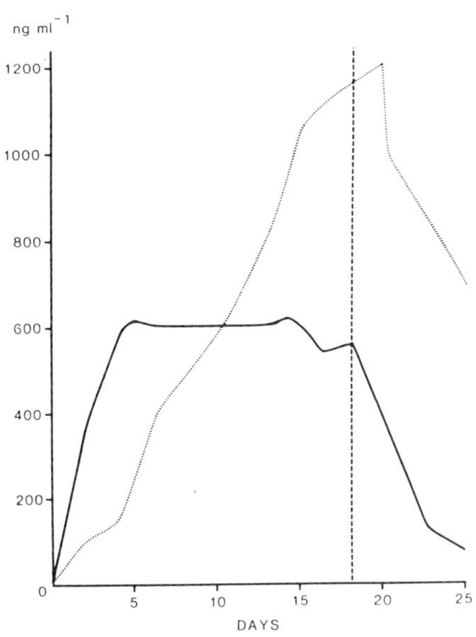

Fig. 12.7 Plasma levels of diazepam (——) and N-desmethyl diazepam (– – –) following administration of 10 mg diazepam 4-hourly for 17 days (Gamble et al, 1976).

and certain oestrogens which are contained in oral contraceptives. In these circumstances, the clearance of the benzodiazepine might be delayed. With the high extraction drugs, liver blood flow is an important factor in determining alterations in the rate of their metabolism. Breakdown may occur to a compound which itself has some hypnotic activity, such as desmethyldiazepam in the case of diazepam. Metabolites might have a longer elimination half-life than the parent compound and this can be of great clinical importance following their repeated use and even more important following their long-term use at short intervals. Gamble et al (1976) have demonstrated a very marked buildup of N-desmethyl diazepam in patients who received the parent compound at 4-hourly intervals for periods of 10–17 days (Fig. 12.7). This slowly eliminated metabolite might result in a very long recovery period.

Diazepam and Midazolam

The physical and pharmacokinetic properties relevant to the fate of diazepam and midazolam in the body are summarised in Table 12.4. These show wide variation between two drugs which have a non-dissimilar clinical profile. Their disposition in the body can be described by a two-compartment open model (Allonen et al, 1981; Klotz & Zeigler, 1982).

The greater lipophilicity of diazepam is compensated for by the increased fraction of free drug in the case of midazolam; this is reflected by a similar volume of distribution of the two drugs and by a similar onset time. The initial redistribution ($t\frac{1}{2}\alpha$) is shorter with midazolam than with diazepam, contributing to a quicker, earlier recovery with midazolam. The main site of metabolism of both drugs is in the liver; clearance is ten times faster with midazolam than diazepam, resulting in a markedly shorter elimination half life ($t\frac{1}{2}\alpha$)-of the latter.

Figure 12.8 shows the metabolites detected in the urine after oral midazolam. The main metabolite, 4-hydroxy-midazolam, has some pharmacological activity, but this is clinically insignificant as it is quickly conjugated in the liver (Heizmann et al, 1983). This contrasts with the main metabolite of diazepam, N-desmethyldiazepam, which, while only having about one-tenth the pharmacological activity of the parent compound, has a very prolonged action. Diazepam has the alternative metabolic pathway of hydroxylation to oxazepam which is used clinically as a night-time hypnotic (Fig. 12.9).

Midazolam is a hiqhly protein bound drug and, as already mentioned, factors influencing protein binding will cause relatively large changes in the free fraction of drug. This affects the potency and pharmacokinetic parameters particularly volumes of distribution with less effect on hepatic clearance. The hepatic elimination of midazolam is

Table 12.4 Physicochemical and pharmacokinetic properties of diazepam and midazolam

Property	*Diazepam*	*Midazolam*
PHYSICOCHEMICAL		
Solubility	Insoluble in water Available in organic solution or lipid emulsion	Solubility in water because of hydrophilic imidazole group
Form of i.v. presentation	Organic solvent Emulsion	Aqueous solution
pKa	3.4	6.2
Lipophilicity Octanol: buffer partition ratio	309	34
PHARMACOKINETICS		
Plasma protein binding	97–99%	94–98%
Volume of distribution (V_d (l kg^{-1}))	0.7–1.6	0.8–1.6
Elimination half life (h) ($t_{\frac{1}{2}}\beta$)	20–70	1.5–5
Clearance *Total body* (ml min^{-1} kg^{-1}) *Plasma* (ml min^{-1})	0.24–0.53 20–47	6.4–11.1 268–630
Metabolism	To desmethyldiazepam and oxazepam Both hypnotically active	Active metabolite α-hydroxymidazolam which is very rapidly conjugated to inactive form ($t_{\frac{1}{2}}\beta < 1$ h)
Second peak	Present at 6–8 h due to enterohepatic recirculation and is of clinical significance	If present, is very small and not clinically significant

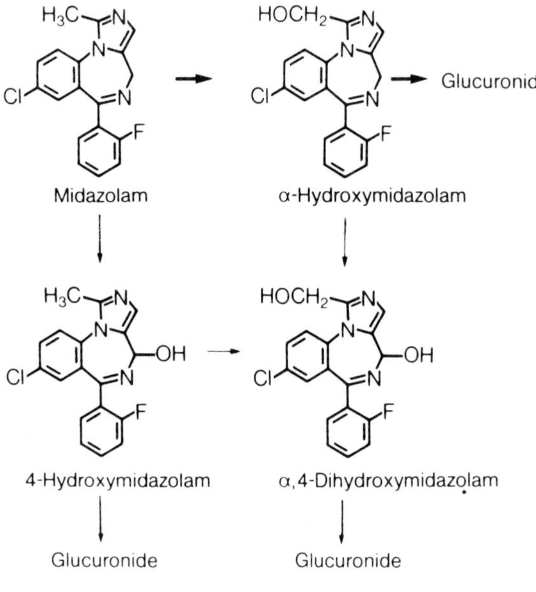

Metabolism of midazolam.

Fig. 12.8 Midazolam and its metabolites (from Gerecke, 1983).

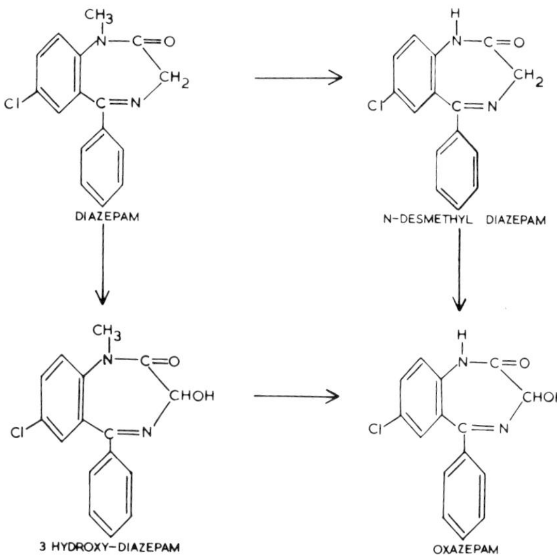

DIAZEPAM

N-DESMETHYL DIAZEPAM

3 HYDROXY-DIAZEPAM

OXAZEPAM

Fig. 12.9 Diazepam and its metabolites.

flow dependent and changes in hepatic blood flow might alter its clearance (Klotz & Ziegler, 1982).

Less than 1% of midazolam is excreted unchanged in the kidneys (Smith et al, 1981), the drug being cleared virtually entirely by liver metabolism. Theoretically liver failure should have a profound effect on its clearance and elimination half-life but this has not been investigated. Renal failure would not be expected to alter the ability of the liver to metabolise free midazolam: more important, Vinik et al (1982) found a three-fold increase in free midazolam in patients with renal failure (88.5% bound instead of 96.4%) leading not only to a greater potency, but possibly to a shorter duration of action. Greenblatt et al (1978) have demonstrated a sex difference in binding of diazepam in patients with chronic renal failure, more free drug being available in women.

As is the case with diazepam (Klotz et al, 1975), $t\frac{1}{2}\beta$ of midazolam is prolonged in elderly patients (Collier et al, 1982; Dundee & Kawar, 1982a). The influence of both age and operation on the pharmacokinetics of midazolam has been studied in detail by Harper et al (1985) in patients receiving an induction dose of 0.3 mg kg^{-1}. With minor operations the short elimination half-life, averaging 2.4 h for patients under 50 years was markedly prolonged with age increasing to 4.1 h for those over 50 years. Figure 12.10 is a combination of data from two identical studies, illustrating the point. In both age groups major surgery increased $t\frac{1}{2}\beta$ to 3.8 and 3.9 h in young and old patients respectively. These were due to changes in both clearance and volume of distribution with age and in volume of distribution with operation. Older patients recovering from coronary artery operations under cardiopulmonary bypass handled the drug similarly to patients of the same age having major operations, showing that the liver can recover rapidly from the effects of hypothermia. An interesting finding in Harper's study was that 6 of 67 patients had an abnormally prolonged terminal half-life which could not be accounted for other than the possibility of a sub-population who oxidize the drug at a slower rate; a similar population has been described for debrisoquine (Evans et al, 1980).

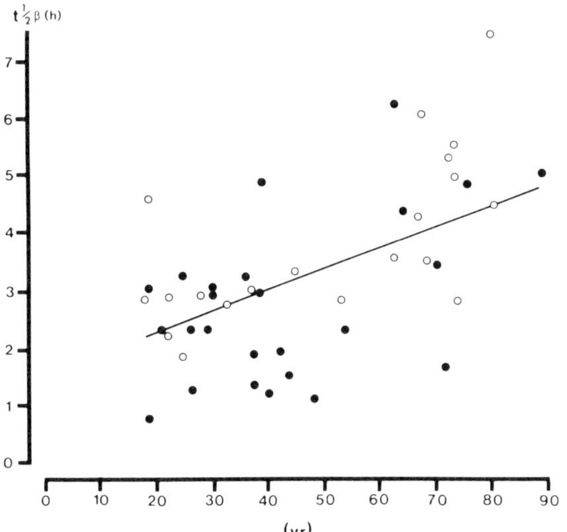

Fig. 12.10 Relationship of elimination half-life of midazolam (0.3 mg kg^{-1}) to age of patients in two series of patients undergoing minor operations [Collier et al, 1982 (●); Harper et al, 1985 (○)].

Midazolam, in normal therapeutic doses, does not cause major changes in routine liver function tests (Kawar et al, 1982) nor is there any evidence of enzyme induction with either drug. Cimetidine and ranitidine might interfere with the metabolism of midazolam by inhibiting the cytochrome P450 oxidising system in the liver, thereby reducing hepatic clearance. This might slightly prolong its action.

Cumulative effect

Reference has been made to the buildup of N-desmethyl diazepam after repeat administration of the parent drug. In a similar study, Lowry et al (1985) gave 5 mg diazepam or 5 mg midazolam two hourly for 12 hours to postoperative patients in a cardiac intensive care unit. Fig. 12.11, which depicts the average 'trough' levels sampled before administration of the next dose, shows the difference between the two drugs. Diazepam levels continued to rise over the period of administration, while those of midazolam levelled off after 8 hours, the eventual decline, and corresponding recovery being much faster with midazolam.

Placental transfer

Being very lipophilic it is not surprising that the benzodiazepines rapidly cross the placental barrier. Plasma diazepam concentrations in infants

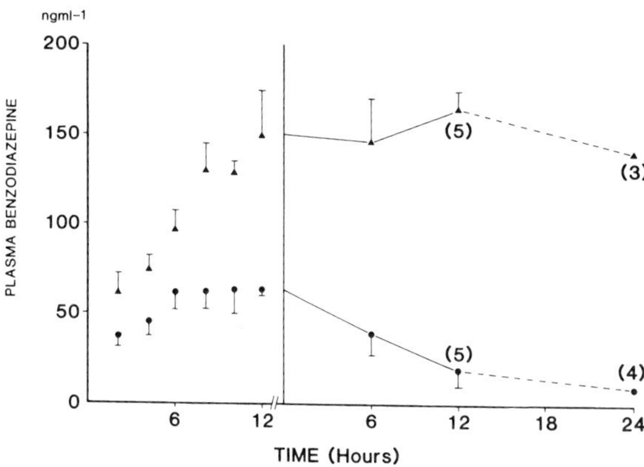

Fig. 12.11 Mean (± SEM) trough plasma levels over a 12 hour period for diazepam (▲) and midazolam (●) following 5 mg i.v. 2-hourly given to patients following cardiopulmonary bypass. The plasma levels for 24 hours following discontinuation are shown on the right. Ten patients received midazolam and nine diazepam. At those times when samples were not available from every patient, the actual number is shown in brackets. (Lowry et al, 1985).

were found to be higher than those in mothers following a single premedicant dose (Erkkola et al, 1974; Gamble et al, 1977). The placental transfer of lorazepam is less marked than that of diazepam (McBride et al, 1979). Evidence from animal studies suggests that the fetal–maternal ratio following a single dose of midazolam is much lower than with the other drugs (Vree et al, 1984). Kanto et al (1983) studied the transfer and kinetics of a single 15 mg oral dose of midazolam given on the night before Caesarean section. The findings, complicated by variations in gastrointestinal absorption in full term pregnant women, suggested that placental transfer takes place more slowly than with diazepam.

Following delivery the plasma diazepam levels fall less rapidly in the fetus than in the mother. Gamble et al (1977) found that the fetal/maternal ratio was 1.46 at birth and 1.64 after 24 hours. This can be attributed to the inability of the neonate to metabolise diazepam as readily as the mother. Of the two pathways of metabolism of diazepam, demethylation and hydroxylation (Fig. 12.9), demethylation is less efficient or sometimes completely non-existent in the neonate (Morselli, 1983).

PHARMACODYNAMICS

As pointed out previously all the benzodiazepines have similar multiple pharmacological actions. These will now be surveyed in general and again with emphasis on diazepam and midazolam.

Central nervous system

As a group the benzodiazepines cause a dose-related depression of the central nervous system (Fig. 12.2). These effects range from mild daytime sedation to full general anaesthesia, depending on the dosage used and the preparation employed.

Animal experiments have demonstrated an anti-conflict action for most of the benzodiazepines with doses that do not produce drowsiness. This is the basis for their anxiolytic action in human which is one of the main clinical indications for their oral use. Even in the absence of any hypnotic effect, small doses of diazepam (0.2 mg kg^{-1}) reduce the MAC for halothane (Perisho et al, 1971).

In larger doses their hypnotic properties predominate and pharmacokinetic differences determine which drug is best suited for this usage. In larger doses, given intravenously, some drugs will induce anaesthesia in 2 to 5 min. There is a wide individual variation in this response and this will be discussed later. Their onset of action does not occur in one arm–brain circulation time as is the case with thiopentone.

Amnesia

The ability to produce amnesia with low doses is one of the desirable effects of the injectable benzodiazepines. It has not been reported with oral medication except with lorazepam (McKay & Dundee, 1980). Figure 12.12 summarises the findings of human experimental amnesic studies with intravenous diazepam, midazolam and lorazepam given in equivalent doses. Subjects who did not lose consciousness were shown objects at varying times following administration and their ability to recall these was tested 6 and 24 hours later. With diazepam and midazolam there was a brief but very intense period of amnesia but this

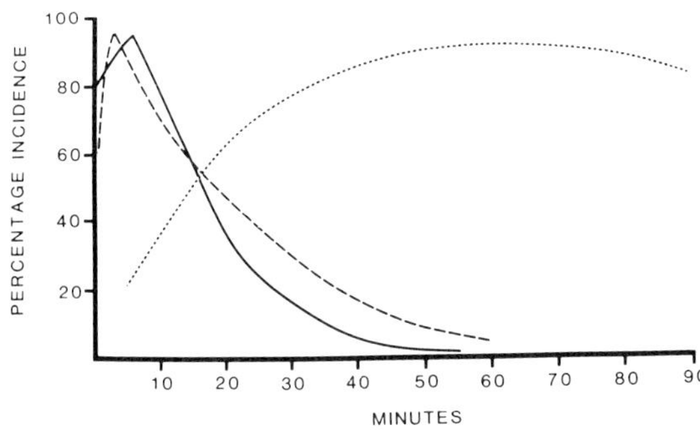

Fig. 12.12 % of patients who could not recall being shown objects at various times following intravenous administration of diazepam 10 mg (– – –), midazolam 5 mg (——) and lorazepam 4 mg (. . .) (from George & Dundee, 1976; Dundee & Wilson, 1980).

effect had mainly passed in 20 to 30 min. In contrast, the onset of amnesic action of lorazepam was very slow and had not reached a peak until about 60 min and was still present in the majority of subjects by 90 min (Dundee & Pandit, 1972; George & Dundee, 1976; Dundee & Wilson, 1980). Flunitrazepam behaves similarly to diazepam in this respect. Heisterkamp & Cohen (1975) have shown that the amnesic action of lorazepam can last up to six hours. Retrograde amnesia was not reported in any patients. A reliable amnesic effect of these benzodiazepines has only been demonstrated following their intravenous use and this effect is variable when given by intramuscular injection or by mouth (Dundee et al, 1970; McKay & Dundee, 1980).

The ability to produce a short period of anterograde amnesia forms part of the basis of the efficacy of both midazolam and diazepam as sedatives for endoscopy and in dental practice. Patients have little or no memory of the unpleasant passage of the endoscope or the injection of local anaesthesia; the quick recovery allows the patient to maintain control of airway and vital functions and remain quietly sedated for the remainder of the procedure.

Anti-convulsant action

All the benzodiazepines possess anti-convulsant properties but not all are used for this purpose. Their action of enhancing the inhibitory neurones in the central nervous system enables them to suppress generalised abnormal activity rather than a primary epileptic focus. Their potency in stopping convulsions is limited in comparison with the intravenous barbiturates or neuromuscular blocking drugs. One preparation, clonazepam (which will not be discussed elsewhere), is specifically used as an anticonvulsant. Like other benzodiazepines it increases the convulsive threshold of the brain and is best used in the prophylaxis of infantile spasm or *petit mal* and myoclonic seizures (Browne, 1978).

Anti-hallucinatory effects

This is the basis for the use of the benzodiazepines in minimising alcohol withdrawal states. If one considers the action of the central nervous system as a balance between inhibition and excitation in normal subjects and that chronic alcoholic intoxication suppresses the normal inhibitory action, then drugs like diazepam might act by increasing or producing inhibitory actions on the neuronal populations of the mesencephalic reticular formation and the limbic system (Kaim, 1973). There might be some relationship between this widely used clinical application and the ability of diazepam, flunitrazepam, lorazepam and midazolam to minimise the emergence sequelae following the use of moderately large doses of ketamine, particularly in unpremedicated patients undergoing minor operations (Coppel et al, 1973). These benzodiazepines also have the ability to ameliorate unpleasant dreams following ketamine.

Analgesia

In clinical doses the benzodiazepines have no analgesic action. More importantly, when used for induction of anaesthesia, small doses do not have the antanalgesic action of the barbiturates.

Muscle relaxant action

Although strictly defined as 'muscle relaxation' this action is due to the effect of the benzodiazepines in suppressing the internuncial neurones of the spinal cord and is different from that of the neuromuscular blocking drugs. The action of the latter is not potentiated to any important degree by benzodiazepines. Neither do they reduce the fasciculations following suxamethonium.

Tolerance

Tolerance to the cerebral depressant effects of the benzodiazepines does occur after long-term use, particularly for night-time sedation. It is not as marked as with the barbiturates when used for the same purpose, but it will induce cross-tolerance to drugs given intravenously for sedation or anaesthesia. A similar cross-tolerance occurs in patients habituated to other depressants such as alcohol or barbiturates.

Cardiovascular system

Even in large doses the benzodiazepines are considered to have less depressant effect on the cardiovascular system than some other intravenous anaesthetics. Combined with high doses of opiate analgesics, diazepam (Knapp & Dubow, 1970) and midazolam (Kawar et al, 1983) have proved very safe in the management of poor risk patients undergoing major heart operations.

Midazolam causes a fall in systemic vascular resistance rather than the rise seen with thiopentone (Al-Khudhairi et al, 1982b). The effects of this are evident when vascular resistance is raised, such as in hypertensive patients and in the stressful period immediately before an operation (Muller et al, 1981). Venous pooling and the fall in the systemic vascular resistance can be helpful in reducing pre-load and after-load performance in the failing heart but this effect will be more marked in hypovolaemic patients (Muller et al, 1981; Schulte-Sasse et al, 1982). In contrast to results in intact persons, in patients on cardiopulmonary bypass diazepam causes more pronounced arterial and venous dilatation than midazolam (Samuelson et al, 1980). Because of the reduction in systemic vascular resistance induced by midazolam (due to vasodilatation) it has been suggested that it might potentiate the hypotensive action of β adrenoreceptor blockers (Schwander & Sansano, 1980).

Some of the early claims by anaesthetists for lesser cardiovascular effects of the benzodiazepines as compared with orthodox induction agents may have been due to their slower onset of action (Clarke & Lyons, 1977). If sufficient time is allowed before tracheal intubation the fall in arterial pressure with equivalent doses of diazepam and thiopentone was similar, but in clinical practice intubation is usually carried out before the maximum depressant effect of the benzodiazepines occurs. Notwithstanding, as a group the injectable benzodiazepines in clinical doses cause less depression of the cardiovascular system than orthodox induction agents and this beneficial effect is more marked when they are combined with large doses of an appropriate opioid.

With marked sedation or loss of consciousness there is the usual peripheral vasodilatation and a slight drop in cardiac output and peripheral resistance but this is of no clinical significance and in anaesthesia these effects are reversed by surgical stimulation.

Sedative doses of the benzodiazepines are sometimes given to patients in the upright or semi-upright position, as in dental surgery, or where there is already marked vasodilatation, as following subarachnoid or epidural analgesia. There have been occasional reports of collapse after subarachnoid block and with epidural analgesia. Their use should be followed by careful observation and adequate fluid therapy. It was recognised early that cardioversion under diazepam carries a high success rate (Vinge et al, 1971). Also the benzodiazepines are associated with fewer ventricular extrasystoles than the barbiturates (Muenster et al, 1967) and this, combined with their minimal cardiovascular depression, has made them the drugs of choice for cardioversion. Tachycardia following these drugs is probably a manifestation of vasodilatation and relative hypovolaemia and is of little clinical importance.

Organ blood flow

The benzodiazepines cause minimal changes in coronary or cerebral blood flow or in myocardial or cerebral oxygen consumption in anaesthetised dogs on mechanical pulmonary ventilation (Hilfiber et al, 1980). Cerebral perfusion pressure is slightly decreased due to a fall in mean aortic pressure. Like other anaesthetics, the benzodiazepines depress renal blood flow and renal function

(Lebowitz et al, 1982). Midazolam has a more profound effect on renal blood flow than equivalent doses of thiopentone although this does not apply to renal vascular resistance. Benzodiazepines reduce liver blood flow in parallel with the small decreases in cardiac output (Gelman et al, 1983).

Respiration

There is nothing to suggest that in the normal therapeutic doses, the oral administration of any of the benzodiazepines is followed by respiratory depression. Their use is not accompanied by bronchoconstriction and they can be given safely to asthmatic subjects.

With intravenous injection one has to consider the dose used, the rate of administration, the concomitant use of opioids and the physical status of the patient. As consciousness is lost so is sensitivity to carbon dioxide and under different circumstances the response to a normal induction dose can vary from no detectable effect to apnoea. The normal effect would be a slight decrease in tidal volume but this might be compensated for by an increase in respiratory rate. The dose–response curve is different from that of the opiates: while both shift the CO_2 response curve to the right (Forster et al, 1980), midazolam and diazepam flatten the slopes, indicating a less profound dose–response effect (Zsigmoid & Shiveley, 1966). Nevertheless, in patients with chronic obstructive airway disease, the respiratory depressant effect of benzodiazepines might be greater than in normal subjects (Catchlove & Hefer, 1971; Gross & Smith, 1981) and as consciousness is lost, so is sensitivity to carbon dioxide.

The liability to produce respiratory obstruction is the most important respiratory effect of sedative doses of diazepam (Healey et al, 1970; Dixon & Thornton, 1973). Both muscle relaxation and central depression may contribute to this event, which is not uncommon in dental practice. Respiratory obstruction rather than depression is more likely to result in the cyanosis which has been noted by a number of workers.

Parenchymatous organs

Alterations in liver or kidney function have not been reported after the intravenous benzodiazepines (Kawar et al, 1982) and any changes associated with their use are the result of the accompanying cardiovascular effects.

Other effects

There is no evidence that the benzodiazepines cause enzyme induction as do the barbiturates. Even after long term administration of clonazepam in epileptics there does not appear to be any stimulation of hepatic microsomal activity (Browne, 1978, 1983).

Despite some early reports to the contrary (Fahmy et al, 1979), pretreatment with diazepam or midazolam does not reduce the myalgia which follows 1 mg kg^{-1} suxamethonium in ambulant patients (Chestnutt et al, 1984). Neither do they affect the onset and offset time of the relaxant.

OVERDOSAGE

Benzodiazepine overdosage, either accidental in the case of children or premeditated in adults, is not uncommon. It is discussed here as many of these patients will be referred to an anaesthetist and their management is that of prolonged profound anaesthesia. Because of the relative lack of cardiovascular depression with these drugs compared with the barbiturates, recovery should occur provided ventilation is maintained and vital functions supported. In many cases patients are very sleepy but respiration is not so depressed as to require assistance: however, the warning regarding the occurrence of respiratory obstruction with the benzodiazepines should be noted and tracheal intubation and assisted ventilation might be the treatment of choice even though this might necessitate the use of a myoneural blocking drug. Physostigmine is a non-specific antidote to benzodiazepine depression (see below) but there are no reports of its use in cases of marked overdosage. Likewise, the antagonist RO 15 1788 has not been studied in this context.

Physostigmine reversal

Physostigmine, being a tertiary amine, crosses the

blood-brain barrier and increases brain acetylcholine concentration by inhibition of cholinesterase. It has been used successfully in ameliorating the 'central cholinergic syndrome' which might be induced by atropine, hyoscine, tricyclic antidepressants and anti-Parkinson drugs (Holzgrafe et al, 1973). There is increasing clinical evidence that it can reverse central depression induced by benzodiazepine tranquillisers.

Little is known about the specificity of this action but several reports show that physostigmine might act as an antidote to the depressant effect of diazepam (Larson et al, 1977). It has also proven effective in one instance of an overdose in a child (DiLiberti et al, 1975). As already stated respiratory arrest following benzodiazepine overdose, while uncommon, is best treated with artificial ventilation but it is useful to have physostigmine available. The adult dose is 1–2 mg given slowly and repeated as required. Delirium following lorazepam has also been treated successfully with physostigmine (Blitt & Petty, 1975).

CLINICAL USES

There is not general agreement as to the role of benzodiazepines in the induction of anaesthesia. Some equate the indications with thiopentone while others reserve their use for sedation only. Part of this might be due to confusing the use of an opiate-benzodiazepine combination with that of a benzodiazepine alone, an analgous situation to neurolept anaesthesia. While it is not possible to reconcile these diverse views, consideration must be given to the three aspects of the use of injectable benzodiazepines:

1. As primary induction agents — their relationship to orthodox induction agents and consideration of any circumstances where they might be specifically indicated.
2. As sedatives and hypnotics in subanaesthetic doses
3. Either of the above in combination with an opioid.

Induction of anaesthesia

Certain aspects of the induction of anaesthesia are peculiar to the benzodiazepines. There is a wide scatter of onset times with both diazepam and midazolam but in no reported incident has this been in the range of the rapidly acting thiobarbiturates. Figure 12.13 shows the onset time, measured from the end of injection until contact was lost with the patient, following an injection of 0.3 mg kg^{-1} midazolam given over a 20 s period in 166 unpremedicated adults. This also shows that younger patients appeared to have more resistance to the drug and that in most of

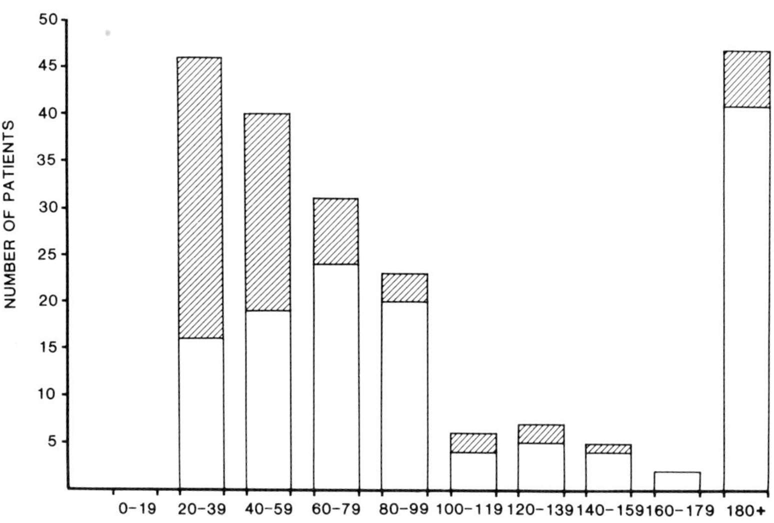

Fig. 12.13 Variability in the time to onset of sleep following the injection of midazolam 0.3 mg kg^{-1} to 200 unpremedicated patients of varying ages (from Dundee et al, 1984a). Patients over 50 years are indicated by hatched area.

the elderly patients the onset time was in the region of 10–40 s. An appreciable number of younger patients did not lose consciousness within three minutes of administration of what is generally considered to be an adequate induction dose. Halliday et al (1984) have demonstrated a direct negative relationship between the age of the patient and induction time. Although similar studies have not been carried out with diazepam a very wide range of doses (0.2 to 2.0 mg kg^{-1}) is required to induce sleep (Brown & Dundee, 1968). Likewise there is a great variation in requirements of flunitrazepam (Dundee et al, 1976).

Benzodiazepines are highly bound to plasma proteins and small changes in binding will lead to a wide variation in the amount of free drug. Halliday and his colleagues (1986) have demonstrated a correlation between plasma albumin and the onset time following 0.3 mg kg^{-1} midazolam and Reves et al (1981) reported a similar observation using varying doses. Clinical reports would suggest that this also applies to diazepam. Thus, where there is a low plasma albumin, as in elderly, undernourished or chronically ill poor-risk patients, there will be a higher concentration of 'free' midazolam available to penetrate the central nervous system. In support of this view is the observation that the onset time of the benzodiazepines can be reduced by drugs, such as probenecid or aspirin, which will affect plasma binding (Halliday et al, 1984).

Given by the intravenous route, midazolam is one and a half times to twice as potent as diazepam (w/w). It is interesting to note that, on clinical grounds, the onset of action of intravenous diazepam and midazolam appears to be similar despite the greater fat solubility of diazepam. This is probably compensated for by the lower plasma binding of midazolam thus leaving more pharmacologically active drug.

The induction of anaesthesia with the benzodiazepines is usually smooth, with little extraneous muscle movement or respiratory upset. Loss of consciousness is a gradual process and the end point is often difficult to define: the loss of eyelid or eyelash reflexes is unsatisfactory as its absence does not necessarily imply loss of consciousness and conversely it might still be present long after contact with the patient is lost. With a balanced technique these points are of little importance except when one might wish to intubate the trachea under suxamethonium paralysis. Fortunately the profound amnesia which follows an induction dose ensures that the patient, if not actually asleep, will not recall the events (Morselli, 1983).

In clinical practice recovery from equivalent doses of midazolam occurs much more rapidly than following diazepam. The effects of diazepam are prolonged both by enterohepatic recirculation and also by the presence of the hypnotically active metabolite nordiazepam, with its long elimination half-life. On theoretical grounds one would not expect the action of diazepam, which has a relatively slow clearance, to be prolonged in the presence of liver damage but this could occur with midazolam. The action of midazolam will be markedly affected by alterations in hepatic blood flow.

There is no suggestion that induction with the benzodiazepines is not compatible with standard techniques for balanced anaesthesia but there has been some difference of opinion as to the relative value of midazolam and thiopentone as routine induction agents (Reves et al, 1982; Dundee & Kawar, 1982b). In the case of thiopentone the advantages are reliability and rapid onset of action. The reliability of midazolam is certainly better in elderly patients and in those given narcotic premedication than in the young (Halliday et al 1985). When used for day case surgery, in combination with fentanyl, recovery was quicker in patients given thiopentone but this was more than compensated for by the lower incidence of nausea in those given midazolam (Crawford et al, 1984). At the time of writing the relative situation of these two drugs as induction agents is in a state of flux. Thiopentone is a well tried drug with known toxic effects on the cardiovascular and respiratory systems: midazolam is less well tried but in certain circumstances the onset of action and unreliability, which can be overcome with the judicious use of narcotics, (q.v.) might more than compensate for the slow onset of action.

The definitive statement that the 'effective induction dose of midazolam (ED_{99}) is

0.23 mg kg^{-1} is at variance with other views (Dundee & Kawar, 1982b) and with Fig. 12.13 as is the statement that, 'apart from a slightly slower onset, 0.2 to 0.4 mg kg^{-1} midazolam is comparable to 3.5 to 4.0 mg kg^{-1} thiopentone' (Sung et al, 1982). It is hard to reconcile the statement of Sarnquist et al (1980) that in unpremedicated subjects, 10 mg midazolam is equivalent in potency to 200 mg thiopentone, with those of Gamble et al (1981) and Dundee et al (1984a) who frequently found this dose of midazolam to be ineffective as an induction agent. The induction dose for fit subjects is in the region of 0.3 mg kg^{-1}; if this is not sufficient, an opioid or other hypnotic should be given–increasing the dose will delay recovery unduly. This dosage can be reduced in the elderly and poor risk patients and particularly in hypoproteinaemia.

The preliminary administration of an opioid makes the induction of anaesthesia with benzodiazepines both more rapid and more reliable. Various clinical papers mention this without supportive data, but studies carried out on young 'resistant' patients under the age of 50 years show that both the reliability and rapidity of induction of anaesthesia with midazolam can be greatly improved by pretreatment with low doses of fentanyl and alfentanil (Table 12.5). These will not make it a 'rapidly acting' drug like thiopentone, but will make it clinically more acceptable.

These findings open up great possibilities for both diazepam and midazolam. As already mentioned there is usually no problem of reliability in elderly and poor-risk patients but if in doubt the benzodiazepines can be combined with an opioid. Judicious choice of drug and dosage can make this an acceptable induction technique and it is very suitable for open heart operations (Reves & Samuelson, 1979). Without the use of an opioid problems can arise in young patients. The benzodiazepines are not suitable as sole anaesthetics for minor procedures and one could best look on these as contributing the hypnotic component in balanced anaesthesia (Reves et al, 1981), for a 'neurolept' technique or with high-dose opiate anaesthesia.

Use as sedative-hypnotic

The use of injectable benzodiazepines in this field stems from their ability to allay apprehension and to produce amnesia in subhypnotic doses. They have no analgesic action but will often 'settle' patients who cannot distinguish between pain and touch sensations. The almost complete short term anterograde amnesia induced by subhypnotic doses of diazepam and midazolam allows a local injection to be carried out without the patient remembering the event. This is particularly important in dental practice. The tiring and often uncomfortable positions on the operating table or dental chair are better tolerated and patients are less aware of the noises going on around them. In addition, patients who might feel nauseated from the use of an opioid or gut traction or even vomit with fear, can be made more comfortable by a moderate degree of sedation.

The main fields for this use are:

a) Oral surgery, usually before injection of the local anaesthetic.
b) Endoscopy following application of often an inadequate topical analgesic.
c) Procedures carried out under regional (usually subarachnoid or epidural) block.
d) In the intensive therapy situation, particu-

Table 12.5 Percentage of pretreated and untreated patients anaesthetized by 1 and 3 min and their mean (±SEM) age (yr) and onset times (s) following midazolam 0.3 mg kg^{-1}.

Pretreatments		*Fentanyl*		*Alfentanil*	
	Nil (*n* = *110*)	*50 μg* (*n* = *52*)	*100 μg* (*n* = *52*)	*150 μg* (*n* = *35*)	*300 μg* (*n* = *35*)
Age (yr)	38	33	34	34	34
Onset time (s)	114 ± 1.1	78 ± 7.1	58 ± 5.7	76 ± 5.1	56 ± 5.4
Percent asleep by 1 min	20	56	85	58	86
Percent asleep by 3 min	60	85	92	86	91

(from Halliday et al, 1986)

larly in patients whose lungs are being mechanically ventilated.

The problem of individual variation in response to the benzodiazepines is less acute with sedative doses (Fig. 12.2). Although it is not possible to quantify this statement more clinical data are becoming available which show a high success rate within a small dose range with diazepam (Litchfield 1980; 1981; Litchfield and Gerrard, 1971) and similar data are accumulating for midazolam. Perhaps this is due to the less easily defined endpoint for sedation and the ability of the operator/administrator to reinforce the pharmacological action by conversation and suggestion. Whatever the explanation, intravenous benzodiazepines can be used with greater confidence in successfully producing sedation, as compared with anaesthesia, even in young patients.

The success of benzodiazepine sedation techniques can be assumed by limiting their use to well motivated, intelligent adults. Unfortunately these are not always the patients who would benefit most from them and so some failure rate must be accepted. This can be minimised by avoiding them in children and in adults with immature personality or low intelligence. They certainly should not be used in the mentally subnormal.

While one uses drug-induced amnesia to advantage in sedative techniques, the operator must always be aware that instructions given to a patient under such sedation may not be recalled. Instructions not to leave unaccompanied should be conveyed to a third person. Clinical experience suggests that amnesia is more intense with midazolam and with more rapid recovery from this agent, this is an important point.

Another problem with benzodiazepine sedation is the risk of producing anaesthesia or too deep a level of sedation. It is essential that the patient keep in verbal contact with the operator or anaesthetist, otherwise there will be a lack of cooperation. Jaw relaxation, leading to respiratory obstruction, might also occur. This can be serious if there is superimposed respiratory depression from either an excessively large dose of benzodiazepine or the concomitant use of an opioid.

Even with sedative doses there might be a considerable time before return of full mental faculties after diazepam. Doses of 0.15 mg kg^{-1} can impair performance for eight hours, as assessed by the deletion of Ps test (Dixon & Thornton, 1973), but more recently Kortilla (1976) found no impairment of other tests of recovery 2.5 hours after this dose. These differences could be due to the use of fit volunteers by Kortilla or less sensitive methods of assessment. By comparison psychomotor performance can be impaired for 12 hours after intramuscular pethidine (Kortilla & Linnoila, 1975).

Recovery is quicker after comparable doses of midazolam as compared with diazepam, but it should be noted that McGimpsey et al (1983) detected measurable quantities of drug (5–61 ng m;$^{-1}$) in venous blood samples in 13 out of 18 ambulant patients about to leave hospital following sedative techniques. This could possibly enhance the soporific effect of alcohol or other sedative drugs and these should be avoided until the day following operation. It is axiomatic that patients are accompanied home after any benzodiazepine; car driving or other tasks requiring discriminative skills should likewise be abstained from until the following day.

Dentistry

There is widespread acceptance of the use of diazepam and this has to some degree replaced intermittent methohexitone, particularly in conservative dentistry. This stems from the work of Main (1968) and his colleagues and the more scientific assessments of Dixon et al (1973) and Healey et al (1970). More recent evaluations of diazepam involved the Diazemuls preparation (Rosenbaum, 1982). McGimpsey and his colleagues (1983) and Parsons (1984) have described the use of midazolam as an alternative to diazepam.

Clearly there have been 'champions' of benzodiazepine sedation techniques over the past decade and one must carefully evaluate their findings. The need for establishing a line is generally accepted and a non-block needle of the Butterfly type is adequate. This should be in a large vein if Valium is to be used. If one remembers the delayed onset time, as compared with thiopentone, an intermittent technique can be used safely.

With any intermittent dosage technique there

must be an end point. Factors which indicate a desired level of sedation are a noticeable reduction of the patient's anxiety and apprehension, some slurring of speech and half-ptosis of the eyelids. The latter, known as Verrill's sign (O'Neill & Verrill, 1969; Verrill, 1970) is a useful guide to adequacy of dosage in dental practice.

Elderly or poor risk patients who are unduly sensitive to the benzodiazepines will have a slower circulation time than young healthy resistant subjects, and this must be remembered in titrating dosage against requirements. Each administrator will develop his own technique but, as a guide, the initial dose should not exceed 0.2 mg kg^{-1} diazepam (as Valium) or 0.1 mg kg^{-1} midazolam and doses in the order of half to three-quarters are preferable. The injection time should not be less than 20 seconds and one minute is preferable.

Having achieved the desired degree of sedation, it is important not to delay the appropriate dental block. Because of the greater initial sedation with midazolam, there might be problems in assessing the adequacy of the local block. McGimpsey et al (1983) recommend splitting the initial dose before carrying out the block and completing the sedation once its efficacy has been established. This is not necessary with simple extractions or for work on the maxilla because of the greater certainty of obtaining effective local anaesthesia. Insertion of mouth props, packs, vacuum suckers etc are not affected by sedation techniques.

In practice, with an adequate local block, once the desired degree of sedation has been obtained and patients are comfortable they might drop off to sleep and the duration of therapeutic effect will bear no relationship to either dosage or drug used. Hiccough is the only drug-induced complication that cannot be avoided. Both respiratory obstruction and depression should be looked for and, together with any evidence of cardiovascular collapse, they should be treated vigorously.

Since all benzodiazepines have a central muscle relaxing action (as evidenced by hypotonia), patients should be asked to 'brace themselves' before leaving the dental chair. Otherwise there is a risk of their 'legs collapsing' as they take their first step. This is an embarrassing and preventable complication.

Intermittent methohexitone has also been used to produce light sedation during dental procedures but its safety has been questioned by workers from Birmingham, England (Wise et al, 1969; Robinson et al, 1969). The latter used somewhat high doses which produced peripheral vasodilatation requiring a greatly increased cardiac output (and tachycardia) to maintain a normal blood pressure. Others have not found intermittent methohexitone to be as toxic (Holden, 1969; Foreman, 1969) but recommend keeping the dose of barbiturate as low as possible.

One way of achieving a low dose of methohexitone is to combine it with diazepam (Holden et al, 1970; Litchfield & Gerard, 1971) and this has met with some success. Any supplementation of benzodiazepines, however, reduces their safety and doses of both drugs must be kept low. With this combination it is not only difficult to maintain the desired level of sedation but the danger of losing contact with the patient is increased.

Supplementation of benzodiazepines with an opioid also reduces their safety; the combination is used more in endoscopy than in dentistry. Pentazocine seems to be the drug of choice for this purpose because of its 'ceiling' effect with respect to respiratory depression and also because its addition to diazepam enables the dose of benzodiazepine to be reduced (Brown et al, 1975) and in a well executed study Corall and his colleagues (1979) showed that if this was done recovery would not be prolonged. Titrating dilute diazepam against patients' needs they found that without pretreatment this averaged 22 mg but this was reduced to 19 mg by preceding it with 15 mg pentazocine and to 18 mg by 30 mg opioid. Sedation was equally good in all these groups. The beneficial effect of an opiate must be considered against the experience of the operator and availability of resuscitation apparatus is essential — a transient respiratory arrest followed the pentazocine-diazepam combination in one of Corall's patients.

Supplementation of midazolam by methohexitone or opioids will undoubtedly be evaluated in due time. Because of its shorter action compared with diazepam they might find a greater place than with diazepam. Furthermore the shorter acting alfentanil might be the drug of choice in this situation.

On the basis of isolated case reports it would appear that a very small number of patients will experience 'fantasies' under benzodiazepine sedation. These can be of a sexual nature and occur in circumstances where there is no possibility of a patient having been assaulted. Present evidence suggests that these are more likely to occur when large doses (the equivalent of 0.1 mg kg^{-1} midazolam) are used (Dundee, 1986). Since all reported cases have occurred in women it is recommended that benzodiazepine sedation should not be used in the absence of a third person in the room.

Endoscopy

Even in experienced hands, fibrelight endoscopy of the upper alimentary tract is an unpleasant experience for patients and benzodiazepine sedation or neurolept analgesia are used almost as a routine for this procedure (Douglas et al, 1980; Ludlam & Bennett, 1971). Techniques vary between deep sedation, often also using an opioid, to light levels which ensure maximum patient cooperation (Nimmo et al, 1978; Le Brun, 1976) In contrast to dental procedures most endoscopists request a preliminary dose of atropine and as this takes time to act it is often given intramuscularly as routine premedication.

Coughing and gagging are reduced by the concomitant use of an opioid (often pentazocine), although a controlled study has shown that the beneficial effects of the opioid are less than expected (Kawar et al, 1984). The inadequacy of topical anaesthesia for endoscopy as compared with oral surgery or conservative dentistry might make the use of an opioid a more essential part of the technique.

Diazepam has been the drug of choice in this field for many years, although recent reports (Brophy et al, 1982; Al-Khudhairi et al, 1982a; Whitwam et al, 1983; Kawar et al, 1984) show the superiority of midazolam with particular emphasis on onset of action and recovery (Bardhan et al, 1984; Green et al, 1984). Since endoscopy is more common in elderly patients caution should be exercised in dosage of both drugs. Initial doses are in the region of those used for oral surgery and one report has emphasised the need to increase this greatly in alcoholics (Kawar et al, 1984). Many patients coming for endoscopy will be receiving H_2 receptor blockers and this can affect the metabolism of both diazepam and midazolam (Fee et al, 1984b) although the clinical significance of this is not clear.

All the precautions concerning respiratory obstruction, amnesia etc. which apply to dental sedation are equally applicable to endoscopy, with the additional factor of oropharyngeal topical analgesia and visual disturbances following atropine. After these procedures patients require the same careful postoperative vigilance, and while the benzodiazepines have made outpatient endoscopy much more acceptable to patients, it is not without its dangers. The precautions mentioned above concerning the need for a third person being present during sedation also apply to endoscopy.

Intensive care

After initial problems of recovery from large doses of diazepam, due to a failure to appreciate its cumulative effect (Gamble et al, 1976) and the possible build up of the hypnotically active N-desmethyl metabolite, diazepam has been the routine for sedation in many intensive care units for many years. It is compatible with opioids, neuromuscular blocking drugs and other agents used in long-term patient care. Surprisingly small doses will produce prolonged periods of sedation and amnesia but with attention to dosage, recovery should not be prolonged.

Midazolam is likely to replace diazepam completely for this purpose but initially it has to be given more frequently at hourly or two-hourly intervals. For assessment of hyperventilated head injury patients the recovery is sufficiently rapid to make this an acceptable agent. Promising results with midazolam infusions for sedation following cardiac surgery (p. 191) suggest its usefulness in the intensive care unit.

BENZODIAZEPINE ANTAGONISTS

The imidazo-benzodiazepine RO 151788 (Fig. 12.14) does not show normal benzodiazepine activity and has been studied as a specific antag-

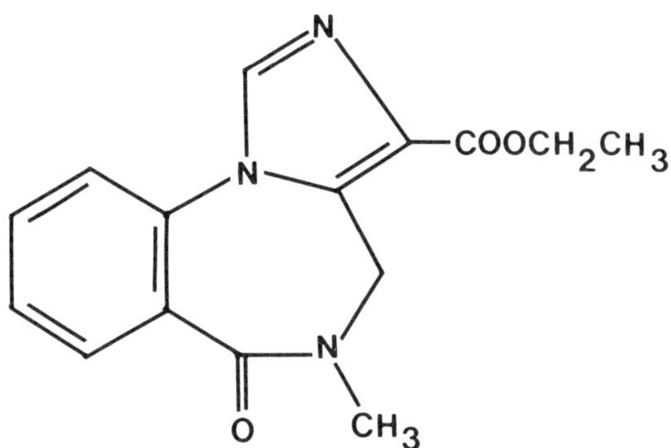

Fig. 12.14 The benzodiazepine antagonist RO 151788.

onist to the acute effects of the benzodiazepines (Hunkeler et al, 1981). In volunteers it has been shown to effectively block the central actions of the potent benzodiazepine 3-methyl clonazepam for up to 2.5 hours. More recently O'Boyle and his colleagues (1983) have shown that RO 151788 antagonises the effects of diazepam in man without affecting its bioavailability. In their study, the drugs were given by mouth and each subject received, in random order, diazepam 20 mg, diazepam 20 mg with RO 151788 200 mg or a placebo. Their study was limited to single dose administration in each of these combinations. RO 151788 antagonised the effect of diazepam on learning capacity and memory recall. The degree of impairment on psychomotor performance and changes in subjective mood induced by diazepam were also antagonised by RO 151 788.

This antagonist is not available at the time of writing. The initial studies were carried out with the oral preparation and they did show that it had a shorter half-life ($t\frac{1}{2}\beta$ 2.5 h) than many of the drugs which it would be used to antagonize. It is insoluble in water and a special injectable form will have to be prepared.

REFERENCES

Al-Khudhairi D, McCloy R F, Whitwam J G 1982a Comparison of midazolam and diazepam in sedation during gastroscopy. Gut 23: A432–463

Al-Khudhairi D, Whitwam J G, Chakrabarti M K, Askitopoulou H, Grundy E M, Powrie S 1982b Haemodynamic effects of midazolam and thiopentone during induction of anaesthesia for coronary artery surgery. British Journal of Anaesthesia 54: 831–835

Allonen N, Ziegler G, Klotz U 1981 Midazolam kinetics. Clinical Pharmacology and Therapeutics 30: 653–661

Bardhan K D, Morris P, Taylor P C, Hinchliffe R F C 1984 Intravenous sedation for upper gastrointestinal endoscopy: diazepam versus midazolam. British Medical Journal 288:1046

Blitt C O, Petty W C 1975 Reversal of lorazepam delirium by physostigmine. Anesthesia and Analgesia . . . Current Researches 54: 607–608

Brophy T O'R, Dundee J W, Heazelwood V, Kawar P, Varghese A, Ward M 1982 Midazolam — a water-soluble benzodiazepine for gastroscopy. Anaesthesia and Intensive Care 10: 344–347

Brown P R H, Main D M G, Wood N 1975 Intravenous sedation in dentistry. British Dental Journal 139:59

Brown S S, Dundee J W 1968 Clinical studies of induction agents. XXV: Diazepam. British Journal of Anaesthesia 40: 108–112

Browne T R 1978 Clonazepam. New England Journal of Medicine 299: 812–816

Browne T R 1983 Enzyme induction and drug interaction. In: Usdin E, Skolnick P, Tallman J F Jr, Greenblatt D, Paul S M (eds) Pharmacology of Benzodiazepines. Macmillan, London, p 330

Catchlove R F H, Hefer E R 1971 The effects of diazepam on respiration in patients with obstructive pulmonary disease. Anesthesiology 34: 14–18

Cheng S–H, Brunner E A 1981 Inhibition of GABA metabolism in rat brain synaptosomes by midazolam (RO 21 3981). Anesthesiology 55: 41–45

Chestnutt N W, Lowry K G, Dundee J W, Pandit S K, Mirakhur R K 1984 Failure of two benzodiazepines to prevent suxamethonium induced muscle pain. Anaesthesia 40: 263–269

Clarke R S J, Lyons S M 1977 Diazepam and flunitrazepam as induction agents for cardiac general surgical operations. Acta Anaesthesiologica Scandinavica 21: 282–292

Collier P S, Kawar P, Gamble J A S, Dundee J W 1982 Influence of age on the pharmacokinetics of midazolam. British Journal of Clinical Pharmacology 13: 602P.

Coppel D L, Bovill J G, Dundee J W 1973 The taming of ketamine. Anaesthesia 28: 293–296

Corall I M, Strunin L, Ward M E, Mason S A, Alcalay M 1979 Sedation for outpatient conservative dentistry. A trial of pentazocine supplementation to diazepam and local analgesic techniques. Anaesthesia 34: 855–858

Crawford M E, Carl P, Andersen R S, Mikkelsen B O 1984 Comparison between midazolam and thiopentone-based balanced anaesthesia for day case surgery. British Journal of Anaesthesia 56: 165–169

Diliberti J, O'Brien M L, Turner T 1975 The use of physostigmine as an antidote in accidental diazepam intoxication. Journal of Pediatrics 86: 106–107

Dixon R A, Day C D, Eccersley P S, Thornton J A 1973 Intravenous diazepam in dentistry: monitoring results from a controlled clinical trial. British Journal of Anaesthesia 45: 202–206

Dixon R A, Thornton J A 1973 Tests of recovery from anaesthesia and sedation: intravenous diazepam in dentistry. British Journal of Anaesthesia 45:207

Douglas J C, Nimmo W S, Wanless R, Jarvie D R, Heading R C, Finlayson N D C 1980 Sedation for upper

gastrointestinal endoscopy. A comparison of oral temazepam and i.v. diazepam. British Journal of Anaesthesia 52: 811–815
Dundee J W 1986 Do fantasies occur with intravenous benzodiazepines? SAAD Digest 6: 173–176
Dundee J W, Halliday N J, Loughran P G 1984a Age and sex as factors influencing the onset of action of intravenous midazolam. Irish Journal of Medical Science 153: 225–226
Dundee J W, Halliday N J, Loughran P G 1984b Variations in response to midazolam. British Journal of Clinical Pharmacology 17: 645P–646P
Dundee J W, Halliday N J, Harper K W, Brogden R N 1984c) Midazolam: a review of its pharmacological properties and therapeutic use. Drugs 28: 519–543
Dundee J W, Haslett W H K, Keilty S R, Pandit S K 1970 Studies of drugs given before anaesthesia. XX: Diazepam-containing mixtures. British Journal of Anaesthesia 42: 143–150
Dundee J W, Kawar P 1982a Benzodiazepines in anaesthesia. In: Usdin E, Skolnick P, Tallman J R Jr, Greenblatt D, Paul S M (eds) Pharmacology of Benzodiazepines. London, Macmillan, p 313–328
Dundee J W, Kawar P 1982b Consistency of action of midazolam (correspondence) Anesthesia and Analgesia 61: 544–545
Dundee J W, Pandit S K 1972 Anterograde amnesic effects of pethidine, hyoscine and diazepam in adults. British Journal of Pharmacology 44: 140–144
Dundee, J W, Varadarajan C R, Gaston J H, Clarke R S J 1976 Clinical studies of induction agents. XLIII: Flunitrazepam. British Journal of Anaesthesia 48: 551–555
Dundee J W, Wilson D B 1980 Amnesic action of midazolam. Anaesthesia 35: 459–461
Erkkola R, Kanto J, Sellman R 1974 Diazepam in early human pregnancy. Acta Obstetricia et Gynecologica Scandinavica 53: 135–8
Evans D A P, Mahgoub A, Sloan T P, Idle J R, Smith R L 1980 A family and population study of the genetic polymorphism of debrisoquine oxidation in a white British population. Journal of Medical Genetics 17: 102–105
Fahmy N R, Malek N S, Lappas D G 1979 Diazepam prevents some adverse effects of suxamethonium. Clinical Pharmacology and Therapeutics 26: 395–398
Fee J P H, Dundee J W, Collier P S, McClean E 1984a Bioavailability of intravenous diazepam. Lancet ii:813
Fee J P H, Dundee J W, Collier P S, McClean E 1984b Diazepam disposition following cimetidine or ranitidine. British Journal of Clinical Pharmacology 17: 617P–618P
Foreman P A 1969 Intermittent methohexitone. British Medical Journal 3:178
Forster A, Gardaz J–P, Suter P M, Gemperle M 1980 Respiratory depression by midazolam and diazepam. Anesthesiology 53: 494–497
Gamble J A S, Dundee J W, Gray R C 1976 Plasma diazepam concentrations following prolonged administration. British Journal of Anaesthesia 48: 1087–1090
Gamble J A S, Kawar P, Dundee J W, Moore J, Briggs L P 1981 Evaluation of midazolam as an intravenous induction agent. Anaesthesia 36: 868–873
Gamble J A S, Moore J, Lamki H, Howard P J 1977 A study of plasma diazepam levels in mother and infant. British Journal of Obstetrics and Gynaecology 84: 588–591
Gelman S, Reves J G, Harris D 1983 Circulatory responses to midazolam anaesthesia: emphasis on canine splanchnic circulation. Anesthesia and Analgesia 62: 135–139
Gerecke M 1983 Chemical structure and properties of midazolam compared with other benzodiazepines. British Journal of Clinical Pharmacology 16: 11S–16S
George K A, Dundee J W 1976 Relative amnesic actions of diazepam, flunitrazepam and lorazepam in man (benzodiazepine amnesia). British Journal of Clinical Pharmacology 3:357
Green J R B, Ravenscroft M M, Swan C H J 1984 Diazepam or midazolam for endoscopy? British Medical Journal 288:1383
Greenblatt D J, Allen M D, MacLaughlin D S 1978 Diazepam absorption: effects of antacids and food. Clinical Pharmacology and Therapeutics 24: 600–609
Greenblatt D J, Divoll M, Abernethy D R, Ochs H R, Shader R I 1983 Benzodiazepine kinetics: implications for therapeutics and pharmaco genetics. Drug Metabolism Reviews 14: 251–292
Greenblatt D J, Harmatz J S, Shader R I 1978 Sex differences in diazepam protein binding in patients with renal insufficiency. Pharmacology (Basel) 16: 26–29
Greenblatt D J, Shader R I, Abernethy D R, Ochs H R, Divoll M, Sellers E M 1982 Benzodiazepines and the challenge of pharmacokinetic taxonomy. In: Usdin E, Skolnick P, Tallman J F Jr, Greenblatt D and Paul S M (eds) Pharmacology of benzodiazepines. Macmillan Press, London p 257–269
Greenblatt D J, Shader R I, Weinberger D R, Allen M D, MacLaughlin D S 1978 Effect of a cocktail on diazepam absorption. Psychopharmacology 57:199
Gross J B, Smith T C 1981 Ventilation after midazolam and thiopental in subjects with COPD. Anesthesiology 55:A384
Haefely W, Kulscar A, Mohler H, Pieri L, Polc P, Schaffner R 1975 In: Costa E, Greengard P (eds) Mechanism of action of benzodiazepines. Raven Press, New York, p 131–151
Halliday N J, Dundee J W, Harper K W 1985 Influence of fentanyl and alfentanil pretreatment on the action of midazolam. British Journal of Anaesthesia 57: 351–352
Halliday N J, Dundee J W, Loughran P G, Harper K W 1984 Age and plasma proteins influence the action of midazolam. Anesthesiology 61:A357
Harper K W, Lowry K G, Elliott P, Collier P S, Halliday N J, Dundee J W 1985 Age and nature of operation influence the pharmacokinetics of midazolam. British Journal of Anaesthesia 57: 866–871
Healey T E J, Robinson J S, Vickers M D 1970 Physiological responses to intravenous diazepam as a sedative for conservative dentistry. British Medical Journal iii: 10–13
Hegarty J E, Dundee J W 1977 Sequelae after the injection of three benzodiazepines — diazepam, lorazepam and flunitrazepam. British Medical Journal ii: 1384–1385
Heisterkamp D V, Cohen J P 1975 The effect of intravenous premedication with lorazepam (Ativan), pentobarbitone or diazepam on recall. British Journal of Anaesthesia 47: 79–81
Heizmann P, Eckert M, Ziegler W H 1983 Pharmacokinetics and bioavailability of midazolam in man. British Journal of Clinical Pharmacology 16: 43S–49s
Hilfiber O, Larsen R, Stafforst D, Kettler D 1980 Midazolam: Wirkung auf allgemeine, coronare und cerebrale Hamodynamik. Anaesthesist 29: 337–338
Holden G G P 1969 Responses to intermittent methohexitone. British Dental Journal 127: 1, 5

Holden G G P, Brett I I, Harrison J P 1970 The value of modern pain control methods in practice. SAAD DIGEST 1: 28–31

Holzgrafe K E, Vandroll J J, Mintz S M 1973 Reversal of postoperative reactions to scopolamine with physostigmine. Anesthesia and Analgesia . . . Current Researches 52: 921–925

Hunkeler W, Mohler H, Pieri L, Polc P, Bonetti E P, Cumin R, Schaffner R, Haefely W 1981 Selective antagonists of benzodiazepines. Nature 290: 514–516

Kaim S C 1973 Benzodiazepines in treatment of alcohol withdrawal states. In: Garattini S, Mussini E, Randall L O (eds) The Benzodiazepines. Raven Press, New York, p 571–574

Kanto J, Sjovall S, Erkkola R, Himberg J–J, Kangas L 1983 Placental transfer and midazolam kinetics. Clinical Pharmacology and Therapeutics 33:786

Kawar P, Briggs L P, Bahar M, McIlroy P D A, Dundee J W, Merrett J D, Nesbitt G J 1982a Liver enzyme studies with disoprofol (ICI 35 868) and midazolam. Anaesthesia 37: 305–398

Kawar P, Carson I W, Clarke R S J, Dundee J W, Lyons S M 1984 Haemodynamic changes during induction of anaesthesia with midazolam and diazepam (Valium) in patients undergoing coronary artery bypass surgery. British Journal of Anaesthesia 56: 767–771

Kawar P, Carson I W, Lyons S M, Clarke R S J, Dundee J W 1983 Comparative study of haemodynamic changes during induction of anaesthesia with midazolam and diazepam in patients undergoing coconary artery bypass surgery. Irish Journal of Medical Science 152:215

Kawar P, Dundee J W 1982 Frequency of pain on injection and venous sequelae following the i.v. administration of certain anaesthetics and sedatives British Journal of Anaesthesia 54: 935–939

Kawar P, Dundee J W, Gamble J A S, Collier P S, Howard P J 1982 Benzodiazepine pharmacokinetics: some observations with midazolam and diazepam. Volume of summaries of VI European Congress of Anaesthesiology, p 245

Klotz U, Avant G R, Hoyumpa A, Schenker S, Wilkinson G R 1975 The effect of age and liver disease on the disposition and elimination of diazepam in adult man. Journal of Clinical Investigation 55: 347–359

Klotz U, Ziegler G 1982 Physiologic and temporal variation in hepatic elimination of midazolam. Clinical Pharmacology and Therapeutics 32: 107–112

Knapp R B, Dubow H 1970 Comparison of diazepam with thiopental as induction agent in cardiopulmonary disease. Anesthesia and Analgesia . . . Current Researches 49: 722–726

Korttila K 1976 Recovery after intravenous sedation. A comparison of clinical and paper and pencil tests used in assessing late effects of diazepam. Anaesthesia 31: 724–731

Kortilla K, Linnoila M 1975 Psychomotor skills related to driving after intramuscular administration of diazepam and meperidine. Anesthesiology 42:685

Larson G F, Hurlbert B J, Wingard D W 1977 Physostigmine reversal of diazepam-induced depression. Anesthesia and Analgesia . . . Current Researches 56: 348–351

Lebowitz P W, Cote M E, Daniels A L, Bonventre J 1982 Comparative renal effects of midazolam and thiopental. Anesthesiology 57:A35

Le Brun H I 1976 Neuroleptanalgesia in upper alimentary endoscopy. Gut 17: 655–658

Litchfield N B 1980 Complications of intravenous diazepam — adverse psychological reactions (an assessment of 16000 cases). Journal of the American Dental Society of Anesthesiology 28: 175–177

Litchfield N B 1981 Complications of intravenous diazepam. Respiratory depression (an assessment of 16000 cases). Journal of the American Dental Society of Anesthesiology 29: 11–17

Litchfield N B, Gerard P 1971 Diazepam intravenous sedation in dentistry. A report of 1557 cases. Australian Dental Journal 1971, 25–33

Lowry K G, Dundee J W, McClean E, Lyons S M, Carson I W, Orr I A 1985 The pharmacokinetics of diazepam and midazolam when used for sedation following cardiopulmonary bypass. British Journal of Anaesthesia 57: 883–885

Ludlam R, Bennett J R 1971 Comparison of diazepam and morphine as premedication for gastrointestinal endoscopy. Lancet ii: 1397–1399

Lyons S M, Clarke R S J 1971 Anaesthesia for cardioversion. British Medical Journal iv:229

McBride R J, Dundee J W, Moore J, Toner W, Howard P J 1979 A study of the plasma concentrations of lorazepam in mother and neonate. British Journal of Anaesthesia 51: 971–978

McGimpsey J G, Mawar P, Gamble J A S, Browne E S, Dundee J W 1983 Midazolam in dentistry. British Dental Journal 155: 47–50

McKay A C, Dundee J W 1980 Effect of oral benzodiazepines on memory. British Journal of Anaesthesia 52: 1247–1257

Main D M G 1968 The use of diazepam in dental anaesthesia. In: Knight P F, Burgess C G (eds) Diazepam in anaesthesia. Wright, Bristol, pp 85–87

Mohler H, Okada T 1978 The benzodiazepine receptor in normal and pathological human brain. British Journal of Psychiatry 133: 261–268

Morselli P L 1983 Clinical pharmacokinetics in neonates. In: Gibaldi M & Prescott L (eds). Handbook of Clinical Pharmacokinetics. ADIS, Auckland, pp 79–97

Muenster J J, Rosenberg M S, Carleton R A, Graettinger J S 1967 Comparison between diazepam and sodium thiopental during d.c. countershock. Journal of the American Medical Association 199: 758–760

Muller von H, Schleussner E, Stoganov M, Kling D, Hempelmann G 1981 Hamodynamische Wirkungen und charakteristika der Narkoseeinbeitung mid Midazolam. Arzneimittel-Forschung/Drug Research 31: 2227–2232

Nimmo W S, Forrest J A, Heading R C, Finlayson N D, Prescott L F 1978 Premedication for upper gastrointestinal endoscopy: a comparative study of flunitrazepam, diazepam and neuroleptanalgesia. Endoscopy 10: 183–186

O'Boyle C, Lambe R, Darragh A, Taffe W, Brick I, Kenny M 1983 RO 151788 antagonises the effects of diazepam in man without affecting its bioavailability. British Journal of Anaesthesia 55: 349–356

O'Neil R, Verrill P J 1969 Intravenous diazepam in minor oral surgery. British Journal of Oral Surgery 7: 12–14

Parsons J D 1984 Some observations on the use of midazolam in conscious sedation. SAAD Digest 5: 220–222

Perisho J A, Buechel D R, Miller R D 1971 The effect of diazepam (Valium) on minimum alveolar anaesthetic requirement (MAC) in man. Canadian Anaesthetists' Society Journal 18:536

Reves J G, Corssen G, Holcomb C 1978 Comparison of two

benzodiazepines for anaesthesia induction, midazolam and diazepam. Canadian Anaesthetists' Society Journal 25: 211–214

Reves J G, Kissin I, Smith L R 1981 The effective dose of midazolam. Anesthesiology 55:82

Reves J G, Newfield P, Smith L R 1981 Midazolam induction time: association with serum albumin. Anesthesiology 3:A259

Reves J G, Samuelson P N 1979 Hemodynamic changes with midazolam anaesthesia induction in patients with ischemic heart disease. Clinical Pharmacology and Therapeutics 25:244

Reves J G, Samuelson J G, Vinik H R 1982 Consistency of action of midazolam (correspondence). Anesthesia and Analgesia 61: 545–546

Robinson J S, Wise C C, Heath M J, Tomlin P J 1969 Responses to intermittent methohexitone. A physiological study. British Dental Journal 126: 499–505

Rosenbaum N L 1982 A new formulation of diazepam for intravenous sedation in dentistry. A clinical evaluation. British Dental Journal 153: 192–193

Samuelson P N, Reves J G, Kouchoukos N T, Dole K, Smith L R 1980 Midazolam versus diazepam: haemodynamic comparison. Anesthesiology 53:S9

Samuelson P N, Reves J G, Smith L R, Kouchoukos N T 1981 Midazolam v. diazepam: different effects on systemic vascular resistance. Arzneimittel-Forschung/Drug Research 32:2268

Sarnquist F H, Mathers W D, Brock-Utne J, Carr B, Canup C, Brown C R 1980 A bioassay of a water-soluble benzodiazepine against sodium thiopentone. Anesthesiology 52: 149–153

Schulte-Sasse U, Hess W, Tarnow J 1982 Haemodynamic responses to induction of anaesthesia using midazolam in cardiac surgical patients. British Journal of Anaesthesia 54: 1053–1058

Schwander D, Sansano C 1980 Cardiovascular changes during intubation with midazolam as anaesthesia inducing agent. Arzneimittel-Forschung/Drug Research 31: 2255–2260

Smith M T, Eadie M J, Brophy T O'R 1981 The pharmacokinetics of midazolam in man. European Journal of Clinical Pharmacology 19: 271–278

Sung Y F, Weinstein M S, Hammond W D, Beny A J, Chari A J 1982 Comparison of midazolam and thiopental for anaesthesia. Anesthesiology 57:A345

Tang M, Soroka S, Falk J L 1983 Agonistic action of a benzodiazepine antagonist: effects of Ro15–1788 and midazolam on hypertonic NaCl intake. Pharmacology, Biochemistry and Behaviour 18: 953–955

Verrill P J 1970 Experiences with diazepam at University College Hospital. SAAD Digest 1: 17–19

Vinge L N, Wyant G M, Lopez J F 1971 Diazepam in cardioversion. Canadian Anaesthetists' Society Journal 18: 166–171

Vinik H R, Reves J G, Greenblatt D J, Nixon D C, Whelchel J D, Luke R, Wright D, McFarland L 1982 Pharmacokinetics of midazolam in renal failure patients. Anesthesiology 57:A366

Vree T B, Reeken-Ketting J J, Fragen R J, Arts T H M 1984 Placental transfer of midazolam and its metabolite 1-hydroxymethyl midazolam in the pregnant ewe. Anesthesia and Analgesia 63: 31–34

Whitwam H G, Al-Khudhairi D, McClay R F 1983 Comparison of midazolam and diazepam in doses of comparable potency during gastroscopy. British Journal of Anaesthesia 55: 773–777

Wise C C, Robinson J S, Heath M J, Tomlin P J 1969 Physiological responses to intermittent methohexitone for conservative dentistry. British Medical Journal 2: 540–543

Zsigmond E K, Shiveley J C 1966 Spirometric and blood gas studies on the respiratory effects of hydroxyzine hydrochloride in the human volunteer. Journal of New Drugs 6:128.

J G Bovill, MD, FFARCSI

The opioids in intravenous anaesthesia

Since the previous edition of this book many significant developments in opioid pharmacology have occurred. These are reflected in the changes in the way anaesthetists now use these drugs. Much less emphasis is now placed on "neuroleptanaesthesia". Indeed few anaesthetists use the technique of pure neuroleptanaesthesia, in which very large doses of droperidol (up to 50 mg) were combined with an opioid (either fentanyl or phenoperidine) to produce surgical anaesthesia. The discovery of the naturally occurring enkephalins and endorphins has resulted in a better understanding of the pharmacodynamics of the opioid drugs. Improvements in analytical techniques have also provided more detailed information on their pharmacokinetic disposition. Partly as a result of this increased knowledge, there has been an extension of the traditional methods of using opioids in anaesthesia. Their epidural and intrathecal administration, that originated from the discovery of opioid receptors in the spinal cord has, despite well recognised side-effects, become popular for the management of postoperative pain. There has also been a reawakening of interest in the use of high doses of opioids to produce anaesthesia, a technique that has become especially popular in cardiac operations In the same period several new opioids, both agonists and agonist-antagonists, have been introduced.

Nomenclature

Various terms are in common use to describe the drugs discussed in this chapter. Many of these terms are used interchangeably and often inappropriately and it is time that some uniformity in nomenclature was introduced. Opiate refers specifically to the products derived from the juice of the opium poppy but has been loosely applied to morphine derivatives. The term opioid refers to any compound directly acting on an opioid receptor, with effects that are stereospecifically antagonised by naloxone. This definition does not exclude the possibility that an opioid may have actions not antagonised by naloxone. By definition, however, these effects are not mediated by opioid receptors. The term 'narcotic' to describe this class of drugs is therefore misleading and should be abandoned.

MODE OF ACTION

The opioids produce a wide spectrum of pharmacological effects, both within the central nervous system and peripherally.

Opioid receptors

The concept that the several pharmacologically distinct actions of the opioids might be due to an interaction with specific receptors developed in the 1960s. The existence of such receptors, both within the central nervous system and elsewhere, was suggested by the following evidence:

1. All opioids are highly stereospecific, with activity exhibited only by the laevorotatory, (−), isomer. The dextrorotatory mirror image of the naturally occurring (−) morphine, (+) morphine, for example, is devoid of analgesic activity (Janssen & van der Eycken, 1968). This stereospecificity strongly supports the

Table 13.1 Agonist responses of the opiate receptors

Mu (μ)	*Kappa* (κ)	*Sigma* (σ)	*Delta* (δ)
Supraspinal analgesia	Spinal analgesia	Dysphoria	Modulates μ-receptors
Respiratory depression	Respiratory depression	Vasomotor stimulation	Supraspinal analgesia
Euphoria	Sedation	Hallucinations	Respiratory depression
Dependance Miosis	Miosis	Mydriasis	

concept of a spatially specific receptor that recognises only one enantiomer.

2. Some opioids are extremely potent. Etorphine, for example, is 1000 times more potent than morphine. Only a selective receptor with high affinity could account for such potency.
3. The existence of drugs such as naloxone which have pure antagonist activity, i.e. they antagonise almost all the effects of opioids but have virtually no pharmacological activity themselves, favours the concept of specific receptors.
4. Many opioids exhibit structural specificity in that small alterations in their chemical structure can alter their pharmacological profile. A basic amino group ($-NCH_3$) appears essential for opioid activity and substitution at this site results in profound alteration in activity (Janssen, 1962). Removal of the nitrogen methyl group of morphine to produce the secondary amine ($-NH-$) normorphine, or substitution of other secondary or quaternary amines results in compounds that are either inactive or very week analgesics. However, substitutions with phenylethyl groups increases potency. When the nitrogen-methyl is replaced with short chain alkyl groups, potent opioid antagonists are produced. Oxymorphone is a pure agonist yet its N-allyl derivative (naloxone) is a pure antagonist.

The existence of stereospecific opioid binding sites in rat brain was demonstrated by three independent groups of researchers in 1973, (Pert & Snyder 1973; Simon et al 1973; Terenius, 1973), using ligands of high specific radioactivity. These sites combined stereospecifically with all known opioid agonists and antagonists. That they were pharmacologically significant was suggested by a high correlation between the affinity that a wide range of opioid-like compounds had for these sites and their pharmacological potency.

Most of the original knowledge about opioid receptors derives from the work of Martin and his colleagues with non-dependent chronic spinal dogs (Martin et al 1976). They found that morphine and allied opioids produced three distinct syndromes which they attributed to separate receptors. They named these receptors after the prototype agonist producing the distinct physiological effect: μ (mu) for morphine, κ (kappa) for ketocyclazocine and σ (sigma) for SKF10 047 (N-allylnormetazocine). The possible role of the various receptors in mediating agonist responses is summarised in table 13.1. More recently other receptors have been identified. A receptor with high affinity for leucine-enkephalin which is preponderant in the mouse vas deferens (δ-receptor), has been described. An ε-receptor, identified in rat vas deferens is thought to be specific for β-endorphin. It is believed that the δ-and μ-receptors coexist within the same physical complex and that endogenous μ-receptor activitation by β-endorphin is regulated by the enkephalins. Binding of enkephalins at the δ-receptor can either promote or inhibit μ-receptor activity (Vaught, et al, 1982) depending on whether leu- or met-enkephalin predominates. Leu-enkephalin potentiates opioid-induced analgesia whereas met-enkephalin antagonises it (Fig. 13.1). The demonstration that the μ- and δ-receptors can interconvert illustrates the close relationship between these two receptor types (Bowen et al, 1981). The μ-receptor is now known to consist of two subtypes, a high-affinity receptor (μ_1) and a low affinity one (μ_2) (Pasternak, 1982). Analgesia is associated with the μ_1 but not the μ_2 receptor. Respiratory depression, an unwanted side-effect of opioid drugs, is not mediated via μ_1-receptors but is probably a property of μ_2 or δ-receptors (Ling et al, 1983). Meptazinol, a μ_1 selective opioid analgesic (Spiegel & Pasternak,

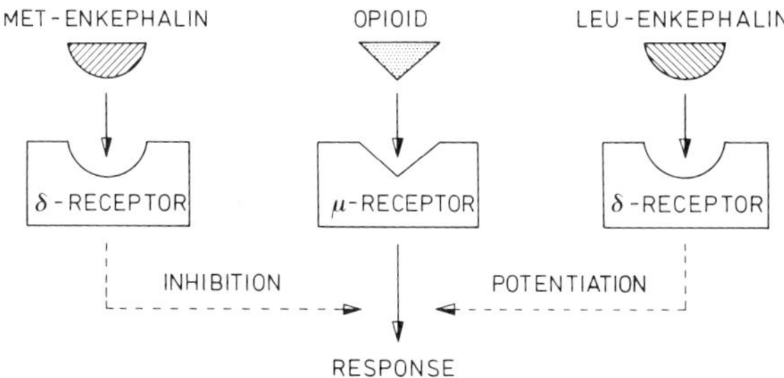

Fig. 13.1 Role of met-and leu-enkephalin in the interaction between δ-and μ-receptors.

1984), causes negligible respiratory depression in conscious volunteers (Jones, 1983) but does produce a dose-related fall in respiratory rate and elevation in end-tidal CO_2 concentration in anaesthetised subjects, reversible with naloxone (Slattery et al 1982).

There is a high correlation between the analgesic potency of opioids and their affinity for the μ-receptor, measured by in vitro inhibition of stereospecific [^{3}H]-sufentanil binding (Fig. 13.2) (Leysen et al, 1983). However, it would appear that only a small proportion of μ-receptors need to be occupied to produce analgesia. Surgical anaesthesia in dogs is produced with doses of opioids that result in only 25% receptor occupancy (Stanley et al, 1983a). This is in marked contrast to the neuromuscular junction, where normal function is maintained until 70–75% of receptors are blocked (Waud and Waud, 1972).

The μ-receptors are also involved in opioid addiction, a phenomenon characterised by tolerance, physical dependence and compulsive drug abuse. Tolerance is the decreasing intensity and shortening of duration of all pharmacological effects produced by a drug after repeated administration of the same dose. Physical dependence

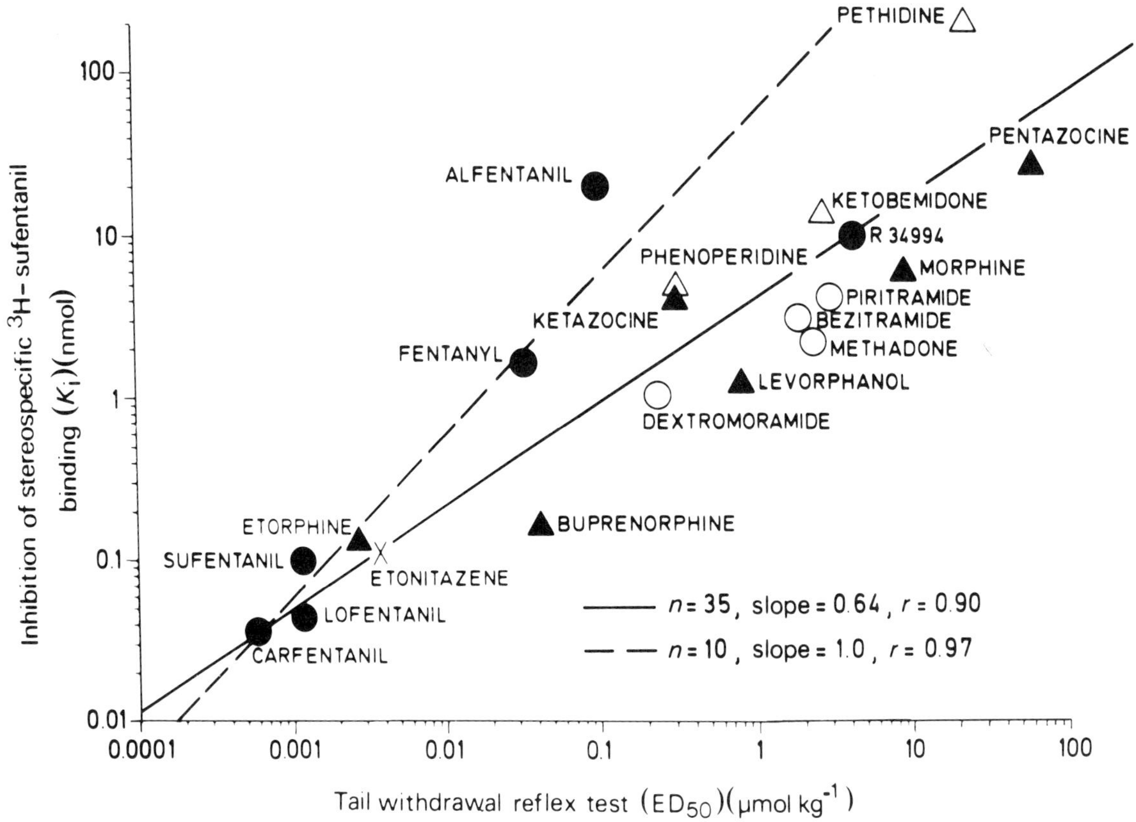

Fig. 13.2 Correlation between inhibition constants measured in vitro for stereospecific sufentanil binding in rat forebrain membranes and analgesic ED_{50} values measured in the rat tail withdrawal test. Lines represent analysis of linear regression. (—— for all compounds, n = 35, r = 0.9; --- for fentanyl analogues, n = 10, r = 0.97). Not all compounds are plotted. (From Leysen et al, 1983).

has been defined as the altered physiological state produced by the repeated administration of a drug which necessitates its continued use to prevent the appearance of a recognisable withdrawal syndrome (Jaffe, 1980). The neuronal mechanism of drug addiction is not fully known, but it probably reflects the adaptation of nerve cells to an altered environment caused by the continuous presence of the drug. Collier (1968) postulated that post-synaptically located receptors became supersensitive on prolonged opioid-induced inhibition of a presynaptically released excitatory neurotransmitter, probably adenylate cyclase. This concept closely resembles the phenomenon of denervation- or disuse-supersensitivity.

The κ-receptor is involved in mediating spinal and supraspinal analgesia, but does so though pathways independent of μ- or δ-receptors (Skingle and Tyers, 1980). Immuno-histochemical studies using dynorphine, a highly selective κ-receptor agonist, have demonstrated the presence of κ-receptors in rat brain and spinal cord. Other receptor binding studies have confirmed the presence of high densities of κ-receptors in the rat spinal cord (Gouardères et al, 1982). It is possible that spinal analgesia is mediated in part by κ-agonists. Unlike μ-receptor agonists, κ-receptor agonists are ineffective against thermal pain except at doses producing sedation and motor impairment (Tyers, 1980).

Several drugs used clinically are κ-receptor agonists. Many of these belong to the mixed agonist–antagonist subclass of opioids i.e. those that show agonist and antagonist action at different receptor subtypes. Nalorphine is the prototype for this group of drugs and shows agonist activity at κ-receptors and antagonist activity at μ-receptors. Others include pentazocine, buprenorphine, butorphanol, and nalbuphine. Although the mixed agonist–antagonists produce respiratory depression at doses above that producing effective analgesia, they all show flat dose–response curves for respiratory depression at higher doses. Whether this is an inherent function of κ-agonist activity or whether it is related to partial antagonist properties of the μ-receptor is unclear. Bremazocine, a benzomorphan derivative, which has been widely studied in animals but not yet in man, appears to be an almost pure κ-agonist. It is twice as potent an analgesic as morphine and appears to be devoid of respiratory depression (Freye et al, 1983).

Although there is general agreement on the function of the μ- and κ-receptors, there is considerable uncertainty as to whether the σ-receptor is a true opioid receptor. SKF10047, the prototype drug for this receptor, is a μ-receptor antagonist that produces delirium and autonomic stimulation in the dog (Martin et al, 1976) and delusional and hallucinatory effects in man (Keats & Telford, 1964). Similar effects are seen with some of the mixed agonist–antagonist drugs e.g., nalorphine and pentazocine, which are thought to be partial σ-receptor agonists. Similarities between the effects of SKF10 047 and phencyclidine, a potent psychomimetic agent related to ketamine, have been demonstrated in animal studies (Shannon, 1981) and in binding assays (Zukin & Zukin, 1979) suggesting that phencyclidine might mediate these effects via the σ-receptor. Stereo-specific binding of ketamine to opioid receptors has been demonstrated by several investigators (Finck & Ngai, 1982). However, others have been unable to demonstrate ketamine binding to opioid receptors, even at very high concentrations (Fratta et al, 1980). Naloxone, a μ-receptor antagonist, has extremely low affinity for σ-receptors (Su, 1982) and only partially antagonises the effects of ketamine. σ-Receptors have been demonstrated in the guinea-pig ileum and brain where highest levels where found in the brain stem, mid brain and cerebellum. This is in contrast to μ-receptors, which are only sparsely present, or absent, in the cerebellum. Phencyclidine-like compounds, which bear structural similarities to the opioids, block low affinity SKF10047 binding sites and it has been proposed that the σ-receptor may represent a composite opioid-phencyclidine receptor complex (Pleuvry, 1983).

The discovery of stereospecific opioid receptors gave an impetus to the search for endogenous ligands. It seemed improbable that such highly specific receptors would have developed in the absence of an endogenous substance that bound to these sites. It was reasoned that the opium alkaloids might be analogous to other plant alkaloids, like nicotine, that mimicked the action of endogenous neurochemicals such as acetylcholine.

Early attempts to isolate an endogenous ligand for the opioid receptors were unsuccessful since it was assumed that it would be chemically similar to morphine. In 1975, Hughes and his colleagues (Hughes et al, 1975) reported the identification of two similar pentapeptides in aqueous extracts of pig brain that produced morphine-like depression of motor activity of the mouse vas deferens and guinea-pig ileum, which was reversible by naloxone. Hughes discovery was confirmed in that same year by Terenius and Wahlström (1975) and Pasternak et al (1975). Hughes and his group identified the two pentapeptides as methionine-enkephalin (H-tyrosine-glycine-glycine-phenylalanine-methionine-OH) and leucine-enkephalin (H-tyrosine-glycine-glycine-phenylalanine-leucine-OH). Simantov and Snyder (1976) confirmed the structure of the same pentapeptides in extracts of bovine brain but noted that bovine brain contained four times more leucine-enkephalin than methionine-enkephalin, the reverse of the ratio in pig brain.

The amino-acid sequence of methionine-enkephalin is identical to the sequence between residues 61 and 65 of β-lipoprotein, a 91-amino acid peptide found in the pituitary. Various fragments of β-lipoprotein possessing opioid activity have been isolated. Residue 61-91, called β-endorphin (*endogenous morphine*) or C-fragment has the greatest activity and has been shown to interact with opioid receptors. α-Endorphin (residue 61–76) and γ-endorphin (residue 61–77) have also been isolated from the pituitary.

The enkephalins appear to have an important function as inhibitory neurotransmitters or neuromodulators within the central and peripheral nervous system. With a fast onset of action and rapid enzymatic termination of activity they are well suited for this role. These peptides constitute a major proportion of the opioid-like activity found in the brain and spinal cord with approximately ten times more enkephalin (300 to 400 pmol g^{-1}) than β-endorphin (30 pmol g^{-1}). They may rival or even exceed the catecholamines in their distribution and physiological importance. The enkephalins are widely but unevenly distributed throughout the central nervous system, their distribution being very similar to that of the opioid receptors. Within the spinal cord, enkephalin-containing neurones are localised in a dense band in the substantia gelatinosa, where initial integration of incoming sensory information takes place. Enkephalin and opioid receptors are also found in the gastrointestinal tract. There is a high association between regions with rich enkephalin innervation and those with high densities of opioid receptors.

Enkephalin and possibly also endorphin has a role in the regulation of pain perception. Modulation of pain is likely to occur at both supraspinal and spinal cord sites. In the spinal cord there is a close relationship between enkephalin and substance P, a polypeptide believed to be involved in excitatory spinal processes specifically associated with nociception (Hökfelt et al, 1977). There is evidence that whereas both β-endorphin and enkephalins participate in analgesic mechanisms centrally, only enkephalins act in the spinal cord. The analgesia produced by morphine-like drugs is thought to occur at both spinal and supraspinal levels.

β-Endorphin is present in high concentrations in the hypothalamus-pituitary axis, where it is thought to mediate control of endocrine function, especially that of prolactin and growth hormone (Rivier et al, 1977). Opioid peptides released from the pituitary may modulate biochemical events at such diverse sites as the adrenal cortex, kidney, pancreas, sex organs and fat cells. Their physiological role thus extends well beyond the pharmacological actions of opioid drugs. Opioid peptides are also involved in homeostatic responses to stress. During operation, ACTH, cortisol and β-endorphin levels increase. This increase can be blocked by moderate doses of fentanyl (Dubois et al, 1982).

Structure-activity relationships

Examination of the large number of naturally occurring, semisynthetic and synthetic compounds with opioid activity reveals an apparently wide diversity in chemical structure. However, it must be realised that molecules exist as three-dimensional structures, which are often difficult to visualise from the conventional two-dimensional representations in textbooks. Closer examination reveals many basic similarities between the

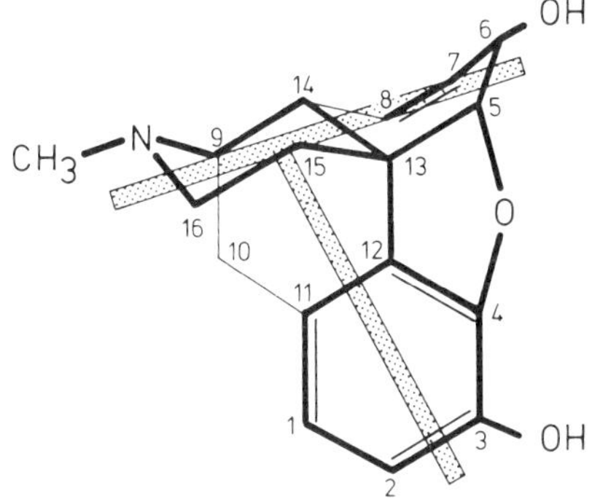

Fig. 13.3 Structure of morphine illustrating the T-shape of the molecule. The bonds C9-C10, C10-C11, and C8-C14 seem not to be essential for opioid activity.

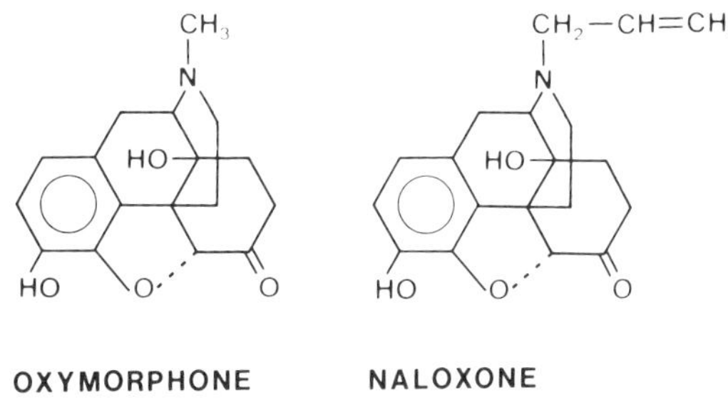

Fig. 13.4 Structure of oxymorphone and naloxone.

various compounds. Two basic opioid structures exist — the rigid molecules of the morphine-like compounds and the more flexible molecules of the phenylpiperidine group, of which pethidine is the prototype.

Morphine consists of a skeleton of five rigidly interlocking rings bearing several peripheral functional groups. This rigid pentacyclic structure has a T-shape with the piperidine ring forming part of the crossbar and a hydroxylated aromatic ring lying in the vertical stem (Fig. 13.3). This rigid T-structure is common to all compounds of this class. Certain portions of the morphine molecule are important for pharmacological activity whereas others play no role in activity and can be removed without altering potency or receptor binding.

The basic amino site in the piperidine ring is essential for opioid activity and substitution at this site profoundly alters activity (Janssen, 1962). In all morphine-like compounds the nitrogen atom is at a constant distance, 0.455 nm, from the centre of the aromatic ring. Replacing the nitrogen methyl with short chain alkyl groups results in potent opioid antagonists. The most effective substitutions have three carbon-chains, e.g. allyl ($-CH_2-CH=CH_2$) or cyclopropylmethyl ($-CH_2-\triangleleft$). Substitution of an antagonist subgroup alone results in compounds with mixed agonist–antagonist properties, e.g. nalorphine, but when this is combined with hydroxylation or bromination at the C-14 position pure antagonists are formed (Osei-Gyimah & Archer, 1981). Hydroxylation alone at the C-14 site confers no antagonist activity (cf. oxymorphone and naloxone, fig. 13.4). Substitution of a phenylethyl group onto the nitrogen increases agonist activity. Fentanyl, which has a phenylethyl subgroup, is six hundred times as potent as pethidine, which has a similar molecular structure but no phenylethyl subgroup.

Dismantling the morphine skeleton by removing the oxide bridge generates more potent tetracyclic compounds known as morphinans. Additional removal of the methylene bridge leaves a phenylpiperidine structure (a phenyl ring connected to a six-membered ring containing 5 carbon and 1 nitrogen atoms), which is the vital part of the morphine molecule. This dismantling results in an unfolding of the molecule so that the aromatic ring reorientates to an equatorial position on the piperidine ring, compared to an axial position in morphine. The distance between the aromatic ring and the piperidine nitrogen increases to 0.566 nm. The phenylpiperidine compounds are an extremely important class of opioids, and include pethidine and fentanyl.

Structural similarity can also be observed between opioids and the endogenous opioid peptides. The enkephalins contain sequences of amino acids in which tyrosine and phenylalanine are separated by two glycine molecules and terminated by either leucine (leu-enkephalin) or methionine (met-enkephalin). Morphine is synthetised by the poppy plant from two molecules of tyrosine (Galt, 1977) and the skeletal backbone of tyrosine is evident in the morphine molecule. Phenylalanine differs from tyrosine by the absence of an hydroxyl group on the phenyl ring. The structure of phenylalanine can be seen in the phenylpiperidine molecule (Thorpe, 1984).

Examination of structure-activity relationships

in opioids and opioid peptides has allowed a model of the opioid receptor to be developed. This receptor model consists of three active sites: an aromatic subsite (T-site) that preferentially binds hydroxylated rings (as in morphine and the tyrosine residue in enkephalin), separated 0.45 nm from an anionic site. A second aromatic site (P-site), 0.55 nm from the anionic site preferentially binds nonhydroxylated aromatic rings (as in the phenylpiperidines and the phenylalanine residue in enkephalin). This P-site also binds the alkyl groups in antagonists and in doing so pulls the bound nitrogen away from the anionic site, thereby interrupting agonist activity. Potent agonists such as fentanyl can bind to both P- and T-sites whereas less potent compounds can only bind to one site. Binding to the P-site seems to play a greater role at the δ-receptor than the μ receptor (Thorpe, 1984).

GENERAL ASPECTS OF OPIOID PHARMACOLOGY

While there are some significant differences in the pharmacological properties of opioids, in general the similarities are greater than the differences. One property where an apparent divergence is obvious is potency. Potency can be defined as the dose or concentration required to elicit a standard response: the more potent a drug the less is needed to produce the response. However, a drug may have different potencies for different types of response, e.g., analgesia and respiratory depression. While an increase in milligram potency by itself may not always be important, potency in terms of receptor affinity is important. The more potent a drug, the fewer molecules are needed to achieve a desired degree of receptor occupancy and less are available to bind to non-specific sites responsible for side-effects (de Castro et al, 1979). Sufentanil, for example, is six to seven hundred times as potent as morphine and has a safety margin (LD_{50}/ED_{50}) in animals of over 25 000 compared to 30 for morphine. In man high doses of sufentanil produce fewer central and peripheral haemodynamic changes than morphine. Some opioids are even more potent. Carfentanil, a fentanyl analogue, is 8000 times as potent as morphine and inhalation of a nebulised solution causes deep surgical anaesthesia in dogs (Port et al, 1982).

In clinical applications, potency is also determined by factors other than receptor affinity. Morphine, for example, is approximately equipotent with fentanyl at the opioid receptor (Table 13.2) (Stahl et al, 1977; Leysen et al, 1983) whereas clinically it is about 60 times less potent. This discrepancy is the result of the very low lipid solubility of morphine, limiting its transport into the CNS.

Table 13.2 Receptor binding characteristics of opioids

	Binding affinity Ki, nM	*Specific binding*
Carfentanil	0.036	80%
Sufentanil	0.1	92%
Fentanyl	1.6	75%
Phenoperidine	4.6	—
Morphine	5.7	60%
Alfentanil	19.0	—
Pethidine	193.0	—

Specific binding is the percentage drug specifically bound to the receptor rather than to non-specific sites. Binding affinity is measured by Ki, the equilibrium inhibition constant for [^{3}H] sufentanil. The lower the value of Ki, the higher the affinity for the receptor. Data for binding affinity from Leysen, et al, 1983.

Respiratory depression

All pure agonist opioids produce a dose-related respiratory depression. The primary effect is a reduction in the sensitivity of the respiratory centre to carbon dioxide so that initially respiratory rate is affected more than tidal volume, which may even increase. With increasing doses respiratory rhythmicity and reflexes are also disturbed resulting in the irregular, gasping characteristic of opioid overdose — 'pharmacological decerebration'. These responses are the result of drug action at centres in the medulla and pons. Several areas on the ventral surface of the medulla contain specific chemoreceptors that, by detecting central changes in [H^+], regulate respiration. Application of opioids directly to the medulla selectively depresses tidal volume and CO_2 response whereas the frequency of respiration is increased (Flórez et al, 1982). Application to the rostral surface of the pons induces a selective depression of frequency without modifying tidal volume, progressing at higher doses to respiratory arrest. On a dose basis, pontine structures are considerably more sensitive to the depressant effects of opioids than the medullary structures. The observed clinical effects are a combination of both medullary and pontine depression.

Maximum respiratory depression occurs within 5–10 min after intravenous injection with most opioids, but depression will last for much longer and may persist beyond the period of effective analgesia. Even with small doses of fentanyl (2–9 μg kg^{-1}), responses to CO_2 may be depressed for 2–4 hours (Kaufmann et al, 1979) whereas the analgesic effect will have subsided by 1–1.5 hours (Kay & Rolly, 1977). This shorter duration of analgesia relative to respiratory depression may be a reflection of the sensitivity of current methods to measure these variables. It may also be a reflection, however, of different affinities for the receptor responsible for analgesia (μ_1) and respiratory depression (μ_2 and/or δ) (McGilliard & Takemori, 1978). Patients who have been given large doses of opioids will often breath on command but when left unstimulated are indifferent to respiration and become apnoeic. Other stimuli, especially pain, are also effective in counteracting opioid-induced depression. A patient who has received intraoperative opioids and is breathing satisfactory at the end of surgery may, when subjected to considerable external stimuli e.g. removal of tracheal tube, transfer to bed etc, relapse into respiratory depression in the recovery room when these stimuli are no longer present. Elderly patients are more sensitive to the respiratory depressant effects of opioids than younger ones and the dose needs to be adjusted accordingly. It is also important to remember that other central nervous system depressants such as barbiturates, alcohol and inhalational anaesthetics also will potentiate the respiratory effects of the opioids.

Reversal of respiratory depression

Opioid-antagonist drugs will reverse both the respiratory depression and analgesia induced by an opioid agonist. Naloxone, a pure antagonist, is the drug most frequently used, but the mixed agonist–antagonists, e.g., nalorphine are equally effective and in some situations may be preferred, since they cause a less abrupt and complete reversal of analgesia due to their inherent analgesic effects. The use of pentazocine to terminate the respiratory depression following large doses of fentanyl intraoperatively was first used by de Castro and Viars (1968), a technique they described as "anesthésie analgésique sequentielle". Others, however, found that whereas pentazocine, 1 mg kg^{-1}, reversed fentanyl induced respiratory depression it did not offer any advantages in comparison with nalorphine or naloxone and did not improve postoperative analgesia (Kaukinen et al, 1981). Recently the use of nalbuphine to reverse respiratory depression in patients given fentanyl 23 μg kg^{-1} intraoperatively for surgical procedures lasting on average 80 min has been described (Latasch et al, 1984). Reversal of respiratory depression was rapid after 20 mg nalbuphine i.v. and the trachea could be extubated within 2 minutes. Postoperative analgesia lasted 3–5 hours.

Extreme caution must be exercised when naloxone is given to reverse respiratory depression when high doses of opioids have been given. There are several reports of intense pressor responses and tachycardia occurring when naloxone was used to reverse the effects of opioids in animals (Freye, 1974; Patschke et al, 1977) and man (Azar & Turndorf, 1979). Attempts to reverse high-dose morphine anaesthesia with intravenous naloxone 0.4 mg caused immediate hypertension and severe pulmonary oedema (Flacke et al, 1977). Large doses of naloxone have been fatal (Andree, 1980). In animals these changes have been associated with sixty percent increases in coronary blood flow and myocardial oxygen consumption (Patschke et al, 1977). Obviously such changes are potentially detrimental for patients with coronary artery disease. They have been attributed to release of catecholamines and sympathetic overactivity resulting from acute reversal of analgesia (Azar et al, 1981). Naloxone administered to subjects who have not been given opioids has no influence on blood pressure or plasma catecholamines (Estilo & Cotrell, 1982). Another explanation for the pressor response after naloxone administration in patients given opioids may be the alteration of baroreceptor reflexes so that an exaggerated haemodynamic response occurs to subsequent stimulation (Montastruc et al, 1981). Naloxone may also have an analeptic action unrelated to opioid receptor antagonism (Kraynack & Gintautas, 1982).

When using antagonists, respiratory depression may recur if the antagonist has a shorter action than the agonist. The elimination half-life of naloxone of 1–1.5 hours (Ngai et al, 1976), is shorter than most opioids with the exception of alfentanil. The duration of the effect of naloxone 0.4 mg 70 kg^{-1} was estimated to be 45 min (Evans et al, 1974). Recurrence of respiratory depression in severely depressed patients may also be due to an overestimation of the potency of naloxone. Naloxone causes a leftward shift of the CO_2 response curve and in the presence of a high $PaCO_2$ will result in marked increase in minute volume. This 'overshoot' will diminish as the $PaCO_2$ falls and if the response curve has not returned to its normal position, ventilation will return to a level that is still depressed with a $PaCO_2$ still higher than normal.

Ideally one should give a dose of naloxone post-operatively that will leave the patient with enough analgesia to be comfortable and a level of respiratory depression compatible with acceptable blood gases. Kaufman has derived a clinical index of naloxone potency which he calls cA_2, derived from morphine–naloxone interaction studies in volunteers (Kaufman et al, 1981). Using this index it is possible to calculate a theoretical dose of naloxone that will reduce the effect of an opioid by a given ratio. This is calculated according to the formula:

$$\text{Dose} = cA_2\ (DR - 1)$$

where DR = dose ratio. Thus, to reduce the effect of 12 mg of morphine to that of 6 mg (DR = 2) requires one cA_2; to reduce the effect to that of 4 mg (DR = 3) requires two cA_2 of naloxone. The cA_2 of naloxone in man is 1.5 $\mu g\ kg^{-1}$

Opioids inhibit the release or acetylcholine from neurons in the central nervous system while direct application of acetylcholine to the floor of the fourth ventricle has been shown to stimulate respiration (Dev & Loeschke, 1979). Physostigmine, an anticholinesterase, increases the level of acetylcholine in the brain and can antagonise morphine-induced respiratory depression in animals without antagonising analgesic activity (Weinstock et al, 1980). Studies in humans have clearly demonstrated that physostigmine, 13–33 $\mu g\ kg^{-1}$ intravenously can rapidly reverse the somnolent effect of morphine and restore ventilation to pre-drug values without altering analgesia (Snir-Mor et al, 1983). The effect lasts approximately 35 to 45 minutes. The use of physostigmine may be accompanied by an increased incidence of nausea and vomiting.

Doxapram, a non-specific respiratory stimulant, may also be used to antagonise opioid-induced respiratory depression. Intravenous doxapram, 1.0–1.5 mg kg^{-1}, administered together with morphine 20 or 40 mg per 60 kg to patients who had undergone upper abdominal operations effectively inhibited morphine-induced depression but had no significant influence on the analgesic effect (Gupta & Dundee, 1974a). Although doxapram is a short-acting drug, when given concurrently with morphine it appears capable of antagonising the respiratory depression caused by the latter for up to 2 hr after administration. Doxapram given as a continuous infusion at a rate of about 3 mg min^{-1} is effective in preventing respiratory depression without antagonising the analgesic effect of morphine (Gupta & Dundee, 1974b).

Cardiovascular effects

All opioids, with the exception of pethidine, produce bradycardia. Pethidine often produces tachycardia, possibly due to the similarities in structure between pethidine and atropine. The mechanism of this bradycardia is not completely understood although it might be due to central vagal stimulation. It is blocked totally by bilateral vagotomy (Reitan et al, 1978) or pharmacological vagal block with atropine (Liu et al, 1976). Morphine, in clinical concentrations has no effect on the sino-atrial node (Urthaler et al, 1975). Tachycardia can occasionally occur with morphine and may be a reflex response to a decreased blood pressure possibly related to histamine release. Tachycardia is the predominant response to morphine in species such as cats, pigs and horses.

Fentanyl-induced bradycardia is more marked in anaesthetised than in conscious subjects

(Tammisoto et al, 1970) although the severity is less when nitrous oxide is used (Prakash et al, 1980). This may be due to the sympathomimetic effect of nitrous oxide. When an opioid is combined with pancuronium, the sympathomimetic effect of the latter can help to minimise bradycardia. The use of the newer muscle relaxants, vecuronium and atracurium, which have no chronotropic activity, may sometimes in combination with opioids result in severe bradycardia. Second and subsequent doses of fentanyl produce less bradycardia than the initial dose (Liu et al, 1976) suggesting a possible tolerance mechanism.

Premedication with atropine can minimise, but may not totally eliminate opioid-induced bradycardia, especially in patients taking β-adrenoreceptor blocking drugs. The speed of injection is important with the more potent drugs, slow administration minimising bradycardia. Although severe bradycardia should obviously be avoided, moderate slowing of heart rate is not harmful and, by reducing myocardial oxygen consumption may be beneficial, especially in patients with coronary artery disease. The negative chronotropic action of fentanyl is an important factor in its protective effect on the heart during periods of ischaemia (van der Vusse et al, 1980).

Isolated heart or heart-muscle studies have demonstrated consistent dose-related negative inotropic effects for morphine (Goldberg & Padget, 1969: Strauer, 1972), pethidine (Strauer, 1972) and fentanyl (Goldberg & Padget, 1969; Strauer, 1972). However all these experimenters used concentrations of the drugs a hundred to several thousand times those found clinically, even during high-dose opioid anaesthesia. With fentanyl 75–100 $\mu g\ kg^{-1}$ peak plasma concentrations are seldom above 100 $ng\ ml^{-1}$ and fall rapidly to about 20 $ng\ ml^{-1}$ within 5 min (Bovill & Sebel, 1980; Sprigge et al, 1982). In the experiments described by Strauer (1972) fentanyl had no significant effect on papillary muscle mechanisms with concentrations up to 1000 $ng\ ml^{-1}$ and a 30% depression when the concentration was 5000 $ng\ ml^{-1}$. Morphine depresses the contractility of the isolated heart only in concentrations equivalent to 285 $\mu g\ ml^{-1}$ (Krishna & Paradise, 1974). Peak concentrations only rarely exceed 1 $\mu g\ ml^{-1}$ immediately after an intravenous dose of 2 $mg\ kg^{-1}$ in man (Hug, 1978).

Peripheral vascular effects

Hypotension can occur after even small (10 mg) doses of morphine intravenously, primarily due to a decrease in systemic vascular resistance. Morphine reduces arteriolar resistance and increases venous capacitance (Hsu et al, 1979). Histamine release appears to be the most important mechanism responsible for these changes. Basic drugs like morphine can displace histamine from its binding sites in mast cells and cause significant elevation in plasma histamine resulting in vasodilatation and hypotension (Moss & Rosow, 1983). Histamine release is reduced by slow administration (<10 $mg\ min^{-1}$). Pretreatment with a histamine H_1 antagonist, diphenylhydramine, or a histamine H_2 antagonist, cimetidine, do not block these reactions but they are significantly attenuated by combined H_1 and H_2 antagonist pretreatment (Philbin et al, 1981). Venodilatation lasts much longer than arteriolar dilation (Hsu et al, 1979) and causes a significant increase in intraoperative fluid requirement during high-dose morphine anaesthesia. Patients receiving a mean of 9.3 $mg\ kg^{-1}$ of morphine needed significantly more blood and crystalloid intra- and postoperatively to maintain filling pressures, blood pressure and urinary output than a similar group given 2.7 $mg\ kg^{-1}$ morphine (Stanley et al, 1973). Postoperatively the patients given the higher dose were described as oedematous, plum-coloured and prone to postural hypotension. These changes are not entirely due to falls in vascular resistance as there is loss of fluid and protein into the interstitial compartment. Henney et al (1966) showed that up to 11 $ml\ kg^{-1}$ blood is pooled or lost from the circulating blood volume in dogs after 1 $mg\ kg^{-1}$ morphine intravenously. Others have reported losses of plasma from the circulation to the interstitial spaces of 17–20% of total blood volume, which they attributed to histamine release (Berthelsen et al, 1980). Neither fentanyl nor sufentanil in high doses release histamine (Rosow et al, 1984), and they have minimal effect on vascular resistance. In isolated vascular tissue studies, neither morphine nor fentanyl, in clinically equivalent concentrations, block α-adrenoreceptors (Rorie et al, 1981; Muldoon et al, 1983) Morphine also may have a direct action on vascular smooth muscle, independent of histamine release (Lowenstein et al, 1972).

Gastrointestinal tract

The gastrointestinal tract is the only system outside the CNS with significant concentrations of opioid receptors. These, together with enkephalin-like immunoreactivity, are distributed throughout the gut, with highest concentration in the upper small intestine and stomach antrum. Morphine and allied drugs delay gastric emptying and the passage of food through the duodenum may be delayed for up to 12 hours after morphine administration. This has important clinical implications for patients presenting for emergency operations, who have received an opioid for either pain relief or premedication. It must always be assumed that they have a full stomach and appropriate steps taken to prevent aspiration during induction of anaesthesia. Opioids also delay transit time through the ileum and colon, by increasing resting tone and diminishing propulsive activity. This latter effect accounts for a major part of the constipating effect of morphine-like drugs, which are frequently used in the treatment of diarrhoea. The use of opioids during anaesthesia and postoperatively can contribute to postoperative ileus.

Opioids also affect the biliary system, increasing common bile duct pressure and decreasing bile production and flow, primarily as a result of spasm of the sphincter of Oddi but also due to increased tone in the bile duct itself (Radnay et al, 1980). Because of its atropine-like activity, pethidine is thought to produce less biliary spasm than other opioids, and to be indicated in patients with biliary colic or in those undergoing operations on the biliary tract involving cholangiography. However, recent evidence suggests that this is not true. When studying changes in biliary mechanics intraoperatively, Radney et al (1980) found that pethidine 1 mg kg^{-1} intravenously caused a 61% increase in common bile duct pressure, compared to a 53% increase after morphine 0.125 mg kg^{-1}. Reversal of biliary spasm with atropine is also unreliable in humans but it is reversible with naloxone (McCammon et al, 1978). Opioids are contraindicated in patients with biliary colic and in those undergoing radiographical investigations of the biliary tract. Spasm of the sphincter of Oddi can be a cause of pain after opioid administration and is difficult to distinguish from angina pectoris.

Emetic effects

Nausea and vomiting are common and undesirable side-effects of opioids, resulting from stimulation of the chemoreceptor trigger zone (CTZ). Emetic effects are more common when opioids are given preoperatively than when given postoperatively — possibly more common in patients not in pain. Fortunately, when given as premedicants they are usually combined with atropine or hyoscine, powerful antiemetics. Nausea and vomiting is more common in ambulatory patients, due to vestibular stimulation of the CTZ, which is sensitised by opioids. Women appear to be more susceptible to the emetic effects of opioids than men. All commercially available opioids cause emetic effects, which vary only in their severity and duration. With pethidine the onset is rapid but of short duration whereas with morphine there is slow onset and a prolonged effect (Morrison et al, 1968). The use of opioids during short operations often leads to prolonged postoperative vomiting. Opioids depress the vomiting centre (Wang, 1963) and with increasing plasma concentrations this effect overcomes the CTZ stimulant effect. Emetic effects are less common after second and subsequent doses and are rare after anaesthetic doses.

Muscle rigidity

All opioids in high doses produce muscle rigidity, a problem first reported during anaesthesia by Hamilton and Cullen in 1953 with levorphanol. It is a particular problem with the lipophylic drugs such as fentanyl. An 80% incidence was reported in patients receiving neuroleptanalgesia with droperidol and fentanyl (Corssen et al, 1964). The phenomenon is characterized by increased muscle tone progressing to severe stiffness, particularly in the abdominal and thoracic muscles; limb muscles are also affected. Rigidity of the thoracic muscles, the 'wooden chest', can cause severe difficulties with ventilation in non-paralysed anaesthetised patients. Chest wall rigidity can occur during recovery from high-dose opioid anaesthesia (Christian et al, 1983). The severity of the rigidity is increased by rapid injection and by concomitant use of nitrous oxide (Sokoll et al, 1972). Fentanyl-induced muscle rigidity is not due to a direct action on muscle fibres since it can be blocked by neuromuscular blocking drugs (Hill et al, 1981) and is not associated with increases in creatinine phosphatase (Georgis et al, 1971). Opioids do not have significant effects on nerve conduction and cause only minimal depression of the monosynaptic spinal reflexes associated with muscle stretch receptors (Georgis et al, 1971). Muscle rigidity is probably a manifestation of the catatonic state, a basic pharmacological property of all opioids, which may be related to enhancement of dopamine biosynthesis in the caudate nucleus (Freye & Kuchinsky, 1976) or an interaction at γ-ergic neurones (Moroni et al, 1979). Morphine-induced catatonia in rats has been ascribed to activation of extensor alpha motor neurones (Jurna et al, 1972).

Tolerance

The development of tolerance, i.e., a decreased intensity and shortened duration of all pharmacological effects with repeated administration of the same dose, is a characteristic feature of all opioid drugs. There is now convincing evidence from animal studies and reports in humans that the onset of tolerance may be very rapid. Acute tolerance to the cardiovascular effects of morphine, developing within a few hours after intravenous administration, has been described (Martin & Eades, 1961). Tolerance to the analgesic effects of fentanyl in rats can develop during a period of 2–4 days (Novack et al, 1978; Colpaert et al, 1980). In dogs, acute tolerance to the effects of fentanyl on the haemodynamic response to radial nerve stimulation occurs within 2.5 h (Askitopoulou et al, 1985). Tolerance to fentanyl has been reported to develop within hours after intravenous administration in man (McQuay et al, 1981) and during prolonged fentanyl infusion (Shafer et al, 1983).

The clinical relevance of the acute onset of tolerance is difficult to ascertain. It is unlikely to be of importance in balanced anaesthesia but may become important when high doses are used to produce anaesthesia. It may be partly responsible for the occasional reports of awareness during fentanyl anaesthesia (Mark & Greenberg, 1983; Hildenberg, 1981; Mummaneni et al, 1980). Mummaneni et al (1980) reported awareness occurred during the second, but not the first, of two fentanyl anaesthetics given 6 days apart. The total doses of fentanyl were similar on both occasions (76 $\mu g\ kg^{-1}$ and 72 $\mu g\ kg^{-1}$), although diazepam was given during the first and not during the second anaesthetic.

PHARMACOLOGY OF INDIVIDUAL OPIOIDS

Morphine is the prototype opioid, although seldom used as the sole opioid drug during balanced anaesthesia, except in high doses to produce anaesthesia (see later). It still remains the standard against which others are compared. Its pharmacology has already been discussed and in this section the pharmacology of other commonly used opioids will be described in so far as they differ from morphine.

Pethidine (meperidine)

Pethidine (Fig 13.5) was the first totally synthetic opioid to be produced. It is the prototype of the phenylpiperidine group of opioids and is structurally similar to atropine. Pethidine is less potent than morphine, 75 mg pethidine being approximately equianalgesic with 10 mg morphine. It produces similar degrees of sedation and euphoria to morphine but, with increasing doses, signs of cerebral excitation — tremors, muscle twitching and eventually convulsions — predominate over depression. This excitatory activity is mainly due to an active metabolite, norpethidine, which has twice the convulsant properties of the parent drug (Kaiko et al, 1983). Although rare, it has been reported in anaesthetic practice (Dundee & Tinckler, 1952). Toxicity is most likely to be seen

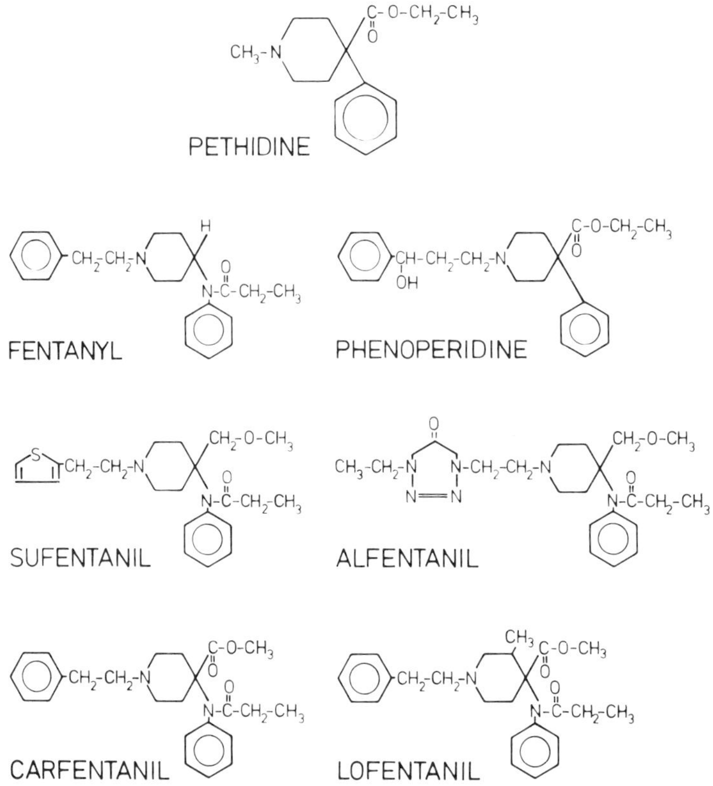

Fig. 13.5 Structure of pethidine and its analogues.

in patients taking pethidine for long periods, those with renal or hepatic disease and when the oral route is used. The latter is due to significant (50%) presystemic metabolism with rapid accumulation of norpethidine. Toxic symptoms may be exacerbated rather than antagonised by naloxone. The elimination half-life of pethidine is 6–8 hours (Verbeeck et al, 1981) but that of norpethidine is considerably longer (14–21 hours).

Since its introduction by Neff and colleagues in 1947 as a supplement to nitrous oxide-oxygen anaesthesia, pethidine 20–50 mg has been popular as the analgesic component of balanced anaesthesia. It is also commonly used for premedication. Pethidine alone is rarely used for the relief of postoperative pain, because of the high incidence of emetic effects. Its use as an intraoperative analgesic has largely been replaced by fentanyl. It is less effective than fentanyl in suppressing the haemodynamic responses to laryngoscopy and intubation and surgical stress (Ghoneim et al, 1984). Recovery, as assessed by performance on psychological tests, is superior with fentanyl than with pethidine. Pethidine causes a higher incidence and magnitude of histamine release than morphine (Flacke et al, 1983).

Pethidine should be avoided in patients taking monoamine oxidase inhibitor drugs as this combination might cause serious adverse reactions, such as excitation, delirium, hypertension, hyperthermia and convulsions. This toxic reaction is probably due to accumulation of norpethidine resulting from modification of the N-demethylase enzyme system responsible for pethidine biotransformation, although firm evidence for this hypothesis is lacking. Although other opioids are probably safe in combination with MAOI drugs, yet caution is advised.

Phenoperidine

Phenoperidine (Fig 13.5), an N-phenylpropyl derivative of norpethidine, was introduced in 1957, three years before fentanyl, to which it is chemically closely related. It has been almost totally restricted to use as a supplement to inhalation anaesthesia (often in combination with droperidol) and in the management of patients requiring prolonged mechanical ventilation. Phenoperidine is approximately 50 times as potent as pethidine. As a supplement during anaesthesia the usual dose is 0.5 to 1 mg intravenously in spontaneously breathing patients and up to 5 mg in those where IPPV is used. For postoperative pain relief 2 mg phenoperidine is equipotent with 10 mg morphine (Morrison et al, 1971). Phenoperidine 2 mg will provide adequate analgesia for approximately 1 hour.

Fentanyl

Fentanyl (Fig 13.5) is a phenylpiperidine of the 4-anilopiperidine series, structurally related to, but not derived from pethidine. It is commercially available as the citrate salt in an aqueous solution containing 50 μg fentanyl base per ml. For many years after its introduction in 1959 the main use of fentanyl was as a component of neuroleptanalgesia in combination with droperidol. In recent years, however, it has become popular as a supplement during balanced anaesthesia and as a total anaesthetic for cardiac operations.

On a weight basis fentanyl is considerably more potent than morphine or pethidine; estimates have ranged from 60 to 270 times as potent as morphine, depending on the species used. In man, fentanyl is between 60 to 80 times as potent as morphine. However, when the intrinsic potencies of these two drugs at the opioid receptor is considered, morphine is only slightly less potent than fentanyl (Stahl et al, 1977: Leysen et al, 1983).

Like all opioid agonists, fentanyl causes a dose-related depression of respiration. With small doses (2 μg kg^{-1}) respiratory rate decreases and there is a compensatory rise in tidal volume. With higher doses tidal volume also decreases leading to irregular periodic respiration and finally apnoea. There is a good correlation between plasma fentanyl concentration and the slope of the CO_2 response curve (Fig. 13.6) (Hug & McClain, 1980). A plasma concentration of around 3 ng ml^{-1} causes a 50% depression of the CO_2 response curve with

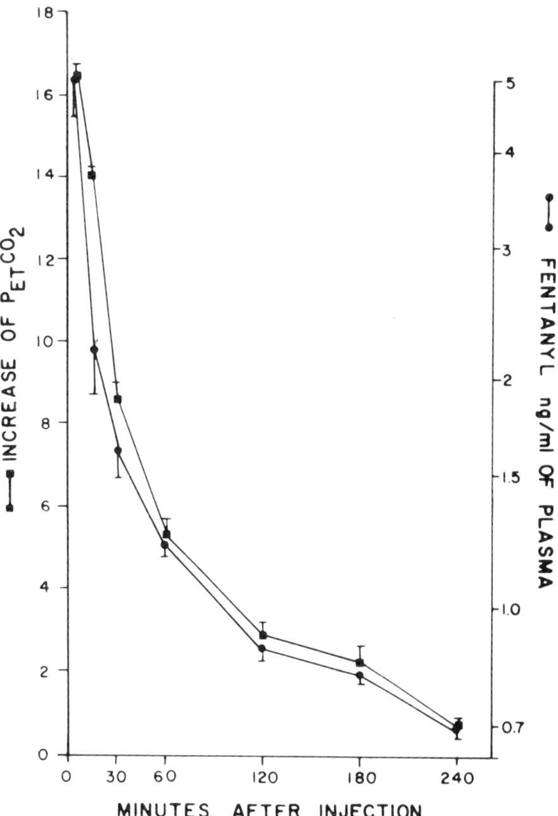

Fig. 13.6 Relationship between plasma fentanyl concentration (●) and recovery from ventilatory depression as measured by end-tidal P_{CO_2} (■), mm Hg, after bolus intravenous injection (From McClain and Hug, 1980).

a resting $PaCO_2$ of about 46 mmHg and provides adequate analgesia in most patients (Gill et al, 1980).

Delayed respiratory depression in the post-operative period has been reported following small intravenous doses of fentanyl during anaesthesia (Adams & Pybus, 1978; Becker et al, 1976). This biphasic respiratory depression may be related to secondary peaks in the plasma fentanyl concentration during the elimination phase (McQuay et al, 1979). Stoeckel et al, (1979) have demonstrated entero-hepatic recirculation of fentanyl with sequestration of fentanyl in the stomach and subsequent reabsorption from the small intestine. These authors have suggested this as an explanation for the secondary peaks in the plasma. This is unlikely since fentanyl undergoes almost complete pre-systemic metabolism and little or none of the absorbed drug would reach the systemic circulation. An alternative explanation is release of fentanyl from body stores, especially muscle, as a result of increased patient activity in the postoperative period.

Fentanyl causes some peripheral vasodilation but much less than is seen with morphine. This may be due partly to the absence of histamine release by fentanyl (Moss & Rosow, 1983). In patients with intracranial space occupying lesions ventilated to normocapnia fentanyl reduces both CSF and intracranial pressure (Misfeldt et al, 1976). In both man and animals fentanyl can cause significant reduction in cerebral blood flow and cerebral oxygen consumption (Vernheit et al, 1978; Carlsson et al, 1982).

Fentanyl produces less sedation than equianalgesic doses of morphine although EEG changes can be observed with doses as low as 2 μg kg^{-1} in human volunteers (Kugler et al, 1977). Nevertheless, large doses of fentanyl will cause unconsciousness in ventilated subjects and doses greater than 75 μg kg^{-1} are regularly used to provide anaesthesia for heart operations. With these doses very striking EEG changes are produced characterized by a progressive slowing in frequency, with ultimately 80–90% of the total power in the EEG contained in the delta (0.5–3.5 Hz) band (Sebel et al, 1981; Smith et al, 1984). Similar changes are seen with sufentanil (Bovill et al, 1982a) and alfentanil (Bovill et al, 1983) (Fig. 13.7).

The relationship between fentanyl and alfentanil serum concentrations during and after slow infusions and EEG changes has been investigated recently (Scott et al, 1985), using the spectral edge parameter as a measure of EEG changes. The spectral edge is the frequency below which 95% of the total power in the EEG occurs, and is a measure of EEG slowing. Spectral edge changes parallelled opioid concentrations but were found to lag between them in time (Fig. 13.8). When concentrations were plotted against spectral edge a well defined hysteresis loop was found, with one arm of the loop representing increasing concentration and the other arm representing changes when concentrations were decreasing (Fig. 13.9). The magnitude of the hysteresis effect was greater for fentanyl than alfentanil and was related to

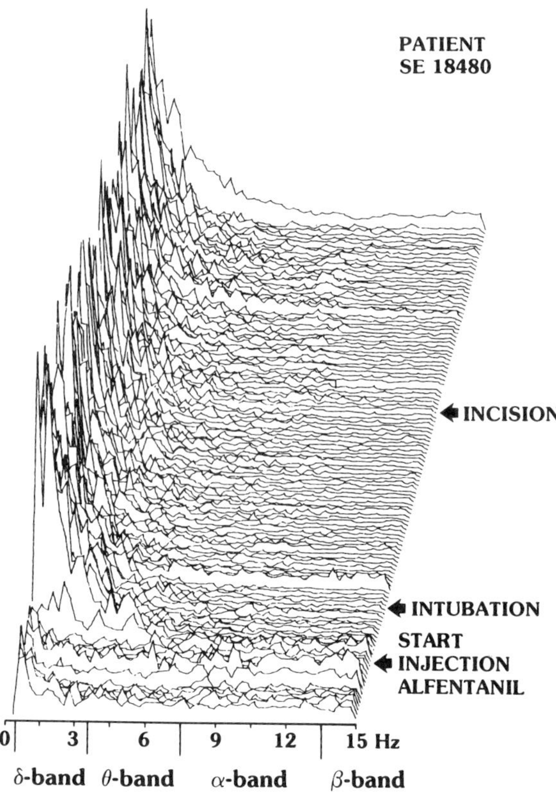

Fig. 13.7 Influence of alfentanil on the compressed spectral array.

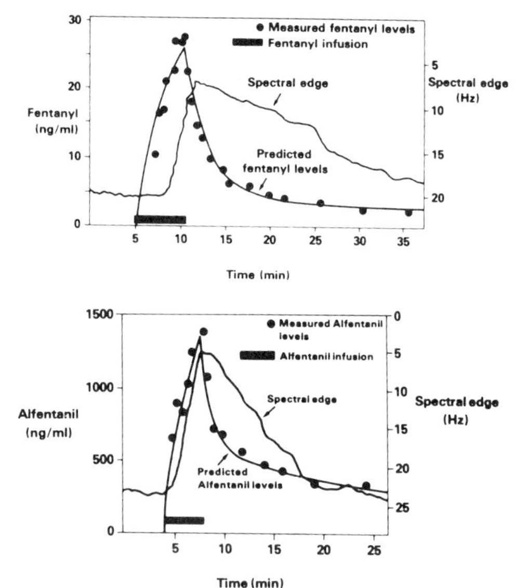

Fig. 13.8 Time course of spectral edge and plasma concentrations during and after infusions of fentanyl and alfentanil. Note the inverted spectral edge axis and how the spectral edge changes lag the concentration changes (From Scott et al, 1985).

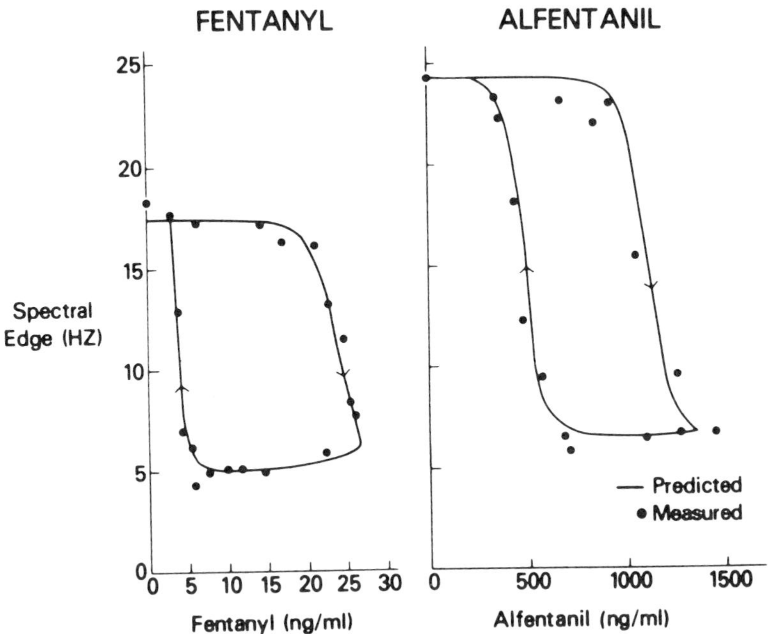

Fig. 13.9 Spectral edge versus serum concentrations of fentanyl and alfentanil, illustrating the hysteresis effect that is greater for fentanyl than for alfentanil. (From Scott et al, 1985).

changes in an 'effect' compartment and to differing pharmacokinetic properties of the two drugs.

Fentanyl is a highly lipophilic substance (Table 13.3), and is rapidly distributed to the tissues after intravenous injection. Large amounts of an administered dose are distributed initially to highly perfused tissues such as muscle, lung and brain. Muscle, because of its large mass, can accumulate up to 55% of an intravenous dose within 5 minutes of administration. In rabbits the brain/plasma ratio is 10.6 for fentanyl compared with 0.046 for morphine after equianalgesic doses (Herz & Teschemacher, 1971). Fentanyl is inactivated almost totally by the liver with only 4–7% excreted unchanged in the urine. In man the primary metabolic pathway is N-dealkylation, which converts fentanyl to norfentanyl (Goromaru et al, 1984). The hepatic intrinsic clearance of fentanyl is higher than liver blood flow so that little of an orally administered dose reaches the systemic circulation. The plasma elimination half-life is approximately 200 minutes (McClain & Hug, 1980; Bower & Hull, 1982) but is prolonged (up to 16 hr) in elderly patients, due to decreased

Table 13.3 Pharmacokinetic parameters

	Morphine	*Pethidine*	*Fentanyl*	*Alfentanil*	*Sufentanil*
pKa	7.9	8.5	8.4	6.5	8.0
% Nonionized of pH 7.4	23.0	7.4	8.5	89.0	19.7
Lipid solubility (octanol—water partition coefficient)	6.0	525.0	816.0	129.0	1757.0
Portein binding (%)	63.0	82.0	84.0	92.0	93.0
Vd_{ss} ($1\ kg^{-1}$)	3.4	4.4	4.0	0.7	1.7
Cl (ml kg^{-1} per minute)	2.3	7.7	12.6	5.1	12.7
$T\frac{1}{2}\beta$ (h)	1.7	6.7	3.6	1.6	2.7

clearance (Bently et al, 1982), and in patients taking cimetidine (Lauven et al, 1981).

Alfentanil

Alfentanil is a new opioid that is structurally related to fentanyl (Fig. 13.5). Initial animal studies have demonstrated that it is approximately one-fourth as potent an analgesic as fentanyl (de Castro et al, 1979; Niemegeers & Janssen, 1981). Potency ratios between fentanyl and alfentanil based on respiratory depression in rabbits varied from 2 : 1 to 3.5 : 1 (Brown et al, 1980). In man, alfentanil is between five and ten times less potent than fentanyl when intravenous doses are compared. However there are marked discrepancies between the potency ratios of fentanyl and alfentanil based on bolus intravenous doses and those based on plasma concentrations at steady state. A 40 : 1 potency difference between the two drugs for analgesia and respiratory depression, derived from plasma concentrations, has been reported (Andrews et al, 1983). The steady state plasma concentration potency ratio derived from EEG responses to infusion of alfentanil and fentanyl was calculated as 75 : 1 (Scott et al, 1985). The differences in potency between bolus dose data and concentration data can be explained by the pharmacokinetc differences between the two drugs.

All animal and human investigations have shown that alfentanil has a much shorter duration of effect than other opioids. This has been confirmed by several pharmacokinetic studies which have demonstrated that alfentanil has an elimination half-life of 75–95 min, a small volume of distribution and low clearance (Mather, 1983). The small distribution volume results from a low lipid solubility and high plasma protein binding (Table 13.3).

Despite low lipid solubility, alfentanil has a rapid onset of action when injected intravenously. This can be explained by several factors. It has a low pKa (6.8) compared to other opioids, all of which have values above 7.4. This results in approximately 85% of unbound alfentanil in plasma being present in the nonionised form compared with only 9% for fentanyl. This high proportion of nonionized molecules allows rapid access to the brain. The lipid solubility of alfentanil, although much lower than that of fentanyl, is probably sufficiently high to allow rapid blood–brain barrier penetration and is thus not a rate-limiting factor in the onset of effect. Differences in the partitioning of the two drugs between blood and brain will also influence the onset of effect. This partition ratio for fentanyl is 1 : 5 (brain concentration = 5 × blood concentration) in the postdistribution phase after intravenous bolus administration (Hug & Murphy, 1981). The blood–brain ratio for alfentanil is 5 : 1, i.e. the reverse of fentanyl (Michiels et al, 1981). These partitioning differences are probably due to increased solution of fentanyl in brain lipid as a result of its higher lipid solubility, thereby limiting the rise of drug concentration at the receptor. Alfentanil, with fewer 'storage' sites to fill, can achieve adequate receptor occupancy more rapidly. This has been compared to differences in alveolar-blood equilibrium between diethyl ether and nitrous oxide (Scott et al, 1985).

Its rapid onset of action has led to alfentanil being investigated as an agent for induction of anaesthesia. Nauta and colleagues (1983) compared anaesthetic induction with alfentanil, thiopentone, etomidate and midazolam in patients premedicated with quinalbarbitone (secobarbital). Alfentanil was given as an infusion (20 μg kg min^{-1}). The average time to loss of consciousness was 93 seconds for alfentanil, 60 seconds for thiopentone and 116 seconds for midazolam. The average induction dose of alfentanil was 173 μg kg^{-1}. Alfentanil was claimed to be superior to the others with respect to cardiovascular stability during induction and tracheal intubation.

Benzodiazepine premedication can significantly reduce induction time. Nauta and colleagues (1982) found that approximately 75 seconds are required to induce anaesthesia in patients premedicated with lorazepam compared with 134 seconds in patients given atropine. The ED_{50} and ED_{90} of alfentanil for unconsciousness and anaesthesia have been determined (McDonnell et al, 1984). Doses of alfentanil from 100 to 250 μg kg^{-1} were given to unpremedicated patients and responses to verbal commands, and response to placement of a nasopharyngeal airway assessed after 90 seconds. The ED_{50} and ED_{90} doses for

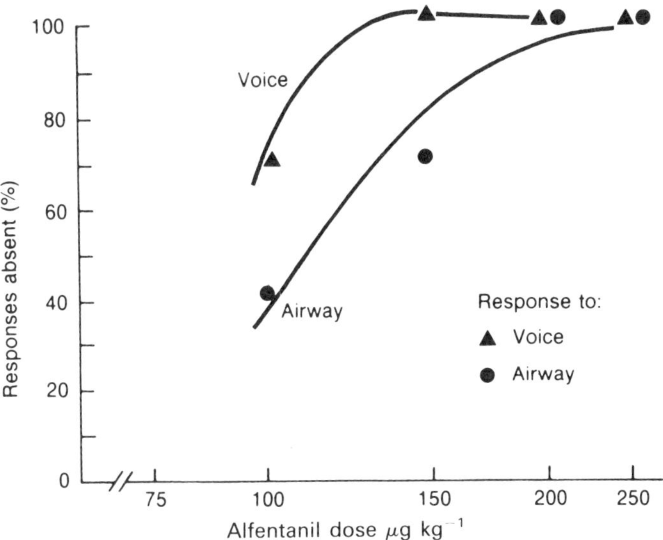

Fig. 13.10 Dose–response curves for loss of response to voice (▲), and insertion of a nasopharyngeal airway (•), 90 sec following alfentanil in unpremedicated patients. (From McDonnel et al, 1984).

loss of voice response were 92 and 111 μg kg^{-1} respectively and for loss of nasopharyngeal airway response 111 and 169 μg kg^{-1} (Fig. 13.10). The eyelid reflex was not abolished completely in any dose group.

A high incidence (55–75%) of muscle rigidity was reported in the above studies. This is reduced by benzodiazepine premedication but this may be secondary to the lower dose requirements of alfentanil.

Alfentanil has been used as a supplement to a variety of induction agents for various (mainly gynaecological) operations (Hug & Chaffman, 1984). It gave good analgesia with rapid recovery, suggesting that this drug may be useful in day-case surgery. For operations lasting longer than 30–60 min, alfentanil is best given with nitrous oxide anaesthesia as a continuous infusion after an initial loading dose. Plasma concentrations needed to suppress responses to surgical stimulation vary with the stimulus (Fig. 13.11) so that a constant rate infusion is not sufficient. However, the rapid onset of effect allows fast control when infusion rates are temporarily increased as during intra-abdominal manipulations. Infusion rates between 0.5 and 1.5 μg kg^{-1} min^{-1} are generally adequate (Ausems & Hug, 1983; Ausems et al, 1983). An infusion scheme designed to initiate and maintain

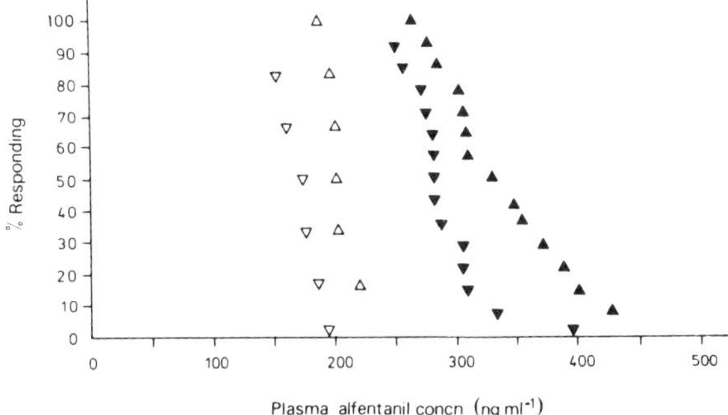

Fig. 13.11 Plasma alfentanil concentrations versus percent of patients responding to surgical stimulation. Open triangles represent responses to microsopic surgery on the fallopian tubes, closed triangles represent responses to intra-abdominal manipulations. (△, ▲ = highest concentration associated with a response; ▽, ▼ = lowest concentration without a response). Patients were ventilated with 66% nitrous oxide in oxygen. (From Ausems et al, 1983).

alfentanil concentrations of approximately 450 ng ml^{-1} has been described (Schüttler et al, 1983). This consists of an initial, rapid infusion of 1.5 mg min^{-1} for 10 min, followed by a 0.15 mg min^{-} maintenance infusion. In order to allow rapid recovery and minimise postoperative respiratory depression, infusion rates should be adjused to the minimum needed to abolish responses to the surgical stimulation and stopped 15–20 min before the end of operation.

Sufentanil

Sufentanil is a thienyl derivative of the 4-amilino-piperidine series, chemically related to fentanyl (Fig. 13.5). It is commercially available as the citrate salt, and has been licenced for clinical use in the USA and some European countries. Animal experiments have shown it to be extremely potent: in the tail-withdrawal test in rats it is more than 4500 times as potent as morphine. It is also very safe; the LD_{50}/ED_{50} ratio in rats being 25111, compared with 69 for morphine and 277 for fentanyl (Niemegeers et al, 1976). Infusions of very high doses of sufentanil (40 μg kg min^{-1}) in atropinised, artificially ventilated dogs causes minimal haemodynamic changes (Reddy et al, 1980). The mechanisms of death following lethal doses of sufentanil in ventilated dogs is cerebral excitation with convulsions (de Castro et al, 1979).

Sufentanil has a very high affinity for the μ-receptor, approximately 10 times that of fentanyl (Table 13.2) (Stahl et al, 1977; Leysen et al, 1983). It is also about 10 times as potent as fentanyl in man. Sufentanil is extremely lipophilic (Table 13.3) with a rapid onset of action. Peak tissues concentrations after 2.5 μg kg^{-1} [^{3}H]-sufentanil administered to rats occurred at 2 min in brain, liver and heart. It is rapidly metabolised in the liver and has an elimination half-life (163 min) intermediate between that of fentanyl and alfentanil (Bovill et al, 1984b).

In man at low doses (0.4 μg kg^{-1}) sufentanil produces more sedation than fentanyl (Kugler et al, 1977). Higher doses (15 μg kg^{-1}) result in surgical anaesthesia with EEG changes similar to these seen with fentanyl (Bovill et al, 1982a). A ceiling effect does not appear to be reached in the cerebral effects of sufentanil whereas this occurs with fentanyl and morphine.

Infusions of sufentanil, 1 μg kg min^{-1}, in rats decreases MAC halothane by more than 90% (Hecker et al, 1983). Similar studies in dogs with fentanyl and morphine resulted in a maximum reduction in MAC of enflurane by only 65% (Fig. 13.12) (Murphy & Hug, 1982a, b). If similar effects occur in man, they could explain the more effective anaesthetic properties of high-dose sufentanil during cardiac operations (Sebel & Bovill, 1982). Sufentanil does not cause histamine release

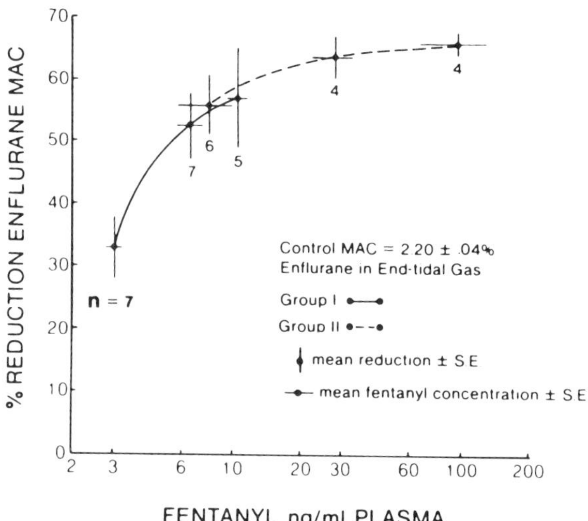

Fig. 13.12 Reduction of enflurane MAC as a function of plasma fentanyl concentration. (From Murphy & Hug, 1982b).

(Rosow et al, 1984). Investigations of the peripheral circulation (Berthelsen et al, 1980; 1981) and central haemodynamics (Eriksen et al, 1981) following sufentanil and morphine anaesthesia in dogs have shown that peripheral perfusion was better maintained with sufentanil and unaltered by β-adrenoreceptor blockade.

Early clinical studies with sufentanil confirmed its effectiveness as an analgesic component of 'balanced anaesthesia' for a variety of surgical procedures (Kalenda & Scheijgrond, 1976; van de Walle et al, 1976; Rolly et al, 1979). More recently, Ghoneim and colleagues (1984) compared sufentanil, fentanyl, pethidine and morphine as supplements to nitrous oxide oxygen anaesthesia. Fentanyl and sufentanil were equally effective and superior to morphine or pethidine. Total doses of 0.1 mg sufentanil and 1.0 mg fentanyl were required for operations lasting 130–150 min. Most publications reporting clinical experience with sufentanil have concentrated on its use in high doses for cardiac surgery or for neurosurgery (Shupak & Harp, 1985). In the latter, doses of 20 μg kg^{-1} produced satisfactory anaesthesia, and the residual opioid effect was reversed in all patients after operation with naloxone, allowing removal of the tracheal tube within one hour from the end of the procedure.

Carfentanil and lofentanil

Carfentanil and lofentanil are novel, ultra-potent members of the fentanyl family of opioids (Fig. 13.5). Carfentanil, one of the most powerful opioids known, is about 8500 times as potent as morphine, and being 3 to 8 times as potent as etorphine (van Bever et al, 1976). It has not been administered to man but has been extensively evaluated as an immobilising agent for free-ranging wild animals, either alone or combined with a potent neuroleptic. It is supplied in 1 ml ampoules at a concentration of 10 mg ml^{-1}. The immobilizing dose for the African elephant is 1 $\mu g\ kg^{-1}$ (1 mg $tonne^{-1}$); for an average elephant weighing 5000 kg less than 1 ml of carfentanil solution is needed (de Vos, 1978). The effects can be rapidly reversed with naloxone or diprenorphine, a specific antagonist developed for use with etorphine. Because of its extreme potency and concentration, personnel handling carfentanil must be very careful since a scratch from a loaded syringe dart could render the victim unconscious and apnoeic. An antagonist must be immediately available and all involved instructed in its use. The potency of carfentanil is such that surgical anaesthesia can be induced in dogs breathing a nebulised solution of the drug (Port et al, 1982).

Lofentanil is 5000–6000 times as potent as morphine (Leysen et al, 1978; de Castro et al, 1979). In contrast to other fentanyl congeners, it has an exceptionally long action, a dose of 0.7 $\mu g\ kg^{-1}$ intravenously causing respiratory depression lasting up to 48 hours (Cookson, 1983). This prolonged effect appears to be due to fixation at the opioid receptor rather than slow metabolism. Lofentanil dissociates from the μ-receptor with a dissociation half-life of 208 min (Gommeren & Leysen, 1982). The equivalent half-lives for fentanyl and sufentanil are 1.2 min and 25 min respectively (Leysen et al, 1983). Although such a potent and long-acting drug might have limited clinical applications, such as in the intensive care unit, lofentanil is unlikely ever to be released for clinical use.

MIXED AGONIST-ANTAGONISTS

The mixed agonist–antagonist drugs produce analgesia by agonist activity at the κ-receptor and are competitive antagonists at the μ-receptor. They will reverse all of the effects of pure agonist opioids, including analgesia and respiratory depression. They all produce respiratory depression, although the dose–response curve is less steep than that of agonists and reaches a plateau as the dose is increased. Nalorphine (N-allylmorphine), the first of this class of drugs to be used clinically, was synthesized in 1942. It is equipotent with morphine as an analgesic and in causing respiratory depression. However analgesic doses produced severe psychotomimetic side-effects, thought to be due to σ-receptor agonism, and its clinical use has been limited to reversal of opioid-induced respiratory depression. Although largely displaced by naloxone, nalorphine is still a valuable drug in this context and its use is associated with fewer haemodynamic disturbances than with naloxone.

Pentazocine

Pentazocine, the n-dimethylallyl derivative of phenazocine (Fig. 13.13), was the first agonist-antagonist to be clinically effective as an analgesic. Its analgesic potency is about one-third to one-fifth that of morphine. Pentazocine increases systemic vascular resistance, pulmonary artery pressure and myocardial work load and decreases myocardial contractility (Jewitt et al, 1971). It is thus contraindicated in the treatment of patients with acute myocardial infarction.

Psychotomimetic side-effects such as hallucinations, bizzare dreams and sensation of depersonalisation occur in about 6–10% of patients (Wood et al, 1974: Hamilton et al, 1967). They are more common in elderly patients and in those who are ambulatory and when doses above 60 mg are given.

Pentozocine has been largely replaced in clinical practice by newer agonist-antagonists, butorphanol, nalbuphine, meptazinol and buprenorphine, that have a lower incidence of these psychotomimetic effects. The introduction of these newer drugs has reawakened interest in the use of agonist–antagonists in anaesthesia.

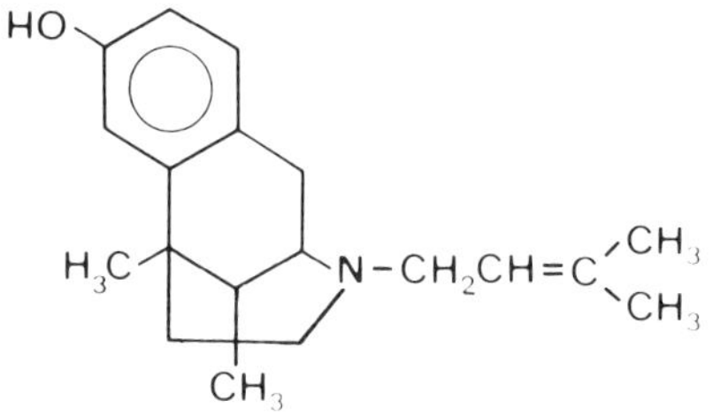

PENTAZOCINE

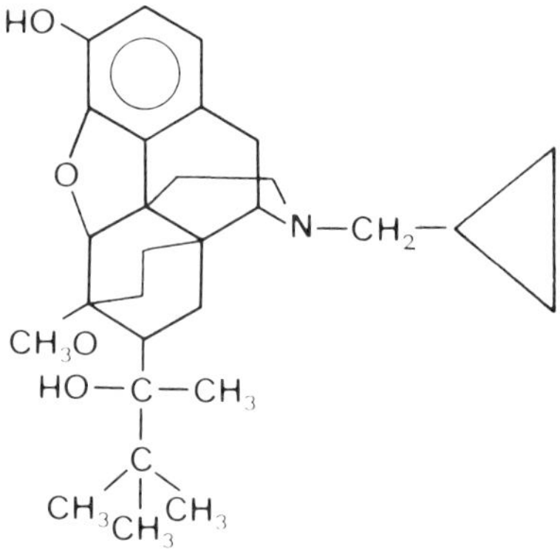

BUPRENORPHINE

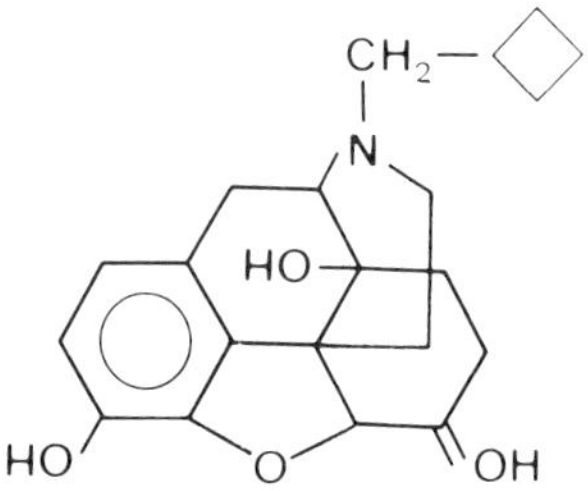

NALBUPHINE

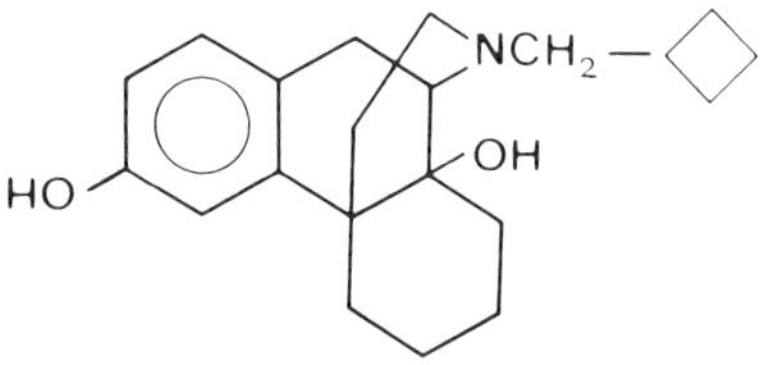

BUTORPHANOL

Fig. 13.13 Structure of four mixed agonist–antagonist drugs.

Butorphanol

Butorphanol tartrate, (Fig. 13.13), is a fully synthetic morphinan derivative 5 to 7 times as potent as morphine. Respiratory depression following butorphanol 2 mg intravenously is similar to that produced by morphine 10 mg. However, maximum depression occurs with doses above 4 mg in adults (Nagashima et al, 1976). A similar ceiling effect also occurs for analgesia (Murphy and Hug, 1982b). Even very high doses fail to provide sufficient analgesia to block responses to intra-abdominal operations (Stanley et al, 1983b). Doses of 0.3 mg/kg (approximately equivalent to 1.5–2.0 mg/kg morphine) do not render patients unconscious (Moldenhauer et al, 1981). Butorphanol is effective as a supplement during balanced anaesthesia, and causes less post-operative depression of respiration than morphine (Del Pizzo, 1978).

In dogs infusions of butorphanol 0.1 and 0.2 mg kg^{-1} min^{-1} produce significant cardiovascular depression, which is exacerbated by addition of nitrous oxide (Sederberg et al, 1981). In healthy humans it causes similar changes in cardiovascular parameters as morphine. However, it does elevate left ventricular preload (Popio et al, 1978) and, like pentazocine, is best avoided in patients with a recent myocardial infarction.

Nalbuphine

Nalbuphine is structurally similar to oxymorphone and naloxone (Fig. 13.13). In low doses it is approximately equipotent with morphine as an analgesic, but a 'ceiling' of analgesic activity is reached with doses above about 0.4 mg kg^{-1} intravenously (Gall, et al, 1982). The ability of nalbuphine to reduce the MAC of inhalational anaesthetics, a measure of analgesic potency, is limited. The maximum reduction of cyclopropane MAC in rats was 22% (Di Fazio, et al, 1981) and of enflurane MAC in dogs 8% (Murphy & Hug, 1982b). This is in contrast to the maximum reduction in MAC produced by morphine of 60%. As with other agonist–antagonists, nalbuphine produces respiratory depression but again a plateau in the dose–effect curve is observed at doses above about 0.4 mg/kg (Romagnoli & Keats, 1980; Gall, et al, 1982).

Nalbuphine causes minimal cardiovascular changes in patients with cardiac disease including those patients undergoing cardiac operations given doses of 2–3 mg kg^{-1} (Lake et al, 1982). In contrast to pentazocine and butorphanol, nalbuphine does not increase cardiac work load or pulmonary artery pressure and is thus safe in the management of patients after acute myocardial infarction. Unlike morphine, nalbuphine does not cause histamine release.

Nalbuphine, being a μ-receptor antagonist, will reverse the effects of agonist opioids. The changes in the pattern and magnitude of activity of medullary inspiratory neurones induced by fentanyl in cats are restored by nalbuphine (Tabatabai, et al, 1983). Nalbuphine is effective in reversing opioid-induced respiratory depression in man (Latasch, et al, 1984). Latasch and colleagues gave a constant dose of 20 mg. nalbuphine intravenously at the end of operation to patients anaesthetised with nitrous oxide and fentanyl (23 μg kg^{-1}) for elective general surgery. Within 2 min of nalbuphine administration all patients had progressed from apnoea to spontaneous respiration and were so alert that they would not tolerate the endotracheal tube. Transient shivering was the only side-effect observed. Analgesia persisted for 3–5 hours. Nalbuphine may prove to be a useful alternative to naloxone for reversal of opioid-induced respiratory depression. The persistence of analgesia should prevent most of the undesirable sympathetic effects which follow the use of naloxone, especially after high doses of opioids. Since nalbuphine has a considerably longer elimination half-life (5 h) than naloxone (1–1.5 h) the risk of recurrence of respiratory depression will be considerably reduced.

Meptazinol

This is another new analgesic which acts as a mixed agonist–antagonist at the opioid receptors. It is approximately equipotent with pethdine. Some features of meptazinol's pharmacology in isolated tissue preparations are untypical of opioids and part of its analgesic effect is thought to be mediated via central cholinergic synapses (Green, 1983). Meptazinol has a high affinity for the μ_1-receptor (Spiegel & Pasternak, 1984) and this can explain its low incidence of respiratory depression. In volunteers meptazinol 1.4 mg kg^{-1} intravenously caused no significant change in the ventilatory response to carbon dioxide compared to demonstrable depression by equivalent doses of morphine and pentazocine (Jordan et al, 1979). Although an opioid devoid of respiratory side-effects should be of interest to anaesthetists, meptazinol has not been widely used during anaesthesia. One reason for this is its relatively potent emetic action, which is marked when it is given as preanaesthetic medication (Chestnutt & Dundee, 1986).

Buprenorphine

Buprenorphine is a semi-synthetic derivative of thebaine, one of the most chemically reactive of the opium alkaloids (Fig. 13.13). It is a potent analgesic, 0.3 mg buprenorphine being approximately equipotent with 10 mg morphine, whether given i.v. or i.m. Early receptor binding studies suggested that buprenorphine was a selective μ-receptor agonist (Martin et al, 1976). However, in rodents, the dose-response curves for buprenorphine induced analgesia and catalepsy are 'bell-shaped' (Dum & Herz, 1981), a finding that is difficult to reconcile with selective agonist activity at one receptor. Subsequent studies have demonstrated that buprenorphine binds to μ-, δ-, and κ-binding sites (Villiger and Taylor, 1981). It has a high affinity for the μ- and δ-receptors and a lesser affinity for the κ-receptor.

Despite being highly lipid soluble, buprenorphine is slow to reach its full effect after intravenous administration. Once established, however. analgesia is maintained for a prolonged period and there is no correlation between plasma concentration and analgesic effect (Bullingham, et al, 1983). This discrepancy between pharmacokinetic and pharmacodynamic effects can be explained by the unique way that buprenorphine binds to the opioid receptor.

Buprenorphine differs from all other opioids in

having very slow rates of both association to and dissociation from the μ-receptor. The differences between buprenorphine and fentanyl binding were studied by Boas and Villiger (1985). Equilibrium for fentanyl binding was achieved within 10 min, whereas buprenorphine binding took 30 min to reach equilibrium. Even greater differences were found for receptor dissociation. The dissociation half-life for fentanyl was 6–8 min, with 100% of the drug being dissociated from the receptor by 60 min. In contrast, the half-life of dissociation of buprenorphine was 160 min, and 50% remained bound at 60 min (Fig. 13.14). This sluggish dissociation of buprenorphine from opioid receptors can account for the prolonged analgesic effect, that persists even when plasma concentrations have fallen below 1 μg ml^{-1} (Bullingham et al, 1983). It might also explain the inability of naloxone to reverse established buprenorphine-induced respiratory depression. On the basis of data reported by Villiger and Taylor (1981) and Villiger and colleagues (1983), 40 times the dose of naloxone would be needed to reverse buprenorphine than fentanyl at comparable concentrations.

Buprenorphine, like other mixed agonist-antagonists, causes respiratory depression. In contrast to the 'bell-shaped' response curves seen for analgesia and some other effects, that for respiratory depression is similar to other drugs in this class with a ceiling effect in animals at about 0.1 mg kg^{-1}, beyond which no further depression occurs. Similar effects occur in Man, with the response curve reaching a plateau at doses between 0.3 and 0.6 mg intramuscularly (Lewis & Rance, 1979). Large intravenous doses, up to 7 mg, given to patients after Caesarean section, do not produce any respiratory depression (Budd, 1981). It is important to realise that, should significant depression occur, no specific antagonist exists, naloxone being relatively ineffective; even doses as high as 14–16 mg will only partially reverse this side-effect. Doxapram might be of value in this situation.

Buprenorphine has minimal effects on the cardiovascular system either in normal patients, or those with cardiovascular pathology. It appears to be a safe analgesic for patients with a recent myocardial infarction (Hayes, et al, 1979).

Buprenorphine has been extensively evaluated as an intra-operative and postoperative analgesic. When compared with fentanyl as a supplement during balanced anaesthesia, it reduces significantly the requirements for inhalation agents (Kay, 1980). The duration of analgesia after

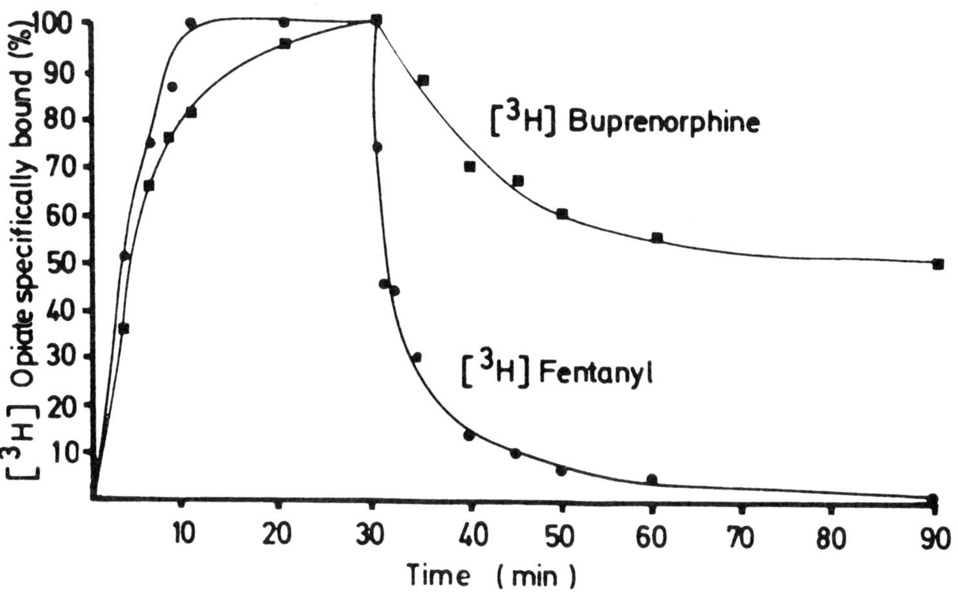

Fig. 13.14 Association and dissociation of fentanyl and buprenorphine to and from the opioid receptor. (From Boas & Villiger, 1985).

surgery is also significantly longer than with other opioids. On average, the time to the first injection of the postoperative analgesic when buprenorphine is used intra-operatively is 10 h compared to 3–5 hr when fentanyl is used (Kay, 1980). Patients receiving buprenorphine were consistently more drowsy after operation than those given fentanyl.

For use as a postoperative analgesic, buprenorphine is effective intramuscularly, sublingually or intravenously. Systemic bioavailability after i.m. administration is greater than 90% and absorption is rapid, with peak concentrations reached within 5 min (Bullingham et al, 1980). Buprenorphine is well absorbed from the buccal mucosa with a systemic availability of about 60% and a transfer half-life of 76 min (Bullingham et al, 1982). Maximum analgesia is reached within 3 hrs. The optimal method of administrations for relief of acute postoperative pain is by the intravenous route, titrating the dose against patient response. Commonly used single bolus doses are 0.3 or 0.6 mg. Not surprisingly the higher dose is more effective but it also seems to result in fewer side effects (Budd, 1981; Watson et al, 1982). Patient-controlled i.v. administration of buprenorphine using an on-demand syringe pump such as the Cardiff Palliator has proved effective, with good quality of analgesia and high patient acceptance (Harmer et al, 1983). Total drug requirements in the first 24 hrs vary from 1 to 1.7 mg. Because of the prolonged duration of action and the lack of correlation between plasma concentration and effect, careful monitoring of ventilation is essential when using repeated doses of buprenorphine. Serious respiratory depression developed in three of 17 patients given 0.3 mg buprenorphine by continuous infusion over 12 h (Fry, 1982). These patients, however, had been given a similar dose of drug intramuscularly at induction of anaesthesia.

PLACE OF INTRAVENOUS OPIOIDS IN ANAESTHESIA

Since the introduction of pethidine supplementation of nitrous oxide anaesthesia, opioids have remained an important element in anaesthetic practice. The anaesthetic state consists of four essential components; narcosis, analgesia, muscle relaxation and abolition of autonomic reflexes to surgery (Gray & Rees, 1952; Woodbridge, 1957). Modern general anaesthesia uses a combination of different drugs to achieve this state, a technique commonly called 'balanced anaesthesia' (pp. 37–38).

The inclusion of an opioid as the specific analgesic component of balanced anaesthesia offers several advantages. When given either as part of the premedication or as a small bolus along with the intravenous induction drug, induction of anaesthesia is smoother, less induction agent is required and the cardiovascular responses to intubation of the trachea are reduced or abolished. The course of anaesthesia tends to be associated with fewer haemodynamic fluctuations and there is a decreased need for inhalation anaesthetics. Dundee and colleagues (1969) gave a single dose of levorphanol, 2 mg, at induction and observed less vasoconstriction and pallor, reduced requirements for neuromuscular blocking drugs, less restlessness after operation and an increased time until the first analgesic was requested after operation. The use of opioids is particularly advantageous in operations that involve sudden painful manipulations, e.g. traction on visceral organs during intra-abdominal operations. Anticipation of these events and prior supplementation with a small dose of an opioid (e.g. 50–100 μg fentanyl) will often suffice to prevent rises of arterial blood pressure and heart rate associated with these manipulations.

The sympathoadrenal responses to laryngoscopy and intubation of the trachea, resulting in hypertension, tachycardia and arrhythmias, are well known (Derbyshire et al, 1983). They are particularly dangerous in patients suffering from hypertension or coronary artery disease. Many different approaches have been tried in order to attenuate these haemodynamic responses, including topical analgesia (Stoelting, 1977), prior administration of β-adrenoreceptor blocking drugs (Prys-Roberts et al, 1973) and the use of vasodilators such as nitroprusside (Stoelting, 1979). Topical analgesia is not always effective and vasodilators, while effective in controlling hypertension, may accentuate tachycardia. The ability of low doses of fentanyl (5–8 μg kg^{-1}), given intravenously at the time of

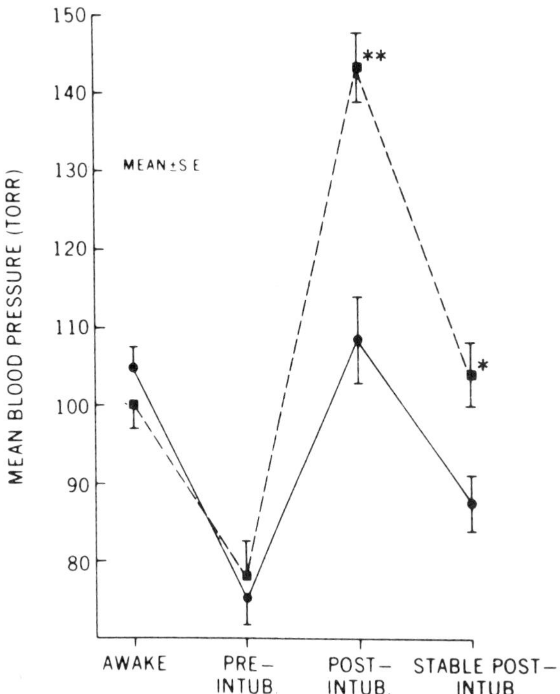

Fig. 13.15 Reduction in blood pressure response during intubation when fentanyl 8 μg kg⁻¹ is given with thiopentone 3 mg kg⁻¹ compared to thiopentone 6 mg kg⁻¹ alone. ●——● = fentanyl-thiopentone; ■——■ = thiopentone. *$P < 0.0005$ **$P < 0.0001$, comparing groups. (From Martin et al, 1982).

induction, to significantly reduce or abolish these haemodynamic responses has been well documented (Martin et al, 1982). This is illustrated in figure 13.15 (Barash et al, 1982). Alfentanil in doses of about 30 μ kg^{-1}, is also effective in reducing the haemodynamic responses to laryngoscopy and intubation (Black et al, 1984).

The cardiovascular changes during laryngoscopy and intubation are a reflex response to stimulation in an area richly innervated by the 9th and 10th cranial nerves. In the rat, high concentrations of opioid receptors are found in the nuclei of these nerves and in the closely associated solitary nuclei (Atweh & Kuhar, 1977). The efficacy of low doses of opioids in suppressing these responses may be due, therefore, to a specific blockade at the level of these nuclei of afferent nerve impulses arising in the pharynx and larynx.

The realisation that opioids could influence the course of inhalation anaesthesia developed early in the history of anaesthesia. Claude Bernard was probably the first to investigate the use of morphine premedication to improve the quality of chloroform anaesthesia (Bernard, 1869). Some 70 years later animal studies demonstrated the ability of opioids to reduce the amount of cyclopropane needed to achieve a given plane of anaesthesia (Robbins et al, 1939). Subsequent investigators have confirmed these findings for diethyl ether (Taylor et al, 1957), halothane (Hecker et al, 1983) and enflurane (Murphy & Hug, 1982a, b). The introduction of the concept of minimum alveolar concentration (MAC) as an index of anaesthetic potency has allowed this opioid effect to be quantified. The anaesthesia-sparing effect of opioids increases in a log-dose fashion. For both morphine (Murphy & Hug, 1982b) and fentanyl (Murphy & Hug, 1982a) there is a limit, or 'ceiling effect,' for their reduction in enflurane MAC, the maximum reduction being about 65% (Fig. 13.12). For sufentanil, such a 'ceiling effect' does not appear to exist, at least for halothane in rats (Hecker et al, 1983). Although the mixed agonist–antagonists also reduce MAC, their effect is less marked, the maximum reduction being only 10–20% (Murphy & Hug, 1982b).

Considerable interest has been expressed in recent years in the possible modification by anaesthesia of the metabolic and endocrine responses to surgical trauma. This so-called stress response consists of increases in plasma concentrations of glucose, cortisol, catecholamines, antidiuretic hormone, lactate and other hormones and metabolites. These responses, part of the body's reaction to trauma, cause a catabolic state designed to stimulate and increase the healing process. This normal physiological response is of obvious benefit to the body when the injury is minor but the response to major surgery may be inappropriate. The profound and often prolonged reaction that results can have undesirable consequences. These include an increased heart work due to hypertension and tachycardia, and vasoconstriction resulting in tissue hypoxia and acidosis. Hormonal responses might depress both inflammatory and immune mechanisms, while excessive protein catabolism can impair tissue repair. The increase in stress hormones is related to the severity of the operative trauma, being much greater during intra-abdominal operations than with body surface procedures (Clarke et al, 1970). Increases in the plasma concentrations of stress hormones and metabolites occur during general anaesthesia with inhalation and intravenous agents. These responses are significantly modified, however, by moderate to high doses of opioids.

Morphine, even in small doses, inhibits ACTH release and blocks at least part of the pituitary-adrenal response to surgical stimulation. Morphine, 1 mg kg^{-1}, suppresses surgically induced increases in plasma cortisol but not human growth hormone during major abdominal surgery (George et al, 1974). Although morphine stimulates antidiuretic hormone (ADH) secretion in dogs and rats (Glariman, et al, 1953) it does not do so in man in the absence of surgical stimulation. Plasma ADH rises significantly during cardiac operations, before cardiopulmonary bypass, in patients anaesthetised with morphine 1 mg kg^{-1} plus nitrous oxide, and further increases occur during bypass (Philbin et al, 1976).

Fentanyl, 50 μ kg^{-1}, given as a supplement to nitrous oxide-oxygen anaesthesia, abolishes the hyperglycaemic response and reduces the cortisol and human growth hormone responses to prolonged microscopic tubal operations more than halothane–nitrous oxide–oxygen anaesthesia (Hall et al, 1978). Similar findings have been reported during gastric operations (Cooper et al, 1981) although a hyperglycaemic response still occurs during other upper abdominal operations (Haxholdt et al, 1981). However, suppression of the stress response is transient and does not compensate for the prolonged postoperative respiratory depression that may occur when doses of a magnitude great enough to effect stress responses are used (Cooper et al, 1981). High doses of fentanyl (50 μg kg^{-1}) are not effective in altering an established metabolic response during surgery (Bent et al. 1984).

High doses of fentanyl, sufentanil and alfentanil sufficient to produce anaesthesia prevent or significantly modify the endocrine changes and metabolic substrate mobilisation during the pre-bypass period of cardiac operations, although significant changes occur during and after bypass (Bovill et al, 1984a). The continued administration of fentanyl, 0.5 μg kg^{-1} hourly for 12–18 hrs after surgery also fails to prevent postoperative endocrine and metabolic responses (Walsh et al, 1981). The mechanism whereby opioids can minimize the endocrine and metabolic stress responses is unknown. It may be related to the resulting analgesia or to a specific effect due to interaction with opioid receptors. The hypothalamus and pituitary, which possess high concentrations of opioid receptors, play a major role in mediation of endocrine and metabolic responses to trauma. The naturally occurring opioid peptides are involved in the modulation of pituitary function by varying dopamine turnover (Gudelsky & Porter, 1979) and it is likely that the interaction of opioid drugs with receptors in that region thereby modifies stress responses. It is known that opioid-peptides stimulate prolactin secretion (Shaar et al, 1977; Rivier et al, 1977), an action that is antagonised by naloxone (Shaar et al, 1977). The release of prolactin from the anterior pituitary is tonically inhibited by tubero-infundibular dopaminergic neurones (Gudelsky & Porter, 1979).

It is of interest that prolactin is the only hormone that significantly increases during anaesthesia with fentanyl or sufentanil (Bovill et al, 1984a). There is experimental evidence that hyperprolactinaemia may be an overt physiological response to stimulation of the the μ_1 sub-type of opioid receptor (Pasternak et al, 1983). Meptazinol, a selective, μ_1 agonist, causes greater elevation of prolactin in postoperative patients than morphine and there is a significant correlation between plasma prolactin and meptazinol concentrations (Kay et al, 1985).

NEUROLEPTANALGESIA

The term neuroleptanalgesia is used to describe the state produced by a combination of potent analgesics, usually fentanyl or phenoperidine, and a tranquilliser or neuroleptic such as droperidol. It is characterized by analgesia, apparent indifference to the surroundings, absence of clinically apparent motor activity, suppression of autonomic reflexes and maintenance of cardiovascular stability. The immediate predecessor of neuroleptanalgesia was the state of "ganglioplegia" or "neuroplegia" (artificial hibernation) induced by a 'lytic cocktail' consisting of chlorpromazine, promethazine and pethidine. This technique of artificial hibernation was associated with considerable cardiovascular instability and frequently with prolonged depression of consciousness. The introduction of droperidol allowed the same degree of neuroleptic activity to be achieved without the unwanted side effects of the haemodynamic instability and prolonged unconsciousness produced by the phenothiazines.

In animals droperidol fulfils the pharmacological profile for neuroleptic activity, viz.

a) Inhibition of motor activity, including both spontaneous movement and learned responses. A state of catalepsy can readily be induced.
b) Antagonism of apomorphine-induced vomiting.
c) Antagonism of amphetamine-induced arousal.

Droperidol is considerably safer than chlorpromazine, the therapeutic ratio being 300 times as great (Shephard, 1964).

The central nervous effects of neuroleptic drugs depend on their ability to decrease the membrane permeability of specific cells excited by dopamine, noradrenaline and 5-hydroxytryptamine (Seeman & Baily, 1963). The permeability of these post-synaptic membranes is regulated by the competitive inhibition of glutamic acid by gamma-aminobutyric acid (GABA). There is a structural similarity between the butyrophenones and GABA. By occupying post-synaptic GABA receptors, neuroleptic drugs decrease synaptic transmission, and inhibit dopamine uptake. Re-uptake of dopamine and noradrenaline into storage granules of the presynaptic terminals also is inhibited (Janssen, 1967). The butyrophenones are also specific dopamine antagonists (Yeh et al, 1969). Neuroleptic drugs are selectively sequestrated in those areas of the brain known to be rich in dopaminergic synapses, particularly those of the chemoreceptor trigger zone (CTZ) and the extrapyramidal motor system related to "operant" (non-Pavlovian, learned) behaviour (Hillarp et al, 1966). Dopamine blockade at the latter in site may be responsible for the extrapyramidal dyskinesia that occurs in a small percentage of patients given small doses of droperidol. This dyskinesia can vary from minor degrees of hypertonus to typical Parkinsonian crises. The onset of severe Parkinsonian rigidity in a patient on levodopa therapy after administration of droperidol has been reported (Wiklund & Ngai, 1971). The incidence of dyskinesia is reduced when droperidol is given concomitantly with an opioid (Morrison, 1970). Such side effects, when they do occur and are troublesome, will respond to atropine, promethazine or other anti-Parkinson therapy with the important exception of levodopa.

In some patients given droperidol alone, e.g., for premedication, the outwardly calm manifestation of the neuroleptic state can mask considerable inner anxiety and discomfort, with hallucinations and bizzare feelings of body transference (Morrison et al, 1970). The patient is usually unable to communicate these feelings at the time but later may be able to recall the unpleasantness of the experience. On occasion erratic behaviour may occur and unwarranted demands by a patient to cancel the operation have been reported after premedication with droperidol (Lee & Yeakel, 1975). This has also been seen with droperidol-nalbuphine.

Droperidol is a potent antiemetic, due to its dopaminergic blockade at the CTZ. It is, however, without effect on vomiting of labyrinthine origin and is thus ineffective for the treatment of motion sickness. The antiemetic effect is particularly useful when droperidol is used in combination with opioids. Very low doses (0.25 mg) are as, or even more effective, as the customary 2.5–5 mg and lack the dyskinetic side-effects associated with the latter (Shelley & Brown, 1978).

Droperidol causes minimal haemodynamic changes in adult volunteers and patients given intravenous doses of 5–20 mg. Transient hypotension can occur associated with a decrease in systemic vascular resistance and an increase in cardiac output (McDonald et al, 1966). Similar changes have been observed when it is given together with other drugs including morphine (Stanley et al, 1976), fentanyl (Stoelting et al, 1975) or inhalation anaesthetics (Stanley, 1978). The hypotension and decrease in vascular resistance probably are due to the combination of central nervous effects and blockade of alpha-adrenoreceptors in vascular smooth muscle (Muldoon et al, 1977). Although the peripheral vascular effects are usually small and transient, profound and dangerous falls in vascular resistance can occur in patients already receiving other vasodilator therapy or in hypovolaemic patients.

Droperidol has antiarrhythmic properties. It increases the threshold for adrenaline-induced arrhythmias during anaesthesia with halothane, cyclopropane or chloroform (Bertolo et al, 1972) and during dental surgery (Whalley et al, 1976). Droperidol has local anaesthetic properties and may stabilise excitable membranes of myocardial cells. Another possible mechanism can be a blood pressure lowering effect on pressure-sensitive arrhythmias (Bertolo et al, 1972).

A commercially available mixture of droperidol and fentanyl (Thalamonal: Innovar), containing 50 μg fentanyl and 2.5 mg droperidol per ml, once gained widespread popularity. Although both drugs have similar elimination half-lives (Cressman et al, 1973), clinical experience has shown that the duration of action of droperidol is considerably longer than that of fentanyl. In the doses commonly used in neuroleptanalgesia, fentanyl (3–5 $\mu g\ kg^{-1}$) has a duration of action of 30–60 min, whereas that of droperidol lasts up to 24 h. On this basis the use of fixed-dose combination is pharmacologically irrational since, although the combinations may provide correct proportions at the first dose, supplementary doses will produce an overdosage of droperidol.

Few anaesthetists now use the classical techniques of pure neuroleptanalgesia, such as described by Nilsson and Janssen (1961). They gave large doses of phenoperidine (up to 20 mg) and droperidol (up to 50 mg) as an infusion to patients premedicated with droperidol 10 mg. Subjects were curarised and the lungs ventilated with air. At the end of the operation respiratory depression was reversed with nalorphine or levallorphan. Today neuroleptanalgesia is more commonly used as the principal component of a balanced anaesthetic technique, which usually employs nitrous oxide and when used in this way, it is associated with intraoperative cardiovascular stability and smooth recovery from anaesthesia. Patients awaken quickly, are cooperative and have a low incidence of emetic symptoms. When used as part of balanced anaesthesias. Thalamonal (Innovar) in doses of 2–4 ml can be given during induction of anaesthesia. If analgesic supplements are indicated during the operation, fentanyl or alfentanil alone should be given rather than additional Thalamonal.

TOTAL INTRAVENOUS ANAESTHESIA

Intravenous infusions of an opioid, often fentanyl, and an hypnotic have been used for maintenance of anaesthesia. Although the term "total intravenous anaesthesia" is often used to describe this technique, it is frequently combined with nitrous oxide or sometimes low concentrations of an inhalation agent, e.g. enflurane. The majority of reports have been of studies using combinations of an opioid with Althesin. (See Chapter 17)

Techniques

Several authors have described total intravenous anaesthesia with etomidate and fentanyl, both for patients breathing spontaneously and those given a muscle relaxant whose lungs were ventilated with oxygen–air mixtures. [Some of these are discussed more fully in Chapter 16.] Lees and colleagues (1981) infused a solution of etomidate 2.5 mg ml^{-1} and fentanyl 7 $\mu g\ ml^{-1}$ to maintain anaesthesia after induction with thiopentone for patients undergoing a wide variety of procedures. The initial infusion rate was 3–4 ml min^{-1} for 2–3 min. after which it was decreased and adjusted according to the patients response to surgical stimulation. The mean total doses were etomidate 20 $\mu g\ kg^{-1}\ min^{-1}$ and fentanyl 0.05 $\mu g\ kg^{-1}\ min^{-1}$. This technique provided satisfactory maintenance of anaesthesia with cardiovascular stability comparable, or superior to, that obtained with halothane. The authors found, however, that the use of a fixed ratio of the two drugs did not allow titration of analgesia and hypnosis in individual patients. They subsequently used separate infusions of etomidate and fentanyl and found that this allowed greater flexibility and greatly decreased the incidence of prolonged recovery that sometimes occurred when using the "fixed dose–ratio" technique (Lees & Antonios, 1984). Intravenous anaesthesia with fixed dose–ratio etomidate-fentanyl infusion has also been described for use in general and gynaecological operations (Jones et al, 1983). These authors used a 'two-step' infusion technique, where etomidate 100 $\mu g\ kg^{-1}\ min^{-1}$ with fentanyl 1 $\mu g\ kg^{-1}\ min^{-1}$ was infused for 10 min, followed by a maintenance dose at a rate of one-tenth this amount. This was sufficient for three quarters of the patients, whereas the remainder needed dose-rate adjustments during operation. Recovery times were less than 10 min in half of the patients.

Other opioid-hypnotic combinations that have been described for total intravenous analgesia include propofol-fentanyl (Major et al, 1982), midazolam–fentanyl (Holmes & Galletly, 1982) and midazolam–alfentanil (de Castro et al, 1981). The combination of midazolam, a water-soluble benzodiazepine, and alfentanil is an interesting and promising one. Both drugs have short half-lives; that of midazolam ranges from 1 to 4 hours, with an average of about 2.5 hours (Table 12.4), and alfentanil has a half-life of about 1.5 hours (Bovill et al, 1982b; Bower and Hull, 1982). The concurrent administration of opioids and benzodiazepines tends to potentiate and prolong the duration of respiratory depression produced by the opioid (Bailey et al, 1984). The authors clinical experience suggests that opioids, including alfentanil, also potentiate and prolong the action of the benzodiazepine, and considerable experience is required to avoid prolonged recovery with combined infusion of midazolam and alfentanil. The possible availability of a specific benzodiazepine antagonist, RO 15–1788, may revolutionise the use of midazolam-opioid combinations. RO 15–1788 rapidly (30–50 sec) awakens subjects receiving a continuous infusion of midazolam, with full orientation returning within 5 min (Lauven et al, 1982).

Intravenous infusions of alfentanil alone have also been used as a supplement to nitrous oxide anaesthesia. A constant infusion rate of 20 $\mu g\ kg^{-1}\ hr^{-1}$ failed to provide satisfactory anaesthesia for patients undergoing body surface operations and supplementation with 0.5% halothane was needed (Andrews et al, 1983). Increasing the infusion rate to 50 or 100 $\mu g\ kg^{-1}\ hr^{-1}$ resulted in satisfactory conditions. With these doses no difficulty was experienced in establishing spontaneous ventilation after reversal of neuromuscular blockade (O'Connor et al, 1983). In this study the alfentanil infusion was continued for 2 hr after operation at a rate of 20 $\mu g\ kg^{-1}\ hr^{-1}$. This provided adequate postoperative pain relief with only moderate effects on minute volume or $PaCO_2$. The carbon dioxide responsiveness was reduced, however, to 50% of the preoperative value.

The use of fixed infusion rates to maintain anaesthesia is illogical (Chapter 17) and is unlikely to provide optimum conditions, particularly during intra-abdominal operations where stimuli of widely varying intensity are encountered. Among the advantages of alfentanil for total intravenous anaesthesia are its rapid onset of action and its short elimination half-life. It would seem, therefore, more logical to adjust the infusion rate to maintain the depth of anaesthesia appropriate to the particular phase of the operation and according to the patients responses to intraoperative events in a manner similar to the adjustments made by an anaesthetist to a halothane vaporizer (Ausems et al, 1983). Ausems and Hug (1983) attempted to define the minimum alfentanil plasma concentration needed to suppress responses of patients to different types of noxious stimuli during lower abdominal operations. Anaesthesia was induced with alfentanil 150 $\mu g\ kg^{-1}$ followed by an initial infusion of alfentanil 50 $\mu g\ kg^{-1}\ hr^{-1}$. The patients lungs were ventilated with 66% nitrous oxide in oxygen. Infusion rates were adjusted during operation between 25 and 150 $\mu g\ kg^{-1}\ hr^{-1}$ and bolus doses of alfentanil, 77 $\mu g\ kg^{-1}$, were given to suppress rapidly any responses indicating inadequate anaesthesia. On the basis of frequently measured plasma alfentanil concentrations, the authors were able to construct concentration response curves for various intraoperative stimuli (Fig. 13.11). By continually adjusting the infusion rate to meet the needs of the patient prolonged recovery resulting from excessive accumulations of drug is prevented.

Cardiac operations

Total intravenous anaesthesia with high doses of opioids is a technique which has recently gained extensive popularity, particularly among cardiac anaesthetists. This technique developed in the 1960s from the observation of Lowenstein and his colleagues in Boston, that patients requiring artificial ventilation after cardiac operations could tolerate intravenous doses of morphine for sedation, exceeding any previously reported in the literature, without detectable circulatory deterioration. This observation led them to administer equivalent doses of morphine as the anaesthetic for these patients. Publication of their results (Lowenstein et al, 1969) stimulated considerable interest and research and today high-dose opioid anaesthesia is extensively used, alone or in combination with other drugs, in cardiac anaesthesia. It soon became apparent, however, that whereas morphine in the doses described by Lowenstein (0.5–3 mg kg^{-1}) was adequate for critically ill patients who often had end-stage valvular heart disease, in other less critically ill patients it did have serious disadvantages. Many problems were reported, including sporadic episodes of incomplete amnesia, occasional histamine-related reactions (cutaneous flushing, hypotension, bronchospasm), hypertension and tachycardia during periods of maximum surgical stimulation and increased intra- and postoperative blood and fluid requirements (Lowenstein, 1971). Attempts to overcome these problems by increasing the dose of morphine were only partially successful, least so in patients undergoing coronary artery operations. These patients, who did not have a history of chronic heart failure and were often relatively young and fit, sometimes were extremely resistant to morphine. Stanley and colleagues (1973) reported requirements of 8–11 mg kg^{-1} and doses of this nature produced further problems. Excessive volumes of blood and fluids were needed to maintain adequate cardiac filling pressures and patients were described as plum-coloured with generalised oedema on return to the intensive care unit. Prolonged respiratory depression was another unacceptable side-effect following large doses of morphine.

A variety of supplements were used in an effort to reduce the incidence of awareness, to control hypertension and reduce the total dose of morphine required and thereby attenuate the extent of postoperative respiratory depression, the most commonly used being nitrous oxide and diazepam. Although by themselves these drugs cause minimal haemodynamic changes, when combined with high-dose morphine they result in significant myocardial depression, with decreases in cardiac output and fall in arterial blood pressure (Stoelting & Gibbs, 1973; Stanley et al, 1976). The addition of halothane after large doses of morphine also produces marked cardiovascular depression in patients with coronary artery disease (Stoelting et al, 1974).

Because of the above problems, several alternative opioids were investigated. Both pethidine and alphaprodine, a methyl-substituted derivative of the reversed ester of pethidine, were studied but caused significant hypotension, tachycardia and marked myocardial depression in anaesthetic doses (Stanley & Liu, 1977; Reddy et al, 1980). Hydromorphone, a hydrogenated ketone derivative of morphine that is 7–10 times as potent and 8–10 times as lipid soluble as morphine has been investigated recently (Welti et al, 1984). Like morphine, hydromorphone did not reliably induce anaesthesia in patients undergoing coronary operations and supplementation with nitrous oxide and halothane were necessary for unconsciousness and complete suppression of sympathetic responses.

Fentanyl, sufentanil and alfentanil have proved to be the most reliable and effective opioids for producing anaesthesia. The use of fentanyl as a total anaesthetic was first reported by Stanley and Webster (1978). They induced anaesthesia in patients undergoing mitral valve replacement operations with fentanyl, 50 $\mu g\ kg^{-1}$, and gave additional fentanyl as needed. The average total dose of fentanyl, 74 $\mu g\ kg^{-1}$, provided complete anaesthesia with minimal haemodynamic disturbances. In a subsequent study involving coronary artery operations, the same group used a total dose of 75 $\mu g\ kg^{-1}$ fentanyl (Lunn et al, 1979). Since then extensive investigations and reports on the use fentanyl in cardiac operations have appeared in the anaesthetic literature. These have been reviewed recently (Bovill et al, 1984a). A major advantage of fentanyl as an anaesthetic for cardiac patients is the cardiovascular stability during induction. In doses of 75 $\mu g\ kg^{-1}$, fentanyl maintains arterial blood pressure, pulmonary capillary wedge pressure, and cardiac index during induction and intubation within the range of control values and preserves the left ventricular ejection fraction, as measured using technetium 99m-labelled red cells and a left ventricular nuclear probe (Barash & Kopriva, 1982). In a subsequent study with a similar group of patients, Barash and colleagues (1982) found 30 μg kg^{-1} fentanyl to be as effective as 75 μg kg^{-1}. The favourable induction properties of fentanyl are due to an absence of histamine release and lack of myocardial depression.

During cardiac operations the doses of fentanyl recommended by Stanley and colleagues have generally been found to be inadequate by other anaesthetists. Waller and colleagues (1981) reported that fentanyl, 50–89 μg kg^{-1}, failed to block the haemodynamic responses to sternotomy in 8 of their 12 patients undergoing elective coronary artery surgery.

Post-sternotomy hypertension is common in patients with coronary artery disease and, in an attempt to prevent it, the recommended doses of fentanyl have steadily increased. Doses of 150 μg kg^{-1} are often given. While doses of this magnitude can provide cardiovascular stability throughout the operation (Zurick et al, 1982), their use can be associated with an unacceptable prolongation of postoperative respiratory depression.

Even with very high doses of fentanyl, total amnesia for the surgical procedure cannot be guaranteed. Two of 10 patients given fentanyl 150μg kg^{-1} could recall sternotomy (Zurick et al, 1982). Other sporadic reports of recall during fentanyl anaesthesia have appeared in the literature. With one exception (Sprigge et al, 1982), they have been associated with non-benzodiazepine premedication. Although the occasional reports of recall have led some to question whether fentanyl (and other opioids) can produce true anaesthesia, the incidence remains considerably less than that reported during general anaesthesia. The electroencephalographic changes produced by high doses of fentanyl and other opioids are certainly consistent with anaesthesia (Sebel et al, 1981; Bovill et al, 1982a; Smith et al, 1984).

Many anaesthetists give fentanyl as a bolus at induction followed by repeated boli as indicated during operations. However, it is pharmacokinetically more logical and efficient if it is administered by continuous infusion. Several such infusion schemes have been described (Sprigge et al, 1982; Wynands et al, 1983a). Basically a loading dose of fentanyl, 30–50 μg kg^{-1}, is followed by an infusion of fentanyl 0.3–0.5 μg kg^{-1} min^{-1} until the start of rewarming on cardiopulmonary bypass or until a predetermined total dose has been given. With these infusion schemes relatively stable plasma concentrations are achieved and they have provided useful information about the steady-state concentrations needed to suppress responses to surgical stimuli. When plasma fentanyl concentrations are 15 ng ml^{-1} or less, 50% of patients will have a hypertensive response to sternotomy (Wynands et al, 1983b). With plasma concentrations above 20 ng ml^{-1}, only 33% develop hypertension at sternotomy (Wynands et al, 1984). Plasma fentanyl concentrations of 20–25 ng ml^{-1} produce optimum anaesthesia for abdominal hysterectomy (Hengstmann et al, 1980).

Supplements

Diazepam is often used as a supplement to fentanyl anaesthesia to ensure amnesia. However, as with morphine, giving diazepam to patients anaesthetised with fentanyl can cause a profound fall in blood pressure and decrease in systemic vascular resistance and cardiac output (Stanley & Webster, 1978; Tomicheck et al, 1983). Neither fentanyl nor diazepam, when given alone, produce important haemodynamic depression. Tomichek and colleagues (1983) found that when fentanyl, 50 μg kg^{-1}, was given after doses of diazepam from 0.125 to 0.5 μg kg^{-1}, plasma concentrations of adrenaline and noradrenaline decreased significantly compared to a control group who received fentanyl only. Urinary levels of adrenaline and noradrenaline have been reported to decrease after anaesthesia with diazepam and fentanyl (Liu et al, 1977). Reduction in plasma catecholamine levels could explain the observed cardiovascular changes. However, in the study by Tomichek, pulmonary capillary wedge pressure did not change, despite a decrease in cardiac output and systemic vascular resistance. This suggests that the diazepam–fentanyl combination caused myocardial depression. In the isolated rat heart preparation, both fentanyl and diazepam have a negative inotropic effect and the combination of the two drugs produces an additive, and not a supraadditive, negative inotropic effect

(Reeves et al, 1984). In this study, however, negative inotropic effects occured at concentrations very considerably in excess of those encountered in patients. This would suggest, therefore, that the haemodynamic changes caused by diazepam and fentanyl in combination are not likely to be the result of significant myocardial depression. The use of midazolam, used in some centres as an alternative to diazepam, results in similar interactions with opioids (Heikkilä et al, 1984).

Addition of nitrous oxide to the inspiratory gas in patients who have been given large doses of fentanyl produces haemodynamic changes similar to those described above with diazepam. Nitrous oxide alone causes myocardial depression in normal volunteers (Eisele & Smith, 1972) and in patients with coronary artery disease (Eisele et al, 1976). In the dog, the myocardial depressant effects of nitrous oxide and fentanyl are additive (Motomura et al, 1984). In patients undergoing coronary artery operations in whom anaesthesia was induced with fentanyl 50 $\mu g\ kg^{-1}$, while breathing 100% oxygen, ventilation with 50% nitrous oxide in oxygen resulted in a significant decrease in cardiac index, an increase in systemic vascular resistance and no change in mean arterial blood pressure in patients with poor left ventricular function. In a similar group of patients with good left ventricular function the addition of nitrous oxide produced no significant haemodynamic changes (Balasaraswathi et al, 1981). The detrimental effect of nitrous oxide in combination with both enflurane and fentany on ventricular function in patients with coronary artery disease has been demonstrated by others (Fig. 13.16) (Moffitt et al, 1984). This has also been confirmed in dogs with coronary constriction anaesthetised with fentanyl (Philbin et al, 1983) or sufentanil (Philbin et al, 1984).

It has been suggested that the reduction in inspired oxygen concentration when nitrous oxide–oxygen is substituted for 100% oxygen in the inspired gas may be partially responsible for the above changes, although the evidence is conflicting. In one study, either 70% nitrous oxide or 70% nitrogen were randomly added 15 min after induction of anaesthesia with fentanyl 100 $\mu g\ kg^{-1}$ and ventilation with 100% oxygen (Michiels et al, 1982). Both resulted in significant reductions in blood pressure and statistical analysis revealed that 50% of the reduction caused by nitrous oxide could be attributed to the reduction in F_IO_2. Conversely, changing the inspired gas mixture from 100% oxygen to 60% helium after administration of fentanyl 75 $\mu g\ kg^{-1}$ produces no significant haemodynamic effects in

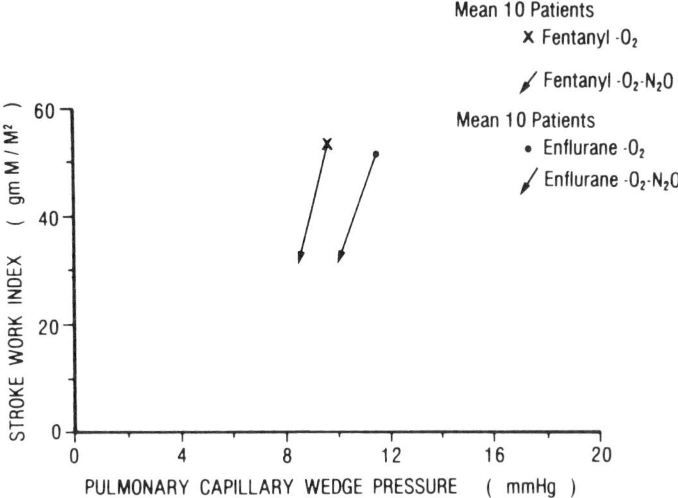

Fig. 13.16 Detrimental effect of nitrous oxide on ventricular function during enflurane or fentanyl anaesthesia. The decrease in stroke work index with little change in wedge pressure indicates depressed left ventricular function. (From Moffitt et al, 1984).

cardiac surgical patients (Lunn et al, 1979). However, when the same patients were ventilated with 60% nitrous oxide, cardiac output decreased by 33% with significant increases in systemic vascular resistance and central venous pressure.

Newer opioids

Sufentanil and alfentanil, the two most recent additions to the fentanyl family, have both been used successfully for cardiac anaesthesia. Although they have different pharmacokinetic properties, both have a faster onset of action than fentanyl (de Lange et al, 1982; Nauta et al, 1982). In ventilated dogs sufentanil in doses up to 3700 $\mu g\ kg^{-1}$ were associated with only minimal changes in cardiovascular parameters (Reddy et al, 1980). Doses of sufentanil (15–30 $\mu g\ kg^{-1}$) have been adminstered to adult patients undergoing a variety of cardiac operations, mainly coronary artery surgery (Sebel and Bovill, 1982; de Lange et al, 1982). With the higher doses, cardiovascular stability during operation appears to be superior to that occurring with fentanyl although post-sternotomy hypertension still occurs in 16% of patients (Griesemer et al, 1982). The elimination half-life of sufentanil is shorter than that of fentanyl (Bovill et al, 1984b) and recovery therefore is more rapid than after equivalent or smaller doses of fentanyl (Table 13.4) (de Lange et al, 1982; Smith et al, Smith et al, 1982).

Alfentanil, because of its rapid elimination, is usually given by continuous infusion. Anaesthesia is induced with alfentanil 100–150 $\mu g\ kg^{-1}$ followed by an infusion at a rate between 5–8 $\mu g\ kg^{-1}\ min^{-1}$ (Sebel et al, 1982). The infusion rate can be adjusted to control haemodynamic reactions to surgical stimuli. When this is not adequate, or not rapid enough, control can usually be achieved by additional 2.5–5 mg alfentanil. Because of the rapid onset of effect with alfentanil, cardiovascular control is superior to that with fentanyl, despite the fact that, experimentally, alfentanil appears to be less efficient at supressing reflex haemodynamic responses to neural stimulation (Askitopoulou et al, 1983). There have been no controlled studies comparing fentanyl, sufentanil and alfentanil as anaesthetics for coronary artery operations. In patients undergoing valve replacement they appear to be equally effective, although sufentanil tends to produce more hypotension during induction (Bovill et al, 1984c). Both sufentanil and alfentanil are superior to fentanyl in reducing the incidence and severity of post-sternotomy hypertension in patients with aortic valve disease.

Paediatrics

Fentanyl and sufentanil anaesthesia has been used also in cardiac operations in children. Robinson and Gregory (1981) gave fentanyl 30–50 $\mu g\ kg^{-1}$ as the sole anaesthetic for transthoracic ligation of patent ductus arteriosus in preterm infants with an average weight of 1123 g. The fentanyl was given over 1 min and the infants were ventilated with oxygen–air. Blood pressure and heart rate decreased by only 5% during induction and thereafter remained stable. Although the infants were electively ventilated for 24 hr postoperatively, they were reported as being awake within 1 hr of the end of the procedure which averaged 47 min.

Table 13.4 Induction and recovery characteristics of morphine, fentanyl and sufentanil in cardiac surgical patients. Approximately equipotent dilutions of each drug were infused at a standard rate. (Data from Smith et al, 1982).

	Morphine	*Fentanyl*	*Sufentanil*
Total dose ($\mu g\ kg^{-1}$)	4400 ± 2100	95 ± 30.0	19 ± 6.5
Time to unconsciousness (min)	15 ± 6.9*	6 ± 2.2.+	3 ± 0.7X
Duration of surgery (h)	5.7 ± 0.9	5.3 ± 1.7	5.9 ± 1.3
Postoperative time to:			
Respond to commands (h)	3.0 ± 2.1*	2.3 ± 1.6	0.6 ± 0.5#X
Adequate spontaneous ventilation (h)	13.1 ± 5.5	9.7 ± 3.3	5.6 ± 3.2#X
Tracheal extubation (h)	18.7 ± 3.1	16.8 ± 3.9	8.9 ± 3.4#X

Values are mean ± SD * = $p < 0.05$ for MvFvS: # = $p < 0.05$ for FvS: + = $p < 0.05$ for MvF: X = $p < 0.05$ for MvS

The safety and efficacy of fentanyl-oxygen (50 and 75 $\mu g\ kg^{-1}$) and sufentanil–oxygen (5 and 10 $\mu g\ kg^{-1}$) have been compared in 40 older infants, average age 8 months and weight 6 kg, undergoing repair of complex congenital heart defects (Hickey & Hansen, 1984). Half of the infants were in compensated congestive heart failure. Fentanyl or sufentanil was given over a period of 5–10 min and caused small but statistically significant decreases in heart rate and falls in diastolic blood pressure, that returned to control values with skin incision and sternotomy. Systolic blood pressure increased after sternotomy in some patients and required nitrous oxide. No significant differences were found between the two opioids although sufentanil was thought to be more effective in blocking haemodynamic response to surgical stimuli. In contrast, Moore and colleagues (1985) found sufentanil in doses up to 20 $\mu g\ kg^{-1}$ a less satisfactory anaesthetic for children aged between 4 and 12 yr undergoing cardiac operations. Significant haemodynamic changes occured during tracheal intubation and to a lesser extent in response to skin incision and sternotomy. All children awakened within 1–2 h after operation although extubation was not possible for 19–24 hrs. One patient, who received 5 $\mu g\ kg^{-1}$ sufentanil, appeared to be aware of the sternotomy.

REFERENCES

Adams A P, Pybus D A 1978 Delayed respiratory depression after use of fentanyl during anaesthesia. British Medical Journal i: 278–279

Andree R A 1980 Sudden death following naloxone administration. Anesthesia and Analgesia 59: 782–784

Andrews C J H, Sinclair M, Prys-Roberts C, Dye A 1983 Ventilatory effects during and after continuous infusion of fentanyl or alfentanil. British Journal of Anaesthesia 55 (Supplement 2): 211S–216S

Askitopoulou H, Whitwam J G, Al-Khudhairi D, Chakrabarti M K, Bower S, Hull C J 1985 Acute tolerance to fentanyl during anesthesia in dogs. Anesthesiology 63: 255–261

Askitopoulou H, Whitwam J G, Sapsed S, Chakrabarti M K 1983 Dissociation between the effects of fentanyl and alfentanil on spontaneous and reflexly evoked cardiovascular responses in the dog. British Journal of Anaesthesia 55: 155–161

Atweh S F, Kuhar M J 1977 Autoradiographic localization of opiate receptors in rat brain. I. Spinal cord and lower medulla. Brain Research 124: 53–67

Ausems M E, Hug C C 1983 Plasma concentrations of alfentanil required to supplement nitrous oxide anaesthesia for lower abdominal surgery. British Journal of Anaesthesia 55: 191S–197S

Ausems M E, Hug C C, de Lange S 1983 Variable rate infusion of alfentanil as a supplement to nitrous oxide anesthesia for general surgery. Anesthesia and Analgesia 62: 982–986

Azar I, Turndorf H 1979 Severe hypertension and multiple atrial premature contractions following naloxone administration. Anesthesia and Analgesia 58: 524–525

Azar I, Patel A K, Phau C Q 1981 Cardiovascular responses following naloxone administration during enflurane anesthesia. Anesthesia and Analgesia 60: 237–238

Bailey P L, Andriano K P, Pace N L, Westenskow D R, Stanley T H 1984 Small doses of diazepam potentiate and prolong fentanyl induced respiratory depression. Anesthesia and Analgesia 63:183

Balasaraswathi K, Kumar P, Rao T L K, El-Etr A A 1981 Left-ventricular end-diastolic pressure (LVEDP) as an index for nitrous oxide use during coronary artery surgery. Anesthesiology 55: 708–709

Barash P G, Kopriva C J 1982 Narcotics and the circulation. In: Kitahata L M, Collins J G (eds); Narcotic Analgesics in Anesthesiology. Baltimore, Williams and Wilkins, pp. 91–132

Barash P G, Giles R, Marx P, Berger H, Zaret B 1982 Intubation: Is low dose fentanyl really effective? Anaesthesia and Analgesia 61: S168–169

Becker L D, Paulson B A, Muller R D, Severinghaus J W, Eger E G 1976 Biphasic respiratory depression after fentanyl–droperidol or fentanyl alone used to supplement nitrous oxide anesthesia. Anesthesiology 44: 291–296

Bent J M, Paterson J L, Mashiter K, Hall G M 1984 Effects of high-dose fentanyl anaesthesia on the established metabolic and endocrine response to surgery. Anaesthesia 39: 19–23

Bentley J B, Borel J D, Nenad R E 1982 Influence of age on the pharmacokinetics of fentanyl. Anesthesia and Analgesia 61: 171–172

Bernard C 1869 Des effects physiologiques de la morphine et de leur combination avec ceux du chloroform. Bulletin General de Therapeutique 77:241

Berthelsen P, Eriksen J, Ahn N C, Rasmussen J P 1980 Peripheral circulation during sufentanyl and morphine anesthesia. Acta Anaesthesiologica Scandinavica 24: 241–244

Berthelsen P, Eriksen J, Ahn N C, Rasmussen J P 1981 Skeletal muscle circulation during sufentanyl and morphine anesthesia in propranolol treated dogs. Acta Anaesthesiologica Scandinavica 25: 6–8

Bertolo L, Novakovic L, Penna M 1972 Antiarrhythmic effects of droperidol. Anesthesiology 37: 529–535

Van Bever W F M, Niemegeers C J E, Schellekens K H L, Janssen P A J 1976 N-4-Substituted 1-(2-arylethyl)-4-piperidinyl-N-phenylpropanamides, a novel series of extremely potent analgesics with unusually high safety margin. Arzneimittel-Forschung 26: 1548–1551

Black T E, Kay B, Healey T E J 1984 Reducing the haemodynamic responses to laryngoscopy and intubation:

A comparison of alfentanil and fentanyl. Anaesthesia 39: 883–887
Boas R A, Villiger J W 1985 Clinical actions of fentanyl and buprenorphine: the significance of receptor binding. British Journal of Anaesthesia 57: 192–196
Bovill J G, Sebel P S 1980 Pharmacokinetics of high-dose fentanyl: A study in patients undergoing cardiac surgery. British Journal of Anaesthesia 52: 795–801
Bovill J G, Sebel P S, Wauquier A, Rog P 1982a Electroencephalographic effects of sufentanil anaesthesia in man. British Journal of Anaesthesia 54: 45–52
Bovill J G, Sebel P S, Blackburn C L, Heykants J 1982b The pharmacokinetics of alfentanil (R 39209): A new opioid analgesic. Anesthesiology 57: 439–443
Bovill J G, Sebel P C, Wauquier A, Rog P, Schuyt C 1983 Influence of high-dose alfentanil anaesthesia on the electroencephalogram: Correlation with plasma concentrations. British Journal of Anaesthesia 55 (Suppl 2): 199–209
Bovill J G, Sebel P S, Stanley T H 1984a Opioid analgesics in anesthesia: With special reference to their use in cardiovascular anesthesia. Anesthesiology 61: 731–755
Bovill J G, Sebel P S, Blackburn C L, Oei-Lim V, Heykants J J 1984b The pharmacokinetics of sufentanil in surgical patients. Anesthesiology 61: 502–506
Bovill J G, Warren P J, Schuller J L, van Wezel H B, Hoeneveld M H 1984c Comparsion of fentanyl, sufentanil and alfentanil anesthesia in patients undergoing valvular heart surgery. Anesthesia and Analgesia 63: 1081–1086
Bowen W D, Gentelman S, Herkenham M, Pert C B 1981 Interconverting μ and δ forms of the opiate receptor in rat striatal patches. Proceedings of the National Academy of Science, USA 78:4818
Bower S, Hull C J 1982 Comparative pharmacokinetics of fentanyl and alfentanil. British Journal of Anaesthesia 54: 871–877
Brown J H, Pleuvry B J, Kay B 1980 Respiratory effects of a new opiate analgesic R 39 209, in the rabbit: comparison with fentanyl. British Journal of Anaesthesia 52: 1101–1106
Budd K 1981 High dose buprenorphine for postoperative analgesia. Anaesthesia 36: 900–903
Bullingham H E S, McQuay H J, Moore R A, Bennnett M R D 1980 Buprenorphine kinetics. Clinical Pharmacology and Therapeutics 28: 667–672
Bullingham R E S, McQuay H J, Porter E J, Allen M C, Moore R A 1982 Sublingual buprenorphine used postoperatively: Ten hour plasma drug concentration analysis. British Journal of Clinical Pharmacology 13: 665–673
Bullingham R E S, McQuay H J, Moore R A 1983 Clinical pharmacokinetics of narcotic agonist–antagonist drugs. Clinical Pharmacokinetics 8: 332–343
Carlsson C, Smith D S, Keykhah M, Englebach I, Harp J R 1982 The effects of high-dose fentanyl on cerebral circulation and metabolism in rats. Anesthesiology 57: 375–380
de Castro J, Viars P 1968 Anesthésie analgésique séquentielle ou ASA. Ars. Med. 23: 121–128
de Castro J, van de Water A, Wouters L, Xhonneux R, Reneman R, Kay B 1979 Comparative study of cardiovascular, neurological and metabolic side-effects of eight narcotics in dogs. Acta Anaesthesiologica Belgica 30: 5–99
de Castro P J, Andrieu A, van Heuneghem L 1981 Etude du midazolam comme inducteur, correcteur et potentialisateur d'une anesthesie analgesique a base d'alfentanil. Arzneimittel-Forschung 31: 2251–2254
Chestnutt W N, Dundee J W 1986 The influence of cyclizine and perphenazine on the emetic effect of meptazinol. European Journal of Anaesthesiology 3: 27–32
Christian C M, Waller J L, Moldenhauer O C 1983 Postoperative rigidity following fentanyl anesthesia. Anesthesiology 58: 275–277
Clarke R S J, Johnston H, Sheridan B 1970 The influence of anaesthesia and surgery on plasma cortisol, insulin and free fatty acids. British Journal of Anaesthesia 42: 295–299
Collier H O J 1968 Supersensitivity and dependence. Nature 220: 228–231
Colpaert F C, Niemegeers C J, Janssen P A J, Maroli A N 1980 The effects of prior fentanyl administration and of pain on fentanyl analgesia: Tolerance to and enhancement of narcotic analgesia. Journal of Pharmacology and Experimental Therapeutics 213: 418–424
Cookson R J 1983 Carfentanil and lofentanil. Clinics in Anaesthesiology 1: 156–158
Cooper G M, Patterson J, Ward L D, Hall G M 1981 Fentanyl and the metabolic response to gastric surgery. Anaesthesia 36: 667–671
Corssen G, Domino E F, Sweet R B 1964 Neuroleptanalgesia and anesthesia. Anesthesia and Analgesia 43: 748–762
Cressman W A, Plosnieks J, Johnson P C 1973 Absorption, metabolism and excretion of droperidol by human subjects following intramuscular and intravenous administration. Anesthesiology 38: 363–369
Del Pizzo A 1978 A double-blind study of the effects of butorphanol compared with morphine in balanced anaesthesia. Canadian Anaesthetists Society Journal 25: 391–397
Derbyshire D R, Chmielewski A, Fell D, Vater M, Achola K, Smith G 1983 Plasma catecholamine responses to tracheal intubation. British Journal of Anaesthesia 55: 855–860
Dev N B, Loeschke H H 1979 A cholinergic mechanism involved in the respiratory chemosensitivity of the medulla oblongata in the cat. Pfluegers Archiv; European Journal of Physiology 379: 29–36
DiFazio C A, Moscicki J C, Magruder M R 1981 Anesthetic potency of nalbuphine and interaction with morphine in rats. Anesthesia and Analgesia 60: 629–633
Dubois M, Pickar D, Cohen M, Gadde P, Macnamara T E, Bunney W E 1982 Effects of fentanyl on the response of plasma beta-endorphin immunoreactivity to surgery. Anesthesiology 57: 468–472
Dum J E, Herz A 1981 In vivo receptor binding of the opiate partial agonist, buprenorphine, correlated with its agonistic and antagonistic effects. British Journal of Pharmacology 74: 627–633
Dundee J W, Brown S S, Hamilton R C, McDowell S A 1969 Analgesic supplementation of light general anaesthesia. Anaesthesia 24: 52–61
Dundee J W, Tinckler L F 1952 Pethidine and liver damage. British Medical Journal 2: 703–4
Eisele J H, Smith N T 1972 cardiovascular effects of 40% nitrous oxide in man. Anesthesia and Analgesia 51: 956–961
Eisele J H, Reitan J A, Massumi R A, Zelis R F, Miller R R 1976 Myocardial performance and N_2O analgesia in coronary artery disease. Anesthesiology 44: 16–20
Eriksen J, Bertelsen P, Ahn N C, Rasmussen J P 1981 Early

response to central haemodynamics to high doses of sufentanil or morphine in dogs. Acta Anaesthesiologica Scandinavica 25: 33–38

Estilo A E, Cotrell J E 1982 Hemodynamic and catecholamine changes after administration of naloxone. Anesthesia and Analgesia 61: 349–353

Evans J M, Hogg M I J, Lunn J N, Rosen M 1974 Degree and duration of reversal by naloxone of effects of morphine in conscious subjects. British Medical Journal i: 589–591

Finck A D, Ngai S H 1982 Opiate receptor mediation of ketamine analgesia. Anesthesiology 56: 291–297

Flacke J W, Flacke W E, William G D 1977 Acute pulmonary edema following naloxone reversal of high dose morphine anesthesia. Anesthesiology 47: 376–378

Flacke J W, van Etten A, Flacke W E 1983 Greatest histamine release from meperidine among four narcotics: Double-blind study in man. Anesthesiology 59: A51

Flórez J, Hurlé M A, Mediavilla A 1982 Respiratory responses to opiates applied to the medullary ventral surface. Life Sciences 31: 2189–2192

Fratta W, Casu M, Balestrieri A, Loviselli A, Biggio G, Gessa G 1980 Failure of ketamine to interact with opiate receptors. European Journal of Pharmacology 61: 389–391

Freye E 1974 Cardiovascular effects of high doses of fentanyl, meperidine and naloxone in dogs. Anesthesia and Analgesia 53: 40–47

Freye E, Kuchinsky K 1976 Effects of fentanyl and droperidol on the dopamine metabolism of the rat striatum. Pharmacology 14: 1–7

Freye E, Hartung E, Schenk G K 1983 Bremazocine: An opiate that induces sedation and analgesia without respiratory depression. Anesthesia and Analgesia 62: 483–488

Fry E N S 1982 Buprenorphine for postoperative analgesia. British Medical Journal 285:1427

Gall J J, DiFazio C A, Moscicki J 1982 Analgesic and respiratory depressant activity of nalbuphine: A comparison with morphine. Anesthesiology 57: 367–374

Galt R H M 1977 The opiate anomalies — another possible explanation. Journal of Pharmacy and Pharmacology 29: 711–714

George J M, Reier C E, Larense R R, Power J M 1974 Morphine anesthesia blocks cortisol and growth hormone response to surgical stress in humans. Journal of Clinical Endocrinology and Metabolism 38: 736–741

Georgis S D, Hoyt J L, Sokoll M D 1971 Effects of Innovar and Innovar plus nitrous oxide on muscle tone and the H-reflex. Anesthesia and Analgesia 50: 743–747

Ghoneim M M, Dhanaraj J, Choi W W 1984 Comparison of four opioid analgesics as supplements to nitrous oxide anesthesia. Anesthesia and Analgesia 63: 405–412

Gill K J, Cartwright D P, Scoggins A, Gray A J, Prys-Roberts C 1980 Ventilatory depression related to plasma fentanyl concentrations during and after anaesthesia. British Journal of Anaesthesia 52:632P

Glariman N H, Mattie L R, Stephenson W F 1953 Studies on the antidiuretic action of morphine. Science 117:225

Goldberg A H, Padget C H 1969 Comparative effects of morphine and fentanyl on isolated heart muscle. Anesthesia and Analgesia 48: 978–982

Gommeren W, Leysen J E 1982 Binding properties of [^{3}H] lofentanil at the opiate receptor. Archives Internationales de Pharmacodynamic et de Therapie 258: 171–173

Goromaru T, Matsuura H, Yoshimura N, et al 1984 Identification and quantitative determination of fentanyl metabolites in patients by gas chromatography — mass spectrometry. Anesthesiology 61: 73–77

Gouardères C, Audiger Y, Cros J 1982 Benzomorphan binding sites in rat lumbo-sacral spinal cord. European Journal of Pharmacology 78: 483–486

Gray T C, Rees G J 1952 The role of apnoea in anaesthesia for major surgery. British Medical Journal ii: 891–892

Green D 1983 Current concepts concerning the mode of action of meptazinol as an analgesic. Postgraduate Medical Journal 59 (Suppl 1): 9–12

Griesemer R W, Moldenhauer C C, Hug C C, Holbrook G W 1982 Sufentanil anesthesia for aortocoronary bypass surgery: 30 μ g/kg vs 15 μ g/kg. Anesthesiology 57:A48

Gudelsky G A, Porter J C 1979 Morphine and opioid peptide induced inhibition of the release of dopamine from the tubero-infundibular neurons. Life Sciences 25: 1697–1702

Gupta P K, Dundee J W 1974a Morphine combined with doxapram or naloxone. A study of post-operative pain relief. Anaesthesia 29: 33–39

Gupta P K & Dundee J W 1974b The effect of an infusion of doxapram on morphine analgesia. Anaesthesia 29: 40–43

Hall G M, Young C, Holdcroft A, Alaghband-Zadeh J 1978 Substrate mobilisation during surgery — a comparison between halothane and fentanyl anaesthesia. Anaesthesia 33: 924–930

Hamilton W K, Cullen S C 1953 Effect of levalorphan tartrate upon opiate induced respiratory depression. Anesthesiology 14: 550–554

Hamilton R C, Dundee J W, Clarke R S J, Loan W B, Morrison J D 1967 Studies of drugs given before anaesthesia. XIII: Pentazocine and other opiate antagonists. British Journal of Anaesthesia 39: 647–656

Harmer M, Slattery P J, Rosen M, Vickers M D 1983 Comparison between buprenorphine and pentazocine given i.v. on demand in the control of postoperative pain. British Journal of Anaesthesia 55: 21–25

Haxholdt O St, Kehlet H, Dyrberg U 1981 Effect of fentanyl on the cortisol and hyperglycemic response to abdominal surgery. Acta Anaesthesiologica Scandinavica 25: 434–436

Hayes M J, Fraser A R, Hampton J R 1979 Randomized trial comparing buprenorphine and diamorphine for chest pain in suspected myocardial infarction. British Medical Journal ii: 300–302

Hecker B R, Lake C L, DiFazio C A, Moscicki J C, Engle J S 1983 The decrease of the minimum alveolar anesthetic concentration produced by sufentanil in rats. Anesthesia and Analgesia 62: 987–980

Heikkilä H, Jalonen J, Arola M, Kauto J, Laaksonen V 1984 Midazolam as adjunct to high-dose fentanyl anaesthesia for coronary artery bypass grafting operation. Acta Anaesthesiologica Scandinavica 28: 683–689

Hengstmann J H, Stoeckel H, Schuttler J 1980 Infusion model for fentanyl based on pharmacokinetic analysis. British Journal of Anaesthesia 52: 1021–1025

Henny R P, Vasko J S, Brawley R K, Oodham H N, Morrow A G 1966 The effect of morphine on the resistance and capacitance vessels of the peripheral circulation. American Heart Journal 72: 242–250

Herz A, Teschemacher H J 1971 Activities and sites of antinociceptive action of morphine-like analgesics. In: Harper N J, Simmonds A B (eds) Advances in Drug Research, New York, Academic Press, pp 79–119

Hickey P R, Hansen D D 1984 Fentanyl- and Sufentanil-oxygen-pancuronium anesthesia for cardiac surgery in infants. Anesthesia and Analgesia 63: 117–124

Hildenberg J C 1981 Intraoperative awareness during high-dose fentanyl oxygen anesthesia. Anesthesiology 54: 341–343

Hill A B, Nahrwald M D, de Rosayro A M, Knight P R, Jones R M, Bolles R E 1981 Prevention of rigidity during fentanyl–oxygen induction of anesthesia. Anesthesiology 55: 452–454

Hillarp N A, Fuxe K, Dahlström A 1966 Demonstration and mapping of central neurones containing dopamine, noradrenaline and 5-hydroxytryptamine and their reaction to psychopharmaca. Pharmacological Reviews 18: 727–741

Hökfelt T, Ljungdahl Å, Terenius L, Elde R, Nilsson C 1977 Immunohistochemical analysis of peptide pathways possibly related to pain and analgesia: Enkephalin and substance P. Proceedings of the National Academy of Science, USA 74: 3081–3085

Holmes C McK, Galletly D G 1982 Midazolam/fentanyl. A total intravenous technique for short procedures. Anaesthesia 37: 761–765

Hsu H O, Hickey R F, Forbes A F 1979 Morphine decreases peripheral vascular resistance and increases capacitance in man. Anesthesiology 59: 98–102

Hug C C Jr 1978 Pharmacokinetics of morphine during cardiac surgery. Anesthesiology 49: 305–306

Hug C C, McClain D B 1980 Ventilatory depression by fentanyl in anesthetized patients. Anesthesiology 53:556

Hug C C Jr, Murphy M R 1981 Tissue redistribution of fentanyl and termination of effect in rats. Anesthesiology 55: 369–375

Hug C C Jr, Chaffman M 1984 Alfentanil: Pharmacology and uses in anaesthesia. Auckland, ADIS Press, pp 71–91

Hughes J, Smith T W, Kosterlitz H W, Fothergill L A, Morgan B A, Morris H R 1975 Identification of two related pentapeptides from the brain with potent opiate agonist activity. Nature 258: 577–579

Jaffe J B 1980 Drug addiction and Abuse. In: Goodman L S, Gilman A (eds) The pharmacological Basis of Therapeutics. 6th ed. Macmillan, New York, pp 245–283

Janssen P A J 1962 A review of the chemical features associated with strong morphine-like activity. British Journal of Anaesthesia 34: 260–268

Janssen P A J 1967 The pharmacology of droperidol. International Journal of Neuropsychiatry 3, supplement 1, 10

Janssen P A J, van der Eycken C A M 1968 The chemical anatomy of potent morphine-like analgesics. In: Burger A (ed). Drugs affecting the central nervous system, vol. 2, pp. 25–60. New York, Marcel Dekker Inc

Jewitt D E, Maurer B J, Sonnenblick E J, Shillingford J P 1971 Pentazocine: Effect on ventricular muscle and hemodynamic changes in ischaemic heart disease. Circulation 44 (supp ii):118

Jones D, Laurence A S, Thornton J A 1983 Total intravenous anaesthesia with etomidate–fentanyl. Use in general and gynaecological surgery. Anaesthesia 38: 29–39

Jones J G 1983 The respiratory effects of meptazinol. Postgraduate Medical Journal 59 (Suppl. 1): 72–77

Jordan C, Lehane J R, Robson P J, Jones J G 1979 A comparison of the respiratory effects of meptazinol, pentazocine and morphine. British Journal of Anaesthesia 51: 497–501

Jurna I Ruzdic N, Nell T, Grossmann W 1972 The effect of α-methyl-ρ-tyrosine and substantia nigra lesion on spinal motor activity in the rat. European Journal of Pharmacology 20: 341–350

Kaiko R F, Foley K M, Grabinski P Y, et al 1983 Central nervous system excitatory effects of meperidine in cancer patients. Annals of Neurology 13: 180–185

Kalenda Z, Scheijgrond H W 1976 Anaesthesia with sufentanil-analgesia in carotid and vertebral arteriography. A comparison with fentanyl. Anaesthetist 25: 380–383

Kaufman R D, Agleh K A, Belville J W 1979 Relative potencies and duration of action with respect to respiratory depression of intravenous meperidine, fentanyl and alphaprodine in man. Journal of Pharmacology and Experimental Therapeutics 208: 73–79

Kaufman R D, Gabathuler M L, Belville J W 1981 Potency, duration of action and pA_2 in man of intravenous naloxone measured by reversal of morphine-depressed respiration. Journal of Pharmacology and Experimental Therapeutics 219: 156–162

Kaukinen L, Kaukinen S, Eerola R, Eerola M 1981 The antagonistic effect of pentazocine on fentanyl induced respiratory depression compared with nalorphine and naloxone. Annals of Clinical Research 13: 396–401

Kay B, Rolly G 1977 Duration of action of analgesic supplement to anesthesia. Acta Anaesthesiologica Belgica 28: 25–32

Kay B 1980 A double-blind comparison between fentanyl and buprenorphine in analgesic-supplemented anaesthesia. British Journal of Anaesthesia 52: 453–457

Kay N H, Allen M C, Bullingham R E S, et al 1985 Influence of meptazinol on metabolic and hormonal responses following major surgery. Anaesthesia 40: 223–228

Keats A S, Telford J 1964 Narcotic antagonists as analgesics. Clinical aspects. In: Gould R F (ed) Molecular modification in drug design: Advances in chemistry series 45. ACS, Washington pp 170–176

Kraynack B J, Gintautas J G 1982 Naloxone: Analeptic action unrelated to opiate receptor antagonism. Anesthesiology 56: 251–253

Krishna G, Paradise R R 1974 Effect of morphine on isolated human atrial muscle. Anesthesiology 40: 147–151

Kugler J, Grote B, Laube M, Doenicke A, Dick E 1977 Die hypnotische Wirkung von Fentanyl und Sufentanil. Anaesthetist 26: 343–348

Lake C L, Duckworth E N, DiFazio C A, Durbin D G, Magruder M R 1982 Cardiovascular effects of nalbuphine in patients with coronary or valvular heart disease. Anesthesiology 57: 498–503

de Lange S, Boscoe M J, Stanley T H, Pace N 1982 Comparison of sufentanil -0_2 and fentanyl -0_2 for coronary artery surgery. Anesthesiology 56: 112–118

Latasch L, Probst S, Dudziak R 1984 Reversal by nalbuphine of respiratory depression caused by fentanyl. Anesthesia and Analgesia 63: 814–816

Lauven P M, Stoeckel H, Schüttler J, Schwilden H 1981 Prevention of fentanyl rebound by administration of cimetidine. Anaesthetist 30: 467–471

Lauven P M, Stoeckel H, Schwilden H, Arendt R, Greenblatt D J, Schuttler J 1982 Application of a benzodiazepine antagonist (RO 15-1788) under steady-state conditions of midazolam. Anesthesiology 57:A325

Lee C M, Yeakel A E 1975 Patient refusal of surgery following Innovar premedication. Anesthesia and Analgesia 54: 224–226

Lees N W, Glasser J, McGroarty F L, Miller B M 1981

Etomidate and fentanyl for maintenance of anaesthesia. British Journal of Anaesthesia 53: 959–961

Lees N W, Antonios W R A 1984 Two-stage infusion of etomidate for the induction and maintenance of anaesthesia. British Journal of Anaesthesia 56: 1239–1242

Leysen J E, Laduron P M, Niemegeers C J E 1978 Receptor binding properties in vitro and in vivo of new long acting narcotic analgesics. In: van Ree, Terenius R (eds) Characteristics and functions of opioids. Elsevier North-Holland, Biomedical Press, Amsterdam, pp 479–482

Leysen J E, Gommeren W, Niemegeers C J E 1983 [^{3}H] Sufentanil, a superior ligand for μ-opiate receptors. Binding properties and regional distribution in rat brain and spinal cord. European Journal of Pharmacology 87: 209–225

Lewis J W, Rance M J 1979 Opioids and the management of pain. Pharmaceutical Journal 222: 61–64

Ling G S F, Spiegel K, Nishimura S L, Pasternak G W 1983 Dissociation of morphine's analgesic and respiratory depressant actions. European Journal of Pharmacology 86: 487–488

Liu W S, Bidwai A V, Stanley T H, Loeser E A 1976 Cardiovascular dynamics after large doses of fentanyl and fentanyl plus N_2O in the dog. Anesthesia and Analgesia 55: 168–172

Liu W, Bidwai A V, Lunn J K, Stanley T H 1977 Urine catecholamine excretion after large doses of fentanyl, fentanyl and diazepam, and fentanyl, diazepam and pancuronium. Canadian Anaesthetists Society Journal 24: 371–379

Lowenstein E 1971 Morphine "anesthesia" — A perspective. Anesthesiology 35: 563–565

Lowenstein E, Hallowell P, Levine F H, Daggett W M, Austen W G, Laver M B 1969 Cardiovascular response to large doses of intravenous morphine in man. New England Journal of Medicine 281: 1389–1393

Lowenstein E, Whiting R B, Bittar D A 1972 Local and neurally mediated effects of morphine on skeletal muscle vascular resistance. Journal of Pharmacology and Experimental Therapeutics 180: 359–367

Lunn J K, Webster L R, Stanley T H, Woodward A 1979 High dose fentanyl anesthesia for coronary artery surgery: Plasma fentanyl concentration and influence of nitrous oxide on cardiovascular responses. Anesthesia and Analgesia 58: 390–395

Major E, Verniquet A J W, Yate P M, Waddell T K 1982 Disoprofol and fentanyl for total intravenous anaesthesia. Anaesthesia 37: 541–547

Mark J B, Greenberg L M 1983 Intraoperative awareness and hypertensive crisis during high dose fentanyl–diazepam anesthesia. Anesthesia Analgesia 62: 698–700

Martin D E, Rosenberg H, Aukbung S J et al 1982 Low-dose fentanyl blunts circulatory responses to tracheal intubation. Anesthesia and Analgesia 61: 680–684

Martin W R, Eades C G 1961 Demonstration of tolerance and physical dependence in the dog following a short-term infusion of morphine. Journal of Pharmacology and Experimental Therapeutics 133: 262–270

Martin W R, Eades C G, Thompson J A, Huppler R E, Gilbert P E 1976 The effects of morphine- and nalorphin-like drugs in the nondependent and morphine-dependent chronic spinal dog. Journal of Pharmacology and Experimental Therapeutics 197: 517–532

Mather L E 1983 Clinical pharmacokinetics of fentanyl and its newer derivatives. Clinical Pharmacokinetics 8: 442–446

McCammon R L, Viegas O J, Stoelting R K, Dryden G E 1978 Naloxone reversal of choledochoduodenal sphincter spasm associated with narcotic administration. Anesthesiology 48: 437–439

McClain D A, Hug C C 1980 Intravenous fentanyl kinetics. Clinical Pharmacology and Therapeutics 28: 106–114

McDonald H R, Baird D P, Stead B R, Crawford I C, Taylor S H 1966 Clinical and circulatory effects of neuroleptanalgesia with dihydrobenzperidol and phenoperidine. British Heart Journal 28: 654–672

McDonnell T E, Bartkowski R R, Williams J J 1984 ED_{50} of alfentanil for induction of anesthesia in unpremedicated young adults. Anesthesiology 60: 136–140

McGilliard K L, Takemori A E 1978 Antagonism by naloxone of narcotic-induced respiratory depression and analgesia. Journal of Pharmacology and Experimental Therapeutics 207: 494–503

McQuay H J, Moore R A, Paterson G M, Adams A P 1979 Plasma fentanyl concentration and clinical observations during and after operation. British Journal of Anaesthesia 51: 543–549

McQuay H J, Bullingham R E S, Moore R A 1981 Acute opiate tolerance in man. Life Science 28: 2513–2517

Michiels I, Kay H, Barash P 1982 Does nitrous oxide or reduced FIO_2 alter hemodynamic function during high dose fentanyl anesthesia? Anesthesiology 57:A44

Michiels M, Hendricks R, Michielsen L, Heykants J, Lenaerts F 1981 Plasma levels and distribution of alfentanil (R 39209) in the male Wistar rat after a single intravenous dose of 0.16 mg/kg. Preclinical Research Report R 39209/13. Janssen Pharmaceutica, Beerse, Belgium

Misfeldt B B, Jörgensen P B, Spotoft H, Ronde F 1976 The effects of droperidol and fentanyl on intracranial pressure and cerebral perfusion in neurosurgical patients. British Journal of Anaesthesia 48: 963–968

Moffitt E A, Scovil J E, Barker R A, et al 1984 The effects of nitrous oxide on myocardial metabolism and hemodynamics during fentanyl or enflurane anesthesia in patients with coronary disease. Anesthesia and Analgesia 63: 1071–1075

Moldenhauer C C, Hug C C, Nagle D M, Murphy M R 1981 High dose butorphanol (Stadol) in anesthesia for aortocoronary bypass surgery. Society of Cardiovascular Anesthesiologists meeting

Montastruc J L, Montastruc P, Morales-Olivas F 1981 Potentiation by naloxone of pressor reflexes. British Journal of pharmacology 74: 105–109

Moore R A, Yang S S, McNicholas K W, Gallagher J D, Clark D L 1985 Hemodynamic and anesthetic effects of sufentanil as the sole anesthetic for pediatric cardiovascular surgery. Anesthesiology 62: 725–731

Moroni F, Peralta E, Cheney D L, Costa E 1979 On the regulation of gamma-aminobutyric acid neurons in the caudatus, pallidus and nigra: Effects of opioids and dopamine antagonists. Journal of Pharmacology and Experimental Therapeutics 208: 190–194

Morrison J D, Hill G B, Dundee J W 1968 Studies of drugs given before anaesthesia. XV: Evaluation of the method of study after 10000 observations. British Journal of Anaesthesia 40: 890–900

Morrison J D 1970 Studies of drugs given before anaesthesia. XXII: Phenoperidine and fentanyl, alone and in combination with droperidol. British Journal of Anaesthesia 42: 1119–1126

Morrison J D, Clarke R S J, Dundee J W 1970 Studies of drugs given before anaesthesia. XXI: Droperidol. British Journal of Anaesthesia 42: 730–735

Morrison J D, Loan W B, Dundee J W 1971 Controlled comparison of the efficacy of 14 preparations in the relief of postoperative pain. British Medical Journal iii: 287–290

Moss J, Rosow C E 1983 Histamine release by narcotics and muscle relaxants in humans. Anesthesiology 59: 330–339

Motomura S, Kissin I, Aultman D F, Reeves J G 1984 Effects of fentanyl and nitrous oxide on contractility of blood-perfused papillary muscle of the dog. Anesthesia and Analgesia 63: 47–50

Muldoon S M, Janssens W J, Verbeuren J J, Vanhoutte P M 1977 Alpha-adrenergic blocking properties of droperidol on the isolated blood vessels of the dog. British Journal of Anaesthesia 49: 211–216

Muldoon S, Otto J, Freas W, Watson R L 1983 The effects of morphine, nalbuphine and butorphanol on adrenergic function in canine saphenous veins. Anesthesia and Analgesia 62: 21–28

Mummaneni N, Rao T L K, Montoya A 1980 Awareness and recall with high-dose fentanyl-oxygen anesthesia. Anesthesia and Analgesia 59: 948–949

Murphy M R, Hug C C Jr 1982a The anesthetic potency of fentanyl in terms of its reduction of enflurane MAC. Anesthesiology 57: 485–488

Murphy M R, Hug C C Jr 1982b The enflurane sparing effect of morphine, butorphanol and nalbuphine. Anesthesiology 57: 489–492

Nagashima H, Karamanian A, Malovany R, Rodnay P, Ang M, Koerner S, Folder F F 1976 Respiratory and circulatory effects of intravenous butorphanol and morphine. Clinical Pharmacology and Therapeutics 19: 738–745

Nauta J, de Lange S, Koopman D, Spierdijk J, van Kleef J, Stanley T H 1982 Anesthetic induction with alfentanil: A new short-acting narcotic analgesic. Anesthesia Analgesia 61: 267–272

Nauta J, Stanley T H, de Lange S, Koopman D, Spierdijk J, van Kleef J 1983 Anesthetic induction with alfentanil: Comparison with thiopental, midazolam and etomidate. Canadian Anaesthetists Society Journal 30: 53–60

Neff W, Mayer E C, Perales M 1947 Nitrous oxide and oxygen anaesthesia with curare relaxation. California Medicine 66: 67–69

Ngai S H, Berkowitz B A, Yang J C, Hempstead J, Spector S 1976 Pharmacokinetics of naloxone in rats and in man. Anesthesiology 44: 398–401

Niemegeers C J E, Schellekens K H L, Janssen P A J, van Bever W F M, 1976 Sufentanil, a potent and extremely safe intravenous morphine-like compound in mice, rats and dogs. Arzneimittel-Forschung 26: 1551–1556

Niemegeers C J E, Janssen P A J 1981 Alfentanil (R 29209), a particularly short-acting intravenous narcotic analgesic in rats. Drug Development Research 1: 83–88

Nilsson E, Janssen P 1961 Neuroleptanalgesia, an alternative to general anaesthesia. Acta Anaesthesiologica Scandinavica 5: 73–84

Novack G D, Bullock J L, Eisele J H 1978 Fentanyl: Cumulative effects and development of short-term tolerance. Neuropharmacology 17: 77–82

O'Connor M, Escarpa A, Prys-Roberts C 1983 Ventilatory depression during and after infusion of alfentanil in man. British Journal of Anaesthesia 55 (Supplement 2): 217S–222S

Osei-Gyimah P, Archer S 1981 Some 14-beta-substitued analogues of N-(cyclo-propylmethyl)normorphine. Journal of Medical Chemistry 24: 212–215

Pasternak G W, Goodman R, Snyder S H 1975 An endogenous morphine-like factor in mammalian brain. Life Science 16: 1765–1769

Pasternak G W 1982 High and low affinity opioid binding sites: Relationship to mu and delta sites. Life Science 31: 1302–1306

Pasternak G W, Gintzler A R, Houghton R A, et al 1983 Biochemical and pharmacological evidence for opioid receptor multiplicity in the central nervous system. Life Sciences 33 (Suppl 1): 167–173

Patschke D, Eberlein H J, Hess W, Tarnow J, Zimmerman G 1977 Antagonism of morphine with naloxone in dogs. Cardiovascular effects with special reference to the coronary circulation. British Journal of Anaesthesia 49: 525–532

Pert C B, Snyder S H 1973 Opiate receptor: Demonstration in nervous tissue. Science 179: 1011–1014

Philbin D M, Wilson N E, Sokoloski J, Coggins C 1976 Radioimmunoassay of antidiuretic hormone during morphine anaesthesia. Canadian Anaesthetists Society Journal 23: 290–295

Philbin D M, Moss J, Rosow C E, Akins C W, Rosenberger J L 1981 The use of H_1 and H_2 histamine antagonists with morphine anesthesia: A double blind study. Anesthesiology 55: 292–296

Philbin D M, Föex P, Lowenstein E, Ryder W A, Jones L A 1983 Nitrous oxide causes myocardial dysfunction. Anesthesiology 57:A44

Philbin D M, Föex P, Drummond G, Ryder W A, Jones L A 1984 Regional ventricular function with sufentanil anesthesia. The effect of nitrous oxide. Anesthesia and Analgesia 63:260

Pleuvry B J 1983 An update on opioid receptors. British Journal of Anaesthesia 55 (Suppl. 2): 143–146

Popio K A, Jackson D H, Ross A M, Schreiner B F, Yu P N 1978 Hemodyamic and respiratory effects of morphine and butorphanol. Clinical Pharmacology and Therapeutics 23: 281–287

Port J D, Stanley T H, Steffey 1982 Narcotic inhalational anesthesia. Anesthesiology 57:A344

Prakash O, Verdouw P D, de Jong J W, et al 1980 Haemodynamic and biochemical variables after induction of anaesthesia in patients undergoing coronary artery bypass surgery. Canadian Anaesthetists Society Journal 27: 223–229

Prys-Roberts C, Foëx P, Biro G P, Roberts J G 1973 Studies of anaesthesia in relation to hypertension V: Adrenergic beta-receptor blockade. British Journal of Anaesthesia 45: 671–680

Radnay P A, Brodman E, Mankiker D, Duncalf D 1980 The effect of equi-analgesic doses of fentanyl, morphine, meperidine and pentazocine on common bile duct pressure. Anaesthetist 29: 26–29

Reddy P, Liu W S, Port D, Gillmor S, Stanley T H 1980 Comparison of haemodynamic effects of anaesthetic doses of alphaprodine and sufentanil in the dog. Canadian Anaesthetists Society Journal 27: 345–350

Reeves J G, Kissin I, Fournier S E, Smith L R 1984 Additive negative inotropic effect of a combination of diazepam and fentanyl. Anesthesia and Analgesia 63: 97–100

Reitan J A, Stengert K B, Wymore M C, Martucci R W 1978 Central vagal control of fentanyl induced bradycardia during halothane anesthesia. Anesthesia and Analgesia 57: 31–36

Rivier C, Vale W, Ling N, Brown M, Guillemin R 1977 Stimulation in vivo of secretion of prolaction and growth hormone by β-endorphin. Endocrinology 100: 238–241

Robbins B H, Baxter J H, Jr, Fitzhugh O G 1939 Studies of cyclopropane. V. The effect of morphine, barbital, and amytal upon the concentration of cyclopropane in the blood required for anesthesia and respiratory arrest. Journal of Pharmacology and Experimental Therapeutics 65: 136–142

Robinson S, Gregory G A 1981 Fentanyl–air–oxygen anesthesia for ligation of patient ductus arteriosus in preterm infants. Anesthesia and Analgesia 60: 331–334

Rolly G, Kay B, Cockx F 1979 A double blind comparison of high doses fentanyl and sufentanil in man. Acta Anaesthesiologica Belgica 30: 247–254

Romagnoli A, Keats A S 1980 Ceiling effect for respiratory depression by nalbuphine. Clincal Pharmacology and Therapeutics 27: 478–485

Rorie D K, Muldoon S M, Tyce G M 1981 Effects of fentanyl on adrenergic function in canine coronary arteries. Anesthesia and Analgesia 60: 21–27

Rosow C E, Philbin D M, Keegan C R, Moss J 1984 Hemodynamics and histamine release during induction with sufentanil or fentanyl. Anesthesiology 60: 489–491

Schüttler J, Stoeckel H, Lauven P M 1983 Pharmacokinetisch begrundete Infusionmodelle für die Narkosefuhrung mit Alfentanil. In: Doenicke A (ed) Alfentanil, Berlin, Springer-Verlag

Scott J C, Ponganis K V, Stanski D R 1985 EEG quantitation of narcotic effect: The comparative pharmacodynamics of fentanyl and alfentanil. Anesthesiology 62: 234–241

Sebel P C, Bovill J G, Wauquier A, Rog P 1981 The effect of high-dose fentanyl on the electroencephalogram. Anesthesiology 55: 203–211

Sebel P S, Bovill J G 1982 Cardiovascular effects of sufentanil anesthesia. Anesthesia and Analgesia 61: 115–119

Sebel P S, Bovill J G, van der Haven A 1982 Cardiovascular effects of alfentanil anaesthesia. British Journal of Anaesthesia 54: 1185–1190

Sederberg J, Stanley T H, Reddy P, Liu W-S, Port D, Gillmor S 1981 Hemodynamic effects of butorphanol-oxygen anesthesia in dogs. Anesthesia and Analgesia 60: 715–719

Seeman P M, Baily H S 1963 The surface activity of tranquillizers. Biochemical Pharmacology 12: 1181–1191

Shaar C J, Fredrickson R C H, Dininger N B 1977 Enkephalin analogues and naloxone modulate the release of growth hormone and prolactin: Evidence for regulation by an endogenous opioid peptide in the brain. Life Sciences 21: 853–860

Shafer A, White P F, Schüttler J, Rosenthal M H 1983 Use of a fentanyl infusion in the intensive care unit: Tolerance to its anesthetic effects? Anesthesiology 59: 245–248

Shannon H E 1981 Evaluation of phencyclidine analogues on the basis of their discriminative stimulus properties in the rat. Journal of Pharmacology and Experimental Therapeutics 216: 543–551

Shelley G S, Brown H A 1978 Anti-emetic effects of ultra-low-dose droperidol. Anesthesiology 1978: 633–634

Shephard N W 1964 The application of neuroleptanalgesia in anaesthetic and other practice. London, Pergamon

Shupak R C, Harp J R 1985 Comparison between high-dose sufentanil-oxygen and high-dose fentanyl-oxygen for neuroanaesthesia. British Journal of Anaesthesia 57: 375–381

Simantov R, Snyder S H 1976 Morphine-like factors in mammalian brain: Structure elucidation and interaction with receptor. Proceedings of the National Academy of Science USA 73: 2515–2519

Simon E J, Hiller J M, Edelman I 1973 Stereospecific binding of the potent narcotic analgesic [^{3}H] etorphine in the rat-brain homogenate. Proceedings of the National Academy of Science USA 70: 1947–1949

Skingle M, Tyers M B 1980 Further studies on opiate receptors that mediate antinociception: Tooth pulp stimulation in the dog. British Journal of Pharmacology 70: 323–327

Slattery P J, Harmer M, Rosen M, Vickers M D 1982 Naloxone reversal of meptazinol-induced respiratory depression. Anaesthesia 37: 1163–1166

Smith N T, Dec-Silver H, Harrison W K, Sanford T J, Gillig J 1982 A comparison among morphine, fentanyl and sufentanil anesthesia for open-heart surgery: Induction, emergence and extubation. Anesthesiology 57:A291

Smith N T, Dec-Silver H, Stanford I J, Westover C J, Quinn M L, Klein F, Davis D A 1984 EEGs during high-dose fentanyl-, sufentanil-, or morphine-oxygen anesthesia. Anesthesia and Analgesia 63: 386–393

Snir-Mor I, Weinstock M, Davidson J T, Bahar M 1983 Physostigmine antagonizes morphine-induced respiratory depression in human subjects. Anesthesiology 59: 6–9

Sokoll M D, Hoyt J L, Georgis S D 1972 Studies in muscle rigidity, nitrous oxide and narcotic analgesic agents. Anesthesia and Analgesia 51: 16–20

Spiegel K, Pasternak G W 1984 Meptazinol: A novel Mu-1 selective opioid analgesic. Journal of Pharmacology and Experimental Therapeutics 228: 414–419

Sprigge J S, Wyands J E, Whalley D G, et al 1982 Fentanyl infusion anesthesia for aortocoronary bypass surgery: Plasma levels and hemodyanic response. Anesthesia and Analgesia 61: 972–978

Stahl K D, van Bever W, Janssen P, Simon E J 1977 Receptor affinity and pharmacological potency of a series of narcotic analgesics. anti-diarrheal and neuroleptic drugs. European Journal of Pharmacology 46: 199–205

Stanley T H, Gray N G, Stanford W, Armstrong R 1973 The effects of high-dose morphine on fluid and blood requirements in open-heart operations. Anesthesiology 38: 536–541

Stanley T H, Bennett G M, Loeser E A, Kawamura R, Sentker C R 1976 Cardiovascular effects of diazepam and droperidol during morphine anesthesia. Anesthesiology 44: 255–258

Stanley T H, Liu W S 1977 Cardiovascular effects of nitrous oxide–meperidine anesthesia before and after pancuronium. Anesthesia and Analgesia 56: 669–673

Stanley T H 1978 Cardiovascular effects of droperidol during enflurane and enflurane–nitrous oxide anaesthesia in man. Canadian Anaesthetists Society Journal 25: 26–29

Stanley T H, Webster L R 1978 Anesthetic requirements and cardiovascular effects of fentanyl–oxygen and fentanyl–diazepam–oxygen anesthesia in man. Anesthesia and Analgesia 57: 411–416

Stanley T H, Leysen J, Niemegeers C J E, Pace N L 1983a

Narcotic dosage and central nervous system opiate receptor binding. Anesthesia and Analgesia 62: 705–709

Stanley T H, Reddy P, Gilmore S, Bennett G 1983b The cardiovascular effects of high-dose butorphanol-nitrous oxide anaesthesia before and during operation. Canadian Anaesthetists Society Journal 30: 337–341

Stoeckel H, Hengstmann J H, Schüttler J 1979 Pharmacokinetics of fentanyl as a possible explanation for recurrence of respiratory depression. British Journal of Anaesthesia 51: 741–744

Stoelting R K, Gibbs P S 1973 Hemodynamic effects of morphine and morphine–nitrous oxide in valvular heart disease and coronary artery disease. Anesthesiology 38: 45–52

Stoelting R K, Creasser C E, Gibbs P S 1974 Circulatory effects of halothane added to morphine anesthesia in patients with coronary artery disease. Anesthesia and Analgesia 53: 449–455

Stoelting R K, Gibbs P S, Creasser C W, Peterson C 1975 Hemodynamic and ventilatory responses to fentanyl, fentanyl-droperidol and nitrous oxide in patients with acquired valvular heart disease. Anesthesiology 42: 319–324

Stoelting R K 1977 Circulatory changes during direct laryngoscopy and tracheal intubation: Influence of duration of laryngoscopy with or without prior lidocaine. Anesthesiology 47: 381–383

Stoelting R K 1979 Attenuation of blood pressure response to laryngoscopy and tracheal intubation with sodium nitroprusside. Anesthesia and Analgesia 58: 116–119

Strauer B 1972 Contractile responses to morphine, piritramide, meperidine and fentanyl: A comparative study of effects on the isolated ventricular myocardium. Anesthesiology 37: 304–310

Su T P 1982 Evidence for sigma opioid receptor: Binding of [^{3}H] SKF 10047 to etorphine-inaccessible sites in guinea-pig brian. Journal of Pharmacology and Experimental Therapeutics 223: 284–290

Tabatabai M, Collins J G, Kitahata L M 1983 Disruption of the activity of the medullary inspiratory neurons by high-dose fentanyl and reversal with nalbuphine. Anesthesiology 59:A485

Tammisoto T, Takki S, Toikka P 1970 A comparison of the circulatory effects in man of the analgesics fentanyl, pentazocine and pethidine. British Journal of Anaesthesia 42: 317–324

Taylor H E, Doerr J C, Gharib A, Faulconer A 1957 Effect of preanesthetic medication on ether content of arterial blood required for surgical anesthesia. Anesthesiology 18: 849–855

Terenius L 1973 Stereospecific interaction between narcotic analgesics and a synaptic plasma membrane fraction of rat cerebral cortex. Acta Pharmacologica et Toxicologica 32: 317–336

Terenius L, Wahlström A 1975 Search for an endogenous ligand for the opiate receptor. Acta Physiologica Scandinavica 94: 74–81

Thorpe D H 1984 Opiate structure and activity: a guide to understanding the receptor. Anesthesia and Analgesia 63: 143–151

Tomicheck R C, Rosow C E, Philbin D M, Moss J, Teplick R S, Schneider R C 1983 Diazepam–fentanyl interaction–hemodynamic and hormonal effects in coronary artery surgery. Anesthesia and Analgesia 62: 881–884

Tyers M B 1980 A classification of opiate receptors that mediate antinociception in animals. British Journal of Pharmacology 69: 503–512

Urthaler F, Isobe J H, James T N 1975 Direct and vagally mediated chronotropic effects of morphine studied by selective perfusion of the sinus node of awake dogs. Chest 68: 222–228

Vaught J L, Rothman R B, Westfall T C 1982 Mu and delta receptors: Their role in analgesia and in the differential effects of opioid peptides on analgesia. Life Science 30: 1443–1455

Verbeeck R K, Branch R A, Wilkinson G R 1981 Meperidine disposition in man: Influence of urinary pH and route of administration. Clinical Pharmacology and Therapeutics 30: 619–628

Vernheit J, Renov A M, Orgogozo J, Constant P, Caille J M 1978 Effect of diazepam–fentanyl mixture on cerebral blood flow and oxygen consumption in man. British Journal of Anesthesiology 50: 165–169

Villiger J W, Ray L S, Taylor K M 1983 Characteristics of [^{3}H] fentanyl binding to the opiate receptor. Neuropharmacology 22: 447–452

Villiger J W, Taylor K M 1981 Buprenorphine: Characteristics of binding sites in the rat central nervous system. Life Sciences 29: 2699–2708

de Vos V 1978 Immobilization of free-ranging wild animals using a new drug. Veterinary Record 103: 64–68

Van de Vusse G J, Coumans W A, Kruger R, Verlaan C, Reneman R F 1980 Effect of fentanyl on myocardial fatty acid and carbohydrate metabolism and oxygen utilization during experimental ischemia. Anesthesia and Analgesia 59: 644–654

Van de Walle J, Lauwers P, Adriaensen H 1976 Double blind comparison of fentanyl and sufentanil in anesthesia. Acta Anaesthesiologica Belgica 27: 129–138

Waller J L, Hug C C Jr, Nagle D M, Craver J M 1981 Hemodynamic changes during fentanyl–oxygen anesthesia for aortocoronary bypass operation. Anesthesiology 55: 212–217

Walsh E S, Paterson J L, O'Riordan J B A, Hall G M 1981 Effects of high-dose fentanyl anaesthesia on the metabolic and endocrine responses to cardiac surgery. British Journal of Anaesthesia 53: 1155–1165

Wang S C 1963 Emetic and anti-emetic drugs. In: Root W S, Hofmann F G (eds) Physiological Pharmacology II. Academic Press, New York, pp 255–328

Watson P J Q, McQuay H J, Bullingham R E S, Allen M C, Moore R A 1982 Single-dose comparison between buprenorphine 0.3 and 0.6 mg. i.v. given after operation: Clinical effects and plasma concentrations. British Journal of Anaesthesia 54: 37–43

Waud B E, Waud D R 1972 The relation between the response to 'Train-of-four' stimulation and receptor occlusion during competitive neuromuscular block. Anesthesiology 37: 413–416

Weinstock M, Roll O, Erez E 1980 Physostimine antagonizes morphine-induced respiratory depression but not analgesia in dogs and rabbits. British Journal of Anaesthesia 52: 1272–1276

Welti R S, Moldenhauer C C, Hug C C Jr, Kaplan J A, Holbrook G W 1984 High-dose hydromorphone (Dilaudid) for coronary artery surgery. Anesthesia and Analgesia 63: 55–59

Whalley D G, Tidnam P F, Tyrrell M F, Thompson D S 1976 A comparison of the incidence of cardiac arrthyhmia during two methods of anaesthesia for dental extractions.

British Journal of Anaesthesia 48: 1207–1210

Wiklund R A, Ngai S H 1971 Rigidity and pulmonary edema after Innovar in a patients on levodopa therapy: Report of a case. Anesthesiology 35: 545–547

Wood A J T, Moir D C, Campbell C 1974 Medicines, evaluation and monitoring. Group: Central nervous system effects of pentazocine. British Medical Journal i: 305–307

Woodbridge P D 1957 Changing concepts concerning depth of anesthesia. Anesthesiology 18: 536–550

Wynands J E, Townsend G E, Wong P, Whalley D G, Srikant C B, Patel Y C 1983a Blood pressure response and plasma fentanyl concentrations of high- and very high-dose fentanyl anesthesia for coronary artery surgery. Anesthesia and Analgesia 62: 661–665

Wynands J E, Wong P, Whalley D G, Sprigge J S, Townsend G R, Patel Y C 1983b Oxygen-fentanyl anesthesia in patients with poor left ventricular function: Hemodynamics and plasma fentanyl concentrations. Anesthesia and Analgesia 62: 476–482

Wynands J E, Wong P, Townsend G E, Sprigge J S, Whalley D G 1984 Narcotic requirements for intravenous anesthesia. Anesthesia and Analgesia 63: 101–105

Yeh B K, McNay J L, Goldberg L I 1969 Attenuation of dopamine renal and mesenteric vasodilation by haloperidol: Evidence for a specific receptor. Journal of Pharmacology and Experimental Therapeutics 168: 303–309

Zukin R S, Zukin S R 1979 Specific [^{3}H] phencyclidine binding in rat central nervous system. Proceedings of the National Academy of Science, USA 76: 5372–5376

Zurick A M, Urzua J, Yared J P, Estafanous F G 1982 Comparison of hemodynamic and hormonal effects of large single-dose fentanyl anesthesia and halothane/nitrous oxide anesthesia for coronary artery surgery. Anesthesia and Analgesia 61: 521–526

Hypersensitivity to intravenous anaesthetics

The problem of hypersensitivity reactions has attracted increasing attention over recent years. This is probably not because of its frequency but rather because the complication can occur suddenly and unexpectedly in an apparently healthy patient and anaesthetists are now aware that it might be the explanation of some mishaps at induction of anaesthesia. As the avoidable complications diminish with better understanding of all the agents used, these adverse reactions assume a disproportionate role. However, hypersensitivity cannot be accepted as an explanation of every episode of hypotension or bronchospasm and more immunological investigations are now being carried out to explore mechanisms and predisposing factors.

The first conclusive case of an allergic or hypersensitivity reaction was reported in 1952 (Evans & Gould). Up to then many writers did not believe in the existence of such reactions but by the time of Clark & Cockburn's paper in 1971 a definite syndrome had been defined. The main features described were hypotension, tachycardia, erythema, cyanosis, bronchospasm, oedema of the glottis, diarrhoea and vomiting. Various combinations of these symptoms and signs have now been seen in most other reports, whatever the agent concerned.

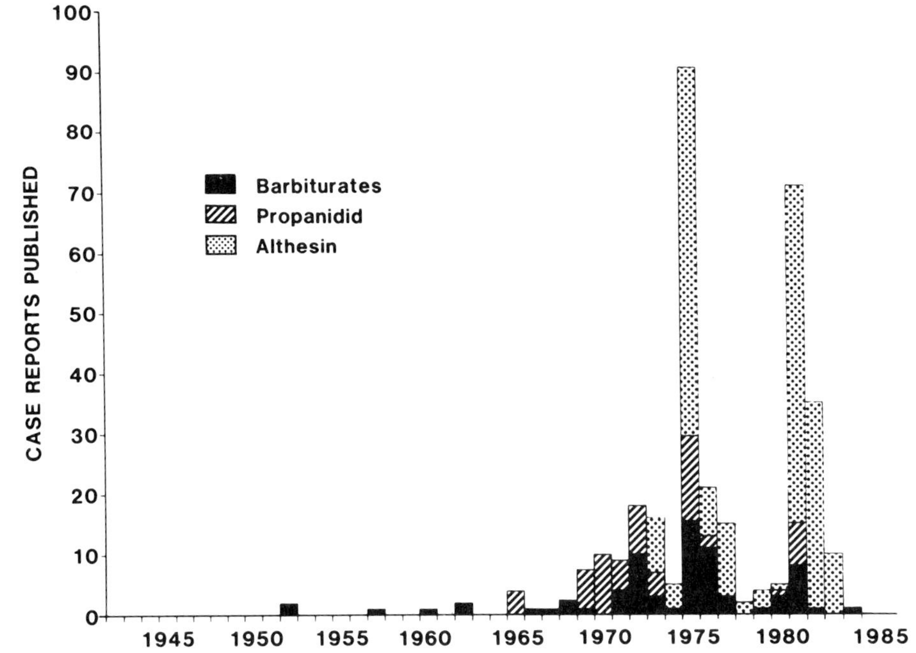

Fig. 14.1 Number of published cases of hypersensitivity reactions to intravenous anaesthetics.

The chronology of published cases, seen in Figure 14.1 appears to show a progressive increase over the past 30 years. This at first involved only the barbiturates but with the advent of Epontol (propanidid in Cremophor EL) in 1965, many more cases were reported and interest in hypersensitivity reactions was stimulated. A further increase occurred after 1973 with the advent of Althesin, also solubilised in Cremophor EL. Figure 14.1 indicates that there are two large

Table 14.1 Summary of published reports of generalised reactions to intravenous anaesthetics (water-soluble group), 1952–1984, with their clinical features and past history where known. A blank in the history columns indicates either none or not known as that it must be regarded as a minimum figure.

Reference	*n*	*Clinical features*				*History*			*Deaths*
		Skin	*CVS*	*RS*	*AS*	*Atopy*	*Allergy*	*Same anaesthetic*	
THIOPENTONE									
Evans & Gould (1952)	2	2	—	—	1	—	—	2	—
Hayward & Kiester (1957)	1	1	—	1	—	—	1	—	—
Kivalo et al (1960)	1	1	1	1	1	—	1	—	—
Strunk (1962)	1	1	1	—	1	—	—	1	—
Currie et al (1966)	1	1	1	1	—	—	1	1	—
Carrie & Buchanan (1967)	1	1	1	—	—	—	1	1	—
Anderton & Hopton (1968)	1	1	1	—	—	—	1	1	—
Cole (1968)	1	1	1	—	1	—	1	—	—
Clark & Cockburn (1971)	1	1	1	1	1	—	—	1	—
Davis (1971)	1	1	1	1	—	—	1	—	—
Fox et al (1971)	1	1	1	—	—	—	1	1	—
Holmes et al (1971)	1	1	1	1	—	—	1	—	1
Barjenbruch & Jones (1972)	1	1	1	—	—	—	1	1	—
Unsworth (1972)	2	2	2	1	—	—	2	2	—
Kelly & Boman (1973)	1	1	1	1	—	—	—	1	—
Wedley (1973)	1	—	—	1	—	—	—	—	—
Dundee et al (1974)	1	1	1	1	—	1	1	1	—
Brown (1975)	1	—	1	—	—	—	—	1	—
Clarke et al (1975)	12	8	8	10	—	5	3	5	4
Callens & Doutriaux (1976)	1	1	1	—	—	—	—	—	—
Chung (1976)	1	1	1	1	—	—	—	1	—
Guilmet & Joue (1976)	1	1	1	—	—	—	1	1	—
Laxenaire et al (1976)	5	4	2	1	1	3	1	—	—
Saint-Maurice et al (1976)	2	2	2	—	—	—	2	1	—
Steiglitz et al (1976)	1	—	1	1	—	—	—	—	1
Evans & Keogh (1977)	3	2	3	2	—	—	2	—	—
Baldwin (1979)	1	1	1	1	—	—	—	1	—
Etter et al (1980)	1	1	1	—	—	—	—	1	—
Lilly & Hoy (1980)	1	1	1	1	—	1	1	1	—
Beamish & Brown (1981)	2	—	—	—	—	—	—	—	—
Fisher & More (1981)	6	4	5	2	1	—	—	6	—
Hirshman et al (1982)	1	1	1	—	—	1	—	—	1
Dueck & O'Connor (1984)	1	1	1	1	—	1	1	—	—
Unpublished	35	23	29	21	2	8	7	18	4
METHOHEXITONE									
Shafto (1969)	1	—	1	—	—	—	—	—	—
Driggs & O'Day (1972)	6	6	6	5	3	3	1	—	—
Reichert & Bassett (1972)	1	1	—	—	1	—	—	—	—
Wyatt & Watkins (1975)	1	1	1	—	—	—	—	—	—
Beamish & Brown (1981)	1	1	1	1	—	—	—	—	—
Unpublished	6	5	4	2	—	0	0	0	0
THIAMYLAL									
Thompson et al (1973)	1	1	1	1	—	—	—	—	—
Dohi et al (1975)	1	1	—	1	—	—	—	—	—
TOTAL BARBITURATES	112	85	88	61	13	23	32	49	11
(% of total)		76	79	54	9	21	29	44	10

Table 14.2 Summary of published reports of generalised reactions to intravenous anaesthetics (group solubilised in Cremophor) 1965–1984.

Reference	*n*	*Clinical features*				*History*			*Deaths*
		Skin	*CVS*	*RS*	*AS*	*Atopy*	*Allergy*	*Same* anaesthetic*	
EPONTOL									
Beck (1965)	2	2	1	—	—	—	—	1	—
Radnay (1965)	1	1	1	—	—	—	—	—	—
Zindler (1965)	1	1	1	—	—	—	—	1	—
Gjessing (1969)	1	—	1	—	—	—	—	—	—
Kay (1969)	2	2	2	1	—	—	—	1	—
Manz & Frank (1969)	2	2	2	—	—	—	—	2	—
Bradburn (1970)	1	1	1	—	—	—	—	1	—
Dannemann & Lubke (1970)	2	2	2	—	—	—	—	2	—
Desai (in Johns, 1970)	1	1	1	—	1	—	—	1	—
Evans (1971)	1	1	1	—	—	—	—	—	—
Johns (1971)	1	1	1	—	—	—	—	1	—
Kruger (1970)	2	1	—	—	—	—	—	2	—
Larard (1970)	1	1	1	—	—	—	—	—	
Milochewsky & Cervenkova (1970)	1	1	1	—	—	—	—	—	
Spreadbury & Marrett (1971)	1	1	1	—	—	—	—	—	—
Stovner & Endresen (1971)	3	3	3	—	—	—	—	3	1
Thornton (1971)	1	1	1	—	1	—	1	1	—
Gotla (1972)	1	1		—	1	—	—	—	—
Jarvis (1972)	1	1	1	—		—	1	1	—
Lorenz et al (1972)	4	4	3	2	1	—	—	3	—
Rozenkranz (1972)	1	1	1	—	—	—	—	—	—
Turner et al (1972)	1	—	1	—	—	—	—	—	—
Harrfeldt (1973)	4	4	4	—	—	—	—	—	—
Clarke et al (1975)	4	4	4	—	1	—	—	3	—
Doenicke (1975)	10	10	10	5	—	—	4	8	—
Laxenaire et al (1976)	2	2	2	1	—	—	—	—	—
Dye & Watkins (1980)	1	1	1	1	—	—	—	—(1)	—
Waldhausen et al (1981)	3	3	3	2	—	—	—	—	—
Fisher & More (1981)	4	3	2	1	1	—	—	2	—
Unpublished	19	19	13	3	1	3	5	9	1
TOTAL EPONTOL	79	75	66	16	7	3	11	42	3
(% of total)		95	84	20	9	4	14	53	4
ALTHESIN									
Avery & Evans (1973)	3	2	1	2	—	—	—	1	—
Crowther (1973)	1	—	—	1	—	—	—	1	—
Healy (1973)	1	—	—	1	—	—	—	1	—
Hester (1973)	1	1	1	1	—	—	—	—	—
Horton (1973)	1	1	1	—	—	—	—	1	—
Mehta (1973)	1	1	1	—	—	—	1	—	—
Notcutt (1973)	1	1	1	—	—	—	—	—(1)	—
Dundee et al (1974)	1	1	1	—	—	1	1	1	—
Kessell & Assem (1974)	1	1	1	—	—	1	—	—	—
Tweedie & Ordish (1974)	2	2	2	2	—	—	—	—(1)	—
Clarke et al (1975)	65	42	43	32	—	6	13	30(35)	—
Bussien et al (1975)	1	—	—	1	—	—	1	—	—
Fisher (1975)	2	2	2	—	2	—	—	2	—
Watt (1975)	4	2	4	3	—	—	—	3	—
Boytell (1976)	1	1	1	—	—	—	—	1	—
Fisher (1976a)	2	2	2	—	2	—	—	2	—
Laxenaire et al (1976)	1	—	1	1	—	1	—	—	—
Monteil et al (1976)	2	2	2	—	—	—	—	—	—
Rawicz et al (1976)	1	1	1	—	—	—	1	—	—
Steel (1976)	1	1	1	1	—	—	—	1	—
Callens & Doutriaux (1976)	1	1	1	1	—	—	—	—	—
Evans & Keogh (1977)	10	8	9	4	1	—	1	3	—

Table 14.2 (continued)

Reference	*n*	*Clinical features*				*History*			*Deaths*
		Skin	*CVS*	*RS*	*AS*	*Atopy*	*Allergy*	*Same** *Anaesthetic*	
Hughes et al (1977)	1	1	1	1	—	—	—	1	—
Jago & Restall (1978)	1	1	1	1	1	—	—	1	—
Watkins et al (1978)	1	1	1	—	—	1	1	1	—
Scott (1979)	2	2	—	2	—	—	—	1	—
Vanezis (1979)	1	1	1	1	—	—	—	—	1
Beamish & Brown (1980)	1	1	—	1	—	—	—	—	—
Beamish & Brown (1981)	12					6		7	—
Waldhausen et al (1981)	3	3	3	2	—	—	—	—	—
Foissac et al (1981)	5	5	5	3	1	—	—	1	—
Michelangeli et al (1981)	16	1	2	14	1	—	4	1(2)	
Zaffiri et al (1981)	3	3	3	—	—	—	1	1	—
Fisher & More (1981) (new cases)	17	13	16	19	3	—	—	8	—
Radford et al (1982)	30	23	10	14	—	4		17	—
Casale (1982)	2	1	2	1	—	—	—	1	1
Howard et al (1982)	2	2	2	—	—	—	—	2	—
Benoit et al (1983)	2	2	2	2	2	—	—	2	—
Brown & Doolan (1983)	1	1	1	—	—	—	—	1	—
Moneret-Vautrin et al (1983)	1	1	1	—	—	—	—	1	—
Sale (1983)	3	3	3	3	—	—	—	—	—
Thompson (1983)	2	2	2	2	—	—	—	1	—
Sear & Prys-Roberts (1983)	1	1	1	1	—	—	—	1	—
Unpublished	134	103	111	59	3	9	18	67	3
TOTAL ALTHESIN	332	233	235	158	16	21	40	157	5
(% of total)		70	71	48	5	6	12	48	2
STESOLID MR									
Falk (1977)	1	1	1	—	1	—	—	—	—
Milner (1977)	1	1	1	—	—	—	1	—	—
Schou Olesen & Huttel (1980)	5								
Huttel et al (1980)	2	2	2	1	1	—	—	1	1
DIPRIVAN									
Briggs et al (1982)	1	1	1	1	—	—	—	—	—
CREMOPHOR EL									
Gjessing & Tomlin (1977)	1	1	1	—	—	—	—	—	—

* Figures in brackets include previous anaesthesia with another cremophor-containing solution.
ˣ The findings in the first 10 reports are also included in the survey by Clarke et al (1975).

peaks, that in 1975 coinciding with the survey from Belfast of 100 alleged reactions (Clarke et al, 1975) and one in 1981 mainly due to the paper by Beamish & Brown (1981) with prospective reporting of a series of 16 reactions. The existence of large numbers of cases when an attempt is made to find them supports the author's belief that there are many that are never described except at hospital morbidity meetings or in conversation among colleagues. Even the figures for unpublished cases in Tables 14.1 and 14.2 are probably only the small group reported to a body outside the hospital. For instance, none of the episodes investigated in Sheffield in 1982–1984 (Fig. 14.2) received detailed published reports and the true incidence of reactions to any one drug is probably more than 10 times that shown.

The most likely explanation for a true increase in reactions, if accepted, is that as more and more drugs are being taken by the patient population there is more likelihood of cross-sensitisation. In addition, as several cremophor-containing anaesthetic solutions were available and some of the non-anaesthetic fat-soluble compounds are also solubilised in cremophor (Lorenz et al, 1981), increasing sensitisation to this organic solvent becomes more likely. Certainly the fact that Harrfeldt (1973) in West Germany had no

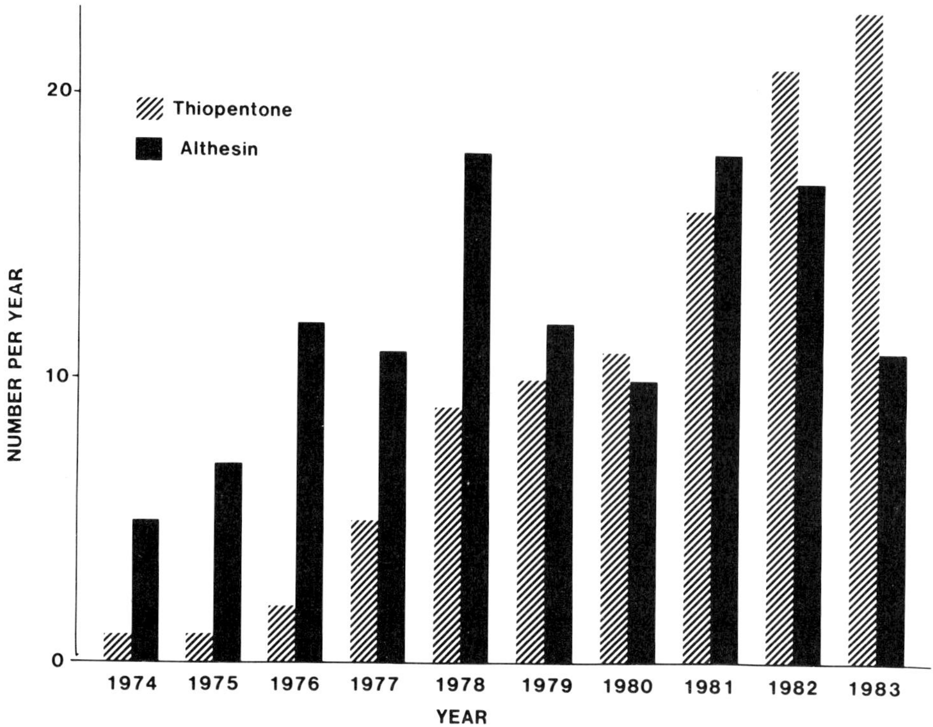

Fig. 14.2 Number of hypersensitivity reactions following thiopentone and Althesin investigated in the Department of Immunology, Royal Hallamshire Hospital, Sheffield, between 1974 and 1983 (J Watkins, personal communication).

reactions with propanidid in cremophor (Epontol) in the first 35 000 administrations and 4 in the next 45 000 supports this suggestion. However, firm evidence in support of this theory is not yet available.

CLINICAL FEATURES OF REACTIONS

Hypersensitivity reactions to anaesthetics take many different forms. Reactions which involve violent movements are difficult to fit into the same pattern and will not be mentioned further. However since histamine liberation accompanies many of the reactions, all episodes with clinical features resembling the effects of histamine will be included.

Contact dermatitis

This is an unusual complication with the intravenous anaesthetics presumably because actual contact can usually be avoided and is limited in quantity. Only two instances have been reported (Sneddon & Glew, 1973; Dundee et al, 1974) and both were with the repeated use of propanidid. They involved anaesthetists and it appears that the main hazard was spraying of fine particles of the anaesthetic solution on to the conjunctiva leading to oedema of the eyelids and face.

Acute cutaneous reactions

These may be divided into a localised reaction with a flare and wheals along the line of the vein and a systemic and generalised response to the injection. Localised reactions are rare with anaesthetic drugs other than pethidine, though bullous eruptions following thiopentone have been described by Hunter (1943) and Fisher (1968). A widespread response is common with tubocurarine, its frequency being estimated as 50% by McDowell & Clarke (1969). Davison described a cutaneous reaction with thiopentone as early as 1943 and this is estimated to occur in 10–20% of patients with Althesin. Its frequency and lack of serious consequences, however, means that it can be accepted as essentially benign. Three typical cases of this type are illustrated by Watkins (1981) and these show the difficulty of defining the cause on the basis of appearances alone: two showed blotchy urticaria following administration of a plasma substitute but only one of these had a raised plasma histamine level. The third followed venepuncture for withdrawal of blood without the administration of any drug; this patient had no other manifestation of anaphylaxis and the plasma histamine level only rose as the cutaneous reaction was fading. Nevertheless, this response might have been attributed to a drug if one had been injected, which shows that cutaneous vasodilatation alone should not be accepted as an adverse response to an anaesthetic. On the other hand, although histamine is liberated in urticarial reactions, the plasma level is not always raised.

The majority of clinically definite and immunologically confirmed reactions have erythema as a main feature. In addition, most have oedema, particularly of the eyelids (Larard, 1970; Spreadbury & Marrett, 1971) and a few have massive wheals (Davis, 1971). When oedema is present it can be calculated that a 1 mm layer of subcutaneous fluid throughout the body represents a circulatory loss of about 1.5 litres. Visible oedema probably involves a much thicker layer than this and might develop within 15 min so that hypotension and circulatory failure are inevitable as an accompaniment. The figure of 1.5 litres is very close to the fluid loss calculated from the haemoconcentration by Fisher (1977a). The most serious form of oedema is that of the glottis but few definite instances have been reported. However many of the reports of coughing, difficulty in breathing and laryngospasm (Clarke et al, 1975) might have been due to incipient laryngeal oedema.

Most of the reactions described have been associated with bright red colouration of the skin or if there was also circulatory failure, with cyanosis. However, in a small proportion of patients there was marked cutaneous pallor accompanied by oedema and severe hypotension (Clarke et al, 1975). These may be described as 'cardiovascular collapse' and although they are hard to include in the same group as the above they should probably be regarded as another manifestation of hypersensitivity.

Cardiovascular changes

Hypotension is the other common feature of the majority of hypersensitivity reactions. Its basis is hypovolaemia from transudation of protein-containing fluid through the capillary wall, as has already been described. The other mechanism, however, is arteriolar vasodilatation, especially in the upper half of the body, and this is a feature of histamine liberation (Dale & Laidlaw, 1919). The severe hypotension, even though it is often mistakenly considered to be a 'cardiac arrest', may return to normal spontaneously as compensatory mechanisms come into play. Rapid infusion of fluid will accelerate the restoration of normal blood pressure but alpha-sympathetic stimulant drugs are often helpful. The action of histamine on capillary permeability appears to be mediated through H_1 receptors and the vasodilator action has been shown in man to involve an early H_1 component, but with larger doses over a more prolonged period H_2 receptors are also stimulated (Boyce, 1982). Effective prevention therefore requires blockade of both groups.

Compensatory tachycardia is an invariable accompaniment of the hypotension, although histamine itself increases both the rate and force of myocardial contraction. These changes are due to an action on H_2 receptors and the H_1 receptors are only responsible for some slowing of A–V conduction which might lead to cardiac arrhythmias (Owen, 1977). In general, bradycardia and asystole are unlikely in such a reaction unless there is marked hypoxia.

Bronchospasm

This occurred in slightly more than half of the published descriptions of reactions, either on its own or as an accompaniment to other changes. However, in clinical practice the term is often loosely used for any unexplained airway obstruction and it should be confined to instances in which other forms of obstruction have been excluded. Furthermore, even true bronchospasm should not be accepted as drug-induced unless one can exclude irritation of the larynx by saliva or gastric juice or by a tracheal tube if this has been inserted. In these circumstances, other symptoms and signs of a hypersensitivity reaction would confirm this explanation of bronchospasm. It is not normally severe but asthmatic patients might be more seriously affected. Certainly coughing is known to be marked even with low levels of plasma histamine. Severe bronchospasm, particularly if accompanied by hypotension, leads rapidly to cerebral hypoxia and this combination has been responsible for most of the deaths which have occurred.

Gastro-intestinal disturbance

Abdominal pain and vomiting have been described during reactions (Cole, 1968; Clarke et al, 1975) and occur in about 10% of published case reports. Increased output of gastric acid has also been reported (Lorenz et al, 1977) in patients having induction doses of propanidid and thiopentone without any clinical adverse reaction. This coincides with the liberation of small but measurable amounts of histamine and the abdominal symptoms after reactions are probably related to the massive histamine liberation which is known to occur.

Clinical course of a reaction

The first event to attract attention is the flush occurring within a minute of completing the drug injection and this is often followed by coughing and bronchospasm. These respiratory disturbances might result in the flushing turning to generalised cyanosis. Marked hypotension usually also occurs in 1–2 min with an impalpable pulse, but the ECG shows a sinus tachycardia. Most patients recover spontaneously but if the patient is in the sitting position (e.g. in a dentist's chair) or has severe bronchospasm accompanying the hypotension, ventricular fibrillation can occur, leading to death in the absence of adequate supportive measures.

An unusual but well-defined group of reactions has similar features but a much slower onset of action. The cutaneous reaction might be delayed for 10 to 90 min and other manifestations such as hypotension, respiratory difficulty and nausea are much less severe. Six such cases following Althesin are summarised by Clarke and his colleagues (1975) and a further one following both methohexitone and Althesin is described by Beamish & Brown (1980). The more prolonged the time course, the more difficult it is to establish a clear causal relationship and episodes with longer delay in onset have not been recorded.

DIFFERENTIAL DIAGNOSIS

The definition of an adverse reaction is quantitative rather than absolute and all the clinical signs mentioned can occur during an otherwise normal anaesthetic induction. It is only when they are life-threatening or require some action on the part of the anaesthetist that they should be described as an adverse or hypersensitivity reaction.

Any discussion of frequency of reactions needs some indication of severity and the grading system in Table 14.3 (Ring & Messmer, 1977) is widely accepted. It must be stressed again that a reaction cannot be defined or graded on the basis of one feature and usually two clinical signs involving different systems are the best criteria for a definition.

The most important differential diagnosis of hypersensitivity is overdosage — actual or relative to the health of the patient; this is uncommon with thiopentone. The anaesthetist is sufficiently familiar with this drug to decide on a dose of 4–5 mg kg^{-1} and to reduce it appropriately in conditions such as hypovolaemic shock, old age, cardiac disease or indeed severe illness of any kind. Furthermore, the large volume of dilute solution encourages slow administration and the effects are readily observed. These considerations also apply to methohexitone. However, the same is not true of propanidid and Althesin. Propanidid is virtually equipotent with thiopentone (Clarke et al, 1968) but because of its short duration of action doses of 6–8 mg kg^{-1} were frequently given. Although both drugs are myocardial depressants and cause peripheral vasodilatation, propanidid has a steeper dose/toxicity curve than thiopentone (Clarke & Dundee, 1970) causing marked hypotension as the dose is increased. In

Table 14.3 Classification of anaphylactoid reactions based on clinical severity modified from Doenicke et al (1972); Ring & Messmer (1977)

Grade	*Cutaneous*	*Cardiovascular*	*Respiratory*	*Gastrointestinal*	*Plasma histamine* ($ng\ ml^{-1}$)
I	Erythema, wheals	—	—	—	0–1
II	Erythema, wheals, oedema	Tachycardia (>20 min) Hypotension (>20 mm Hg)	Dyspnoea	Nausea	1–10
III	Erythema, wheals, oedema	Shock	Bronchospasm, cyanosis	Vomiting, defaecation, abdominal cramps	10–100
IV	Erythema, wheals, oedema	Cardiac arrest	Respiratory arrest	Vomiting, defaecation, abdominal cramps	100+

addition, Soga and his colleagues (1973) compared propanidid with methohexitone and found it to be more depressant to the myocardium. Finally, as will be shown below, propanidid can liberate histamine in some patients by a direct pharmacological action, and this is broadly related to dose and rate of injection.

Soon after the first reports of collapse following propanidid, the suggestion of possible overdosage was made (Clarke & Dundee, 1969) and Grimmeisen (1971) and Zindler (1975) have supported this view. However, overdosage is not the whole explanation and Doenicke (1975) has confirmed this from an analysis of dose against frequency of reactions to propanidid. The most frequently administered adult dose was 500 mg and no severe reactions occurred with this dose. Neither the occurrence rate nor the severity of reactions appears to be dose-dependent.

The situation with Althesin was different since it had a high therapeutic index in animals (Child et al, 1971) and man (Clarke et al, 1972) causing little hypotension or myocardial depression in doses up to 150 $\mu l\ kg^{-1}$. However the small dose volume of the Althesin solution encouraged overdosage and too rapid administration, in spite of its viscosity. Early studies indicate that 50 $\mu l\ kg^{-1}$ is approximately equipotent with thiopentone 4 $mg\ kg^{-1}$ (Carson et al, 1975) but the dose required to induce anaesthesia is more variable than with the barbiturate. Certainly Mathieu & Grilliat (1976), Sutton (1976) and Mehta (1981) have suggested that overdosage and/or rapid injection are factors in adverse reactions and the incidence and severity of non-anaphylactoid hypotension are reduced by slow administration (Samuel & Dundee, 1973; Fantera & Maurina, 1976).

Overdosage is a likely cause of profound hypotension during induction with any intravenous anaesthetic except ketamine, but it is very unlikely to cause erythema, oedema, weals or bronchospasm. It is therefore in the patients presenting with marked pallor and cardiovascular collapse that overdosage should be seriously considered.

Other syndromes, such as acute intermittent porphyria (with barbiturates), pulmonary embolism, myocardial infarction and carcinoid tumour can cause cardiovascular collapse but can be excluded in retrospect. Gastric aspiration is probably the commonest cause of bronchospasm during induction of anaesthesia and can only be confirmed by testing with litmus paper the acidity of the fluid aspirated from the tracheal tube.

MECHANISMS OF HYPERSENSITIVITY REACTIONS

The phenomena described above are broadly similar and all have features of histamine liberation. They might therefore be thought to have a common mechanism. However, analysis of the plasma of reactors has shown that there are different types with different predisposing factors and pathways. It might be useful first to list the standard classification of drug reactions, although only the first appears to be truly applicable to intravenous anaesthetic drugs.

Type I reactions

These require previous exposure with production of specific IgE antibodies, though the general level of plasma IgE is usually raised also. These antibodies become firmly fixed to mast cells and basophils and subsequent exposure to the antigen results in rapid degranulation of these cells with liberation of vasoactive substances, particularly histamine. Although IgE is most commonly involved and complement plays no part in these reactions, IgG might be concerned instead and in these patients complement C4 is probably involved. In general this mechanism is uncommon with drugs, except those given by the intravenous route, including all dextrans, gelatins and the induction agents. Type 1 reactions, although rare, occur more frequently with thiopentone than following Althesin (Table 14.4).

Type II reactions

These involve antigens which are transmitted on the surface of a host or foreign cell.

Type III reactions

These involve soluble antiqens and any circulating antigen–antibody complex is normally destroyed by complement fixation and phagocytosis. In certain circumstances the complexes can be deposited in skin, kidneys and central nervous system and the process of inactivation liberates vasoactive amines. These are responsible for certain immune complex diseases (eg: SLE) and drug-induced haemolytic anaemias (eg: those caused by aspirin, sulphonamides etc) but not for reactions to anaesthetic agents.

Type IV reactions

These are T-lymphocyte-mediated with delayed hypersensitivity and are concerned with allergic responses to bacteria and rejection of transplanted organs. Skin sensitivity or contact dermatitis, chemicals, cosmetics, dyes, metals etc also fall into this group. Finally it could also include certain reactions to cremophor-containing anaesthetics, but this has not been confirmed.

Classical complement-mediated reactions

These result in the activation of the complement cascade Cl to C9 with consumption of C4 and C3 and liberation of C3a (anaphylatoxin) and C3b (Fig. 14.3). Previous exposure to the drug is obligatory. The amount of C3 conversion is generally below 30% in this type of reaction but since the complement proteins form almost 10% of the plasma globulins (C3 is approximately 1 g l^{-1}), the amount of anaphylatoxin formed is quite sufficient to liberate histamine from the mast cells. C4 is consumed and plasma C4 level is lowered in this type of reaction.

Alternate pathway

Activation of C3 with or without previous exposure involves conversion of a high proportion of the C3 (30–70%) but not the C4. The majority of Althesin reactions fall into this group (Table 14.4).

Pharmacological responses to the drug

These include the relative overdose and the genuine drug (dose-related) hypersensitivity in a patient. Such reactions might simply resemble the

Table 14.4 Reaction mechanisms in 'immediate adverse' reactions involving Althesin and thiopentone alone (Sheffield study for 1974–83, adapted from Watkins, 1985).

Drug	n	*Severe anaphylactoid reactions involving*			
		immune mechanisms		*non-immune mechanisms*	
		Type I	*involving complement*	*complement (C3)*	*Others (histaminoid)*
Althesin	118	1 (1%)	43 (36%)	47 (40%)	27 (23%)
Thiopentone	98	20 (20%)	10 (10%)	4 (4%)	64 (65%)

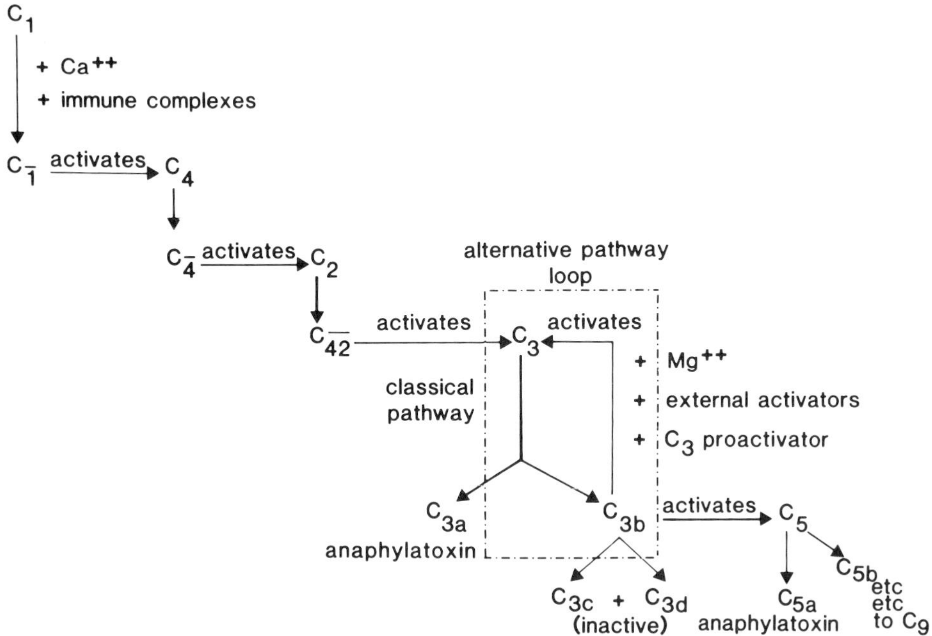

Fig. 14.3 Main pathways of complement activation. Activation is of the cascade type producing considerable enhancement of a small initial 'signal'. Positive feedback loops, such as the alternative (C_3) pathway enhance the effect and action of this inflammatory response system.

effects of histamine liberation or might actually involve histamine liberation as an intermediary. In the absence of a histamine assay all reactions which after analysis do not fit into the antibody or complement groups must be included here.

Histamine

This is the most important substance liberated from the mast cells during anaphylactic reactions and its presence has been shown on many occasions (Lorenz et al, 1972; 1976; 1981). However, serotonin, bradykinin, slow reacting substance (SRS-A) and prostaglandins have been suggested as possible accessories. While complement proteins are present in the plasma in mg ml^{-1} quantities, normal histamine concentration is less than 1 ng ml^{-1}, rising to perhaps 100 ng ml^{-1} during an anaphylactic reaction (Lorenz et al, 1972). Analysis of its concentration is made particularly difficult since it can be liberated from platelets or tissues in vitro if sampling technique is not standardised. Accurate estimates of plasma histamine have therefore rarely been made during reactions and only when the episode was anticipated and preparations for collecting samples had been made. The action of histamine is to cause profound dilatation of the capillaries in all vascular beds but particularly in the skin of the upper half of the body (Dale & Laidlaw, 1919). There is also an increase in capillary permeability not only in the capillary but in the whole range of vessels from terminal arteriole to small venule (Douglas, 1975). The vessels become permeable to plasma proteins, as shown by studies with attached dyes such as Evans blue, and this accentuates the fluid loss. Histamine has little direct action on the heart but failure of venous return lowers the cardiac output. Tachycardia, which is a reliable indication of histamine release (Lorenz et al, 1981), is probably due to sympathetic stimulation and release of adrenaline from the adrenal medulla.

Cellular changes

During administration of Althesin these occur even in the absence of clinical manifestations. These seem to result from a sharp rise in C3 breakdown products which have a chemotactic

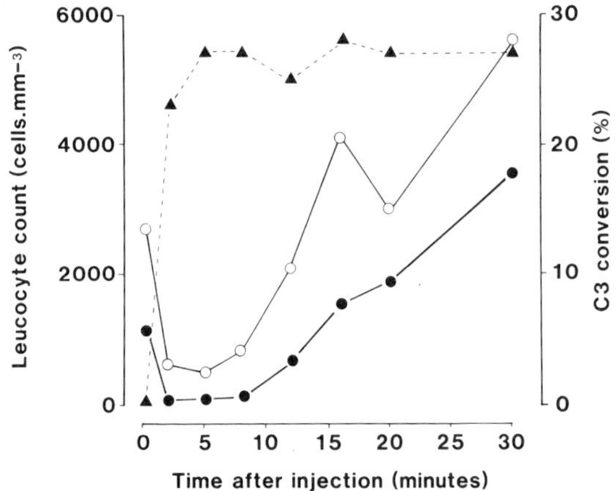

Fig. 14.4 Changes in polymorph (●-●-●) and leucocyte (○-○-○) count and complement conversion (▲-▲-▲) in a patient showing a minor but clinically significant adverse response after a second exposure to Althesin (reproduced from Watkins et al, 1978).

effect on leukocytes, particularly polymorphs. On first exposure the typical pattern is a slight rise in numbers continuing for about 10 min. However, second exposure after an interval of a few days results in a sharp fall in leukocyte and platelet count due to margination lasting for approximately 5 min followed by a rise to about double the normal count (Watkins et al, 1976; 1978) (Fig. 14.4). Similar changes in the polymorph leukocytes have been observed in the mini pig following a second exposure (Glen et al, 1979).

FREQUENCY OF REACTIONS

Barbiturates

Thiopentone

Published reports of reactions to thiopentone are few but the number is increasing as Figure 14.1 and Table 14.1 show. Perhaps a better indication of the number of possible reactions is the group of figures analysed by the Department of Immunology in Sheffield (Fig. 14.2). The number has risen steadily between 1974 and 1984 and the figures for the mechanism, discussed later, confirm that these are true anaphylactoid responses and not simply anaesthetic mishaps. The numbers for recent years are also far in excess of the number of published cases, in Table 14.1. As stated earlier this is probably mainly due to increasing awareness of the problem but a true rise in incidence cannot be ruled out.

Figures for numbers alone do not allow the estimation of reaction frequency and this can only come when the total of anaesthetics given is also known as in the studies listed in Table 14.5. These give an approximate figure of 1 in 30 000.

The individual reports do not reveal any reaction characteristics peculiar to thiopentone. For instance the frequency of cardiovascular collapse, bronchospasm or gastrointestinal symptoms is similar after the various anaesthetics listed in Tables 14.1 and 14.2. Only in the mortality is there a marked difference between drugs, for death in the thiopentone group is much more common than following propanidid or Althesin.

The reason for this might well be in the mechanism since the majority of thiopentone reactions are antibody-mediated or pharmacological and the prolonged life of thiopentone in the body extends the period of danger. Reactions to Althesin, and probably propanidid, are largely complement-mediated and because of the rapid metabolism of these drugs, most reactions are short-lived and eventually harmless (Watkins, 1981).

Methohexitone

This has been implicated in 16 reactions (Table 14.1) and the report by Driggs & O'Day (1972) suggests a reaction incidence of 1 in 7000.

Table 14.5 Estimates of frequency of hypersensitivity reactions following intravenous anaesthetics.

Anaesthetic	*Reference*	*Frequency*
Thiopentone	Shaw (1974)	1 in 36 000
	Evans & Keogh (1977)	1 in 29 000
	Beamish & Brown (1981)	1 in 23 000
Methohexitone	Driggs & O'Day (1972)	1 in 7 000
Epontol	Danneman & Lubke (1970)	1 in 800
	Kay (1972)	1 in 1 700
	Doenicke (1975)	1 in 170
Althesin	Clarke et al (1975)	1 in 11 000
	Watt (1975)	1 in 900
	Fisher (1976)	1 in 900
	Evans & Keogh (1977)	1 in 1 900
	Scott (1979)	1 in 430
	Beamish & Brown (1981)	1 in 600
	Howard et al (1982)	1 in 7 000
Stesolid MR	Schou Olesen & Huttel (1978)	1 in 1 000

Beamish & Brown (1981) had one delayed reaction in 630 administrations of methohexitone. This seems to be higher than clinical experience or other published reports with this drug would suggest and the Department of Anaesthetics in Belfast has records of over 25 000 administrations of methohexitone without any kind of hypersensitivity incident. Pharmacologically also it is unlikely that this drug would cause more anaphylactoid reactions than thiopentone, especially as its destruction in the body is more rapid. There have been no deaths reported with this agent.

Thiamylal

Two reactions have been reported with thiamylal (Thompson et al, 1973; Dohi et al, 1975) in the USA and Japan.

Ketamine

Only one hypersensitivity reaction has been described following the use of ketamine (Mathieu et al, 1975) and it consisted only of a rather severe macular rash. It was therefore merely a more severe form of the erythema commonly seen with many agents and was probably due to an exaggerated pharmacological liberation of histamine.

Etomidate

This is one of the few intravenous anaesthetics which does not cause liberation of histamine to any measurable extent (Doenicke et al, 1973) but when suxamethonium is given in association, even etomidate can be shown to liberate histamine (Lorenz & Doenicke, 1975). There have been five episodes possibly due to reaction to etomidate, reported to Sheffield (Watkins, 1983), but they differ from those described earlier in having been mainly cutaneous or gastrointestinal, rather than of the more hazardous cardiovascular type. None involved C3 or C4 and all must be classed as non-immune. Two other episodes were reported by Sold (1985) in which etomidate appeared to be responsible for acute erythema, tachycardia and hypotension. In spite of this, etomidate together with ketamine and the benzodiazepines must be regarded as the safest intravenous anaesthetics from the standpoint of causing anaphylactoid reactions.

Cremophor-containing solutions

Propanidid (Epontol)

Reactions following this drug have been reported since 1965, that is, even before its widespread clinical use. The annual numbers of published cases show little because of the fluctuating number of administrations (Table 14.2). The figures of Harrfeldt (1973) of only four cases in 80 000 administrations suggest a low incidence and in the author's first 3000 patients receiving the drug (1964–7) there were no reactions. More recently Beamish & Brown (1981) reported 629 administrations without a reaction. Certainly no deaths have been reported (Table 14.2). However, there are controlled series over the same period showing a different picture (Table 14.5). Doenicke (1975), in particular, tabulates two series from different hospitals with incidences for severe reactions of 1 in 200 and 1 in 84 (regardless of premedication or previous anaesthesia). The predisposing factors will be discussed below but there is still no firm explanation for the variation in reported frequency of reactions. It need only be said that they were too frequent to justify the continued clinical use of this drug. It is surprising that the drug was only withdrawn from the market in 1983 but it seems that many physicians and dentists were not aware of its dangers and one dentist who reported 'seven anaphylactic reactions' to the Committee on Safety of Medicines presumably thought the risks an acceptable price to pay for the rapid recovery. This does not appear to be a rational view considering the much better safety record of methohexitone.

Althesin

There are more published reports of reactions following this drug than after any other (Table 14.2), presumably because of the interest generated from its first use (Avery & Evans, 1973). The survey by Clarke and colleagues (1975), although prospective, was based on voluntary reporting of cases set against the amount of drug distributed, and the figure of 1 in 11 000 must now be accepted as an underestimate. The figures from other surveys (Table 14.5) suggest a much higher figure of about 1 in 1000. As with propanidid, reported deaths are few if we exclude those probably due to the poor health of the patient. It lacks the cardiovascular toxicity of propanidid and has a high therapeutic index (Clarke et al, 1972; Soga et al, 1973) but it is not followed by the very rapid recovery which gave propanidid a special place in outpatient anaesthesia. Therefore, even if reactions are somewhat less common than with propanidid there would appear to be no indications for using this steroid combination as a conventional induction agent unless a new formulation becomes available.

Diazepam in Cremophor EL (Stesolid MR)

Diazepam in its Valium formulation (Chapter 12) is irritant whether given intramuscularly or intravenously. Both routes of administration lead to local pain and intravenous injection is followed by a high incidence of venous thrombosis during the first two weeks (Hegarty & Dundee, 1977). Dilution of Valium with cremophor was tried by Burton and his colleagues (1974) with the virtual elimination of pain and venous thrombosis. However, they abandoned the technique (Burton, personal communication) after an anaphylactoid reaction. A new preparation of diazepam in cremophor was introduced into Scandinavia in 1977 and reports of anaphylactoid reactions were circulated very quickly (Milner, 1977; Falk, 1977) with an analysis of 5200 administrations by Schou Olesen & Huttel (1978). There were five reactions in this latter group, against no published reports of such reactions following the use of diazepam as Valium, pointing strongly to the involvement of Cremophor EL. There have, however, been reports of reactions to the sodium benzoate in Valium (Moneret-Vautrin et al, 1982) and to diazemuls (Nielsen, 1984) so that all available formulations of the drug carry some risk.

Propofol (Diprivan; ICI 35 868)

This is a phenol derivative which is sparingly soluble in water: a form solubilised in Cremophor EL was introduced into clinical practice by Kay & Rolly in 1977. From the outset it led to a high incidence of pain on injection (which is not a feature of other preparations in cremophor). In addition, during clinical trials in 1981 there was one typical reaction with erythema, hypotension, mild bronchospasm and oedema of the eyelids (Briggs et al, 1982). The patient had no history of atopy or allergy and no previous exposure, as far as is known, to a cremophor-containing anaesthetic. At that time less than 1000 anaesthetics with the drug had been given so that it seemed that reactions with this preparation were to be expected as with the other similar anaesthetics. In 1984 the drug was re-introduced in an emulsion and clinical trials over two years have not revealed any hypersensitivity reactions in this formulation.

The role of Cremophor EL

This is a mixture of higher fatty acids of molecular weight approximately 3170 (Scholtan & Lie, 1966) which has been used for solubilising some of the newer intravenous anaesthetics. It has also been used in solubilising vitamin preparations and cosmetics and for reducing the irritant qualities of Valium, so that it is not always possible to be certain whether a patient has been previously exposed to the substance.

It is not a single compound but has hydrophilic and hydrophobic components varying with temperature and with different preparations from year to year. A major change in the preparation was made c. 1972 in order to reduce the frequency or severity of adverse reactions. However in a blind retrospective study no significant difference in the effects on cardiovascular or respiratory systems could be detected between the old and new forms of propanidid (Doenicke, 1975).

The early studies suggested that Cremophor EL was almost without pharmacological action. For instance the LD_{50} in the mouse is 6500 mg kg^{-1} (Child et al, 1971). It does not cause histamine liberation in man (Lorenz et al, 1972; Doenicke et al, 1973), nor does it depress the cardiovascular system (Savage et al, 1973).

Evidence against Cremophor EL is still accumulating. For instance a reaction to Althesin has been described two weeks after exposure to propanidid (Notcutt, 1973) and one patient has been found to be sensitive to Epontol, Althesin and Cremophor on skin testing (Kessell & Assem, 1974). At least 5 patients out of 70 having reactions following Althesin had been previously exposed to propanidid (Tweedie & Ordish, 1974; Clarke et al, 1975). The reverse situation has also been reported by Dye & Watkins (1980), with a patient having a reaction to Epontol one week after an uneventful exposure to Althesin.

The possible role of Cremophor EL in hypersensitivity reactions was studied by Glen and his colleagues (1979) in the miniature pig. This species exhibits a reaction on repeated exposure to certain substances which is characterised by hypertension instead of collapse. However, liberation of histamine is still a feature in the majority of cases. The experiments showed that while the reactions following second exposure occurred with propanidid in Cremophor EL, they did not when ethyl alcohol and propylene glycol were used as solvents. The situation was not as clear-cut with Althesin for, even in the absence of cremophor, alphaxalone and alphadolone acetate induced some reactions. No reactions occurred in the miniature pig when thiopentone was given.

One reaction to cremophor alone has been reported (Gjessing & Tomlin, 1977) with the typical features of erythema, facial oedema and hypotension. The solvent was being given in this instance as a placebo control for diazepam in cremophor. In addition one patient has been shown to have reacted specifically to Cremophor EL in a reaction to a small dose of Althesin given by infusion.

With each of the above Cremophor EL preparations there is a reaction incidence of approximately 1 in 1000 which is much higher than with the barbiturates or other anaesthetics. The involvement of this solubiliser is particularly striking in the case of Stesolid MR where two formulations have had extensive clinical use. In addition to the reaction frequency, reactions to Epontol and Althesin differ from those following barbiturates in the high proportion which are complement-mediated (Table 14.4). The explanation for the role of cremophor is still uncertain but perhaps its surfactant properties enhance the immunogenicity of propanidid or alphaxalone, thereby rendering the clinical effects potentially more dangerous (Watkins et al, 1976; Padfield & Watkins, 1977). Alternatively in some cases there might be a true anaphylactic reaction to cremophor itself (Dye & Watkins, 1980).

PREDISPOSING FACTORS

Age and sex

Reactions occur throughout the age range and variations in frequency probably reflect the requirements for surgery. However there is a suggestion (Fisher & More, 1981) that the average age of reactors is lower than that of a control group of patients. There does not appear to be any difference between the sexes in reaction frequency following induction agents though there is a female preponderance in reactions to muscle relaxants (Fisher, 1978; Lim & Churchill-Davidson, 1981).

Infection, *carcinoma* and even *stress* can predispose to a hypersensitivity reaction by causing enhanced reactivity of Complement C3 (Watkins, 1982). A patient who, when ill, has reacted adversely to a drug might therefore have no response to the same drug after recovery from the immunopathology.

Dose and rate of injection

The question of dose has been discussed under the differential diagnosis and the difference between the effects of overdosage and an anaphylactoid reaction have been stressed. It appears likely on theoretical grounds, that an anaphylactoid reaction could occur with any significant dose or indeed with a slow infusion since the cascade is self-generating once it has been activated. Published reports (Clarke et al, 1975; Fisher & More, 1981; Benoit et al, 1983; Sear & Prys-Roberts, 1983) indicate that reactions can occur with a test dose of 0.5 ml and there are unpublished reports of reactions with an Althesin infusion (J G Whitwam and R J McBride, personal communications), contrary to the oft-stated belief (Saady, 1982) that infusions are safer than bolus injections.

Atopy

The survey by Clarke and his colleagues (1975) indicates a figure of approximately 15% of reactors having an atopic history (asthma, hay fever or eczema). This is probably a minimum figure and those in Table 14.5 and 14.6 are probably also underestimates. However, when analysing all these reports it is apparent that a history of atopy is approximately three times as common in barbiturate reactors than in those reacting to propanidid or Althesin. The incidence of an atopic history in patients reacting to intravenous anaesthetics must be compared with that in the general population to determine whether it is a true predisposing factor. The survey by Dundee and his colleagues (1978) of 10 000 preoperative surgical patients showed that the incidence in this group was 8.5%. This is not significantly different from the overall figure or that for the Althesin reactors but is significantly less than that for the barbiturate reactors (20%).

Allergy

A history of allergy to food or drugs is found in 19% of patients having reactions to intravenous anaesthetics (Clarke et al, 1975) and again is much higher in the barbiturates than in the Althesin group (Table 14.6). The incidence of a history of allergy in the general surgical population is 13.5% (Dundee et al, 1978) and the incidence in reactors in general is significantly higher than this. When reactors are divided into those to barbiturates and to other anaesthetics, it appears that the incidence is highest with the barbiturate group in whom almost one-third give a history of allergy.

The basis for a history of atopy or allergy might appear rather indefinite and an attempt has been made (Watkins et al, 1981) to determine whether there might be any immunological basis for such a history. Figure 14.5 shows the IgE levels in two groups of preoperative patients, one 'normal' and the other with a history of atopy or allergy. In general the levels in the 'normal' group fall below 200 IU ml^{-1} with a mean of 52.5, whereas the 'hypersensitive' patients had values up to 1000 IU ml^{-1} with a mean of 182.3. In addition those with an allergy to penicillin or who were atopic had the highest values, while those with allergies to food, miscellaneous drugs or skin contact had often a low IgE level. Nevertheless, it must be said that the correlation noted previously between allergy and reactions to intravenous barbiturates applies to any allergy and there is no reason to suppose that only those patients with raised IgE levels are involved. It might be that the patients with raised IgE levels have mainly type 1 reactions whereas those producing contact and other allergies which are T-lymphocyte-mediated fall into the type IV group.

It appears therefore that a history of atopy or allergy is a predisposing factor to barbiturate reactions though not to Althesin or propanidid reactions. However, Doenicke (1975) did find that patients with a history of allergy had more severe reactions to propanidid than those who had no such history. This is the main reason for withholding the cremophor-based anaesthetics in such patients, but even the barbiturates can probably be given safely since the incidence of reactions to this group of drugs in both atopic or non-atopic patients is so low.

Table 14.6 Anaesthetic-related history (%) in reactors to various intravenous anaesthetics and in the general surgical population.

	n	*Atopy*	*Allergy*	*Exposure to:*		
				Barbiturates	*Epontol*	*Althesin*
Reactors to						
barbiturates*	112	20	29	44	—	—
Epontol*	79	4	14	—	53	—
Althesin*	332	6	12	—	—	46
General surgical population†	10 000	8.5	13.5	54	Not known	12

* Data from Tables 14.1 and 14.2. Figures for history are all minimum figures because of incomplete information.
† Data from Dundee et al (1978) and Fee et al (1978); the figures for anaesthetic history were obtained by extrapolation.

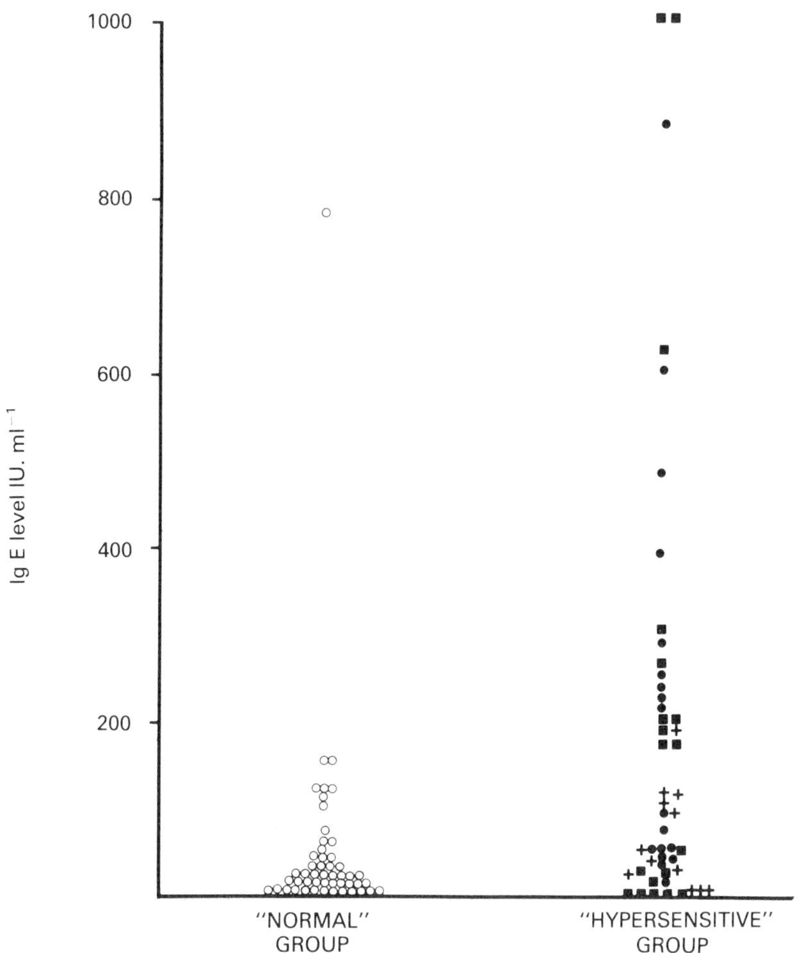

Fig. 14.5 IgE levels in two groups of preoperative patients. 'Normal' group — open circles; 'Hypersensitive' group: atopic — closed circles; allergic to penicillin — closed squares; other allergies — crosses. (Watkins et al, 1981).

Previous anaesthetics

The figures in Table 14.6 show that approximately 50% of patients reacting to intravenous anaesthetics have been previously exposed to the same drug and these are minimum figures because of inadequate questioning of some reactors. It is difficult to determine the anaesthetic history of a typical surgical population but Fee and his colleagues (1978) found that as many as 67% of such patients had previously been given an anaesthetic. Exact details of the drug received were not available in all cases but extrapolation from the information given suggested that 80% of patients previously anaesthetised had had thiopentone and 18% had received Althesin (unfortunately propanidid was not included in the survey). The figure of 80% for thiopentone is similar to that observed in a previous survey of UK hospitals by Dundee (1956) and by Evans & Keogh (1977). This suggests that approximately 54% of the total surgical population have previously received thiopentone which is approximately the same percentage as in barbiturate reactors. There is no evidence from these figures that previous exposure to thiopentone predisposes to a reaction or sensitises a patient to the drug.

The figures for Althesin indicate a different pattern, since only 18% of those previously anaesthetised and 12% of the total surgical population would have received Althesin. This is significantly less than the 46% of reactors in Table 14.5 and suggests that previous exposure is a

Table 14.7 Percentage incidence of clinical signs in 301 reactions following Althesin (information supplied by Glaxo Group Laboratories Limited)

	Previous exposure to Althesin		
Clinical manifestation	*Yes* (*151 cases*)	*No* (*75 cases*)	*Unknown* (*75 cases*)
Hypotension	76	71	59
Cardiac arrest	10	13	5
Flushing	54	51	44
Cyanosis	60	51	41
Bronchospasm	40	45	45
Laryngospasm	6	7	3
Facial oedema	22	25	19

predisposing factor in reactions to Althesin, as suggested also by the findings of Glen and colleagues (1979) in the mini-pig. Doenicke (1975) concluded that the same was true for propanidid since his retrospective figures showed that 22% of reactions occurred during first propanidid exposures and 78% during those who had one or more previous exposures.

It must also be said that there are reports of multiple uneventful anaesthetics with Althesin over 10 years (Cooper, 1972; Howard et al, 1982), one involving 84 anaesthetics. However, the correspondence after the latter article indicated that the use of Althesin in this way must be regarded as unsafe.

It might be thought that there might be a difference in reaction severity between those patients previously exposed to the drug and those having non-immune reactions. However, analysis by Glaxo Group Laboratories of the records of 301 reactors (Table 14.7) shows that the clinical pattern is similar whatever the previous history.

The interval since the previous exposure to Althesin is also relevant, according to unpublished figures supplied by Glaxo Laboratories. While 67% of the general population have had an anaesthetic in the past, the great majority of these were anaesthetised at least 12 months previously (Figure 14.6) and only 19% in the previous one month. Among Althesin reactions on the other hand 49% had received Althesin within the past

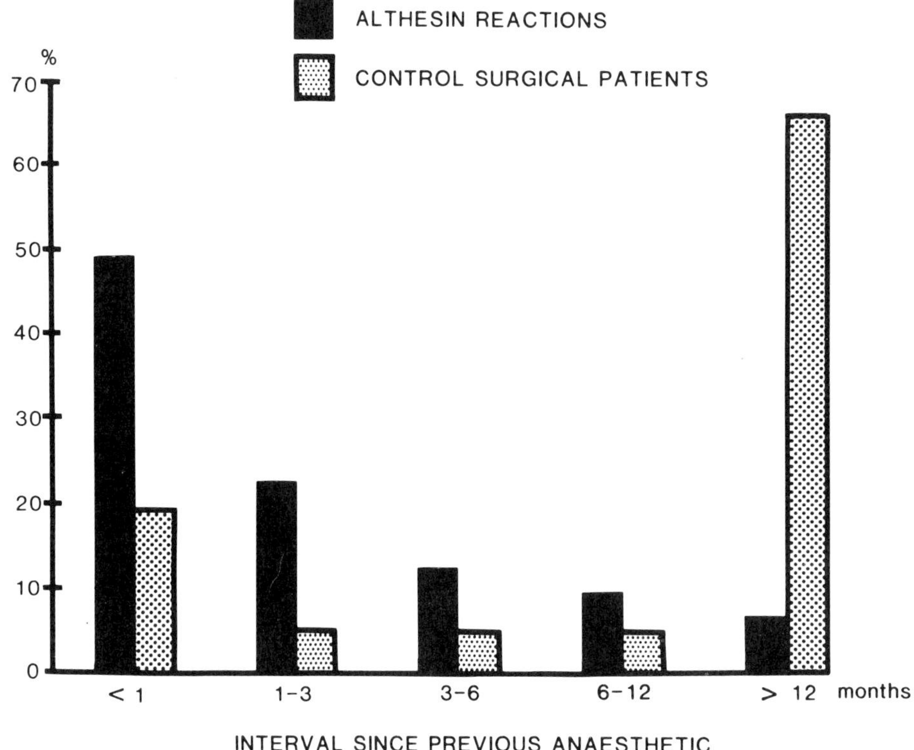

Fig. 14.6 Interval since previous anaesthetic in a group of reactors to Althesin (information supplied by Glaxo Group Research Limited), compared with a control group of surgical patients (Fee et al, 1978).

month. The figures therefore indicate that the first month after Althesin is a time of particular vulnerability in humans to reactions with subsequent exposure, but the whole of the first year must also be considered as within the danger period — unlike the mini-pig, in which the period of risk appears to be no more than 21 days (Glen et al, 1979).

INVESTIGATION OF REACTORS

It is clear from the above analysis that many anaphylactoid reactions can be partly identified for what they are by diverse physical signs indicative of widespread histamine release. The episode can thus be distinguished from an overdose phenomenon but cannot be defined as Type I, complement-mediated or due to pharmacological liberation of histamine. These distinctions are not simply academic but have a bearing on management. A true immunological or Type I reaction will, of necessity, be exacerbated if the causative agent or a related cross-reacting antigen is presented to the patient in the future. On the other hand complement-mediated reactions, particularly to short-acting anaesthetic drugs, are most unlikely to be exacerbated by further exposure of the patient, who later will probably show little specificity for the supposed causative agent. He might in fact either react in a similar manner to a different type of drug at a later date, or even not react at all to the original drug, if a temporary causative factor such as underlying infection, is no longer operative.

Immunological investigation

The first stage of investigating a reaction is therefore to obtain a history of atopy, allergy, previous exposure to the same drug (or solvent) or evidence of an acute viral infection. The exact timing of the phases of the reaction in relation to drug administration should be noted as soon as possible. The most important step then is to take serial venous blood samples at the following times (ideally into EDTA tubes): prereaction, 30 min, 3, 6 and 24 h and 5 days postreaction (Watkins et al, 1979). The plasma is separated, deep-frozen and later the batch is analysed for complement C3, C4, C3 proactivator and Cl inhibitor) as well as calculation of C3 conversion. IgA, IgE, IgG and IgD are measured in a control sample which is prereaction if possible, but if this is not available (e.g. from a sample stored in the blood bank) the 5-day sample is adequate. The great advantage about this procedure for investigation is that no specific mechanism is assumed and it is relatively simple. On the other hand it can only identify plasma events and is of poor sensitivity for marginal adverse reactions (Watkins, 1981).

Simultaneous haematological samples will give information about haemodulution (see under Treatment, p. 266) but leukocyte counts, preferably with differential, also help to identify the mechanism.

Intradermal testing

This has been strongly advocated by Fisher (1976b; 1979; 1981) and has the advantage of being simple and possibly leading to an identification of the causative agent which is not obtained from the complement analysis. On the other hand it does assume an immune mechanism and one must wait four weeks before testing to avoid a false negative response or a dangerous challenge reaction. It is probably only justified if the reaction appears to be IgE mediated.

The technique recommended by Fisher (1984) is as follows: prepare fresh solutions of all drugs and solvents that are relevant, dilute them to 1:100 (1:1000 for muscle relaxants) and inject 0.01–0.02 ml intradermally on the anterior surface of the forearm after cleaning with alcohol. (*Note*: many workers use 0.1 ml for the intradermal injection). A positive reaction is a flare with a wheal of at least 1.0 cm appearing within 30 min and persisting for 30 min. If there is a reaction with more than one drug, both should be tested in a higher dilution. Resuscitation facilities should always be available though Fisher (1975) states that the risks of provoking a generalised reaction by skin testing in this way are small.

Other investigative techniques such as the Prausnitz–Kustner and specific cellular tests require to be carried out in laboratories specialising in the field. They can however provide confirmatory evidence.

PREVENTION

It is not possible to prevent adverse reactions completely since almost any drug can cause one, even with a test dose, and even skin testing of every patient would not exclude all types. However, the severity of the reaction can be reduced by administering only moderate doses of the drug and doing so slowly. There is no evidence that any particular drug ought to be avoided in patients with a general atopic or allergic history. If a patient is known to be sensitive to a particular drug this should obviously not be given. However, it is not easy to incriminate one agent with certainty when two are given together. A patient who has had a reaction to one agent can probably be anaesthetised safely with another but he is still at considerable risk. Such patients should probably have both H_1 and H_2 receptor blocking drugs (promethazine 50 mg with cimetidine 400 mg or ranitidine 150 mg) two hours before anaesthesia. Similar combinations have been shown to be effective in preventing reactions to cross-linked gelatin (Haemaccel), histamine infusion and morphine administration and presumably are effective against drug-related reactions generally (Lorenz et al, 1980; Kaliner et al, 1982; Philbin et al, 1981). However, cimetidine administration itself causes some release of histamine and disturbance of blood coagulation (Serlin et al, 1979) so that it cannot be recommended as a general prophylactic. Disodium chromoglycate has been shown to block signs of immune recognition in vitro (Watkins et al, 1976) and will prevent bronchospasm in susceptible individuals but its value in preventing hypersensitivity reactions is still unknown. The prophylactic dose is 200 mg by mouth.

TREATMENT

Anaesthesia should only be undertaken where facilities for resuscitation are available. This seems axiomatic but the criteria listed must be regarded as minimum and are not always followed where the anaesthetic is considered 'minor'.

1. Indwelling needle/cannula — ideally an infusion running.
2. A table which permits the head-end to be lowered below the horizontal.
3. Means of inflating the lungs with oxygen: a demand type of anaesthetic machine is not sufficient.
4. Drugs: chlorpheniramine, adrenaline, hydrocortisone, metaraminol, aminophylline.
5. Infusion fluids: a synthetic plasma expander or human plasma protein fraction (albumin).
6. Tracheal tubes and laryngoscope.

The commonest manifestations of a hypersensitivity reaction are vasodilatation and extravasation of fluid into the tissue spaces. The logical treatment is therefore the administration of fluid, preferably a synthetic plasma expander such as low-molecular weight dextran, cross-linked gelatin or human plasma protein fraction. Fisher (1977a) has calculated that the volume lost is 1–2 litres and this volume should be rapidly infused. Progress can be monitored by the central venous pressure but urgent restoration of the circulating volume should not wait for this. Tilting of the table into the head-down position is also a useful first-aid measure to counteract the tendency to venous pooling in the legs. The trachea will also need to be intubated if this has not already taken place and inhalational anaesthesia should, of course, be replaced by oxygen. This will be valuable whether or not there is bronchospasm or laryngeal oedema.

Adrenaline is valuable for its positive inotropic action to raise the blood pressure in spite of peripheral vasodilatation. In addition, by its action on beta-adrenergic receptors it increases the level of cyclic AMP, inhibits degranulation of mast cells and thereby prevents further liberation of histamine (Stoelting, 1983). Many workers (Larard, 1980; Runciman, 1980; Sage, 1985) now believe that this is the most effective drug for treating both circulatory and respiratory problems in a reaction and that its efficacy outweighs the risk of inducing ventricular fibrillation. However, a defibrillator should be readily available when a reaction is being treated. To be effective in shock adrenaline must be given intravenously and this necessitates dilution of the standard 1:1000 solution to 1:10 000 and administration in approximately 1 ml increments. The alpha stimulators such as metaraminol 1–10 mg may have a place if the heart rate is already rapid, which is a likely consequence of the action of histamine. A theoretical disadvantage of the use of alpha-adrenergic and cholinergic drugs is that they might actually stimulate histamine production by reducing the mast cell content of cyclic AMP.

Adrenaline has an additional advantage of being a potent bronchodilator but slow intravenous injection of aminophylline 250 mg is probably safer if this is the main problem. Hydrocortisone 100–250 mg i.v. is beneficial to counteract both the bronchospasm and the cardiovascular collapse and antihistamines such as chlorpheniramine 10 mg i.v. might also help to terminate the reaction but both these drugs are less urgent and have a slower action.

The patient will probably require continued observation with supportive treatment but reactions, especially those following Althesin, are often surprisingly brief and it might be possible to proceed with the operation. Since most anaesthetists only experience one or two of these reactions in a career, it is surprising that treatment is so effective and complete recovery occurs in about 95% of cases.

REFERENCES

Anderton J M, Hopton D S 1968 Thiopentone anaphylaxis: a hazard of multiple cystoscopic examinations under general anaesthesia. Anaesthesia 23: 90–93

Avery A F, Evans A 1973 Reactions to Althesin. British Journal of Anaesthesia 45: 301–303

Baldwin A C 1979 Thiopentone anaphylaxis. Anaesthesia 34: 333–335

Barjenbruch K P, Jones J R 1972 Thiopental anaphylaxis: a case report. Anesthesia and Analgesia . . Current Researches 51: 113–116

Beamish D, Brown D T 1980 Delayed adverse responses to both methohexitone and Althesin. Anaesthesia 35: 279–281

Beamish D, Brown D T 1981 Adverse responses to i.v. anaesthetics. British Journal of Anaesthesia 53: 55–58

Beck L 1965 Podiumgesprach uber das Kurznarkotikum Propanidid. In: Horatz K, Frey R, Zindler M (eds) Die intravenose Kurznarkose mit dem neuen Phenoxyessigsaure-derivat Propanidid (Epontol), Springer, Berlin, p 307

Benoit Y, Chadenson O, Ducloux B, Veysseyre C M, Bringuier J P, Veysseyre C Descotes J 1983 Hypersensitivity reactions to Althesin infusion: measurement of complement involvement. Anaesthesia 38: 1079-1081

Boyce M J 1982 Pharmacological characterisation of cardiovascular histamine receptors in man in vivo. Klinische Wochenschrift 60: 978–982

Boytell K A 1976 Anaphylactic reaction to Althesin. Anaesthesia and Intensive Care 4: 362–363

Bradburn C C 1970 Severe hypotension following induction with propanidid. British Journal of Anaesthesia 42: 362–363

Briggs L P, Clarke R S J, Watkins J 1982 An adverse reaction to the administration of disoprofol (Diprivan). Anaesthesia 37: 1099–1101.

Brown T P 1975 Thiopentone anaphylaxis — case report. Anaesthesia and Intensive Care 3: 257–259

Burton G W, Lenz R J, Thomas T A, Midda M 1974 Cremophor EL as a diluent for diazepam (letter). British Medical Journal iii:258

Bussien R, Rybaric E, Thurler B 1975 Crise d'asthme apres induction avec l'alfatesine (CT 1341). Anesthesie, analgesie, reanimation 32: 147–148

Callens J, Doutriaux J 1976 Deux cas d'allergie severe en anesthesiologie. Journal des sciences medicales de Lille 94: 293–295

Carrie L E S, Buchanan R L 1967 Thiopentone anaphylaxis. Anaesthesia 22: 290–295

Carson I W, Dundee J W, Clarke R S J 1975 The speed of onset and potency of Althesin. British Journal of Anaesthesia 47: 512–515

Casale F F 1982 Multiple general anaesthesia with Althesin. British Medical Journal 285:378

Child K J, Currie J P, Davis B, Dodds M G, Pearce D R, Twissell D J 1971 The pharmacological properties in animals of CT 1341, a new steroid anaesthetic agent. British Journal of Anaesthesia 43: 2–13

Chung D C W 1976 Anaphylaxis to thiopentone: a case report. Canadian Anaesthetists' Society Journal 23: 319–322

Clark M M, Cockburn H A 1971 Anaphylactoid response to thiopentone. British Journal of Anaesthesia 43: 185–189

Clarke R S J, Dundee J W 1969 Hypotensive reaction after propanidid and atropine. British Medical Journal iv:369

Clarke R S J, Dundee J W 1970 Toxic effects of intravenous anaesthetics: a comparison of propanidid with thiopentone. In: Boulton T B, Bryce-Smith R, Sykes M K, Gillett G B, Revell A L (eds) Progress in Anaesthesiology. Proceedings of the 4th World Congress of Anaesthesiologists, Excerpta Medica, Amsterdam, p 1189–1191

Clarke R S J, Dundee J W, Barron D W, McArdle L 1968 Clinical studies of induction agents. XXV: The relative potencies of thiopentone, methohexitone and propanidid. British Journal of Anaesthesia 40: 593–601

Clarke R S J, Dundee J W, Carson I W 1972 Some aspects of the clinical pharmacology of Althesin. Postgraduate Medical Journal 48 (Suppl 2): 62–65

Clarke R S J, Dundee J W, Garrett R T, McArdle G K, Sutton J A 1975 Adverse reactions to intravenous anaesthetics: a survey of 100 reports. British Journal of Anaesthesia 47: 575–585

Cole F 1968 Sensitivity to thiopental. Nebraska State Medical Journal 53:478

Cooper J 1972 Althesin in outpatient psychiatric practice. Postgraduate Medical Journal 48 (Suppl 2): 115–116

Crowther A N 1973 Bronchospasm following Althesin anaesthesia. British Medical Journal 2:775

Currie T T, Whittingham S, Ebringer A, Peters J S 1966 Severe anaphylactic reaction to thiopentone: case report. British Medical Journal 1: 1460–1463

Dale H H, Laidlaw P P 1919 Histamine shock. Journal of Physiology 52: 355–390

Dannemann H, Lubke P 1970 Komplikationen wahrend Narkosen mit Epontol. Zeitzchrift fur praktische Anaesthesiol und Wiederbelebung 5: 273–277

Davis J 1971 Thiopentone anaphylaxis. Case report. British Journal of Anaesthesia 43: 1191–1193

Davison T C 1943 Intravenous anesthesia in modern surgery (sodium-pentothal-oxygen). Anesthesia and Analgesia . . . Current Researches 22: 52–56

Doenicke A 1975 Propanidid. In: Arias A, Llaurado R, Nalda M A, Lunn J N. Recent Progress in Anaesthesiology and Resuscitation. Excerpta Medica, Amsterdam, p 107–113

Doenicke A, Lorenz W, Beigl R, Bezecny H, Ulig G, Malmar L, Praetorius B, Mann G 1973 Histamine release after intravenous application of short-acting hypnotics: a comparison of etomidate, Althesin (CT 1341) and propanidid. British Journal of Anaesthesia 45: 1097–1104

Dohi S, Naito H, Takahashi T 1975 A case of anaphylactoid reaction to thiamylal. Japanese Journal of Anesthesiology 24: 743–748

Douglas W W 1975 Histamines and antihistamines. In: Goodman L S and Gilman A (eds) The pharmacological basis of therapeutics, 5th edn. Macmillan, New York

Driggs R L, O'Day R A 1972 Acute allergic reaction associated with methohexital anesthesia: report of six cases. Journal of Oral Surgery 30: 906–909

Dundee J W 1956 Thiopentone and other thiobarbiturates. Livingstone, Edinburgh, p 9–10

Dundee J W, Assem E S K, Gaston J M, Keilty S R, Sutton J A, Clarke R S J, Grainger Ð 1974 Sensitivity to intravenous anaesthetics: a report of three cases. British Medical Journal i: 63–65

Dundee J W, Fee J P H, McDonald J R, Clarke R S J 1978 Frequency of atopy and allergy in an anaesthetic patient population. British Journal of Anaesthesia 50: 793–798

Dueck R, O'Connor R D 1984 Thiopental: false-positive RAST in patients with elevated serum IgE. Anesthesiology 61: 337–338

Dye D, Watkins J 1980 Suspected anaphylactic reaction to Cremophor EL. British Medical Journal 280:1353

Etter M S, Helrich M, MacKenzie C F 1980 Immunoglobulin E fluctuation in thiopental anaphylaxis. Anesthesiology 52: 181–183

Evans A 1971 Reaction to propanidid. British Journal of Anaesthesia 43:802

Evans F, Gould J 1952 Relation between sensitivity to thiopentone, sulphonamides and sunlight. British Medical Journal i: 417–419

Evans J M, Keogh J A M 1977 Adverse reactions to intravenous anaesthetic induction agents. British Medical Journal ii: 735–736

Falk R H 1977 Allergy to diazepam. British Medical Journal i:287

Fantera A, Maurina M 1976 Impiego dell' Althesin dell' introduzione endovenosa dell' anestesia generale e valutazione dei suoi effetti cardicircolatori e respiratori. Acta anaesthesiologica Italia 27: 241–256

Fee J P H, McDonald J R, Dundee J W, Clarke R S J 1978 Frequency of previous anaesthesia in an anaesthetic patient population. British Journal of Anaesthesia 50: 917–920

Fisher M M 1975 Severe histamine mediated reactions to intravenous drugs used in anaesthesia. Anaesthesia and Intensive Care 3: 180–197

Fisher M M 1976a Severe histamine-mediated reactions to Althesin. Anaesthesia and Intensive care 4: 33–35

Fisher M M 1976b Intradermal testing after severe histamine reactions to intravenous drugs used in anaesthesia. Anaesthesia and Intensive Care 4: 97–104

Fisher M M 1977 Blood volume replacement in acute anaphylactic cardiovascular collapse related to anaesthesia. British Journal of Anaesthesia 49: 1023–1026

Fisher M M 1978 Anaphylactic reactions to gallamine triethiodide. Anaesthesia and Intensive Care 6: 62–65

Fisher M M 1979 Intradermal testing in the diagnosis of acute anaphylaxis during anaesthesia — results of five years experience. Anaesthesia and Intensive Care 7: 58–61

Fisher M M 1981 The diagnosis of acute anaphylactoid reactions to anaesthetic drugs. Anaesthesia and Intensive Care 9: 235–241

Fisher M M 1984 Intradermal testing after anaphylactoid reaction to anaesthetic drugs: practical aspects of performance and interpretation. Anaesthesia and Intensive Care 12: 115–120

Fisher M M, More D G 1981 The epidemiology and clinical features of anaphylactic reactions in anaesthesia. Anaesthesia and Intensive Care 9: 226–234

Fisher T 1968 Allergies ignored: routine versus thought. Canadian Medical Association Journal 99: 854–855

Foissac J, Jaboeuf R, Coulon C, Verret J, Baguet G 1981 Chocs anaphylactoides a l'Alfatesine. Cahiers d'Anesthesiologie 29: 249–255

Fox G S, Wilkinson R D, Rabow F I 1971 Thiopental anaphylaxis: a case and a method for diagnosis. Anesthesiology 35: 655–657

Gjessing J 1969 Hypotension, hypoventilation and delayed recovery after propanidid. British Journal of Anaesthesia 41:1012

Gjessing J, Tomlin P J 1977 Intravenous sedation and regional analgesia. Anaesthesia 32: 63–69

Glen J B, Davies G E, Thomson D S, Scarth S C, Thompson A V 1979 An animal model for the investigation of adverse responses to i.v. anaesthetic agents and their solvents. British Journal of Anaesthesia 51: 819–827

Gotla D W 1972 Apparent anaphylactic reaction to propanidid. Anaesthesia 27: 16–17

Grimmeisen H 1971 Epontol anaesthesia. Medizinische Klinik 66:1417

Guilmet C, Jove P 1976 Un choc anaphylactique au Pentothal a l'induction. Annales de l'Anesthesiologie Francaise 17: 77–80

Harrfeldt H P 1973 10 Jahre Kurznarkosen mit Propanidid. In: Zindler M, Yamamura H, Wirth W (eds) Intravenose Narkose mit Propanidid, Springer, Berlin, p 234–242

Hayward J R, Kiester G L 1957 Severe allergic reactions during thiopentone sodium anaesthesia. Journal of Oral Surgery 15: 61–63

Healy T E J 1973 Bronchospasm following Althesin induction. Lancet ii:975

Hegarty J E, Dundee J W 1977 Sequelae after the intravenous injection of three benzodiazepines, diazepam, lorazepam and flunitrazepam. British Medical Journal ii: 1384–1385

Hester J B 1973 Reaction to Althesin. British Journal of Anaesthesia 45:303

Hirshman C A, Peters J, Cartwright-Lee I 1982 Leukocyte histamine release to thiopental. Anesthesiology 56: 64–67

Holmes R P, Ross J W, Williams E R 1971 Acute anaphylaxis under anaesthesia. Anaesthesia 26: 363–367

Horton J N 1973 Adverse reaction to Althesin. Anaesthesia 28: 182–183

Howard D J, Farag S, Liscombe R M 1982 Multiple general anaesthesia with Althesin. British Medical Journal 285: 99–100

Hughes R L, Inglis M, Campbell D 1977 Althesin reactions. Anaesthesia 32: 910–911

Hunter A R 1943 Dangers of pentothal sodium anaesthesia. Lancet 1: 46–48

Huttel M S, Schou Olesen A S, Stoffersen E 1980 Complement-mediated reactions to diazepam with cremophor as solvent (Stesolid MR). British Journal of Anaesthesia 52: 77–79

Jago R H, Restall J 1978 Sensitivity testing for Althesin. Anaesthesia 33: 644–645

Jarvis C A N 1972 Reaction to propanidid. British Journal of Anaesthesia 44:989

Johns G 1970 Cardiac arrest following induction with propanidid. British Journal of Anaesthesia 42: 74–77

Kaliner M, Shelhamer J H, Ottesen E A 1982 Effects of infused histamine: correlation of plasma histamine levels and symptoms. Journal of Allergy and Clinical Immunology 68:283

Kay B 1969 Hypotensive reaction after propanidid and atropine. British Medical Journal iii:413

Kay B 1972 Brietal sodium in children's surgery. In: Lehmann C (ed) Das Ultrakurznarkoticum Methohexital, Springer, Berlin, p 149–158

Kay B and Rolly G 1977 ICI 35 868, a new intravenous induction agent. Acta Anaesthesiologica Belgica 28: 303–316

Kelly A J, Boman A 1973 Anaphylaxis under anaesthesia. Anaesthesia and Intensive Care 1: 322–323

Kessell J, Assem E S K 1974 An adverse reaction to Althesin. British Journal of Anaesthesia 46:209

Kivalo I, Wist A, Mustakallio M 1960 Anaphylactic shock in thiopental anesthesia. Duodecim (Helsinki) 76: 509–510

Kruger H W 1970 Anaphylaktischer Schock nach Epontol-Kurznarkosen. Geburtshilfe und Frauenheilkunde 30:37

Larard D G 1970 Cardiac arrest following induction with propanidid. British Journal of Anaesthesia 42:652

Larard D G 1980 Treatment of anaphylactic reactions. Anaesthesia 35: 1011–1012

Laxenaire M C, Sigiel M, Moneret-Vautrin D A, Mueller R, Chastel A 1976 Accidents anaphylactoides lies a l'emploi de produits anesthesiques et adjuvants. A propos de 18 cas. Annales de l'anesthesiologie francaise 17: 85–90

Lilly J K, Hoy R H 1980 Thiopental anaphylaxis and reagin involvement. Anesthesiology 52: 335–337

Lim M, Churchill-Davidson H C 1981 Adverse effects of neuromuscular blocking drugs. In: Thornton J A (ed) Adverse reactions to anaesthetic drugs, North-Holland Biomedical Press, Elsevier, p 65–136

Lorenz W, Doenicke A 1975 Anaphylactoid reactions and histamine release by intravenous drugs used in surgery and anaesthesia. In: Watkins J, Ward A M (eds) Adverse response to intravenous drugs, Academic Press, London, p 83–112

Lorenz W, Doenicke A, Dittman I, Hug P, Schwarz B 1977 Anaphylaktoide Reaktionen nach Applikation von Blutersatymitteln bim Menschen: Verkinderung dieser Nebenwirkung von Haemaccel durch Pramedikation mit H_1 und H_2 Rezeptorantagonisten. Anaesthesist 26: 644–648

Lorenz W, Doenicke A, Messmer K, Reimann H-J, Thermann M, Lahn W, Berr J, Schmal A, Dormann P, Regenfuss P, Hamelmann H 1976 Histamine release in human subjects by modified gelatin (Haemaccel) and dextran: an explanation for anaphylactoid reactions observed under clinical conditions? British Journal of Anaesthesia 48: 151–165

Lorenz W, Doenicke A, Meyer R, Reimann J, Kusche J, Barth H, Geesing H, Hutzel M, Weissenbacher B 1972 Histamine release in man by propanidid and thiopentone: pharmacological effects and clinical consequences. British Journal of Anaesthesia 44: 355–369

Lorenz W, Doenicke A, Schoning B, Mamorski J, Weber D, Hinterlang E, Schwarz B, Neugebauer E 1980 H_1 + H_2-receptor antagonists for premedication in anaesthesia and surgery: a critical view basing on randomized clinical trials with Haemaccel and various anti-allergic drugs. Agents Actions 10: 114–124

Lorenz W, Doenicke A, Schoning B, Neugebauer E 1981 The role of histamine in adverse reactions to intravenous agents. In: Thornton J A (ed) Adverse reactions to anaesthetic drugs. North-Holland Biomedical, Elsevier, p 169–238

McDowell S A, Clarke R S J 1969 A clinical comparison of pancuronium with tubocurarine. Anaesthesia 24: 581–590

Manz R, Frank G 1969 Zur Frage allergischer Reaktionen nach Epontol. Anaesthesist 18:223

Mathieu A, Goudsouzian N, Snider M T 1975 Reaction to ketamine: anaphylactoid or anaphylactic? British Journal of Anaesthesia 47: 624–627

Mathieu A, Grilliat J P 1976 Correspondence. British Journal of Anaesthesia 48: 49–50

Mehta S 1973 Anaphylactic reaction to Althesin. Anaesthesia 28: 669–672

Mehta S 1981 Adverse responses to i.v. anaesthetics. British Journal of Anaesthesia 53:1005

Michangeli F, Donsa E, Feyler C, Maestracci P 1981 L'alfatesine en perfusion controlee en geronta-anestesie incidence des reactions anaphylactoides. Mediterranee Medicine 239: 29–36

Milner L 1977 Allergy to diazepam. British Medical Journal i:144

Miloschewsky D, Cervenkova M 1970 Cardiovascular collapse following induction with propanidid. British Journal of Anaesthesia 42:833

Moneret-Vautrin D A, Laxenaire M C, Viry-Babel F 1983 Anaphylaxis caused by anti-Cremophor EL IgG STS antibodies in a case of reaction to Althesin. British Journal of Anaesthesia 55: 469–471

Moneret-Vautrin D A, Moeller R, Malingrey L, Laxenaire M C 1982 Anaphylactoid reaction to general anaesthesia: a case of intolerance to sodium benzoate. Anaesthesia and Intensive Care 10: 156–157

Monteil A, Navarrot P, Kiencen J, Du Cailar J 1976 A propos de deux observations de reaction de type anaphylactique a l'alfadione (Alfatesin-Althesin CT 1341). Annales de l'anesthesiologie francaise 17: 71–76

Nielsen F-B 1984 Anaphylactoid reaction to Diazemuls. British Journal of Anaesthesia 56:1179

Notcutt W G 1973 Adverse reaction to Althesin. Anaesthesia 28: 673–674

Owen D A 1977 Histamine receptors in the cardiovascular system. General Physiology 8: 141–156

Padfield A, Watkins J 1977 Allergy to diazepam. British Medical Journal i: 575–576

Philbin D M, Moss J, Akins C W, Rosow C E, Kono K, Schneider R C, Verlee T R, Savarese J J 1981 The use of H_1 and H_2 histamine antagonists with morphine anaesthesia: a double-blind study. Anesthesiology 55: 292–296

Radford S G, Lockyer J A, Simpson P J 1982 Immunological aspects of adverse reactions to Althesin. British Journal of Anaesthesia 54: 859–863

Radnay P A 1965 Cardiovascular effects of propanidid. Acta anaesthesiologica Scandinavica 17:49

Rawicz M, Rondio Z, Cwizewicz-Adamska J 1976 Anaphylactic shock following Althesin. A case report. Anaesthesia, Resuscitation and Intensive Therapy 4: 65–69

Reichert E F, Bassett P A 1972 A rare allergic reaction to sodium methohexital. Journal of Oral Surgery 30:910

Ring J, Messmer K 1977 Incidence and severity of anaphylactoid reactions to colloid volume substitutes. Lancet 1: 466–469

Rozenkranz I 1972 Cardiovascular collapse after propanidid. British Journal of Anaesthesia 44:1332

Runciman W B 1980 Sympathomimetic amines. Anaesthesia and Intensive Care 8: 289–309

Saady A 1982 Anaesthetic anaphylactoid reactions. Anaesthesia and Intensive Care 10: 90–91

Sage D J 1985 Anaphylactoid reactions in anesthesia. International Anesthesiology Clinics 23: 175–186

Saint-Maurice C, Daihle-Dupont D, Roche M, Rulin M, Viallard C 1976 Deux cas de reactions de type anaphlactique en rapport avec l'anesthesie. Annales de l'anesthesiologie francaise 17: 81–84

Samuel I O, Dundee J W 1973 Clinical studies of induction agents. XLII: Influence of injection rate and dosage on the induction complications with Althesin. British Journal of Anaesthesia 45: 1215–1216

Savege T M, Foley E I, Simpson B R 1973 Some cardiorespiratory effects of Cremophor EL in man. British Journal of Anaesthesia 45: 515–517

Scholtan W, Lie S Y 1966 Kolloid-chemische Eigenschaften eines neuen Kurznarkoticums. Arzneimittel-Forschung 16: 679–691

Schou Olesen A, Huttel M S 1978 Circulatory collapse following intravenous administration of Stesolid MR. Ugeskrift for Laeger 140:2644

Scott P V 1979 Sensitivity testing for Althesin. Anaesthesia 34: 86–87

Sear J W, Prys-Roberts C 1983 Hypersensitivity reactions to infusions of Althesin. Anaesthesia 38:1223

Serlin M J, Sibeon R G, Mossman S, Breckenridge A M, Williams J R B, Atwood J L, Willoughby J M T 1979 Cimetidine: interaction with oral anticoagulants in man. Lancet 2:317

Shafto C E 1969 Continuous intravenous anaesthesia for paediatric dentistry. British Journal of Anaesthesia 41: 407–416

Shaw H 1974 Anaesthetic complications. New Zealand Society of Anaesthetists Newsletter 21:144

Sneddon I B, Glew R C 1973 Contact dermatitis due to propanidid in an anaesthetist. Practitioner 211: 321–323

Soga D, Beer R, Bader B, Andrae J, Gotz E 1973 Die Beeinflussung der linksventrikularen. Myokardkontraktilitat und Haemodynamik durch Propanidid beim Menschen. In: Zindler M, Yamamura H, Wirth H (eds) Intravenose Narkose mit Propanidid. Springer, Berlin, p 78–87

Sold M J 1985 Etomidate: an 'immunologically safe' anaesthetic agent? Anaesthesia 40: 1014–1015

Spreadbury T H, Marrett H R 1971 Cardiovascular collapse after propanidid. British Journal of Anaesthesia 43:925

Steel G C 1976 Reaction to Althesin. British Journal of Anaesthesia 48:50

Stieglitz P, Jacquot C, Riondel J P 1976 Accidents d'histamino-liberation per anesthesique. Annales de l'Anesthesiologie Francaise 17: 91–94

Stoelting R K 1983 Allergic reactions during anesthesia. Anesthesia and Analgesia 62: 341–356

Stovner J, Endresen R 1971 Repeated propanidid in cancer. British Journal of Anaesthesia 43: 207–208

Strunk H A 1962 Reaction to thiopental. Anesthesiology 23:271

Sutton J A 1976 Mechanism of a reaction to Althesin. British Journal of Anaesthesia 48: 711–712

Thompson D S, Eason C N, Flacke J W 1973 Thiamylal anaphylaxis. Anesthesiology 39: 556–558

Thornton H L 1971 Apparent anaphylactic reaction to propanidid. Anaesthesia 26: 490–493

Turner K J, Keep V R, Bartholomaeus N 1972 Anaphylaxis induced by propanidid and atropine. British Journal of Anaesthesia 44: 211–214

Tweedie D G, Ordish P M 1974 Reactions to intravenous agents (Althesin and pancuronium). British Journal of Anaesthesia 46:244

Unsworth I P 1972 Thiopentone anaphylaxis. Anaesthesia and Intensive Care 1: 79–80

Vanezis P 1979 Death after Althesin. Practitioner 222: 259–261

Waldhausen E, Marquardt B, Helms U 1981 Erfahrungen aus 31 anaphylaktoiden Reaktionen. Anaesthesist 30: 47–51

Watkins J 1981 Mechanisms and factors predisposing towards adverse response to intravenous anaesthetic substances. In: Thornton J A (ed) Adverse reactions to anaesthetic drugs. North-Holland Biomedical Press, Elsevier, p 137–167

Watkins J 1982 'Hypersensitivity response' to drugs and plasma substitutes used in anaesthesia and surgery. In: Watkins J, Salo M (eds) Trauma, stress and immunity in anaesthesia and surgery. Butterworth, London, chapter 9

Watkins J 1983 Etomidate: an 'immunologically safe' anaesthetic agent. Anaesthesist 38 supplement, 34–38

Watkins J 1985 Allergic and pseudoallergic mechanisms in anaesthesia. In: Sage D J (ed) Anaphylactoid reactions in anaesthesia. International Anesthesiology Clinics 23: 17–40

Watkins J, Clark A, Appleyard T N, Padfield A 1976 Immune-mediated reactions to Althesin (Alphaxalone). British Journal of Anaesthesia 48: 881–886

Watkins J, Clarke R S J, Fee J P H 1981 The relationship between reported atopy or allergy and immunoglobulins: a preliminary study. Anaesthesia 36: 582–585

Watkins J, Padfield A, Alderson J D 1978 Underlying immunopathology as a cause of adverse responses to two intravenous anaesthetic agents. British Medical Journal i: 1180–1181

Watkins J, Thornton J A, Clarke R S J 1979 Adverse reactions to i.v. agents (letter). British Journal of Anaesthesia 51:469

Watkins J, Udnoon S, Taussig P 1978 Mechanisms of adverse response to intravenous agents in man. In: Watkins J, Milford Ward A (eds) Adverse response to intravenous drugs. Academic Press, London

Watt J M 1975 Anaphylactic reactions after use of CT 1341 (Althesin) British Medical Journal iii: 205–206

Wedley J R 1973 Thiopentone-induced bronchospasm. Anaesthesia 28: 318–319

Wyatt R, Watkins J 1975 Reaction to methohexitone. British Journal of Anaesthesia 47: 1119–1120

Zaffiri O, Marchetti G, Perani R, Giuntelli V, Sandalvadore G, Pinsoglio M, Scarella M R, Bonardi C, Borsatti T 1981 Le reazione da ipersensibilita agli agenti anestetici endovenosi e lora prevenzione. Minerva Anestesiologica 47: 127–135

Zindler M 1965 Allergic and anaphylactic reactions, decrease in blood pressure. Acta anaesthesiologica Scandinavica, Suppl 17: 79–80

Zindler M 1975 Propanidid (Epontol): reappraisal of its present position. In: Arias A, Llaurado R, Nalda M A, Lunn J N (eds) Recent progress in anaesthesiology and resuscitation. Excerpta Medica, Amsterdam, p 114–117

15

Clinical aspects of intravenous anaesthetics

This chapter reviews the clinical aspects of intravenous anaesthesia and of necessity covers topics which are discussed in more detail elsewhere. References are only included if they do not appear in the specific chapters. Readers are reminded that there are many currently available intravenous anaesthetics, listed in Table 15.1. This chapter deals only with widely used drugs.

INDUCTION OF GENERAL ANAESTHESIA

This is the obvious principal indication for intravenous anaesthesia, and there are those who claim that the drugs in Table 15.1 should be reserved for this purpose only, with gaseous or volatile agents for maintenance and the appropriate use of neuromuscular blocking drugs and parenteral opioids as required. In practice, induction of anaesthesia means more than the production of unconsciousness and is usually taken to include preparing the patient fully for a surgical incision or similar assault. This might involve both an induction agent and parenteral opioid.

Table 15.1 Classification of intravenous anaesthetics available by the end of 1986

Rapidly acting (primary induction) *agents*
1. Thiobarbiturates: thiopentone, thiamylal Barbiturates: methohexitone
2. Imidazole compounds: etomidate*
3. Sterically hindered alkyl phenols: propofol

Slower acting agents: basal hypnotics
4. Ketamine
5. Benzodiazepines: diazepam, midazolam, flunitrazepam
6. Large dose opioids: fentanyl, alfentanil, sufentanil
7. Neurolept combinations: opioid + neuroleptic

* Not used as an infusion;

Dosage

While the term 'induction dose' is generally reserved for that amount of drug which, if given over 20–30 s, will result in loss of consciousness and contact of the patient with their surroundings, in practice one usually gives more than the minimal induction dose so as to 'cover' the period before the subsequent agents take effect. This might be necessary to ensure that the anaesthesia does not lighten to the extent that the patient will recall unpleasant procedures such as suxamethonium fasciculations or tracheal intubation.

To complicate matters it is now established practice to precede an intravenous induction agent with an intravenous dose of an opioid, the preliminary administration of which makes 'induction' possible with what would normally be subhypnotic doses of induction agents. This is the logical extension of opioid premedication, which not only reduces the induction dose but also, by reducing the frequency of extraneous muscle movement, has made the use of excitatory drugs such as etomidate and methohexitone acceptable as part of a balanced induction sequence (Dundee, 1979). The extent to which a low dose of opioid (which will permit spontaneous respiration) will reduce the dose of thiopentone required to induce anaesthesia in fit patients is shown by the study of Dundee et al (1986). Using a standard method of administration, the induction dose of 4.6 mg kg^{-1} was significantly reduced to 3.3 mg kg^{-1} by the prior administration of 100μg fentanyl and to 3.8 mg kg^{-1} when 300μg alfentanil was given. Doses of opioids greater than these caused marked respiratory depression.

The general health of the patient will also have

a marked effect on induction dose: that this decreases with age has been very clearly demonstrated with propofol (Fig. 11.3) and would appear to apply to all rapidly acting induction agents. The slower circulation time in elderly patients has to be remembered: when a fixed rate of injection technique is used patients could easily be given an overdose, with consequent cardiovascular and respiratory depression. This in turn could reduce the initial redistribution of the drugs and prolong both their hypnotic and toxic effects.

Acquired tolerance to sedatives and hypnotics, including alcohol, is the most common cause of a high induction dose. This can cause problems in clinical practice as the tolerance only applies to the cerebral effects of the drugs — one might encounter poor-risk or elderly alcoholics to whom, one would hesitate to administer the large dose of thiopentone or similar drugs required to induce anaesthesia because of their effects on the cardiovascular system. This can best be overcome by generous preanaesthetic medication and/or pretreatment with a rapidly-acting opioid.

Drugs must not be given on a weight-related basis to morbidly obese patients, as this will result in an overdose, with attendant problems of delayed recovery and prolonged respiratory depression. The latter can be disastrous in patients who already have ventilatory perfusion abnormalities (Key & Newmark, 1984).

It is more difficult to comment on the induction dose of the slower acting agents, ketamine and the benzodiazepines (diazepam and midazolam). One normally injects a predetermined dose and waits for at least one minute with ketamine and two minutes with the benzodiazepines. With ketamine, in particular, the dose given is usually in excess of the minimum induction dose. In practice it is more appropriate to add a narcotic or small dose of a rapidly-acting drug rather than 'top up' with further benzodiazepines. Table 15.2 shows that with midazolam the 'onset time' can be considerably shortened by prior administration of fentanyl or alfentanil and this can be achieved with doses of opioids which allow spontaneous respiration.

Opioids can also reduce the requirements of benzodiazepines but, to achieve absolute certainly of inducing anaesthesia, one would require doses of opioids which would depress respiration. The use of opioids and benzodiazepines as part of a 'balanced' technique is discussed in Chapter 13.

Table 15.2 Mean induction times and percentage of patients asleep by 3 min following intravenous midazolam 0.3 mg kg^{-1} in fentanyl, alfentanil and unpretreated groups of fit young patients.

Pretreatment	*n*	*Mean induction time (s)*	*Percent asleep at 3 min*
	110	114	60
Fentanyl 50 μg	52	78	60
100 μg	52	58	92
Alfentanil 150 μg	40	76	85
300 μg	40	56	90

Dundee et al (1986)

Because of its profound analgesic action, it is unlikely that opioids will enhance the action of ketamine to the same extent as with the benzodiazepines. Their influence on dosage and onset time has not been studied but this is less important as an effective dose of ketamine can be expected to induce anaesthesia within one minute.

INJECTIONS

Site

There is an increasing tendency to give injections into small veins on the back of the hand and avoid the larger vessels at the wrist and antecubital fossa. This stems from the dangers of arterial thiopentone and the occurrence of aberrant vessels at the elbow or injection into forearm nerves. These are minimised but not entirely removed by the use of dilute solutions, and there does not appear to be a problem with other induction agents. In view of the high incidence of injection pain one cannot recommend these small vessels for routine use, particularly with etomidate, methohexitone and propofol. Of these three agents, etomidate causes most pain and this can occur even with injection into a large vessel.

Injection into a long-term infusion increases the risk of phlebitis to the extent that Friedland (1985) recommends the use of in line filters (0.22 μm). Falchuk et al (1985) found about a 58% incidence of phlebitis after 3 days of infusion, which was reduced to 25% by the filter. Some of the drug combinations used in intravenous anaesthesia might produce particulate matter in the infusion tubing. A separate infusion set should be used for continuous intravenous anaesthesia and when various substances are to be transfused, it might be advisable, where possible to use a separate infusion set for the intravenous anaesthetic.

Subcutaneous injections

These should not be ignored and infiltration of the site with a dilute solution of a local anaesthetic not only relieves the pain, but might prevent the vicious circle of reflex spasm. The local anaesthetic solution must not contain adrenaline and if a large volume has been injected outside the vein hyaluronidase added to the local anaesthetic will help disperse the irritant.

Intra-arterial

The local effects of intra-arterial thiopentone have been dealt with in Chapter 8, and this section is limited to a brief recapitulation of the clinical picture and the treatment recommended. It is pertinent to re-state that the incidence and severity of sequelae increases with the concentration of the solution injected (Table 8.5).

The intra-arterial injection of thiopentone and other alkaline intravenous anaesthetics is usually accompanied by immediate intense pain distal to the site of injection, which might cause involuntary withdrawal of the arm in an attempt to remove the offending needle. The pain might be of short duration or last for several hours; it might be continuous or intermittent returning several times, presumably because of recurrence of vascular spasm. On rare occasions there might be no pain, yet tissue damage might be extensive. Concurrently with the pain there is blanching in the hands and fingers and disappearance of peripheral pulsation. The severity of the pain might lead to vasomotor collapse, if a large dose has been injected, while onset of unconsciousness might be somewhat delayed because of the circuitous route which the drug must take to reach the central nervous system. Blanching might be followed by cyanosis, followed in turn by gangrene or, in more favourable circumstances, by reactive hyperaemia if spasm is controlled.

Ideally, if the complication is recognised while injection is in progress, the needle should be kept in the artery and vasodilator drugs injected direct into the artery. Papaverine in doses of 40–80 mg in 10–20 ml of saline is the vasodilator of choice, but the drug is rarely available instantaneously in the operating room. Rather than delay treatment until it can be procured, 5–10 ml of any readily available non-adrenaline containing local anaesthetic solution is injected into the artery to produce both vasodilation, relieve spasm, and neutralise the alkalinity of the barbiturate. Failing even the availability of a local anaesthetic without adrenaline, a slightly warmed solution of normal saline injected into the artery might be of some benefit. Heparin might additionally be injected to prevent clotting within the damaged arterial tree. If the needle has been removed from the artery, no time should be lost in attempts to repeat arterial puncture, as this will be extremely difficult to accomplish in the presence of the existing spasm, and indeed might be impossible, leading merely to a loss of precious time. Subclavian artery puncture should be attempted, as this is a much easier procedure under the circumstances. The artery lies posteriorly in the immediate vicinity of the scalenus anterior muscle. At the same time vasodilation should also be attempted by chemical sympathectomy of the affected limb. In the case of the hand and arm this means performing a brachial plexus block, preferably with a stellate ganglion block. These manoeuvres not only relieve the spasm in the affected vessels, but also open up available collateral channels. This hopefully will prevent or at least minimize any tissue damage that might otherwise occur. Immersion of the opposite limb into hot water or placing it into a heat cradle might assist in the opening up of the collateral circulation. If nerve blocks are contemplated these need not be delayed because heparin has been injected into the artery, since the dose is unlikely to be sufficient to cause systemic heparinisation and the danger of bleeding is not great. For long-term anticoagulant therapy one of the coumarin drugs might be given orally. Venous and lymphatic drainage of the affected limb should be assisted by elevation up to, but not above, the heart level. The limb should be wrapped in sterile towels and kept warm but must not be overheated.

Even with injections of small amounts of solution, if the patient has complained of pain then there is likely to be spasm or damage and ideally the patient should be heparinised and any non-urgent operation postponed for 2 to 3 days.

With the absence of pain in some patients and the necessity for the patient to complain of pain before a diagnosis is made, intra-arterial injection cannot be taken as indicating negligence on the part of the anaesthetist. Negligence would rather be implied if the injection was continued in the present of pain and if no steps were taken to treat the sequelae.

Injection into nerves

Reference has been made in Chapter 2 to the anatomical relationships of the structures in the antecubical fossa. From this it is obvious that the nerve most likely to be injured in the course of an intravenous injection made in that region is the medial nerve. If an injection must be made at this site, accidental damage to the median nerve could occur by mischance even though prudence were exercised. Here then is another reason why the medial aspect of the antecubital fossa should not be used for the injection of drugs if at all avoidable.

The most prominent sign of injection into the median nerve is an intense shooting pain with sudden flexion of the wrist and thumb. The distribution of pain following an injection into a nerve is determined by the sensory distribution of that nerve, and so differs from the pain which follows intra-arterial injection since that is general over the entire area distal to the site of injection.

Treatment must be prompt, and does not differ substantially from that described for extravascular injection. It is helpful if the needle has not been moved, so that injection of the local anaesthetic is made into the exact site of injury, but if the needle is no longer in place, generous infiltration of the area is the best alternative under the circumstances. Injury caused by injection into a nerve is a serious complication; a neurologist should be consulted to establish the extent of damage and to advise on long-term treatment.

DRUGS

Table 15.3 gives the comparative properties of the available intravenous induction agents.

Barbiturates

All barbiturates (Table 15.4) are unstable highly alkaline solutions and extravenous injection should be avoided, although the sequelae appear to be less with the more dilute methohexitone. They are also antanalgesic (hyperalgesic) in low doses: lightly anaesthetised patients will over-react to somatic stimuli. This, and their inability to produce muscle relaxation in safe doses, makes them unsuitable for use as sole agent except for very short procedures. Here one might use the technique of producing a high plasma (and hence brain) concentration by the rapid injection of a small dose, from which recovery is usually quick. The absence of any analgesic action from small doses of any of the barbiturates is again stressed and the concomitant use of nitrous oxide produces marked potentiation of effect.

Finally, no barbiturate should be given to a patient with suspected porphyria. With other safe drugs available, this contraindication should apply to any form of porphyria.

Thiopentone and thiamylal

Table 15.3 shows thiopentone to be a very reliable rapidly-acting induction agent which, even in unpremedicated patients, will produce a smooth induction of anaesthesia, with few excitatory effects. However, it can cause severe hypotension and some respiratory depression. Both of these will be minimised by slow injection of small doses; pretreatment with an opioid is valuable where one is concerned about the cardiovascular status of the patient. Recovery from normal induction doses is not too rapid to lead to concern about awareness of suxamethonium fasciculations or tracheal intubation and uptake of volatile agents is usually smooth. Eventual recovery from the drug is moderately slow and outpatients given thiopentone (in any dosage) should not be allowed to leave hospital unaccompanied and should not attempt discriminating tasks until the following day.

Table 15.3 Comparative properties of intravenous anaesthetics.

Property	*Barbiturates*		*Non-barbiturates*			*Benzodiazepines*	
	Thiopentone	*Methohexitone*	*Etomidate*	*Propofol*	*Ketamine*	*Diazepam*	*Midazolam*
Aqueous solution	+	+	–	–	+	–	+
Solvent			Organic	Emulsion		Organic and emulsion	
Available in solution	–	–	+	+	+	+	+
Pain on injection	–	+	++	±	–	+	–
Venous thrombosis	–	–	+	–	–	+	–
Analgesic action	–	–	–	±	++	–	–
Rapidly acting	+	+	+	+	–	–	–
Normal induction dose for fit unpremedicated adults (mg kg^{-1})	4–5	1.5	0.3	2.0–2.5	1.5–2.0		
Reliable	++	++	+	+	+	–	–
Smooth induction	++	±	–	+	+	+	+
Respiratory upset	–	+	±	–	–	–	–
Respiratory depression	+	+	±	++	–	–	±
Cardiovascular depression	++	+	–	++	–	±	±
Rapid recovery	–	±	+	++	–	–	–
Smooth recovery	+	+	–	+	–	±	±
Suitable for infusion	–	+	*	+	±	–	±
Safe in porphyria	–	–	–	?	+	?	?

* *Pharmacokinetically suitable: adrenocortical suppression may make this use undesirable*

Table 15.4 Undesirable features of injectable barbiturates

Unstable in aqueous solution
High pH and irritant on extravenous injection
Antanalgesic effect (hyperalgesia) in lower doses
Absence of analgesic action in clinical doses
Do not produce muscle relaxation in safe doses
Porphyrogenicity

(Dundee, 1985)

Table 15.5 Some properties of methohexitone compared with thiopentone

More pain on injection
2–3 times more potent (w/w) than thiopentone
Clear less-irritant solution
Higher incidence of excitatory movements and of cough and hiccough
Shorter elimination half-life
More rapid recovery

Thiamylal is clinically indistinguishable from thiopentone.

Methohexitone

Methohexitone, the other barbiturate, produces a less smooth induction than thiopentone (Table 15.5) and causes more pain on injection. Its side effects can be markedly reduced by opioid premedication or pretreatment, and also by slow injection of small doses. The lesser cardiovascular depression, compared with thiopentone, is probably due to the compensatory tachycardia and one recent comparative study (Table 15.6) showed a 25% average increase in heart rate with normal induction doses. It has however, a more rapid recovery than thiopentone, which ensures it a place in current practice, particularly in outpatient procedures, although at the time of writing this use is being challenged by propofol. Methohexitone is pharmacokinetically very suitable for infusion, but the high incidence of excitatory effects, particularly with large doses, makes it clinically unacceptable as sole agent for this use. Its future here depends on the evolution of a technique in which it is combined with a short-acting opioid.

Etomidate

The cardiovascular stability which accompanies

Table 15.6 Comparative effects of 4 induction agents, injected over 20 s to groups of 50 fit patients (McCollum et al, 1986)

Agent	*Dose mg kg*$^{-1}$	*Anaesthesia induced*$^{+}$	*Induction complications*				*Induction acceptable to anaesthetist*
			SBP fall 20+ mmHg	*Apnoea 30+ s*$^{++}$	*Excitatory effects*	*Respiratory disturbances*	
Thiopentone	4.0	45(6)	3	11(1)	4	4	38
	5.0	50(5)	10	19(1)	4	4	43
Methohexitone	1.5	48(2)	1*	10(1)	18	10	37
Etomidate	0.3	50(0)	4	0	35	5	36
Propofol	2.0	45(5)	10	12(5)	16$^{\times}$	2	35
	2.5	50(0)	19	22(6)	12$^{\times}$	3	43

$^{+}$ Figures in brackets: rapid lightening of anaesthesia
$^{++}$ Figures in brackets: apnoea lasting over 1 min
* average of 25% increase in heart rate (3–9% with other agents)
$^{\times}$ very minor in nature, compared with methohexitone and etomidate

the induction of anaesthesia with etomidate is its most desirable property and its use in subjects with a compromised cardiovascular system is its most common indication for its use in clinical practice. It can be seen from Table 15.3 that in unpremedicated patients induction is often complicated by excitatory effects which can be troublesome at times. In healthy patients Giese et al (1985) found no significant difference between the cardiovascular effects of etomidate and thiopentone as induction agents and apart from the excitatory side effects associated with the etomidate their actions were similar. Recent complex EEG studies (Arden et al, 1985) showed that a dose of thiopentone must be 20 times as large as that of etomidate to produce a similar EEG effect, although in clinical practice we normally use a 12–15:1 potency ratio. Perhaps we could use smaller doses of etomidate although these have not been studied in clinical practice.

As shown in Table 15.6, the normal recommended induction dose of 0.3 mg kg^{-1} is reliable in action and induced anaesthesia in all of the unpremedicated patients studied. Like methohexitone, the excitatory side effects can be reduced by opiate premedication but more reliably so by pretreatment with small doses of fentanyl or alfentanil. Neither of these opioids cause problems in patients with cardiac disease and this sequence is widely used for such subjects.

The injection of etomidate into small veins on the back of the hand is unacceptably painful and is followed by a high incidence of venous thrombosis. The drug should be injected into a moderately-sized forearm or antecubital vein or else into a rapidly-running infusion. While pharmacokinetically etomidate is very suitable for use in an infusion (see Ch. 17), this cannot be recommended as a routine because of the undesirable effects of large doses on adrenocortical function (Ch. 10) although there might occasionally be circumstances when the lack of cardiovascular toxicity more than outweighs the risk of inhibiting adrenal steroidogenesis. There is a suggestion that normal induction doses can cause a temporary suppression of function and the drug is better avoided in circumstances where this would be considered undesirable. Like the barbiturates, etomidate is not recommended in patients with suspected porphyria.

Propofol

This rapidly-acting new agent, available as an easily injectable emulsion, causes pain when injected into small veins, but is well tolerated in forearm and antecubital vessels. In effective doses, induction is smooth with very minor muscle movements and no respiratory upset. There is, however, a higher incidence of apnoea and hypotension (Table 15.6) than with other agents. Apnoea is not a problem in clinical practice, but one must administer the drug slowly, particularly in poor-risk patients, to minimise the fall in blood pressure. Elderly patients are more susceptible to both the hypnotic and other depressant effects of propofol and the induction dose is in the region of 1.75 mg kg^{-1} in patients over 60 yr compared with 2 to 2.5 mg kg^{-1} in younger patients. In clinical use the absence of an antanalgesic action such as occurs with thiopentone, is most useful and patients readily tolerate a pharyngeal airway in light anaesthesia. This might make it a useful drug to use as sole agent for minor procedures.

Propofol is compatible with the available myoneural blocking drugs and it can be used as an induction agent before volatile agents as well as in balanced anaesthesia. The smoothness of recovery differs little from thiopentone. Early recovery is faster than from equivalent doses of methohexitone: patients feel much better in the first postoperative hour and return to full activity (including eating) is quicker with propofol. Postoperative vomiting is rare after its use.

Care is required in interpreting the literature on propofol, as it was originally available in a cremophor solution. This was referred to as ICI 35868, di-isopropyl phenol or disoprofol. This formulation was abandoned because of risk of anaphylactoid reactions. It was slightly more potent w/w than the current emulsion preparation.

It is too early to comment on the use of propofol infusions, but its pharmacokinetic profile favours this use. It cannot however be diluted or mixed with opioids so that a syringe pump is needed for its use. It does not appear to have an advance effect on cortisol synthesis such as occurs with etomidate (Stark et al, 1985).

Ketamine

This unique drug can be given by the intramuscular (6–8 mg kg^{-1}) and intravenous (1.5–2.0 mg kg^{-1}) routes. In contrast to the standard induction agents it causes a slight rise in blood pressure and a variable degree of tachycardia and has a good analgesic action. Skeletal muscle (including jaw) tone is well maintained during anaesthesia. The main drawback with ketamine is the high incidence of emergence delirium and later psychotic sequelae.

Sequelae are particularly likely to follow minor operations in unpremedicated women. They can be reduced by benzodiazepine (lorazepam preferred) premedication or by a small intravenous dose of diazepam or midazolam given near the end of the operation. The administration of a small dose of thiopentone (150 mg) at the end of minor operations will also reduce the incidence and severity of emergence reactions and in this dose of thiopentone usually does not produce respiratory depression. (Magbagbeola & Thomas, 1974).

Because of its slow onset of action ketamine is not used as a routine induction agent but generally for situations where its unique properties more than outweigh the disadvantages of psychotic sequelae. These include repeat administration, radiotherapy or burns dressings and its use in children. However, Byer & Gould (1981) have noted the development of tolerance on repeat administration. Many favour ketamine in shocked patients. Small doses have a potential in producing total (or at least adequate) analgesia in circumstances where a trained anaesthetist is not available.

Economically ketamine is not really expensive compared with, say, the cost of a course of certain antibiotics, modern inhalation anaesthetic agents or indeed, a surgeon's presterilised sutures. It would help if the manufacturers supplied it in only the 100 mg ml^{-1} strength: this is the least bulky strength for intramuscular injection, it is cheapest, and it can be easily diluted if required.

Benzodiazepines

These are usually limited to diazepam and midazolam; flunitrazepam is available in some centres. All have a delay in onset of action and are much less reliable than the other drugs discussed here. Where available diazepam is most commonly used in its non-irritant emulsion form (Diazemuls), while midazolam is soluble in water. All cause a short period of anterograde amnesia.

The main use of benzodiazepines as induction agents is in the elderly, where their reduced requirements and greater reliability contrast with young patients in whom induction of anaesthesia is unsatisfactory unless they are pretreated with an opioid. More valuable is their use as sedative-hypnotic to 'cover' unpleasant local procedures such as dental treatment or oral endoscopy.

Recovery from all doses of these drugs is much longer than after the standard induction agents. Diazepam has a hypnotically active metabolite which will prolong its action after large doses.

Midazolam is shorter acting and less cumulative than diazepam.

BALANCED ANAESTHESIA

This term is used to describe anaesthesia in which three separate components of surgical anaesthesia are produced by drugs with different action. Intravenous anaesthetics are used principally to produce loss of consciousness and analgesia is produced with nitrous oxide–oxygen or a parenteral opioid. Specific myoneural blocking drugs are used to produce muscular relaxation, the choice depending on the length of the procedure and whether the patients are breathing spontaneously or respiration is controlled. Volatile supplements can be used to produce all three parts of this triad, depending on the agent used. For example trichloroethylene has a profound analgesic action but does not produce any muscular relaxation whereas isoflurane does have a marked relaxant component in its action.

One of the problems, already referred to, is the need to ensure that patients will remain unconscious during the procedure except in certain rare circumstances. If return of consciousness is desirable or if it is felt that the risk of this happening is less than the risk to the patient then there must be a major analgesic component in the technique so that patients will not feel pain. If told that they might begin to regain consciousness this does not usually upset the patient and all the fears occur when this occurs without prior warning.

Preanaesthetic medication can play a major part in balanced anaesthesia though the benzodiazepines have no analgesic action but will contribute to the hypnotic component of the technique, whereas the longer-acting opioids (morphine, pethidine), having little hypnotic effect will contribute to the analgesia.

While benzodiazepines can be used to induce anaesthesia for a balanced technique tracheal intubation is not so easily performed after these drugs as after orthodox induction agents. When suxamethonium is used one must ensure that patients are fully asleep as fasciculations can be unpleasant. Bali & Dundee (1985) found that, when using alcuronium or atracurium, intubation was not as easy after midazolam as after thiopentone but a minute 50 mg dose of thiopentone given with the benzodiazepine produced very good intubating conditions.

The combination of an induction agent with suxamethonium and ventilation of the patient's lungs by injection apparatus can be considered another form of balanced anaesthesia, in which nitrous oxide–oxygen should be avoided. In this circumstance thiopentone, although very reliable, might be followed by some degree of bronchospasm on recovery which can lead to an appreciable degree of oxygen desaturation. It will particularly cause problems where biopsy has led to some bleeding in the lungs. Aghdmi et al (1985) consider that etomidate is superior to thiopentone under these circumstances because of rapidity of recovery. Bronchospasm is rare after etomidate but the absence of pain on injection when using large veins and also the smooth induction points to a preference for the new phenol derivative and propofol might eventually prove to be the drug of choice for these procedures.

USE IN PATHOLOGICAL STATES

Cardiovascular disease: shock

Consideration will be given initially to those conditions in which there is primary disease of the cardiovascular system leading to decreased efficiency of the myocardium. In 'shock' the vulnerability of the myocardium is secondary to extra-cardiac factors and many of the principles which apply to the administration of intravenous anaesthetics to patients with primary cardiovascular disease also apply in the presence of shock. Anaesthesia for cardiac operations is not specifically considered here.

The safe administration of thiopentone or other intravenous anaesthetics except ketamine to persons with cardiovascular disease requires the proper appreciation of the following:

1. Peripheral vasodilatation occurs with anaesthetic doses.
2. Intravenous barbiturates in particular are direct myocardial depressants.
3. Any fall in cardiac output is in proportion to the concentration of the drug in contact with the heart.

4. The unhealthy myocardium is more susceptible to the effects of these drugs than the healthy heart muscle.
5. The depressant effects of repeated doses on the myocardium are cumulative.
6. The arm-brain circulation time is prolonged in some types of heart disease and the onset of sleep therefore might be delayed.
7. Many other drugs used for the maintenance of anaesthesia as adjuvants are also myocardial depressants, and their effects then are additive to those of the barbiturates. However, in general, the shorter-acting opioids cause minimal cardiovascular depression.
8. Hypoxia and hypercarbia, secondary to overdosage, respiratory depression, or laryngeal spasm must be avoided at all costs since they contribute to the depression of the myocardium and predispose to arrhythmias.
9. Coughing and straining also must be avoided as they result in increased intrathoracic pressure with consequent reduction of venous return to the heart and decreased cardiac output.

It is essential that every patient be assessed individually and the degree of cardiovascular impairment be determined. Some conditions are mild and there is then no need to exercise care other than ordinarily required. Beyond this there is a vast spectrum of conditions varying from mild through moderate to exceedingly severe abnormalities requiring increasingly rigorous care. The degree of severity of the heart disease is related to the reserve which the myocardium can muster to compensate for the effects of the injection of the intravenous anaesthetic. If the drug is given slowly, in minimum doses and in dilute solution, with frequent pauses to observe its effects, and if the myocardial disease is not extreme, few ill-effects should result. If, on the other hand, the dose, concentration and speed of injection are excessive for the particular cardiovascular condition, then severe, if not irreversible, consequences might ensue. In connection with the response capability of the myocardium one must bear in mind not only intrinsic myocardial disease and coronary perfusion but also the presence or absence of extraneous factors which might influence myocardial response. Here one thinks of constrictive pericarditis, a condition where the myocardium itself might be quite healthy but where it is rigidly encased and thus incapable of adjusting and other conditions of fixed cardiac output e.g. severe aortic or mitral valve stenosis. Coronary perfusion is a function of mean aortic pressure, and where this is allowed to fall significantly, as in aortic valvular disease, severe myocardial ischaemia might result with catastrophic consequences. Great care, therefore, must be exercised during induction of anaesthesia in such patients.

Shock, when fully established, might be described as failure of the 'micro-circulation'. Such failure in turn leads to tissue hypoxia with the accumulation of fixed acid metabolites. If not remedied early, it becomes self-perpetuating and eventually leads to death. Failure of the micro-circulation might be due to oligaemia, to primary myocardial failure, to interference with autonomic balance or it might be on a toxic basis. Be that as it may, the full-blown oligaemic form is characterized by hypotension, tachycardia, sweating, air-hunger, listlessness and a sluggish capillary refill time.

The concern of the anaesthetist with the shocked patient, however, begins at a much earlier stage. Since all intravenous agents are to a greater or lesser degree peripheral vasodilators, as well as central nervous system and myocardial depressants, and since many other anaesthetics possess all or some of these properties as well, any discrepancy between the capacity of the circulatory tree and the blood volume becomes of great importance. In order to overcome this imbalance a number of compensatory mechanisms come into play, including peripheral vasoconstriction. Because of the tachycardia, cardiac output increases despite a reduction in stroke volume, while return of blood to the heart is assisted by the constriction of the peripheral veins, a fact well known to the physician who attempts venepuncture in such individuals. Because of these compensatory mechanisms discrepancies between circulating volume and circulatory tree capacity might well exist long before the classical picture of shock becomes apparent. This has been referred to as 'compensated shock' a condition which might be acute or chronic.

Where blood loss has not been overwhelming

the circulatory tree will be capable of adapting to the reduced volume until obligatory fluid shifts from the extravascular to the intravascular compartment have taken place or volume has been replaced from external sources. This compensation occurs at the expense of the microcirculation, but if correction takes place rapidly no ill-effects need follow. In this situation the heart rate is invariably higher than the systolic blood pressure which itself might have remained unchanged or might even be elevated. The pulse rate indeed might be the only sign that all is not well. Whenever this picture is encountered, compensated shock must be excluded before the patient is exposed to anaesthesia, and particularly to the administration of an intravenous barbiturate.

If hypovolaemia has come about over a period of many weeks or even months, in consequence of debilitating disease or inability to maintain an adequate fluid intake the picture of relative tachycardia might or might not present itself, but the general condition of the patient, the history of the disease and the low skin turgor might provide valuable warning signs. Once suspicion has been aroused, the diagnosis can be confirmed by blood volume or central venous pressure estimation.

If the existing compensation is destroyed through the injudicious administration of barbiturates, or any agent which has a similar potential when given too fast or in too large an amount, re-establishment of compensation might be very difficult or indeed impossible, largely because a vicious circle has been set up. As blood pressure falls, myocardial hypoxia is increased which in turn leads to further hypotension. The hypoxia, affecting blood vessels as well as all other tissues, destroys the integrity of the capillary wall with consequent increase in permeability which then leads to further depletion of the circulating blood volume and increasing haemoconcentration. A further hazard associated with intravenous anaesthesia in shock is the slow circulation time; consequently the effect of the agent is not apparent as promptly as would be the case were circulation time not impaired. The unwary anaesthetist might be tempted to inject a further dose in the mistaken assumption that the first injection has been inadequate when in fact he is now administering an overdose.

Much of our knowledge of the dangers of intravenous barbitutate anaesthesia has come to us through military experiences, and the lessons learned in war must not be forgotten by civilian practitioners, who are faced to an increasing degree with anaesthetic problems involving severely traumatised patients, those of advanced age and the chronically ill. Therefore the descriptions of fatalities in the early days of intravenous anaesthesia in emergency situations retain their pertinence even today and warrant quotation. Referring to the Pearl Harbour experience in 1941, Halford (1943) writes thus:

> 'A number of patients were given evipal by competent anaesthetists only to have respiratory failure, some of which ended in death. After several such fatalities, pentothal sodium was used, and again respiratory failures occurred and, as in the case of evipal, death ensued in enough cases to cause us to abandon it as too dangerous. In several cases when as small an amount as 0.5 g of pentothal sodium solution had been administered, there suddenly appeared a "cyanosis decollatage" predecessor of death.'

Halford points out that the wounded were all 'healthy young adult males with adequate lung volume and unbelievable morale'. He continues,

> 'The injuries were all severe, the list of wounds consisted mainly of traumatic amputations of one or more extremeties often in the same patient, compound comminuted fractures penetrating chest and abdominal wounds, head and jaw injuries.
>
> 'That we were attending patients in severe shock there can be no denial. These patients were prepared with perhaps a minimum of plasma and whole blood transfusions. There was a definite lack of oxygen and equipment for administering continuous oxygen therapy.'

This report condemns the use of intravenous anaesthesia in the presence of shock, referring to it as 'an ideal form of euthanasia'. No suggestion is made that the technique of administration was at fault, and no part of the blame is put on the *competent* anaesthetists. An Editorial (1943) appearing in the same issue of *Anesthesiology* as Halford's paper makes the following pertinent comment:

> 'Direct and indirect information from Pearl Harbour would lead to the belief that administration of both evipal and pentothal sodium to severely wounded casualties is extremely hazardous. Both drugs are said to have produced sudden and often irreversible respiratory failure in a number of cases. While it would be reasonable to assume that these occurrences were directly attributable to the barbiturates, it would be instructive to know more concerning how rapidly and in what amounts the barbiturates were administered and what concentration of solution was employed.'

It concludes,

> 'When pentothal sodium is administered intravenously to patients who are in a state of shock, the lessened tolerance of these patients must be kept in mind. Small doses (1 to 2 ml of a 2.5% solution) administered slowly, with intervals between injections of sufficient length to allow the full effect to take place, is the only rational scheme of dosage. It is amazing how little of the drug will provide anaesthesia and relaxation for such patients. Oxygen is an important adjunct to many patients in shock who are under intravenous anaesthesia and when shock is present it should be available for use if required.'

Although not the first choice, intravenous barbiturates can be administered safely to individuals in shock (Adams & Gray, 1943) or with severe cardiovascular disease of any nature, as long as due care is being exercised, circulatory effects borne in mind, and it is realised that the amount appropriate to induce anaesthesia in a healthy individual might be quite deleterious or even lethal when administered in a similar concentration, amount and rate of injection to a person in shock. However the availability of other agents and analgesic techniques make it unwise to place sole reliance on one group of drugs, requiring so much skill and experience for their safe use in these circumstances. Therefore one should consider drugs with less potent effect on the cardiovascular tree, be they intravenous or inhalational.

In 'shock' patients appear to be less aware of pain. Since the clinical level of narcosis is related to the intensity of stimulation reaching the central nervous system, shocked patients might be induced at lower plasma levels of drugs than normal subjects. After prolonged hypotension the cerebral cells themselves might be more susceptible to the effects of depressant drugs.

Patients in shock with reduced circulation volume and derangement of tissue perfusion are also less able to redistribute an induction dose of an induction agent. Whereas under normal conditions, the plasma concentration of thiopentone falls to less than 20% of its peak level within 15 min of injection, in shock the reduction will be much less and the desired effect can require much smaller amounts of the drug. Reliance is placed more on detoxication than on diffusion for removal of thiopentone from the blood stream but this is a slow process even in fit patients. In moderate degrees of shock the portal blood flow is reduced by about half and the deleterious effects of hypotension and the resulting hypoxia and hepatic function must be appreciated.

Renal circulation is particularly sensitive to changes in blood pressure and renal vasoconstriction might persist for a long time after the blood pressure has been restored to normal.

Bearing the above in mind, the following principles are useful in the use of intravenous agents in patients with a compromised cardiovascular system or in a state of shock:

1. Maximum replacement of the blood or fluid where required and appropriate medical treatment (vasoactive drugs) to achieve the optimum condition of the cardiovascular system.
2. Preoxygenation and correction of metabolic acidosis.
3. Slow injection of appropriate dose of a short-acting opioid such as fentanyl or alfentanil, the dose depending on whether the patient is to breathe spontaneously or not.
4. Preference to etomidate over thiopentone, where there is cardiac disease.
5. Where appropriate, prior injection of about one-quarter of the expected dose of long-acting myoneural blocking drug: avoidance of tubocurarine and alcuronium.
6. Slow injection of the induction agent, bearing in mind the possibility of a slow circulation time.
7. Attainment of an adequate degree of anaesthesia and relaxation before tracheal intubation (to minimise pressure rises).
8. In appropriate cases to consider the use of an opioid as the sole, or main, anaesthetic. This could be combined with a benzodiazepine if necessary.

The deleterious effects of thiopentone on the cardiovascular system are paralleled by its effects on the respiratory system. Depression of respiration, or even apnoea, follows the administration of small doses to shocked patients. There might be a true sensitivity of the respiratory centres resulting from prolonged hypoxia, either the result of arterial hypotension or due to an increased intracranial pressure following injury to the head. The stimulating effects of carbon dioxide will be very much reduced or even completely abolished.

Respiratory disease

The potential ability of the barbiturates to cause bronchoconstriction had led one to prefer other agents in asthmatics. Etomidate does not appear to cause bronchoconstriction but ketamine may be the agent of choice although its other effects must be remembered. There is an impression that the respiratory disturbances (cough and hiccough) caused by methohexitone are more frequent in patients with upper respiratory tract disease.

Of the available agents propofol would appear to cause the greatest degree of respiratory depression followed by thiopentone, with lesser effects from both etomidate and ketamine.

RESPIRATORY OBSTRUCTION

The problems which are associated with the use of general anaesthesia of any kind in respiratory obstruction are mostly of a purely mechanical nature and are related to the degree of obstruction. In severe cases, adequate respiratory exchange can only be maintained with help of the accessory muscles of respiration and these are under voluntary control. When consciousness is lost, their activity is abolished, and the intercostal muscles and the diaphragm, which are of course still functioning, are unable to draw sufficient gas past the obstruction to maintain adequate respiratory exchange. In less severe cases, abolition of the use of the accessory muscles will result in hypoxia which, at least for a short period, can be counteracted by the inhalation of oxygen.

The difference between intravenous and inhalation anaesthesia in this respect lies in the fact that intravenous anaesthesia will abolish the use of the accessory muscles almost instantaneously upon injection since consciousness is lost very quickly. This may then result in either complete obstruction or severe limitation of respiratory exchange, necessitating immediate re-establishment of an airway. This may be very difficult indeed to accomplish. In contrast, consciousness is lost more slowly with inhalation anaesthesia and as respiratory exchange becomes less adequate with the progressive weakening of the accessory muscles, completion of induction may not be possible, and the increasing obstruction may become quite obvious. The attempt at induction can then be abandoned.

Nevertheless, it is axiomatic that in the presence of upper airway obstruction general anaesthesia is contraindicated unless a patent airway has been previously assured. This can be done in one of two ways: tracheal intubation may be carried out before induction, preferably by the nasal route and under adequate topical anaesthesia, or if the introduction of a tracheal tube, either by the nasal or the oral route, proves impossible, a preliminary tracheostomy must be carried out. In acute situations such as Ludwig's angina, epiglottitis, etc., tracheal intubation is preferred since the artificial maintenance of an airway will be required for a short period only. In conditions in which airway impairment is likely to persist for a matter of days, such as in severe facial smashes, fractured larynx and similar conditions, pre-anaesthetic tracheostomy is recommended since that operation may be required in any case in the postoperative period.

The following anonymous case report taken from the *British Journal of Anaesthesia* (1953) will serve to illustrate some of the problems which can be encountered:

> An African male, aged 18 years, was admitted with severe Ludwig's angina, but no evidence of any respiratory obstruction. The patient was premedicated with atropine 0.65 mg and a sterile tracheostomy set made readily available in the operating room. Thiopentone 400 mg was given followed by 75 mg suxamethonium chloride. On laryngoscopy there was marked oedema of the whole of the pharynx, and the glottis could not be visualised. A tube was passed, but on squeezing the reservoir bag it became evident that it was in the oesophagus. Further manipulation of the tube precipitated severe laryngospasm and respiration became completely obstructed. The patient became deeply cyanosed and ceased to make any respiratory efforts. The pulse became almost imperceptible. Tracheostomy was performed and a tracheal tube inserted through the stoma and the lungs inflated with oxygen. The patient recovered consciousness in 15 minutes and was discharged from hospital two weeks later none the worse for his ordeal.

In minor degrees of respiratory obstruction adequate pre-oxygenation of the lungs may be all that is necessary, but the intravenous barbiturate must be given in such a way as to minimise respiratory depression. There are many degrees of obstruction and each case must be judged on its own merits and a decision be made whether awake intubation of the trachea is required or not. The following report illustrates this:

A woman, aged 42, suffering from a mild quinsy which was rapidly becoming worse and causing some obstruction to respiration. There was no improvement with intensive chemotherapy and it was considered necessary to relieve the tension as the patient had become very distressed. Oxygen was administered without any improvement and on several occasions trichloroethylene was added to the oxygen in an attempt to produce anaesthesia, but each time it only increased the restlessness.

When seen by an anaesthetist, the patient was extremely apprehensive, severe trismus and slight cyanosis were present, the accessory muscles were being used to their full extent, the pulse was rapid and bounding and the blood pressure 185/110 mmHg. Inhalation of 79 per cent helium and 21 per cent oxygen immediately improved her condition, the distress became less and the pulse rate slowed. Because of a shortage of supply it was only possible to continue this administration for 10 minutes, but during this time a spray was passed through the nostril and the pharynx and larynx sprayed with two per cent amethocaine and 1:200 000 adrenaline. Two minutes later a nasal tracheal tube was passed blindly, and after a brief period of coughing the patient's condition improved and cyanosis was not present when air was inhaled. Anaesthesia was induced with thiopentone and continued with nitrous oxide and oxygen, the patient was put in the head-down position, a sucker placed in the pharynx and a large peritonsillar abscess incised. The tracheal tube was left in position until the patient opened her eyes, and on its removal breathing was satisfactory.

Renal disease

This does not cause any particular problems as regards induction agents except to bear in mind that patients who come for transplant operation without the benefit of haemodialysis will be unduly susceptible to intravenous anaesthetics. An exaggerated response to barbiturates, due to decreased protein binding and deficiencies in the blood brain barrier, may occur in uremic patients.

Liver disease

This has often been quoted as a contraindication to intravenous barbiturates but this misconception stems from the lack of understanding of the basis for their short duration of action. The liver has a great reserve potential so that even moderate doses of drugs can be disposed of in patients with severe liver damage. However, one must be aware of the dangers of hypoxia to these patients. With the small doses of thiopentone and other drugs now in common use, the deleterious effects of liver dysfunction can be ignored. However, should proloned coma follow the injudicious use of thiopentone, the treatment should be no different from that of any other case of barbiturate poisoning — tracheal intubation, assistance of respiration and adequate administration of oxygen with appropriate treatment for depression of the cardiovascular system where this has occurred. One can state categorically that there is no place for the administration of analeptic drugs here. They do not increase the breakdown of any induction agents and they may lead to coughing which, in itself, can cause disturbances of the vascular system.

The full stomach

The importance of the full stomach lies in the fact that material from it may find its way up the oesophagus and into the respiratory tree where it may cause acute obstruction, chemical irritation or reflex cardiac inhibiton. All these are very serious complications which must be avoided at all costs. While the end results are little different, nevertheless vomiting must be distinguished from regurgitation. Vomiting is an active process initiated by the emetic trigger zone in the medulla which, in turn, may have been activated by nervous or chemical stimuli. Regurgitation, on the other hand, is passive, and is due to relaxation of the cardiac sphincter mechanism which occurs *pari passu* with the establishment of general anaesthesia. While vomiting is easily detected, passive regurgitation may be insidious and hence prevention of aspiration from this cause is more difficult.

Morton and Wylie (1951) have classified the circumstances under which material may be present in the oesophagus and stomach as follows:

Material in the oesophagus — Oesophageal obstruction or pouch. Pyothorax with oesophageal fistula.

Material introduced into the stomach from above — Food and drink given, i.e. lack of preoperative preparation. Fluids given for medical reasons, e.g. to diabetic patients or stomach washouts not completely removed. Swallowed blood. Bleeding from nose, mouth or pharynx due to accident or operation.

Material introduced into the stomach from below — Intestinal obstruction. Ileus.

Material from stomach itself — Normal or

hypersecretion. Bleeding from ulcer, neoplasm or site of operation.

Prolonged emptying-time of the stomach:

(*a*) Pyloric obstruction (including congenital pyloric stenosis).

(*b*) Dilatation of the stomach.

(*c*) Reflex:

1. Emotional states, pain, women in labour, shock, accidents, e.g. cuts, fractures, burns.
2. Peritoneal irritations, e.g. perforated ulcer, twisted ovarian tumour.

(*d*) Abdominal distension, e.g. large tumours, pregnancy at term, gross ascites.

(*e*) Severe illness. Toxaemia. Moribund patients.

(*f*) Drugs: opioids, hyoscine, atropine. Most anaesthetic agents.

Several causes are often present together, e.g. a patient brought to the theatre for resuture of a burst abdomen may be in very poor general condition and may have taken food or fluids just before the incident. There will be shock, emotional disturbance and peritoneal irritation, and morphine may have been given.

Ideally the stomach should be emptied before an operation but none of the methods in vogue are foolproof whether they be the passage of a large bore stomach tube, an indwelling small bore tube or the administration of an emetic. Much more satisfactory is to use a 'crash induction' in which an appropriate dose of an induction agent is followed immediately by a large dose of suxamethonium and cricoid pressure (Sellick's manoeuvre) applied before intubation. There is a problem in the use of opioids in these patients because of delayed onset of action. An alternate technique is the passage of a tracheal tube under topical anaesthesia/analgesia but this also has a risk of aspiration before the tube is inserted.

Alcoholics

Those patients also presents problems with induction of anaesthesia because of the high drug requirement. Moreover, chronic alcoholism is often accompanied by malnutrition and a poorly functioning cardiovascular system. Rather than give a large bolus dose of an induction agent it is preferable to pretreat the patient, either with 'heavy' opioid premedication and a benzodiazepine or to give a relatively large dose of fentanyl or alfentanil immediately before the induction agent. The usual precautions to minimise cardiovascular depression should be taken and when the patient is adequately pretreated there should be no problems. Delirium on recovery may occur and while this can be attributed to the anaesthetic there are occasions when the patient is already beginning to show withdrawal symptoms from alcohol, having been in hospital for 3–4 days without any supply. A slow infusion of a 10% alcohol in Hartmann's solution will quickly correct the situation (this is simple to prepare by adding 55 ml of absolute alcohol to the standard 500 ml infusion pack).

Drug abusers

Two problems arise here. First there is the acquired tolerance to hypnotics, sedatives, tranquillizers and opioids which will lead to high barbiturates requirements. These can be treated as with the alcoholic patient. Perhaps more important is the fact that many patients who are abusing these drugs are in poor nutritional states and may have septicaemia and paucity of usable veins. Pretreatment with an opioid will again be of use here and, depending on the condition of the patient, the dose of the induction agent should be as low as possible.

Porphyria

Porphyria variegata (South African genetic porphyria) and acute intermittent porphyria are probably the only two absolute contraindications to the use of the intravenous barbiturates. Their deleterious effects in these two related conditions have been described in detail in Chapter 8 and Appendix 5. The importance of recognising porphyria is illustrated by the following cases reported by Dean (1953).

> A woman, aged 29, with no relevant history, became paralysed three days following a uterine curettage under thiopentone anaesthesia. Recovery took seven months. Two years later, after a dental extraction for which thiopentone was administered, paralysis again occurred, recovery taking five months.
>
> After hysterectomy, for which a barbiturate was admin-

istered, the patient was unable to walk for six months. Nineteen years later she received thiopentone and the resulting paralysis proved fatal in six weeks. Dean found a family history of skin sensitivity in this patient, who had previously been regarded as a neurotic.

A girl of 19, having had several attacks of paralysis following oral barbiturates, had thiopentone for an exploratory laparotomy. Within three days complete paralysis had occurred and this proved fatal five days later.

A family history of five relatives who died from general paralysis after drugs and anaesthetics was present in a woman who herself suffered from skin blisters. After two operations at which thiopentone was administered, she suffered from paralysis and delirium but eventually recovered.

These are examples of porphyria variegata and the following case report by Dundee, et al (1962) is an example of acute intermittent porphyria.

A young woman attended the outpatient department complaining of 'haematuria'. Preliminary investigations proving negative, she was admitted to hospital for cystoscopy, by which time discoloration of the urine had ceased. The examination was carried out under thiopentone sodium (550 mg in all), nitrous oxide and oxygen anaesthesia. No abnormality was observed, the anaesthesia was uneventful, and recovery was prompt.

Following this, she passed reddish-coloured urine and complained of acute abdominal pain. Two days later, a second cystoscopy, under thiopentone sodium–nitrous oxide–oxygen anaesthesia again revealed no vesical abnormality. However, recovery was not so prompt on this occasion.

Forty-eight hours later she presented with a clinical picture of an acute abdominal emergency and at this stage the possibility of acute porphyria was considered, as she was still passing dark red-coloured urine; later this diagnosis was confirmed by biochemical tests. Unfortunately paralysis occurred and resulted in a fatal outcome.

Although porphyria is a rare disease in Britain and in North America, being more prevalent in the Scandinavian countries and South Africa,

It can be seen that the anaesthetist may encounter porphyria at any stage of the disease. In the latent phase there are some guides to its detection, such as a history of paralysis from a previous operation or after taking sedatives. The skin changes of the cutaneous variety may be obvious as scars from previous blisters of the hands, or the patient may volunteer the history of a sensitive skin. There may be a history of relatives having died after anaesthetics, and while this may have no relationship to porphyria, at least it should arouse suspicion and lead to a more detailed questioning of the patient. A history of passing red urine would be of most positive value but except in the case of an elective operation such information is unlikely to be volunteered by patients as they could see no relationship between this and their present complaint.

Porphyria has been described as the 'little simulator' and the most difficult case to detect is the 'acute abdomen of unknown aetiology'. That there is no previous history of porphyria is apparent from the fact that a laparotomy is contemplated and the stage of porphyrinuria may not have been reached. Whereas in the case of an elective operation it seems clear that thiopentone can precipitate an attack of acute porphyria with resulting paralysis, in the emergency operations the acute attack has already started and the chances of a patient having paralysis are already great, whether thiopentone be given or not. There seems little justification in withholding thiopentone from every patient having an emergency laparotomy in whom the exact diagnosis has not been made, on the remote chance that the abdominal pain may be due to acute porphyria.

At the time of writing it appears that both propofol and the benzodiazepines can be safely given to patients with porphyria.

Other conditions

The familial disease *dystrophia myotonia* may render patients more susceptible to the depressant effects of induction agents on respiration. This has only been shown to apply with thiopentone (Dundee, 1952; Hewer, 1957; Kaufman, 1960). It is worth noting that suxamethonium and neostigmine may increase the degree of myotonia, whereas other muscle relaxants will block neuromuscular transmission without necessarily overcoming the myotonia.

Patients with *myasthenia gravis* will react normally provided that the appropriate care has been taken in adjusting the dose of anticholinesterase. However, the respiratory depressant effects of thiopentone and similar drugs will be more marked and it is often possible to carry out an atraumatic intubation without any difficulty, and without any muscle relaxant in these patients.

One must be prepared for a period of respiratory depression lasting up to 15 or 20 min if a 'normal' dose of thiopentone is given to a patient with *severe* myasthenia gravis. Where the operation is for removal of the thymus this is not a serious mishap as a cuffed tracheal tube will be passed in case the pleura is opened during the splitting of the sternum. However, for minor procedures, such as opening of an abscess, only sufficient drug should be given to produce loss of consciousness and maximum use be made of agents which have little effect on the myoneural junction. On the other hand, because of its curarising action, a minute dose of barbiturate may result in the loss of eyelash and other reflexes without actual loss of consciousness, or with only a very brief period of narcosis. This had led to patients recalling events during 'anaesthesia' and can best be avoided by the use of inhalational agents.

Patients with Addison's disease or other types of *adrenocortical insufficiency* may be very susceptible to thiopentone and similar drugs, particularly if substitution therapy has not been given preoperatively. This sensitivity may be manifest in the form of prolonged narcosis, hypotension or an excessive degree of respiratory depression. These patients are susceptible to all forms of stress and for suggested regimen of treatment for preoperative preparation one is referred to the surveys of Plumpton et al (1969a, b).

CLINICAL SITUATIONS

Paediatrics

Children, especially those between 1 and 5 years, are often distressed when forced to leave the security of their home and family to enter hospital. The induction of anaesthesia by inhalation can be a traumatic experience, producing psychological changes, resulting in enuresis, temper tantrums and other behavioural problems and it is surprising that intravenous induction of anaesthesia is not more widely used in these situations. Except in large paediatric centres, anaesthesia, especially for younger age patients, is still induced with inhalation agents and this may be partly due to difficulties associated with venepuncture in small children by anaesthetists whose practice is not devoted exclusively to dealing with children. However, the skilful induction of anaesthesia by the intravenous route can be of great advantage to the child: a rapid smooth induction is assured and the child is spared the relatively slow onset of anaesthesia which occurs even with modern inhalation agents.

An assessment of the physical and emotional state of the child should be made preoperatively and the presence of veins suitable for venepuncture should be noted. The emotional state of the child should be assessed and particular attention paid to those children having repeated procedures. Children under 5 years suffer greatly from lack of security due to separation from their parents, while older children fear the pain and suffering from the operation they are about to undergo. Simple honest explanations as to the nature of the procedure and how they will be put to sleep do much to reassure the older child. However, calming the upset preschool child is much more difficult. Premedicant drugs and the presence of a parent during the induction of anaesthesia can help to alleviate the emotional disturbances of this age group.

The stomach should be empty prior to the induction of anaesthesia but prolonged fasting should be avoided. Hypoglycaemia can occur, especially in children under 5 years. Clear fluids with glucose added should be allowed up to 4 hours before surgery in infants under 6 months and up to 6 hours in children between 6 months and 5 years.

It is widely accepted that infants under 1 year do not need preoperative sedation. Older infants and children are usually given some form of medication. Many drugs have been used for preanaesthetic medication and their number testify to their relative ineffectiveness. Morphine provides a reliable sedative effect and its analgesic action is of value postoperatively. A wide variety of oral sedatives has been used such as trimeprazine tartrate, diazepam and temazepam. In the agitated preschool child, rectal diazepam, thiopentone or methohexitone can induce sleep within 5 min prior to transfer to the operating room. However, the presence of an anaesthetist is necessary both to administer the drug and to supervise transfer of the child. Most anaesthetists administer an anticholinergic agent to children to provide a vagolytic effect and to prevent the bradycardia which can occur in response to painful surgical stimuli or after the administration of agents such as suxamethonium, halothane or ketamine.

Intravenous induction

Induction by the intravenous route can be a relatively painless procedure if fine, 27 gauge needles are used. This requires dexterity on behalf of the anaesthetist and skilled assistance from the nursing staff. Suitable veins can be found on the dorsum of the hand or foot, the volar aspect of the wrist, the antecubital fossa or on the scalp. However, care should be exercised when injecting irritant drugs into scalp veins as accidental intra-arterial injection can occur. When attempting venepuncture the child should be gently but firmly held by an assistant who also compresses the arm. In small infants it is relatively easy to stop the arterial inflow by pressure, and blanching of the hand will occur. This should be avoided as venepuncture is made more difficult. The anaesthetist should firmly grip the arm or hand and stretch the skin over the venepuncture site. Older children are told that they are to have a 'little scratch' and at the moment of venepuncture have their attention distracted by the nurse, or is asked to give a cough or a grunt.

Thiopentone (2.5% solution) is still the most popular agent for induction of anaesthesia in children but methohexitone (1% solution) has been widely used for outpatient anaesthesia. However, children frequently complain of pain along the course of the vein during its injection and there is a high incidence of muscle twitching and respiratory upset. One must realise that it is very easy to overdose a patient of small body mass by adding 10 or 25 mg to the intended dose of thiopentone, an amount which one would normally consider insignificant. This is especially likely to occur with injections made into a slow-running intravenous infusion at a site remote from the vein itself. For this reason many will substitute a 1% solution for the customary 2.5% when dealing with young children and many will avoid it altogether in infants weighing less than 5 kg. As pointed out previously (p. 81) the required dose of thiopentone for these children is much greater on a mg kg^{-1} basis than in adults.

Ketamine has had widespread use in paediatric practice, particularly since the psychomimetic side effects so commonly seen in adults appear to be a less frequent occurrence in children. It can be given intravenously or intramuscularly, producing analgesia without cardiovascular or respiratory depression and the airway is well maintained on most occasion.

Intravenous administration of 2 mg kg^{-1} ketamine (1% solution) will produce unconsciousness within 30 s. Vertical or horizontal nystagmus may be noted initially and when the eyes become central the patient is ready for surgery. This dose will last about 5–10 min. Muscle tone is enhanced and the airway is usually well maintained. There is little respiratory depressant effect and bronchodilation has been noted which may be of assistance when anaesthetising children with asthma. Salivation can cause a problem and, unless an antisialogogue has been administered preoperatively, laryngeal spasm occurs. Contrary to popular belief the laryngeal reflexes are depressed and pulmonary aspiration has been reported. Instrumentation of the upper airway should be avoided because laryngeal spasm is likely to occur under ketamine anaesthesia. The intracranial pressure is greatly increased and ketamine is contraindicated when it is raised.

In early infancy (3–6 months) the effects of ketamine are very unpredictable. Large doses may be needed to produce satisfactory operating conditions and it is often associated with periods of apnoea and laryngospasm. Nevertheless ketamine is a valuable drug in paediatric practice. It is especially useful for burn dressing and surgery, minor therapeutic procedures such as bone marrow aspirations, and radiological investigations. In most circumstances it is the drug of choice for repeat anaesthetics although Byer & Gould (1981) have described the development of tolerance in an infant undergoing repeat anaesthesia. It has the advantage that it can also be given intramuscularly but care should be exercised to ensure that the injection is not too superficial.

Obstetrics

Despite the increasing use of extradural blocks for pain relief for operative obstetrics general anaesthesia still has a place. It may be the patient's preference or may be necessitated by the inexperience of the anaesthetist. On occasions a rapid induction may be required and this necessitates the use of intravenous agents. Following their introduction it was advocated that the surgeon-operator should be scrubbed and ready for any procedure before the drug was given and that the infant should be extracted in the shortest possible time. However it was gradually realised that thiopentone rapidly crosses the placenta and that undue haste is not only not necessary but inadvisable as it will lead to the infant being born with a relatively high drug concentration; but neither should there be too much delay as a prolonged induction–delivery interval leads to delivery of a drowsy child irrespective, of the technique of anaesthesia used. As all patients at term must be considered to have a potentially full stomach the 'crash induction' technique as described previously is popular.

Thiopentone is the most widely used induction agent and it is usually mixed with atropine and given in doses adequate to obtund the eylash reflex. This is usually followed by a paralysing dose of suxamethonium and rapid tracheal intubation. If this proves difficult and further inflation with oxygen is necessary, the risk of 'aware' intubation is greatly increased. Maintenance of 'light' anaesthesia continues until delivery of the baby is completed, the contribution of the induction agent to anaesthetic 'sleep' decreasing as the induction–delivery interval is prolonged.

Awareness may be a problem in some patients, particularly if nitrous oxide is not given until the infant is born. It can be avoided by the use of low concentrations of inhalational agents. The suggestion that intravenous diazepam given at this stage will reduce recall only applies to events following its administration and not to the period prior to delivery. This complication is also more frequent in the unpremedicated patient for elective surgery and is rare in the parturient who has received sedative — analgesic treatment.

Active vomiting following intravenous anaesthetics is much less common than with inhalation agents. However, regurgitation of gastric contents can occur especially when suxamethonium is given as this increases intragastric pressure. The induction agents depress the protective laryngeal reflex and this effect is enhanced by sedative-analgesic premedication. The danger to the obstetric patient of soiling the lung with highly acid gastric contents is well known, hence most authorites now recommend tracheal intubation when intravenous anaesthesia is used.

The supine hypotensive syndrome (Scott, 1968) is a well recognised problem in late pregnancy. All intravenous induction agents, except ketamine, depress the cardiovascular system and will accentuate existing hypotension or, by impairing compensatory mechanisms, unmask the syndrome. Lateral tilting will remove the pressure effect of the pregnant uterus on the inferior vena cava, restoring venous return, cardiac output, blood pressure and placental perfusion. Ketamine, because of its cardiostimulatory effects, may be used to induce anaesthesia in patients with pre-existing supine hypotension (Bunodiere et al, 1977).

None of the currently available intravenous agents depress uterine function or increase the incidence of placental retention or third stage blood loss. Ketamine may increase uterine tone and make intrauterine manipulation more difficult (Dick et al, 1973).

Intravenous induction agents, because of their sedative and anticonvulsant actions are sometimes used in the management of eclamptic states. The aim is to induce a light plane of narcosis where the patient is just rousable and supports her own airway. Rapid administration will produce deep sedation, hypotension and respiratory depression. Chlormethiazole and diazepam are the most commonly used drugs. Duffus et al (1969) reported good maternal effects from chlormethiazole without associated severe infant depression. Diazepam, whilst producing satisfactory sedative effects in the mother can, even in moderate doses, cause infant hypotonicity, hypothermia, respiratory depression and exacerbation of neonatal jaundice (Moir, 1976). Midazolam may be preferred for this purpose, but when given to women in labour the plasma concentration does not fall as rapidly as in non-parturient patients (Wilson et al, 1986).

The intravenous induction agents have contributed greatly to patient acceptability of anaesthesia in obstetrics. Their safe use demands expert anaesthetic care so that mother and infant are spared the harmful effects of mismanagement or overdosage.

Outpatient or day case operations

These are increasing in frequency and patients are usually allowed to go home 4–6 hours after the procedure accompanied by a responsible adult. They will normally not return to active work until the following day. At first one might think that the very short-acting drugs such as methohexitone and etomidate were essential components for day case anaesthesia but in practice a delay in recovery is not usually a problem and drowsiness is more likely to be associated with the use of inappropiate premedication than with thiopentone. Likewise, these patients being ambulant may suffer more ill effects from the use of fentanyl and alfentanil to reduce doses of intravenous anaesthetics and prolonged vomiting is a distressing complication. The use of anti-emetics in outpatients must be very judicious as drugs like perphenazine can themselves have marked side effects. This applies even to metoclopramide and a useful compromise between efficacy and side effects is probably cyclizine, although even this can cause some residual drowsiness.

The absence of changes in environment the night before operation may make patients less apprehensive than in hospital but a good night's sleep is desirable and an end-product benzodiazepine such as tempazepam would seem to be the drug of choice. This may be repeated on the morning of anaesthesia but only when the patients have someone to accompany them to the hospital.

Patients selected for day case operations must be reasonably fit and this excludes diabetics and those with other metabolic upset. For this reason the choice of anaesthetic agent will probably be more determined on the type and duration of the procedure than on the fitness of the patient.

Post-suxamethonium myalgia is a distressing complication of outpatient anaesthesia and although this is reduced slightly by the use of thiopentone this attenuation is not of any great clinical importance. It is recommended that, where possible, the fasciculations and sequelae should be attenuated by the prior use of a non-depolarising muscle relaxants. Gallamine has much to recommend it for this purpose as it can be mixed with thiopentone and in doses of 20 mg its action is usually transient, although it does increase the requirement of suxamethonium. Vercuronium can also be recommended.

Crawford and colleagues (1984) have suggested that midazolam will be useful for outpatient anaesthesia but this does not seem a very rational choice as they say that patients require at least 4 hours to recover. Propofol will find a useful place in this field, not only because of the rapidity of recovery but because of the potential anti-emetic action.

There is a place for supplementation of local anaesthesia by low doses of midazolam as in dental procedures in outpatients and here one must realise that although patients may seem to be fully awake, full recovery from even hypnotic doses of midazolam usually takes as long as after a full induction dose.

Dentistry

Since most chairside dentistry is conducted on an outpatient basis what has been said above about choice of agents, recovery and the need for proper attention to patients in the immediate postoperative phase applies equally to dentistry.

Chairside anaesthesia can be induced with any of the intravenous anaesthetics and continued with nitrous oxide and most inhalation agents. Methohexitone and etomidate are probably preferred to thiopentone because of their rapidity of action and lesser cardiovascular effects. This latter is important as many of these patients will be in a semi-upright position and will not have the same preoperative evaluation as would inpatients. The troublesome muscle movements can be minimised by slow injection of small doses.

Intermittent methohexitone had a period of popularity as a means of producing very light anaesthesia or 'deep sedation' for prolonged conservative and restorative procedures. Ideally patients were kept in verbal contact with the operator and deep anaesthesia was avoided. It was essential to make sure that there was a good local anaesthetic in combination with methohexitone as the barbiturates have no analgesic action. This technique has lost popularity because of the dangers of anaesthesia developing rather than sedation, with the risk of respiratory obstruction and minor degrees of hypoxia. It is very much a technique for the expert who is using it frequently. Some operators combine this with an intravenous injection of pentazocine which gives the additional analgesia.

There has been a trend against the 'operator-anaesthetist' in recent years and in certain countries, including Britain, this is no longer allowed.

This has also contributed to the abandonment of the intermittent methohexitone technique and a replacement with light-sedation produced by a benzodiazepine in combination with good local anaesthesia. Midazolam is the benzodiazepine of choice for this work because of the ease of administration and the more rapid recovery as compared with diazepam. Initial doses are in the region of 0.05 to 0.07 mg kg^{-1} with supplements as required. Midazolam also produces a temporary period of amnesia so that if the local is injected within 2 min of its administration there is little chance of the patient remembering it. This is very important with apprehensive patients who have reacted badly to local anaesthesia on previous occasions. Many dentists will be very aware that these sedation techniques have now made conservative dentistry acceptable to many patients who would otherwise have been too apprehensive to have the procedures carried out under local anaesthesia alone.

OTHER ROUTES OF ADMINISTRATION

Rectal use

Rectal thiopentone has enjoyed a certain popularity for the psychologically atraumatic induction of anaesthesia in children and indeed no supplement may be required for minor surgical procedures involving minimal painful stimulation.

The usual dose is 1 g per 25 to 35 kg body weight depending upon the depth of narcosis desired in a normally active robust child, but it is recommended that a total dosage of 1 to 1.5 g should not be exceeded in children. Rectal thiopentone may be prepared as a 2.5 or 5 per cent solution, but it is also available as a commercial suspension containing 400 mg of sodium thiopentone buffered with 24 mg of anhydrous sodium carbonate as a buffer in a water-miscible suspension of mineral oil and dimethyldioctyldecylammonium bentonite. Is is supplied in a disposable plastic syringe, ready for injection. The advantage of this much more concentrated suspension lies in the fact that the amounts administered are very much smaller than with the aqueous solutions thus minimising the likelihood of the substance being expelled.

Although rectal administration does not alter the basic pharmacological effects of thiopentone, the slowness of absorption into the bloodstream reduces the impact of its depressant effects and the interposition of the liver between the site of absorption and the cerebral circulation reduces the amount of drug which actually reaches the brain, in comparison with all other routes of administration; yet in the presence of marked stimulation laryngospasm may still occur. The protective airway reflexes are obtunded and airway obstruction therefore may occur, so that the patient must never be left unattended. The effects of rectal thiopentone become readily apparent within 8 to 10 minutes and maximal effects may be expected to last for 20 to 30 minutes. Awakening is relatively slow and this constitutes one of the definite disadvantages of this mode of administration.

Although Kraus et al (1984) found only 17% bioavailability after rectal methohexitone, rectal induction with 10% methohexitone (25 mg kg^{-1}) is safe and effective in young children. Goresky & Stewart (1979) found this to be especially valuable in the 3-months to 4-year age group and recovery was not unduly delayed after a 30 min operation. However, Liu et al (1980) have not found this dose of methohexitone to be 100% effective and occasionally a patient will not fall asleep even after 30 min. In subsequent studies Liu et al (1985) have correlated the effect with peak plasma concentrations. The mean time to onset of sleep was 8.3 min at which time the mean plasma concentration was 4.4 μg ml^{-1}. The mean peak concentration was 4.7 μg ml^{-1} which was achieved on the average in 14 min. Three of the 20 children they studied failed to lose consciousness and the achieved plasma concentration in these was never greater than 2 μg ml^{-1}. Thus the emptiness of the rectum and the position of the catheter (too high may lead to a marked first pass effect) are more likely causes of variation in effect than individual response by the patient.

The contraindications to rectal barbiturates are those which have already been described for their intravenous use. In addition, situations where rectal administration of drugs is contraindicated or undesirable, where adequate supervision of the patient is impossible, or when prompt return of protective reflexes is desired constitute further contraindications to this method.

Recently the use of rectal barbiturates has lost much of its popularity, largely because of the introduction of new agents and in particular because of the rapidity of onset of intramuscular ketamine which also can be given rectally.

The rectal administration of diazepam (organic solvent preparation) has been studied in some detail. Absorption occurred more rapidly than after oral or intramuscular administration but when given in a suppository form absorption was slow (Moolenaar et al, 1980). Knusden (1977) found that when the solution was given rectally anticonvulsant plasma levels ooourred within 4 to 5 min and in subsequent clinical studies (Knusden, 1979; 1981) he found very few side effects and recommended this as an alternative to intravenous administration. The solution used was similar to that for intravenous injection and doses were in the region of 5 to 7.5 mg for children up to 3 years with 7.5 to 10 mg for older children. This was given both therapeutically and prophylactically to children with temperatures of 38.5°C or above, every 8–12 hours with total doses as high as 2.7 mg kg^{-1} in 24 hours.

The use of rectal diazepam as premedication has not been studied in detail but it has been used in dentistry (Lundgren, 1983). Although it is difficult to record amnesia in children the authors thought that this was a valuable aspect of its use. Slezak (1983) likewise found the drug to be useful as premedication for gastroscopy in providing relief of anxiety and relaxation in two-thirds of the patients who required no other form of sedation.

Intramuscular administration

Most barbiturates can be administered by the intramuscular route, provided injection is made deep into the muscle. This applies particularly to methohexitone which is probably less irritant than thiopentone and has 100% bioavailability (Kraus et al, 1984). Intramuscular etomidate does not appear to have been used. Ketamine has been referred to above.

All available preparations of diazepam cause too much pain on injection to recommend their use. Midazolam, although not painful on injection, has not been studied in detail as an intramuscular injection, but would appear to have a potential use in this field.

REFERENCES

Adams R C, Gray H K 1943 Intravenous anesthesia with pentothal sodium in the case of gunshot wound associated with accompanying severe traumatic shock and loss of blood: report of a case. Anesthesiology 4: 70–73

Aghdami A, Ellis R, Estes M D 1985 Anesthesia for bronchoscopy and mediastinoscopy: a comparison between etomidate and pentothal. Anesthesiology 63:A367

Anonymous 1953 Nothing but the truth. Lancet 1: 585–586

Arden A R, Holly F O, Stanski B R, Ebling W F 1985 Dose potency comparison of thiopentone and etomidate. Anesthesiology 63:A286

Bali I M, Dundee J W 1985 Effect of i.v. induction regimens on endotracheal intubation with alcuronium and atracurium. British Journal of Anaesthesia 57: 830–831P

Bunodiere M, Green M, Bunodiere N, Ravaud Y, Guilmet C, Deligne P 1977 Ketamine hydrochloride and obstetric anesthesia. In: Clinical use of ketamine in obstetric and gynecological indications. Selected proceedings of the Sixth World Congress of Anaesthesiology, Mexico City, April 24–30 1976. Excerpta Medica, Amsterdam. p 27–33

Byer D E, Gould A B 1981 Development of tolerance to ketamine in an infant undergoing repeated anesthesia. Anesthesiology 54: 255–256

Crawford M E, Carl P, Anderson R S, Mikkelsen B O 1984 Comparison between midazolam and thiopentone-based balanced anaesthesia for day-case surgery. British Journal of Anaesthesia 56: 165–169

Dean G 1953 Porphyria. British Medical Journal 2: 1291–1294

Dick W, Borst F, Fodor H, Haug H, Milewki H, Schumann R, Traub E 1973 Ketamine in obstetrical anesthesia: clinical and experimental results. Journal of Perinatal Medicine 1: 252–262

Duffus G M, Tunstall M E, Condie R G, McGillivray I 1969 Chlormethiazole in the prevention of eclampsie and the reduction of perinatal mortality. Journal of Obstetrics and Gynaecology of the British Commonwealth 76: 645–651

Dundee J W 1952 Thiopentone in dystrophia myotonia. Anesthesia and Analgesia, Current Researches 31: 257–262

Dundee J W 1985 Intravenous anaesthesia and the need for new agents. Postgraduate Medical Journal 61: (suppl. 3) 3–6

Dundee J W, Halliday N J, McMurray T J, Harper K W 1986 Pretreatment with opioids. The effect on thiopentone requirements and on the onset of action of midazolam. Anaesthesia 41: 159–161

Dundee J W, McCleery W N C, McLoughlin G 1962 The hazard of thiopental anaesthesia in porphyria. Current Researches in Anesthesia 41: 567–574

Falchuk K H, Peterson L, McNeil B J 1985 Microparticulate-induced phlebitis: its prevention by in-

line filters. New England Journal of Medicine 312: 78–82
Friedland G 1985 Infusion-related phlebitis — is the in-line filter the solution? New England Journal of Medicine 312: 113–114
Giese J L, Stockham R J, Stanley T H, Pace N L, Nelissen R H 1985 Etomidate versus thiopental for induction of anesthesia. Anesthesia and Analgesia 64: 871–876
Goresky G V, Stewart D J 1979 Rectal methohexitone for induction of anaesthesia in children. Canadian Anaesthetists' Society Journal 26: 213–215
Halford F J 1943 A critique of intravenous anesthesia in war surgery. Anesthesiology 4: 67–69
Hewer C L 1957 Thiopentone and dystrophia myotonia. British Journal of Anaesthesia 29:180
Kaufman K 1960 Anaesthesia in dystrophia myotonia. Proceedings of the Royal Society of Medicine 53: 183–188
Key J C, Newmark S R 1984 Surgery in the obese patient. Journal of the Oklahoma State Medical Association 77: 345–347
Knudsen F U 1977 Plasma-diazepam in infants after rectal administration in solution and by suppository. Acta Paediatrica Scandinavica 66: 563–567
Knudsen F U 1979 Rectal administration of diazepam in solution in the acute treatment of convulsions in infants and children. Archives of Disease in Childhood 54: 855–857
Knudsen F W 1981 Successful intermittent diazepam prophylaxis in febrile convulsions: preliminary results of a prospective, controlled study. In: Dam M, Gram L, Penry J K (eds) Advances in Epileptology: XIIth Epilepsy International Symposium. Raven Press, New York
Kraus G, Frank S, Knoll R, Prestele H 1984 Pharmacokinetic analysis of intravenous, intramuscular and rectal application of methohexitone in children. Anaesthesist 33: 266–271
Liu L M P, Gaudreault P, Friedman P A, Goudsouzian N G, Liu P L 1985 Methohexital plasma concentrations in children following rectal administration. Anesthesiology 62: 567–570
Liu L M P, Goudsouzian N G, Liu P L 1980 Rectal methohexital premedication in children, a dose-comparison study. Anesthesiology 53: 343–345
Lundgren S 1983 Rectal diazepam as premedication in dentistry. In: Breimer D D (ed) 1st International Symposium on rectal diazepam for acute therapy. Zuckschwerdt, Munich. p 43–45
Magbagbeola J A O, Thomas N A 1974 Effect of thiopentone on emergence reactions to ketamine anaesthesia. Canadian Anaesthetists' Society Journal 21: 321–324
Moir D D 1976 Obstetric anaesthesia and analgesia, 1st edn. Balliere Tindall, London. p 49
Moolenaar F, Bakker S, Visser J, Huizinga T 1980 Biopharmaceutics of rectal administration of drugs in man. IX: Comparative biopharmaceutics of diazepam after single rectal, oral, intramuscular and intravenous administration in man. International Journal of Pharmaceutics 5: 127–137
Morton H J V, Wylie W D 1951 Anaesthetic deaths due to regurgitation or vomiting. Anaesthesia 6: 190–205
Plumpton F S, Besser G M, Cole P V 1969a Corticosteroid treatment and surgery. 1: An investigation of the indications for steroid cover. Anaesthesia 24: 3–11
Plumpton F Sh, Besser G M, Cole P V 1969b Corticosteroid treatment and surgery. 2: The management of steroid cover. Anaesthesia 24: 12–18
Scott D B 1968 Inferior vena caval occlusion in late pregnancy and its importance in anaesthesia. British Journal of Anaesthesia 40: 120–128
Slezak P 1983 Rectal diazepam premedication in gastroscopy. In: Breimer D D (ed) 1st International Symposium on rectal diazepam for acute therapy. Zuckschwerdt, Munich. p 46–48
Stark R D, Binks S M, Dutka V N, O'Connor K M, Arnstein M J A, Glen J B 1985 A review of the safety and tolerance of propofol (Diprivan). Postgraduate Medical Journal 61 (Suppl 3): 152–156
Wilson C M, Dundee J W, Moore J 1986 Plasma midazolam levels in non-pregnant and parturient women. Anesthesia and Analgesia 65: S 167

Prevention and treatment of brain ischaemia

PREVENTION AND TREATMENT OF BRAIN ISCHAEMIA

Few topics have aroused as much interest in recent years as the therapeutic role of barbiturates in the management of brain ischaemia. This might in part be due to a complete absence of any glimmer of hope from other forms of therapy in a condition with an otherwise hopeless prognosis. A full discussion of this topic is impossible in this chapter which concentrates on current views, but a bibliography of some relevant earlier publications on the subject is appended. The subject has been reviewed recently in an educational issue of the British Journal of Anaesthesia (Smith & McDowall, 1985).

The action of the barbiturates in increasing survival time of mice breathing 5% oxygen was demonstrated by Wilhjelm & Arnfred (1965) and Wilhjelm & Jacobson (1970). The clinical application of this finding is derived from the observation by Michenfelder (1974) that barbiturates, in doses which render the EEG isoelectric, reduce the cerebral metabolic rate ($CMRO_2$) by about half, but additional doses have no further effect. Michenfelder & Theye (1973) had previously demonstrated cerebral protection by thiopentone in dogs subjected to hypoxia, induced by acute haemmorhage or an abrupt decrease of FIO_2 to zero. Where hypoxia was associated with continued cerebral function (active EEG), earlier administration of thiopentone offered some protection against cerebral ATP depletion and lactate accumulation, but there was no protection in the presence of a flat EEG. Another early study by Goldstein et al (1966) indicated the value of pentobarbitone pretreatment in giving protection from global brain ischaemia, but these results could not be reproduced by Steen & Michenfelder (1979). Another early relevant observation was that of Meyers (1975) who demonstrated that fetal distress in the offspring of asphyxiated monkeys could be ameliorated by pentobarbitone administration to the mother.

The most convincing early study on the protective role of barbiturates was by Bleyaert and colleagues (1978). They induced global ischaemia for 16 min in monkeys by application of a high pressure neck tourniquet and systemic hypotension and demonstrated that a major portion of the permanent brain damage which occurred after restoration of the circulation was amenable to therapy with thiopentone. In discussing this work Rockoff & Shapiro (1978) asked the question as to whether barbiturates had real therapeutic value or represented Pandora's box. They did not doubt the protective action of the barbiturates in experimental focal ischaemia and suggested that this might be due to decreased cerebral metabolic demand and vasoconstriction of normal cerebral vessels shunting blood from healthy brain to an ischaemic area. Reviewing the literature they concluded "there has not been any definitive study clearly proving a specific protective action of barbiturates in global ischaemia." They pointed out the severe cardiovascular depressant effects of these doses, particularly in elderly subjects, adding "anyone who has treated patients with massive barbiturate overdose does not need to have the dangers emphasised further." The latter anxiety has been justified by the finding of Rogers et al (1981) of an increased myocardial infarct size produced by the dose of barbiturates used for brain protection after cardiac arrest. Despite the enthusiasm of some Continental workers (Belopavlovic & Buchthal, 1980) and the encouraging preliminary results from a multinational randomised trial (Breivik et al, 1978) Aitkenhead (1981) in an editorial expressed doubt about whether babiturates protect the brain in humans, and also whether they are the most appropriate drugs to use in view of their associated severe metabolic depression and prolonged metabolism. Similar views have been expressed at a later date by Michenfelder (1982) and by Shapiro (1984). At the time of writing we eagerly await the findings of the collaborative randomised study of cardiopulmonary-cerebral resuscitation, described by Detre and her colleagues in 1981. However, a recent paper from the Medical College of Virginia (Ward et al, 1985) entitled "Failure of prophylactic barbiturate coma in the treatment of severe head injury" gives the findings of another randomised study. This consisted of 27 barbiturate-treated and 26 control patients, all of whom had the same vigorous resuscitation, prompt diagnosis and treatment of mass lesions and intensive care with close follow-up monitoring. The outcome was essentially the same in each group. Arterial hypotension occurred in about half the treated group and in only 7% of the untreated group. On the basis of this study the authors cannot recommend the prophylactic use of pentobarbitone coma in the treatment of patients with severe head injury; they also believe that its use is accompanied by significant side effects which can potentially worsen the condition of the patient.

While it appears that barbiturates have no specific beneficial effects in ameliorating the sequelae of global ischaemia (Gisvold et al, 1984) the situation appears to be different in patients with post-hypoxia convulsions. Post-ischaemic seizures increase the cerebral metabolic rate at a time when compensatory increases in cerebral blood flow might be limited by intrinsic pathological responses involving the vasculature as well as the haemodynamics of the systemic circulation (Shapiro, 1984). Seizure prophylaxis and/or prompt effective anticonvulsant therapy in the post arrest period would appear to be beneficial, but hypo and hypertension should be avoided. It is interesting to note that, in an uncontrolled clinical study with phenytoin after cardiac arrest Aldrete et al (1981) reported complete recovery in 9 out of 10 patients, all of whom were comatose with dilated pupils before treatment. This approach warrants further study.

OVERVIEW

In a recent review on therapy for the ischaemic brain, Dearden (1985) lists the following reasons for the beneficial effects of the barbiturates:

1. Reduction of cerebral metabolic rate, especially in areas of high activity, to the level of EEG suppression.
2. Diversion of blood from areas of high perfusion into ischaemic areas by cerebral vasoconstriction (inverse steal), which should increase penumbral flow in focal ischaemia.
3. Reduction of intracranial pressure and improvement of cerebral perfusion pressure by cerebral vasoconstriction, secondary to metabolic depression. This mechanism of action provides a rationale for barbiturate infusion to reduce intracranial pressure after head injury.
4. Anticonvulsant actions is independent of the sedative effects of the barbiturate.
5. Stabilisation of lysosomal membranes.
6. Free-radical scavenging — a property confined to thiopentone.

He summarizes the views expressed above that 'after cardiac arrest, investigations in animals and humans have consistently shown an absence of benefit from barbiturates' (Gisvold et al, 1984).

Discussing head injury and brain ischaemia, Miller (1985) stressed the importance of avoiding an increase in intracranial pressure. He lists (Table 16.1) five steps and only includes infusions of barbiturates as one of them. It is becoming clear that some of the benefits originally attributed to the barbiturates might have been due to better all-round care including adequate ventilation and the avoidance of hypoxia and hypotension, and other forms of supportive therapy (Gisvold & Steen, 1985). Miller commented on an unpublished study that allowed some temporary control of intracranial pressure with pentobarbitone but no long term benefit and pointed out the dangers of hypotension with this therapy.

In a related field it has been demonstrated by

Table 16.1 Methods of controlling increased intracranial pressure

Treatment	*Limitations*	*Risks*
Hyperventilation	Blood vessels must be responsive to changes in PCO_2	Vasoconstriction might produce brain ischaemia (although structural damage has never been shown to occur
CSF drainage	From ventricular catheter only	Leakage of CSF might interfere with ICP recording. Haemorrhage in track of cannula through brain
Mannitol	Serum osmolality must be less than 320 mosmol litre^{-1}	Fluid and electrolyte disturbance and renal failure
Barbiturates	Loss of neurological responsiveness	Arterial hypotension (especially in hypovolaemic patients); increased risk of infection
Gammahydroxybutyrate	Irritant solution, needs central venous line	Production of seizure-like EEG activity

from Miller (1985)

Nussmeier and colleagues (1986) that the administration of sufficient thiopentone (by intermittent administration or by infusion) to maintain EEG silence reduced the frequency and duration of neuropsychotic problems following cardiopulmonary bypass. It is interesting to note that Michenfelder (1986), who was among the first to study the potential therapeutic effect of barbiturates on brain protection, heralds this as a breakthrough which should be applied clinically.

PREVENTION

Brain protection against focal ischaemia during extra and intracranial revascularisation procedures is the most frequent indication for the use of intravenous barbiturates. Most procedures are carried out under general anaesthesia for which a barbiturate can be given and alterations in the technique are all that is necessary with the provision of a high plasma concentration for a period less than the total operating time. Moffatt et al (1983) have shown that 4–5 mg kg^{-1} thiopentone, administered just before internal carotid artery occlusion during carotid endarterectomy will result in around 5 min of EEG burst suppression which is much less than the total period of arterial occlusion. Local metabolic depression might, however, persist in the poorly perfused brain areas and extend the period of potentiation.

More prolonged high blood barbiturate concentrations are required for intracranial microvascular procedures, with their longer occlusion periods and less compensatory collateral circulation (Hoff et al, 1977). Spetzler et al (1982) recommended a dose of 10 mg kg^{-1} thiopentone and advocated EEG monitoring. Shapiro (1985) advocates a trial vascular occlusion of at least 5 min with subsequent barbiturate therapy if this occlusion results in EEG abnormalities. If abnormalities occur which do not resolve on re-establishment of the circulation, then an embolic episode must be suspected and high dose barbiturate therapy started. Others will routinely give an additional dose of barbiturate, but with EEG monitoring.

Bendsten et al (1984) report their clinical experience with supplementary thiopentone loading in 30 patients undergoing operations for intracranial aneurysm after a recent episode of intracranial haemorrhage. As a standard they induced balanced anaesthesia with pentobarbitone and as the aneurysm was approached they obtained satisfactory hypotension with thiopentone (with or without sodium nitroprusside). Intermittent doses of 100–200 mg barbiturate were given to a total of approximately 20 mg kg^{-1}. Uncontrolled hypotension did not occur. Recovery was slow, most patients requiring pulmonary ventilation during the first few hours after operation and the time to tracheal extubation varied from 20 min to 40 h. This can be explained by the altered pharmacokinetics of the large dose of thiopentone (Stanski et al, 1980) discussed in Chapter 6. Cerebral metabolism was already low due to the pentobarbitone–fentanyl–relaxant–hyperventilation anaesthetic sequence; thiopentone loading reduced this by only a further 15% and the blood flow by 16.5% (Astrup et al, 1984). Nevertheless, these Danish workers felt that this method, although requiring intensive postoperative care, not only produced excellent operating conditions but contributed to the favourable outcome of the operation. Despite the enthusiasm of these workers one can still echo the view of Yatsu (1982) that a prospective study is needed to establish the intraoperative efficacy of barbiturate protection in these situations.

The increase in blood pressure and associated elevation in incracranial pressure associated with laryngoscopy and tracheal intubation under light anaesthesia could have a disastrous effect in patients with an already compromised cerebral circulation. Bedford et al (1980) found pretreatment with lignocaine to be effective in preventing this, while Prys-Roberts et al (1973) and Greenbaum (1976) recommend pretreatment with a beta-adrenoreceptor blocking drug. A simple and effective method is recommended by Unni and his colleagues (1984). They follow an initial dose of 5 mg kg^{-1} thiopentone by a long-acting myoneural blocking drug with a further 2.5 mg kg^{-1} thiopentone given after 3 min. Laryngoscopy and topical analgesia to the larynx follow the second dose of thiopentone and are immediately followed by tracheal intubation which can be carried out with minimal upset to cerebral dynamics. When it was available, Althesin would probably have been as effective as thiopentone in this situation (Moss et al, 1978; Unni et al, 1983).

Another interesting concept is the infusion of a mixture of 1.5 g thiopentone and 200 mg lignocaine (in 500 ml solution) for pneumoencephalography (Raudzens & Cole, 1974). This requires careful attention to detail and the services of an experienced anaesthetist.

McDowall (1982) in discussing the use of induced hypotension in brain ischaemia comments that cerebral metabolic depressant drugs such as thiopentone might have a place in clinical techniques of induced hypotension, but he favours the use of isoflurane which might itself produce satisfactory hypotension.

Thiopentone appears to inhibit the response of both the renin–angiotensin system and particularly the autonomic nervous system to hypotension (Spring et al, 1983). This is a beneficial effect in neurological patients undergoing procedures under controlled hypotension as, by preventing the increase in plasma adrenaline, it minimises rebound hypertension.

THERAPY

Various regimes of barbiturate therapy have been described (Marshall et al, 1979; Rockoff et al, 1979; Shapiro, 1984; 1985) but as emphasised above these must be part of intensive patient management with avoidance of hypoxia and hypotension and with continuous monitoring of intracranial pressure and periodic estimations of blood barbiturate levels. The continuous administration of barbiturates has been discussed in Chapter 17; the following techniques have been recommended by experts in this field.

Pentobarbitone (Shapiro, 1985)

The objective is to maintain a mean arterial pressure in excess of 70 mm Hg and cardiac filling pressure sufficient to produce a cardiac index of 2 l min^{-1}m^{-2} and a blood barbiturate concentration of 3–4 mg dl^{-1}.

- Loading dose 10 mg kg^{-1}, administered over 30 min, with subsequent doses depending on the cardiovascular response
- Pentobarbitone 5 mg kg^{-1}h^{-1} for the next 3 hours (20–25 mg kg^{-1} should be given over the first 4 h of treatment, giving a blood concentration of 2 mg dl^{-1})
- Maintenance dose of 2.5 mg kg^{-1}h^{-1} to achieve levels of 3–4 mg dl^{-1}
- If hypotension occurs: dopamine infusion and volume expansion
- If intracranial pressure exceeds 20 mm Hg and blood level is under 3 mg dl^{-1}, give an additional dose of 5 mg kg^{-1}

Another approach is simply to titrate the dose of barbiturate until a burst suppression pattern is present on the EEG and then keep the bursts and suppressions of equal length (Bruce et al, 1978). This usually occurs at serum levels of 2.5–5 mg dl^{-1}.

Thiopentone (McDowall, 1982).

The use of thiopentone involves the precautions and monitoring referred to above, but reliance is placed on intracranial pressure readings rather than blood levels and the intracranial pressure must not rise above 20 mm Hg. The following regimen is suggested:

- 1 g thiopentone over 1st hour
- 600 mg thiopentone over 2nd hour
- 300 mg thiopentone over 3rd hour
- Thereafter adjust to maintain intracranial pressure at a low level
- Treat falls or rises in blood pressure
- Lower blood viscosity with dextran, reducing Hb to 10 g dl^{-1}
- Avoid hyperglycaemia (No 50% dextrose)
- Controlled ventilation and relaxants to suppress convulsive activity
- Mannitol 0.5 g kg^{-1} at 6 and possibly at 12 hours

Other workers have suggested plasma levels similar to those for pentobarbitone. These concentrations are usually well tolerated unless the patient is hypovolaemic. Thiopentone must not be combined with nitrous oxide which increases both cerebral glucose utilisation and cerebral oxygen consumption and minimises the protective effect of the barbiturates (Hartung & Cottrell, 1985).

It is interesting to note that Sawada et al (1982) found acute tolerance developing to high-dose barbiturates (thiamylal). After 15 min of therapy the plasma concentration required to maintain a burst suppression pattern on the EEG averaged 21.0 mg ml^{-1}, at 25 h this was 30 mg ml^{-1}, reaching 41 at 48 h and 48 by 72 h. This could be a clinical manifestation of the phenomena discussed on p. 75.

Barbiturates and hypothermia

Since the barbiturates will only affect the cerebral metabolic rate in the presence of neuronal electrical activity, and hypothermia works independently of brain activity, the effects of the two are not simply additive (Steen et al, 1983) and the action of barbiturates will vary at different temperatures. Clearly the two techniques can be combined but lower doses of barbiturates are required than at normothermia. In the general management of such patients it should be noted that large doses of barbiturates will render the patients poikilothermic (Domingues de Vilotta et al, 1981) and active steps might be needed to keep the core temperature at the desired level.

Other drugs

Althesin, a rapidly acting anticonvulsant which decreases cerebral metabolic rate and blood flow (Rasmussen et al, 1978; Sari et al, 1976) and intracranial pressure (Pickerodt et al, 1972; Turner et al, 1973) was a promising alternative to thiopentone and was preferred by some for neuroanaesthesia. Etomidate, which is equally effective in lowering intracranial pressure (Cunitz et al, 1978; Schulte am Esch et al, 1978), likewise was preferred by many, particularly in view of its lesser cardiovascular toxicity (Dearden & McDowall, 1985). While methohexitone will cause a comparable reduction in cerebral blood flow and intracranial pressure, its action is very short lived (Herrschaft & Schmidt, 1974) and this, combined with its tendency to produce tachycardia, has not commended its use in this field.

Lignocaine has also been recommended for the rapid lowering of intracranial pressure and Bedford et al (1980) claimed that it appears to be as effective as thiopentone in this respect. It is not discussed among recommended drugs in recent papers on this topic and presumably did not live up to initial expectations.

Midazolam appears to have all the desired properties of the barbiturates with regard to intracranial pressure (Cottrell et al, 1982; Nugent et al, 1982) but has not offered any competition to thiopentone in the current context. Delay in recovery might be a problem here, but increasing familiarity with infusion techniques might overcome it.

It is too early to assess the potential role of propofol in this field (Ch. 11). Preliminary infusion data suggest that hypotension might be a problem with large doses or prolonged administration, but rapidity of recovery might more than compensate for this.

It has been suggested that, since isoflurane decreases cerebral metabolism and maintains the cerebral energy state during minimal suppression of cortical electrical activity (Newberg et al, 1983), it might offer an alternative to thiopentone, but animal experiments have not confirmed its therapeutic index (Bendo et al, 1985).

REFERENCES

Aitkenhead A R 1981 Editorial. Do barbiturates protect the brain? British Journal of Anaesthesia 53: 1011–1013

Aldrete J A, Romo-Salas F, Mazzia V D B, Tan S L 1981 Phenytoin for brain resuscitation after cardiac arrest: an uncontrolled clinical trial. Critical Care Medicine 9: 474–477

Astrup J, Rosenorn J, Cold G E, Bendsten A O, Sorensen P M 1984 Minimum cerebral blood flow and metabolism during craniotomy: effect of thiopental loading. Acta Anaesthesiologica Scandinavica 28: 478–481

Bedford R F, Persing J A, Pobereskin L, Butler A 1980 Lidocaine or thiopental for rapid control of intracranial hypertension? Anesthesia and Analgesia 59: 435–437

Belopavlovic M, Buchtal A 1980 Barbiturate therapy in the management of cerebral ischaemia. Anaesthesia 35: 271–278

Bendo A A, Kass I S, Cottrell J E 1985 Comparison of the protective effect of thiopental and isoflurane against anoxic damage in the rat hippocampal slice. Anesthesiology 63:A411

Bendsten A O, Cold G E, Astrup J, Rosenorn J 1984 Thiopental loading during controlled hypotension for intracranial aneurysm surgery. Acta Anaesthesiologica Scandinavica 28: 473–477

Bleyaert A L, Nemoto E M, Safar P, Stezoski S W, Mickell J J, Moossy J, Rao G R 1978 Thiopental amelioration of brain damage after global ischemia in monkeys. Anesthesiology 49: 390–398

Breivik H, Safar P, Sams P, Fabritius R, Lind B, Lust T, Mullie A R M, Renck H, Sneider J V 1978 Clinical feasibility trials of barbiturate therapy after cardiac arrest. Critical Care Medicine 6: 228–244

Bruce D A, Gennarelli T A, Langfitt T W 1978 Resuscitation from coma due to head injury. Critical Care Medicine 6: 254–269

Cottrell J E, Griffin J P, Lim K, Milhorat T, Stein S, Shwiry V 1982 Intracranial pressure, mean arterial pressure and heart rate following midazolam or thiopentone in humans with intracranial masses. Anesthesiology 57:A323

Cunitz G, Dannhauser I, Wickbold J 1978 Comparative investigations on the influence of etomidate, thiopentone and methohexitone on the intracranial pressure of patients. Anaesthesist 27: 64–70

Dearden N M 1985 The ischaemic brain. Lancet 2: 255–259

Dearden N M, McDowall D G 1985 Comparison of etomidate and Althesin in the reduction of increased intracranial pressure after head injury. British Journal of Anaesthesia 57: 361–368

Detre K, Abramson N, Safar P, Snyder J, Reinmuth O, Bitsko J, Kelsey S, Mullie A, Hedstrand U, Tammisto T, Lund I, Breivik H, Lind B, Jastremski M 1981 Collaborative randomized clinical study of cardiopulmonary-cerebral resuscitation. Critical Care Medicine 9: 395–396

Dominques de Vilotta E, Mosquerrar J M, Stein L, Shubin H, Wild H M 1981 Normal temperature control after intoxication with short-acting barbiturates. Critical Care Medicine 9: 662–666

Gisvold S E, Safar P, Hendrickx H L L, Rao G, Moossy J, Alexander H 1984 Thiopental treatment after global brain ischemia in pigtailed monkeys. Anesthesiology 60: 88–96

Gisvold S E, Steen P A 1985 Drug therapy in brain ischaemia. British Journal of Anaesthesia 57: 96–109

Goldstein A, Wells B A, Keats B S 1966 Increased tolerance to cerebral anoxia by pentobarbital. Archives Internationales de Pharmacodynamie et de Therapie 161: 138–143

Greenbaum R 1976 General anaesthesia for neurosurgery. British Journal of Anaesthesia 48: 773–781

Hartung J, Cottrell J E 1985 Does nitrous oxide preclude the protective effect of barbiturates? Anesthesiology 63:A413

Herrschaft H, Schmidt H 1974 The effect of methohexitone sodium on global and original cerebral blood flow in man. Anaesthesist 23: 340–344

Hoff J I, Pitts L H, Spetzler R F 1977 Barbiturates for protection against cerebral aneurism surgery. Acta Neurologica Scandinavica 56:158

McDowall D G 1982 Protection of the ischaemic brain. Lecture at 6th European Congress of Anaesthesiology, London.

Marshall L F, Smith R W, Shapiro H M 1979 The outcome with aggressive treatment in severe head injuries. Part II: Acute and chronic barbiturate administration in the management of head injury. Journal of Neurosurgery 50: 26–30

Meyers R 1975 Material psychological stress and fetal asphyxia: study in the monkey. American Journal of Obstetrics and Gynecology 122: 47–59

Michenfelder J D 1974 The interdependency of cerebral functional and metabolic effects following massive doses of thiopental in the dog. Anesthesiology 41: 231–236

Michenfelder J D 1982 Barbiturates for brain resuscitation: yes and no. Anesthesiology 57: 74–75

Michenfelder J D 1986 A valid demonstration of barbiturate-induced brain protection in man — at last. Anesthesiology 64: 140–141

Michenfelder J D, Theye R A 1973 Cerebral protection by thiopental during hypoxia. Anesthesiology 39: 510–517

Miller J D 1985 Head injury and brain ischaemia — implications for therapy. British Journal of Anaesthesia 57: 120–129

Moffatt J A, McDougall M J, Brunet B, Saunders F, Shelley E S, Cervenko F W, Milne B 1983 Thiopental bolus during carotid endarterectomy — rational drug therapy. Canadian Anaesthetists' Society Journal 30: 615–619

Moss E, Powell D, Gibson R M, McDowall D G 1978 Effects of tracheal intubation on intracranial pressure following induction of anaesthesia with thiopentone or Althesin in patients undergoing neurosurgery. British Journal of Anaesthesia 50: 353–360

Newberg L A, Milde J H, Michenfelder J D 1983 The cerebral metabolic effects of isoflurane at and above concentrations that suppress cortical electrical activity. Anesthesiology 59: 23–28

Nugent M, Artru A A, Michenfelder J 1982 Cerebral metabolic, vascular and protective effects of midazolam maleate. Anesthesiology 56: 172–176

Nussmeier N A, Arlund C, Slogoff S 1986 Neuropsychiatric complications after cardiopulmonary bypass: cerebral protection by a barbiturate. Anesthesiology 64: 165–170

Pickerodt V W A, McDowall D G, Coroneos N J, Keaney N P 1972 Effect of Althesin on cerebral perfusion, cerebral metabolism and intracranial pressure in the anaesthetised baboon. British Journal of Anaesthesia 44: 751–757

Prys-Roberts C, Foex P, Biro G P, Roberts J G 1973 Studies

of anaesthesia in relation to hypertension. V. Adrenergic beta-receptor blockade. British Journal of Anaesthesia 45: 671–681

Rasmussen N J, Rosendal T, Overgaard J 1978 Althesin in neurosurgical patients. Effects of cerebral hemodynamics and metabolism. Acta Anaesthesiologica Scandinavica 22: 257–269

Raudzens P, Cole A F D 1974 Thiopentone/lidocaine anaesthesia for pneumo-encephalography. Canadian Anaesthetists' Society Journal 21: 1–14

Rockoff M A, Marshall L F, Shapiro H M 1979 High dose barbiturate therapy in man. A clinical review of sixty patients. Annals of Neurology 6: 194–199

Rockoff M A, Shapiro H M 1978 Barbiturates following cardiac arrest: possible benefit or Pandora's box? Anesthesiology 49: 385–387

Rogers M C, Jugdutt B, Hutchins G M, Becker L C 1981 Increased myocardial infarct size by barbiturates used for brain protection after cardiac arrest. Critical Care Medicine 9: 184–188

Sari A, Maekawa T, Tohjo M, Okuda Y, Takeshita H 1976 Effects of Althesin on cerebral blood flow and oxygen consumption in man. British Journal of Anaesthesia 48: 545–550

Sawada Y, Sugimoto H, Kobayashi H, Ohashi N, Yoshioka T, Sugimoto T 1982 Acute tolerance to high dose barbiturate treatment in patients with severe head injuries. Anesthesiology 56: 53–54

Schulte am Esch J, Pfeifer G, Thiemig G 1978 Effects of etomidate and thiopentone on the previously elevated intracranial pressure. Anaesthesist 27: 71–75

Shapiro H M 1984 Brain resuscitation: the chicken should come before the egg. Anesthesiology 60: 85–87

Shapiro H M 1985 Barbiturates in brain ischaemia. British Journal of Anaesthesia 57: 82–95

Smith G, McDowall D G 1985 A symposium on brain ischaemia. British Journal of Anaesthesia, Postgraduate Medical Education issue 57: 1–130

Spetzler R F, Sellman W R, Roski R A, Bonstelle C 1982 Cerebral revascularisation during barbiturate coma in primates and humans. Surgical Neurology 17: 111–115

Spring A, Spring G, Liebau H, Kirchner H 1983 The effect of thiopental on plasma renin and noradrenaline during neurological procedures with hypotension. Anaesthesist 32: 12–17

Stanski D R, Mihm F G, Rosenthal M H, Kalman S M 1980 Pharmacokinetics of high dose thiopental used in cerebral resuscitation. Anesthesiology 53: 169–171

Steen P A, Michenfelder J D 1979 Barbiturate protection in tolerant and nontolerant hypoxic mice: comparison with hypothermic protection. Anesthesiology 50: 404–408

Steen P A, Newberg L, Milde J H, Michenfelder J D 1983 Hypothermia and barbiturates: Individual and combined effects on canine oxygen consumption. Anesthesiology 58: 527–532

Turner J M, Coroneos N J, Gibson R M, Powell D, Ness M A, McDowall D G 1973 The effect of Althesin on intracranial pressure in man. British Journal of Anaesthesia 45: 168–171

Unni V K N, Johnston R A, Young H S A, McBride R J 1984 Prevention of intra-cranial hypertension during laryngoscopy and endotracheal intubation: use of a second dose of thiopentone. British Journal of Anaesthesia 56: 1219–1223

Unni V K N, Young H S A, Johnston R A 1983 Anesthetic induction with Althesin infusion. Prevention of ICP changes during laryngoscopy and intubation. In: Ishii S, Nagai H, Brock M (eds) Intracranial Pressure V. Springer-Verlag, Berlin, 838–841

Ward J D, Becker D P, Miller J D, Choi S C, Marmarou A, Wood C, Newlon P G, Keenan R 1985 Failure of prophylactic barbiturate coma in the treatment of severe head injury. Journal of Neurosurgery 62: 383–388

Wilhjelm B J, Arnfred I 1965 Protective action of some anesthetics against anoxia. Acta Pharmacologica Toxicologica 22: 93–98

Wilhjelm B J, Jacobson E 1970 The protective effect of different barbiturates against anoxia in mice. Acta Pharmacologica Toxicologica 28: 203–208

Yatsu F M 1982 Pharmacological protection against ischaemic brain damage: need for prospective human studies. Stroke 13:745

ADDITIONAL READING

Bleyaert A, Safar P, Nemoto E, Mussie J, Sasano J 1980 Effect of post-circulatory arrest life support on neurological recovery in monkeys. Critical Care Medicine 8: 153–156

Fitch W 1981 Protection of the brain from ischaemia. British Journal of Anaesthesia 53: 201–202

Freeman R B, Scheff M F, Maher J F, Schrenir G E 1962 The blood–cerebro spinal fluid barrier in uremia. Annals of Internal Medicine 56: 233–240

Gisvold S E, Safar P, Alexander H, Thompson M 1981 Cardiovascular tolerance of thiopental anesthesia for brain resuscitation in monkeys. Journal of Cerebral Blood Flow Metabolism 1: Suppl 1, S264–265

Hoffmann L, Gethmann J W, Schmidt B, Schwarz M, Rating D 1979 High-dose thiopentone therapy for post-ischaemic brain hypoxia. A case report. Anaesthesist28: 339–342

Koch K A, Jackson D J, Schmiedl M, Thompson W L, Rosenblatt J I 1984 Effect of thiopental therapy on cerebral blood flow after total cerebral ischemia. Critical Care Medicine 12: 90–95

McDowall D G 1985 Induced hypotension and brain ischaemia. British Journal of Anaesthesia 57: 110–119

Magalini S I, Bondoli A, Corrado M 1981 Protective effect of phenobarbital on amino-acid cerebral metabolism on experimental acute hypoxia. Critical Care Medicine 9: 249–253

Marshall L F, Shapiro H M, Rauscher A, Kaufman N M 1978 Pentobarbital therapy for intracranial hypertension in metabolic coma. Reye's Syndrome. Critical Care Medicine 6: 1–5

Michenfelder J D, Theye R A 1971 The effect of anesthesia and hypothermia on canine cerebral ATP and lactate during anoxia produced by decapitation. Anesthesiology 33: 430–439

Michenfelder J D, van Dyke R A, Theye R A 1970 The effects of anesthetic agents in techniques on canine

cerebral ATP and lactate levels. Anesthesiology 33: 315–321
Miller J R, Meyers R E 1970 Neurological effect of systemic circulatory arrest in the monkey. Neurology 20: 715–724
Nemoto E M 1977 Post-ischaemic amelioration of brain damage. In: Zulch K J (ed) Brain and heart infarcts. Springer, Berlin. p 73–80
Nemoto E M 1978 Pathogenesis of cerebral ischaemia-anoxia. Critical Care Medicine 6: 203–212
Nemoto E M, Kofkaew A, Kessler T 1977 Studies on the pathogenesis of ischaemic brain damage and mechanism of its amelioration by thiopental. Acta Neurologica Scandinavica 56: Suppl 64:142
Nordstrom C H, Siesjo B K 1978 Effects of phenobarbital in cerebral ischemia Part I: Cerebral energy metabolism during pronounced incomplete ischemia. Stroke 9:327
Safar P 1978 Introduction on the evolution of brain resuscitation. Critical Care Medicine 6: 199–202
Safar T, Stezoki W, Nemoto E M 1976 Amelioration of brain damage after 12 minutes cardiac arrest in dogs. Archives of Neurology 33: 91–95
Shiu G K, Nemoto E M, Bleyaert A L, Nemmer J 1981 Comparison of pentobarbital, etomidate and halothane in attenuation of brain-free fatty acid liberation during complete global ischemia. Critical Care Medicine 9:184

17

Infusion anaesthesia

An increasing awareness of the danger of chronic exposure to low concentrations of gaseous or volatile anaesthetic agents and their adverse effects on health has been the main stimulus for the development of total intravenous anaesthesia. This is coupled with the fact that in certain operations, for example neurosurgical procedures, the volatile and gaseous anaesthetics do not provide the best or safest operating conditions. Another possible reason for this interest is that, on theoretical grounds, the apparatus used for total intravenous anaesthesia should be much simpler and also much less expensive than that used for inhalation agents as one could possibly dispose of bulky cylinders or pipe line gases.

If high frequency jet ventilation achieves wide acceptance this would provide another field for the use of total intravenous anaesthesia. Nitrous oxide or volatile agents cannot be used with this technique, partly because of the high volume discharged into the atmosphere and the high drug usage and also because currently available machines are calibrated for air and oxygen.

At the time of writing most anaesthetists will consider total intravenous anaesthesia as the avoidance of volatile supplements although many will still use nitrous oxide-oxygen as the carrier gas. The technique does not necessitate continuous infusion as most people will give the drugs by intermittent administration. There have, however, been developments in shorter-acting opioids (Ch. 13) and drugs like alfentanil can only be used for long procedures if given by infusion. In North America, but not in Britain, infusions of suxamethonium are commonly used, though in practice many anaesthetists would use intermittent doses of longer-acting drugs and even start with a long-acting drug and finish with a short-acting one if necessary.

For most anaesthetists total intravenous anaesthesia implies the intermittent injection of either the drug used for induction, or of a potent analgesic, combined with a longer-acting myoneural blocking agent. This has the advantage over an infusion in that one can be more aware of the condition of the patient and of changes in the 'depth of anaesthesia', although this might be difficult with total paralysis. It does, however, require constant attention and might result in uneven anaesthesia. In practice it is very valuable for short operations lasting 10–15 min but for longer procedures one is more likely to use a single dose of an induction agent and supplement this with opioids, usually given by intermittent injection, although they can be administered by infusion. This form of balanced technique is described more fully in Chapter 13. In this section emphasis is placed on the intermittent or continuous use of induction agents rather than opioids.

DRUGS

For infusion anaesthesia the drug used should ideally be soluble in water so that the toxicity of the solvent can be ignored and should be capable of being given in a concentrated solution if one wishes to avoid excess fluid load to the patient. The solution should be stable for the duration of the infusion and stability should also include absence of deterioration on exposure to light. There should be no absorption into plastic so that amounts of the active drug do not vary over the infusion period (Morgan, 1983). With the use of large veins and plastic cannulae, venous damage is not a major problem with dilute solutions but the drug should not be irritant if injected extravascularly.

Since one might wish to make moment-to-moment variations in delivered concentrations the ideal drug should induce sleep in one arm-brain circulation time. By virtue of the fields in which this technique is likely to be used it would be important not to have a drug where there is prolonged action due to accumulation of metabolites. Intravenous anaesthetics all have some respiratory depressant effects but this is usually less marked than with equivalent doses of volatile agents (Sear, 1983). The cardiovascular effects of the drugs might be a problem with prolonged use where the direct myocardial depressant action can become evident. However, there is a sufficiently large range of drugs available to minimise this problem, particularly as the new short-acting opioids produce very little hypotension.

Thiopentone

Thiopentone can be used as sole anaesthetic but its cumulative properties make it unsuitable for prolonged use as delayed recovery can occur. It has also a marked cardiovascular depressant effect in high doses.

Methohexitone

Methohexitone has a more rapid recovery than thiopentone and its pattern of distribution in the body favours its use by infusion (Table 6.3). The fact that the early recovery from this drug, like thiopentone, is mainly due to redistribution does mean that with prolonged use one can get cumulative effects and this should be borne in mind when it is infused. Its intermittent use is very popular for minor procedures and it has also been used as a supplement to nitrous oxide. Experience has shown that the excitatory effects are a major problem with this drug in subjects who have not been premedicated with an opioid and this places severe limitations on its use.

Etomidate

Etomidate would seem to be an ideal drug for continuous infusion anaesthesia. Although there is a high incidence of involuntary muscle movement this is not as marked as with methohexitone. Its pharmacokinetic properties suggest that it is non-cumulative and causes minimal organ toxicity and minimal effects on the cardiovascular and respiratory systems. In its commercially available form (propylene glycol solvent) one has to limit the dosage because of the potential haemolytic effect of the latter. However, there is a preparation prepared specially for infusion.

At the time of writing the continuous use of etomidate is limited in some countries because of its depressant effect on adrenocortical function (Ch. 10). This situation might be resolved in time with the possibility of replacement therapy. Etomidate alone is not a good drug for non-paralysed patients and when used for a continuous infusion with spontaneous respiration it must be accompanied by an opioid.

Propofol

Propofol has only recently become available commercially and its use in this field has not been adequately explored. Its pharmacokinetic properties suggest that it might be very useful here and it does not cause the same degree of excitatory effects as methohexitone and etomidate. Like thiopentone it has a cardiovascular depressant effect in large doses and more information is needed before one can recommend its use for total intravenous anaesthesia.

Opioids

Opioids used as sole intravenous anaesthetic are discussed in detail elsewhere (Ch. 13). It would seem that of the available drugs sufentanil is the most likely to achieve long-term usage in this field.

Ketamine

Ketamine has a slower onset of action and its relatively prolonged duration coupled with a high incidence of adverse reactions during recovery would seem to make this agent unsuitable for continuous intravenous infusion. Nevertheless it is a very potent analgesic if compared with the drugs previously mentioned. A full understanding of its pharmacokinetics when used as an infusion (Idvall et al, 1979), however, shows that it can be given (Lilburn et al, 1978) in dilute solution and since propanidid and Althesin have been withdrawn from clinical use there might be a need to look at ketamine in more detail.

Midazolam

Despite its longer action than other intravenous drugs, midazolam is being investigated as a sedative for long-term use in the intensive care unit or other similar situations. It has proved safe and effective in controlling agitation in a small group of critically ill patients and it did not appear to inhibit adrenal steroidogenesis as did etomidate (Shapiro et al, 1985).

A fixed non-weight-related dose of 2 mg h^{-1} following an initial bolus of 2 mg has provided very good sedation for adults following open heart operations, but it requires a generous use of small intravenous doses of opioids (Carson et al, 1986). Plasma concentrations levelled off around 100 $\mu g\ ml^{-1}$ and although this is much lower than that suggested by others (Dirksen et al, 1986) it proved adequate. Even after 14 hours of infusions the elimination half life of midazolam was not unduly prolonged. However, one must be on the look-out for patients, possible 1:20, in whom midazolam will have a prolonged elimination half life and an exaggerated action (Ch. 12).

Individual response to drugs

Before discussing techniques it is important to stress that even apparently normal individuals vary greatly in their requirements of drugs. This is well known with induction doses but the importance of this variation still applying when intravenous drugs are used as sole agent for maintaining unconsciousness has not been adequately stressed.

The degree of variation is best illustrated by looking at dose requirements when intravenous drugs are given by intermittent injection to maintain an adequate depth of surgical anaesthesia in non-relaxed patients, with supplementary doses being given on any evidence of lightening of anaesthesia. While this has been studied with a number of drugs the most recent data were obtained with methohexitone (McMurray et al, 1982, 1986) and with propofol (Wright et al, 1984; Robinson 1985, Robinson & Dundee 1986). The cumulative dose requirements of methohexitone in 50 unpremedicated patients is shown in Figure 17.1, while Figure 17.2 shows the skew distribution of total doses of propofol at 40 min in 19 patients. Wright and his colleagues (1984) found a similar variation in dosage to those in Figure 17.2. At 45 min their range of cumulative doses of propofol in 50 patients was 2.7 to 11.2 mg kg^{-1}. This represents 60–200 $\mu g\ kg^{-1}\ min^{-1}$ with a mean value of 100 $\mu g\ kg^{-1}\ min^{-1}$ which was less than the median of 130 $\mu g\ kg^{-1}\ min^{-1}$. These patients also had nitrous oxide oxygen and one can imagine that the variations would have been greater had the propofol been given alone.

When one is relying on the intravenous anaesthetic to ensure that the patient is not aware of his surroundings, then the average or even the median dose would leave some patients at risk of awareness, yet to give the largest required dose would overdose many others. Herein lies the weakness of the concept of minimum infusion rate (q.v.). It also shows the need for a drug which can be given safely in doses well above the average requirements to ensure that anaesthesia is adequate in all patients. In practice, this variation in response to drugs is best dealt with by using a combination of an intravenous anaesthetic and an injectable opioid, or less satisfactorily by heavy opiate premedication.

TECHNIQUES

With total intravenous anaesthesia all the techniques used aim at acquiring a cerebral concentration which will render patients unaware of their surroundings and maintain this concentration until the end of the procedure. Clearly the target concentration will depend on the concomitant use of opioids or myoneural blocking drugs but one

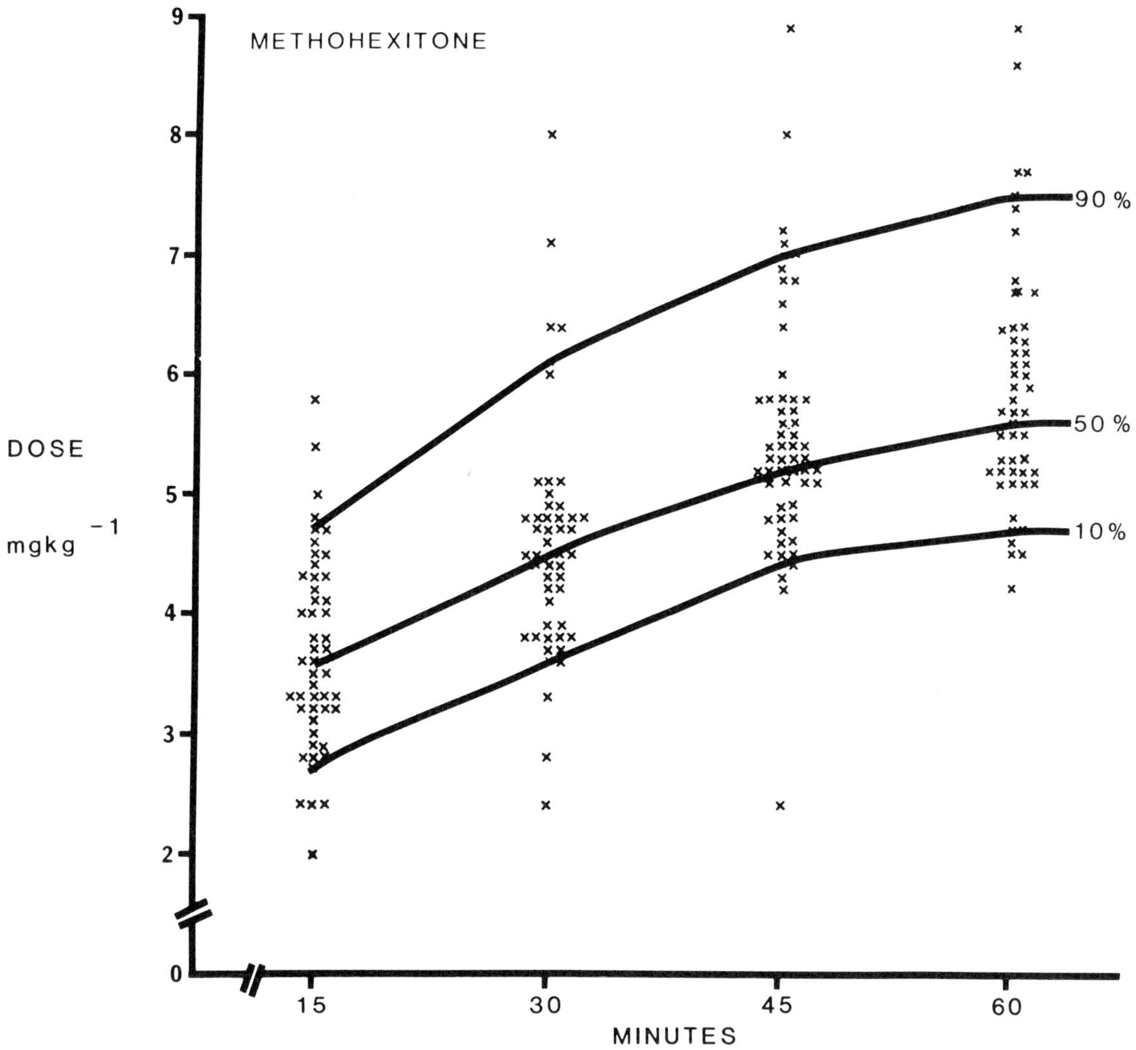

Fig. 17.1 Cumulative dose requirements of methohexitone in 50 unpremedicated patients as anaesthesia progressed (Dundee & McMurray, 1984; Wright et al, 1984)

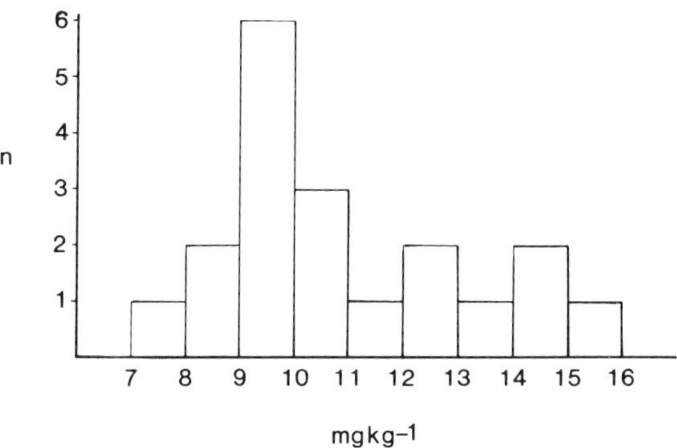

Fig. 17.2 Total dose requirements of propofol at 40 min in 19 unpremedicated fit patients to whom the drug was given as main hypnotic for body surface operations

would feel unhappy with their use unless there was a certainty that the administered concentration would retain unconsciousness. Fortunately with the drugs available today there is a fairly large margin between the dose required to produce anaesthesia and that which will result in patients being aware of their surroundings. In a relaxed patient one can produce satisfactory anaesthesia with a plasma concentration of the drug which, if given alone or with nitrous oxide, would be inadequate. Use of nitrous oxide as an analgesic has been mentioned already and with all the agents which are used there is evidence that this will markedly reduce the requirements. Savege et al (1975) have shown that supplementation by 67% nitrous oxide in oxygen will reduce the requirements of Althesin by 60%.

The application of any drug to infusion anaesthesia necessitates an understanding of its relevant pharmacokinetics (Ch. 4). This has also been discussed by Schwilden et al (1983) and by Sear (1983). A steady plasma concentration of a drug given by infusion will not be reached until it has been infused for 3–5 times its elimination half-life. This means that infusions alone are not satisfactory for induction of anaesthesia. One normally relies on the usual bolus induction dose but even if that is followed immediately by an infusion there will be a 'dip' in plasma concentration for some time and this makes the induction unsatisfactory. This lowering of concentration occurs at a time when the surgical stimulus is maximal and unless this is 'covered' by a large dose of an opioid some other method of achieving a heightened plasma concentration is needed. The ideal intravenous drug input (Kruger-Theimer, 1968) is a single loading dose in combination with an infusion the rate of which declines exponentially towards that required to maintain the desired plasma concentration. Wagner (1974) achieved this with multiple small bolus injections along with a constant rate infusion and by initially using a fast constant rate infusion and then decreasing this to a slower maintenance rate. More recently Schuttler et al (1983) have described computer-assisted total intravenous anaesthesia (CATIA) in which a programmed infusion pump delivered exponentially decreasing concentrations of the drug: they have used this satisfactorily with etomidate and alfentanil. The same end can also be achieved by a 'two-bottle' technique as described by Dundee & McMurray (1984) and McMurray et al (1984; 1985). This technique has been used for infusions of lignocaine by Riddell and his colleagues (1984): its application in anaesthesia was with methohexitone (McMurray et al, 1986) which however is not an ideal drug for this purpose.

The concept of minimum infusion rate (MIR) has been described by Sear & Prys-Roberts (1979), by Prys-Roberts (1980) and by Sear (1983). This is an attractive way of comparing the potency of different drugs but as a practical means of applying intravenous anaesthesia it has the disadvantage that one must use frequent opioid supplementation during the first half hour of anaesthesia.

The proposed concept of MIR is comparable to that of ED_{50}, i.e. the infusion rate of an intravenous anaesthetic which will prevent movement in response to surgical stimuli in 50% of patients. This allows comparison under conditions of equipotency of different intravenous anaesthetic infusion rates. There appears to be a 1:1 relationship between infusion rate and total drug plasma concentration up to twice the MIR (Hebron, 1983; Prys-Roberts et al, 1983). This does not apply to Althesin with which Sear & Prys-Roberts (1979) showed that by administering the drug in multiples of MIR up to 5 MIR there was only a doubling of the total plasma alphaxalone concentration.

From a practical point of view it is important to appreciate that premedication with morphine (0.15 mg kg^{-1}) reduces the ED_{50} of Althesin and methohexitone as compared with patients premedicated with 10 mg diazepam (Sear, 1983). Sear et al (1984a) have studied the influence of age on the MIR in a series of 210 patients. They found about one third reduction in dosage for the 55–80 age group as compared with younger subjects (20–40 yr).

ILLUSTRATIVE TECHNIQUES

Savege et al (1975) reported on their use of Althesin infusions in anaesthesia for routine operations, analgesia being provided by intravenous narcotics using neuromuscular blockade where appropriate. They found the technique to be difficult with a high (15%) incidence of unsatisfactory anaesthetics, and occasional prolonged recovery. Nevertheless, until its withdrawal Althesin proved to be the most popular drug for infusion anaesthesia. It has been used with jet ventilation (Rogers et al, 1985), for neurosurgery and in cases of brain damage (Bendsten et al, 1985; Dearden & McDowell, 1985), for sedation in the intensive care unit (Ramsay et al, 1974) and for operations on the trachea (Vyas et al, 1983).

As pointed out previously etomidate would appear at first glance to be a near-ideal agent for use by infusion — it is rapidly-acting with a high therapeutic index, gives good cardiovascular stability, the recovery phase is rapid due to metabolism by liver esterases and it is unlikely to release histamine.

However, despite these almost ideal pharmacokinetic properties, difficulties have been encountered by many workers in the practical application of the agent to infusions in patients. Kay (1977) used etomidate infusions in children and found, as did Savege, that it was a difficult technique with a 15% incidence of unsatisfactory anaesthetics. The initial infusion rate was 0.04–0.05 mg kg^{-1} min^{-1}, slowing as the operation progressed. It was impossible to prevent movement in response to skin incision without using a neuromuscular blocking drug and in the presence of these maintenance of unconsciousness became a cause for concern. When these workers (Kay and Rolly, 1977) used etomidate infusions in adults using a bolus injection of 0.3 mg kg^{-1} for induction and 0.03 mg kg^{-1} min^{-1} for maintenance of anaesthesia, they had to abandon the technique due to myoclonic movements and pain on injection (even with concomitant use of opioids). Sear et al (1984b) also found that these adverse effects were a major disadvantage in the use of etomidate infusions for neuroanaesthesia.

Lees and Antonios (1984) were able to overcome these problems to some extent by the use of a 2-stage infusion technique (similar to that of Wagner). Induction of anaesthesia was by a rapid infusion of etomidate at a rate of 100 μg kg^{-1} min^{-1} for 10 min, reducing it to 10 μg kg^{-1} min^{-1} for maintenance. This method gave good cardiovascular stability, with reduced pain on injection and muscle movement. They attribute these findings to either the administration of fentanyl before the start of the etomidate infusion, or because by giving the 'induction dose' as a rapid infusion (rather than as a bolus), there is effectively both a decreased rate of administration and a decreased concentration of drug.

It is interesting that in certain situations where total intravenous anaesthesia offers positive advantages over inhalational agents, workers tend to be more enthusiastic about it. Versichelen et al (1983) reported the use of etomidate infusion in a dose of 30 μg kg^{-1} min^{-1} following an induction dose of 300 μg kg^{-1} supplemented by alfentanil in small bolus doses as required for endolaryngeal microsurgery. They considered that this technique was ideal in that it allowed smooth awakening, with a rapid recovery of the cough reflex and a low incidence of nausea and vomiting, and also permitted ventilation of the patient's lungs with air when necessary to avoid the danger of fire during the use of the laser. Oduro et al (1983) also considered etomidate infusion a suitable technique for cardiopulmonary bypass in that it provided unconsciousness, was simple and easily controlled.

Two-bottle technique

The principle of this method (Riddell et al 1984) can be seen from Figure 17.3. Its application to anaesthesia has only been described with methohexitone (McMurray et al, 1986). The apparatus consists of a 250 ml bottle containing dilute methohexitone (0.76%) connected to a vented intravenous giving set, a peristaltic pump and a narrow bore needle to a 50 ml bottle containing a 1.8% solution. The induction dose of 180 mg is divided into a bolus of half this amount given over 20 s and the remainder over the next 2–3 min. These concentrations while calculated for a 70 kg subject in practice are suitable for most patients. A target plasma concentration of 10 mg ml^{-1} is achieved within 10 min but there might be a slight tendency for cumulation after 45–60 min.

Methohexitone, although pharmacokinetically suitable for this technique, is not the ideal drug to use in the absence of opioid premedication or supplementation. However this technique could clearly be used to advantage for an opioid and perhaps for infusion of an opioid and hypnotic. It could also be used with a myoneural blocking drug where one could guarantee that whatever happened the patients would not regain consciousness during the operation.

The principles employed with the adjuvants are similar to those described above and the technique has the advantage of using inexpensive apparatus and being independent of a power supply. It does, however, require a drug which is soluble in water

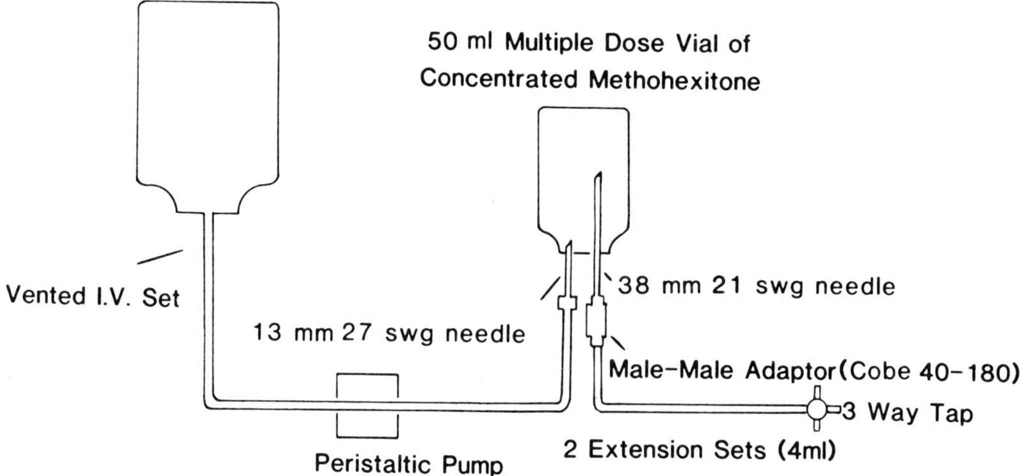

Fig. 17.3 Schematic representation of the 'two bottle' method of delivery of solution of exponentially decreasing concentration of methohexitone (McMurray et al, 1986).

over a wide range of concentrations and it cannot be used with chemically unstable emulsions.

Computer assisted total intravenous anaesthesia (CATIA)

Computer assisted total intravenous anaesthesia, in which the delivered dose is regulated by a microprocessor controlled infusion system which is able to generate arbitrary drug concentrations or amounts of the drug in the central or peripheral compartment using pharmacokinetic data, has been described by Schuttler et al (1983). They used etomidate as the hypnotic and alfentanil as the narcotic. The infusion scheme (BET) is made up of three factors: a bolus (B) to fill the central volume of distribution, the maintenance infusion rate which compensates for elimination (E) and the exponentially decreasing infusion rate compensating for transfer into the peripheral compartment until saturation (T). The infusion pumps required must be capable of being controlled independently and manually: since one cannot exclude inter-individual variations of kinetic data there must be means of giving supplementary doses of narcotics.

This question of interindividual variations of kinetic data is one which cannot be avoided with any of these techniques and both this one and the 'two-bottle' technique are based on average plasma concentration requirements. With experience it might be possible to scale down or increase dosage in patients with different degrees of fitness.

Constant infusion

Kay (1984) described a technique based on etomidate and alfentanil in which, following an induction dose of 0.2 mg kg^{-1} etomidate and 0.8 mg kg^{-1} alfentanil, the infusion rate was not changed. Such a technique is only applicable when one is using drugs such as etomidate and alfentanil where exceeding the therapeutic range will have minimal effects on the cardiovascular system. With this technique it is also advisable to have some method of monitoring the depth of anaesthesia. Although there was no awareness during operation this technique was marred by postoperative nausea and vomiting and by the unacceptably high incidence of postoperative twitching.

At the time of writing the future of infusion anaesthesia is uncertain. Clearly the advent of isoflurane and alfentanil together with the shorter acting neuromuscular blocking drugs (atracurium and vecuronium) has maintained the interest in inhalational techniques and the introduction of effective scavenging methods has reduced the risk of atmospheric pollution. Withdrawal of Althesin and etomidate for use in this field has left a gap which might eventually be filled with propofol, but as yet it is not available for use as an infusion. An increasing use of parenteral opioids (Ch. 13) has improved the situation and reduced the need for large doses of conventional agents, and eventually techniques might evolve with a major analgesic component and a lesser part played by conventional intravenous anaesthesia.

REFERENCES

Bendsten A, Kruse A, Madsen J B, Astrup J, Rosenorn J, Blatt-Lyon B, Cold G E 1985 Use of a continuous infusion of Althesin in neuroanaesthesia. British Journal of Anaesthesia 57: 369–374

Carson I W, Collier P S, Dundee J W, Howard P J, Lyons S M, Mathews H M L, Orr I A 1986 Pharmacokinetics of midazolam sedation following open heart surgery. British Journal of Pharmacology 89:474P

Dearden N M, McDowall D G 1985 Comparison of etomidate and Althesin in the reduction of increased intracranial pressure after head injury. British Journal of Anaesthesia 57: 361–368

Dirksen M S C, Vree T B, Driessen J J 1986 Clinical pharmacokinetics of long-term infusion of midazolam in critically ill patients — preliminary results. Workshop on Midazolam and Ro 15–1788 in ICU, Basle, 30 January 1986. Editiones (Roche), Basle.

Dundee J W, McMurray T J 1984 Clinical aspects of total intravenous anaesthesia: discussion paper. Journal of the Royal Society of Medicine 77: 669–672

Hebron B S 1983 Plasma concentrations of etomidate during intravenous infusion over 48 hours. Anaesthesia 38: 39–43

Idvall J, Ahlgren I, Aronsen K F, Stenberg P 1979 Ketamine infusions: pharmacokinetics and clinical effects. British Journal of Anaesthesia 51: 1167–1172

Kay B 1977 Total intravenous anesthesia with etomidate. 1. A Trial in children. Acta Anaesthesiologica Belgica 28: 107–113

Kay B 1984 Etomidate and alfentanil infusion for major surgery. Acta Anaesthesiologica Belgica 35: 19–24

Kay B, Rolly G 1977 Total intravenous anesthesia with etomidate III: Some observations in adults. Acta Anaesthesiologica Belgica 28: 157–164

Kruger-Theimer E 1968 Continuous intravenous infusion and multi-compartment accumulation. European Journal of Pharmacology 4:317

Lees N W, Antonios W R A 1984 Two stage infusion of etomidate for the induction and maintenance of anaesthesia. British Journal of Anaesthesia 56: 1239–1241

Lilburn J K, Dundee J W, Moore J 1978 Ketamine infusions: observations on technique, dosage and cardiovascular effects. Anaesthesia 33: 315–321

McMurray T J, Wright P J, Dundee J W, Clarke R S J, Greenfield A A 1982 Problems in determining the dosage of continuous intravenous infusion anesthetics. British Journal of Intravenous Therapy 3:34

McMurray T J, Riddell J G, Dundee J W, McAllister C B 1984 A new simple method for rapidly achieving and maintaining constant methohexitone concentrations. British Journal of Anaesthesia 56: 429P–430

McMurray T J, Robinson F P, Dundee J W, Riddell J G, McClean E 1986 A new method for producing constant plasma drug levels: application to methohexitone. British Journal of Anaesthesia 57: 1085–1090

Morgan M 1983 Total intravenous anaesthesia. Anaesthesia 38: 1–9

Oduro A, Tomlinson A A, Voice A, Davies G K 1983 The use of etomidate infusions during anaesthesia for cardiopulmonary bypass. Anaesthesia 38: 66–69

Prys-Roberts C 1980 Practical and pharmacological implications of continuous intravenous anesthesia. Acta Anaesthesiologica Belgica 31: 225–230

Prys-Roberts C, Davis J R, Calverley R K, Goodwin N W 1983 Haemodynamic effects of infusion of di-isopropyl phenol (ICI 35 868) during nitrous oxide anaesthesia. British Journal of Anaesthesia 55: 105–111

Ramsay M A E, Savege T M, Simpson B R J, Goodwin R 1974 Controlled sedation with alphaxalone-alphadolone. British Medical Journal 2: 656–659

Riddell J G, McAllister C B, Wilkinson G R, Wood A J J, Roden D M 1984 A new method for constant plasma drug concentrations: application to lidocaine. Annals of Internal Medicine 199:25

Robinson F P 1985 Propofol ('Diprivan') by intermittent bolus with nitrous oxide in oxygen for body surface operations. Postgraduate Medical Journal 61: 116–119

Robinson F P, Dundee J W 1986 Dose requirements of propofol as main agent for body surface surgery. British Journal of Clinical Pharmacology 21:612P

Rogers R C, Gibbons J, Cosgrove J, Coppel D C 1985 High-frequency jet ventilation for tracheal surgery. Anaesthesia 40: 32–36

Savege T M, Ramsay M A E, Curran J P J, Cotter J, Walling P T, Simpson B R 1975 Intravenous anaesthesia by infusion: a technique using alphaxalone/alphadolone (Althesin). Anaesthesia 30: 757–764

Schuttler J, Schwilden H, Stoekele H 1983 Pharmacokinetics as applied to total intravenous anaesthesia: practical implications. Anaesthesia 38: 53–56

Schwilden H, Schuttler J, Stoekele H 1983 Pharmacokinetics as applied to total intravenous anaesthesia: theoretical considerations. Anaesthesia 38: 51–52

Sear J W 1983 General kinetic and dynamic principles and their application to continuous infusion anaesthesia. Anaesthesia 38: 10–25

Sear J W, Prys-Roberts C 1979 Plasma concentrations of alphaxalone during continuous infusions of Althesin. British Journal of Anaesthesia 51: 861–865

Sear J, Prys-Roberts C, Phillips K C 1984a Age influences the minimal infusion rate (ED_{50}) for continuous infusion of Althesin and methohexitone. European Journal of Anaesthesiology 1: 319–325

Sear J W, Walters F J M, Wilkins D G, Willatts S M 1984b

Etomidate by infusion for neuroanaesthesia kinetic and dynamic interactions with nitrous oxide. Anaesthesia 39: 12–18

Shapiro J M, White P F, Sladen R N, Westphal L M, Rosenthal M H 1985 Midazolam infusion in critically ill patients: effect on adrenal function. Anesthesiology 63:A149

Versichelen I, Rolly G, Beerens J 1983 Alfentanil/etomidate anaesthesia for endolaryngeal microsurgery. Anaesthesia 83: 57–60

Vyas A B, Lyons S M, Dundee J W 1983 Continuous intravenous anaesthesia with Althesin for resection of tracheal stenosis. Anaesthesia 38: 132–135

Wagner J G 1974 A safe method for rapidly achieving plasma concentration plateaus. Clinical Pharmacology and Therapeutics 16: 691–700

Wright P J, Clarke R S J, Dundee J W, Briggs L P, Greenfield A A 1984 Infusion rates for anaesthesia with propofol. British Journal of Anaesthesia 56: 613–616

Drugs of historical interest

THE VOLATILE INHALATION ANAESTHETICS

In the early years of this century the first attempts were made by Burkhardt (1909) to administer inhalation anaesthetics by the intravenous route. After first using **chloroform**, which proved unsatisfactory, he turned to diethyl ether. The use of the intravenous route was considered to be of advantage, in that it circumvented the slow induction by the inhalation of **diethyl ether**, which was so often a stormy and thoroughly unpleasant affair. Elimination of the agents via the respiratory tract was believed to provide a certain measure of controllability and safety, especially in view of the fact that it was thought that inhalation agents were not metabolised within the body.

Diethyl ether was administered as a 5 per cent solution, warmed to 29.3°C (85°F) and shaken until all ether was completely dissolved. Subsequent administration was by intravenous drip infusion. Induction, as a rule, was complete within one to five minutes, was smooth and usually devoid of excitement and struggling. As anaesthesia became established the rate of infusion was slowed. Emphasis was placed on not exceeding the 5 per cent concentration lest haemoglobinuria be produced. The occurrence of phlebitis at the site of infusion was a definite disadvantage.

This type of anaesthesia played some limited role for a time, but with the more common use of tracheal intubation and the advent of more refined methods of inducing anaesthesia, intravenous diethyl ether fell into disuse.

In 1961 Krantz and associates revived the intravenous administration of a volatile anaesthetic by investigating the feasability of intravenous **methoxyflurane** as an emulsion. They based their investigations on the theoretical consideration that a potent anaesthetic with a low vapour pressure would require only relatively small amounts to achieve anaesthesia by the intravenous route since it can exert its powerful effect without being easily eliminated by the lungs (Krantz et al, 1962). Despite their early optimistic reports they finally had to concede that the high incidence of severe phlebitis made this route of administration of methoxyflurane impractical. They did show clearly that the venous reaction depended upon the concentration of methoxyfluence and was not caused by the emulsion itself or any of its constituents (Cascorbi et al, 1968).

The intravenous injection of **halothane** in dogs is followed by acute pulmonary damage including severe haemorrhage and oedema (Sandison et al., 1970). The manifestations are of such severity as to preclude further investigation of its use. However, Sutton et al (1971) have described the accidental intravenous injection of halothane in a 16-year-old girl. The dose given was such as to result in peak blood levels several times higher than would be achieved during clinical anaesthesia. As in animals, severe pulmonary oedema and right heart failure occurred and hypoxaemia was very marked with transient mild changes in hepatic, renal and haemopoietic function. The administration of positive-pressure oxygen therapy via a tracheal tube saved the patient's life, but only after six days of very intensive treatment.

Burkhardt L 1909 Die intravenose Narkose mit Aether and Chloroform. Münchener medizinische Wochenschrift 2:2365

Cascorbi H F, Helrich M, Krantz J C, Baker L R, Rozman

R S, Rudo F G 1968 Hazards of methoxyflurance emulsions in man. Anesthesia and Analgesia, Current Researches 47: 557–559

Krantz J C Jr, Cascorbi H F, Helrich M, Burgison R M, Gold M I, Rudo F G 1961 A note on the intravenous use of anesthetic emulsions in animals and man with special reference to methoxyflurance. Anesthesiology 22: 491–492

Krantz J C Jr, Cascorbi M F, Rudo F G 1962 Anesthesia. LXIV: The intravenous administration of methoxyflurane (Penthrane) emulsions in animals and man. Anesthesia and Analgesia, Current Researches 41: 257–262

Sandison J W, Sivapragasam S, Hayes J E, Woon-Ming M O 1970 An experimental study of pulmonary damage associated with intravenous injection of halothane in dogs. British Journal of Anaesthesia 42: 419–424

Sutton J, Harrison G A, Hickey J B 1971 Accidental intravenous injection of halothane: case report. British Journal of Anaesthesia 43: 513–520

BROMETHOL

Bromethol (Avertin) contains 66.7 per cent (w/w) of tribromethyl alcohol ($CHBr_3CH_3OH$) dissolved in amylene hydrate; 1 ml solution contains 1 g of tribromethyl alcohol. It should be kept in a dry, well-closed container, protected from light as it is rapidly decomposed by moisture (British Pharmacopoeia. 1953). Tribromethanol itself is a white crystalline substance, soluble in water up to 3.5 per cent. This agent was primary introduced as a basal narcotic to be administered by the rectal route, but in 1929 and 1930 Kirschner reported the intravenous administration of bromethol. Macintosh and Pask reported the use of a 1 per cent solution at Oxford in 1941 and in 1945 Thornton and Rowbotham described its use in a military maxillofacial surgical unit.

Tribromethanol is detoxicated in the liver by conjugation with glycuronic acid and is then excreted in the urine. Bromethol fluid 4 to 5 ml is added to 150 ml of 5 per cent dextrose solution. The resultant 3 per cent solution is tested with Congo red to guard against formation of toxic disintegration products. On the average a normal dose is 1 ml kg^{-1} of the 3 per cent solution.

The calculated dose is administered over a period of 30 to 45 seconds. Induction is usually complete within one and half to two minutes and as soon as the a patient is asleep the administration is discontinued, regardless of whether or not all the calculated predetermined dose has been administered. If, on the other hand, anaesthesia has not resulted from the calculated dose, an additional amount may be administered, but a total of 1.5 ml kg^{-1} should not be exceeded. By and large, systemic effects from intravenous bromethol are rare, but the incidence of venous thrombosis is high and haematuria has occurred.

In 1953 Dwyer, Strout and Thomas re-evaluated intravenous bromethol in a series of patients, but considered the incidence of superficial phlebitis unacceptable and concluded that intravenous tribromethanol in amylene hydrate was unsuitable as an intravenous analgesic or basal anaesthetic.

Dwyer C S, Strout W G, Thomas P B 1953 Intravenous Avertin Anesthesia. Anesthesiology 14: 291–298

Kirschener M 1929 Eine psychenschonende and steuerbare Form der Allgemein-betauburg. Chirurg 1:672

Kirschner M 1930 Erfahrungen mit der intravenosen Avertinnarkose. Langenbecks Archiv für klinische Chirurgie 162:361

Macintosh R R, Pask E A 1941 Improved apparatus for continuous intravenous anaesthesia. Lancet ii:10

Thornton H L, Rowbotham E S 1945 Anesthesia in a mixillo-facial surgical unit with the British Liberation Army. Anesthesiology 6: 580–596

DOLITRONE

Dolitrone was first reported by Thompson and associates in 1954, under the code MRB-125. Chemically it is in a class on its own, being 5-ethyl-6-phenyl-m-thiazane-2, 4-dione.

It is a white crystalline powder with a melting point of 159°C. The sodium salt is soluble in water and the 2.5 per cent solution has a pH of 11.5 to 12.

The original work by Thompson in animals showed that respiration was not seriously depressed by this drug, but that laryngeal reflexes were markedly diminished. Abdominal relaxation was good and the margin of safety was shown to be greater than with the barbiturates. The ratio of LD_{50} to minimal hypnotic dose in rabbits was 16 as compared with 5 for sodium thiopentone. Again, in contradistinction to the barbiturates, there appeared to be no cumulative effect with repeated doses and recovery from the effects of the drug was rapid. Duration of hypnosis with a single 60 per cent LD_{50} dose was 53 minutes as compared with 20 minutes for sodium thiopentone. The acute LD_{50} for Dolitrone was approximately three times that of sodium thiopentone, while minimal hypnotic doses were similar for both agents. In dogs, the blood pressure was not appreciably altered with repeated, rapid intravenous injection until the stage of respiratory arrest was reached.

Seldon (1940) remarked that the capillaries in the rabbit ear as seen through a Clarke window were smaller with Dolitrone than with diethyl ether, cyclopropane, ethylene or thiopentone, and somewhat resembled the state seen under nitrous oxide-oxygen anaesthesia. Cotten and Bay (1956) found that in dogs Dolitrone had only a limited effect on blood pressure, force of ventricular contraction and on the electrocardiogram, but produced marked tachycardia, and concluded that in all these effects it behaved similar to thiopentone. On the other hand, after Dolitrone adrenaline-induced arrhythmias were fewer than after thiopentone. In contradistinction to Thompson et al, they found that with equivalent anaesthetic doses the duration of anaesthesia was approximately identical for both drugs. After pre-treatment with morphine, Dolitrone was well tolerated whereas sodium thiopentone frequently produced fatal respiratory arrest under identical experimental conditions. Twenty per cent of the dogs studied by Cotten and Bay showed intense excitement during emergence from anaesthesia.

Lundy (1954a, b, 1955a, b, c, d) was much impressed by the general analgesic properties of this new drug. Wyant et al. (1956), in comparing the agent with sodium thiopentone in man, found that Dolitrone had marked respiration sparing properties and caused practically no apnoea in double the sleep dose; neither was there any significance hypotension. Muscle relaxation for procedures such as pelvic examination was often satisfactory but unpredictable, and they corroborated Lundy's observation that the agent had definite analgesic properties, although this was subjectively less pleasant than that induced with either nitrous oxide, trichloroethylene or intravenous procaine. No amnesia could be demonstrated. Spontaneous and often uncontrollable movements made the agent unsuitable for maintenance of anaesthesia even when large doses were used. However, the major and insuperable disadvantage of the drug which eventually led to its abandonment was the high incidence of phlebitis, ranging from mild to very severe, and which occurred whenever more than a single injection was given.

The agent is of historical interest only, but being the first tentative venture into intravenous analgesia for surgical procedures by an agent specifically designed for the purpose, it deserves a place in the history of the development of general intravenous analgesia.

Cotten M De V, Bay E 1956 Comparison of the cardiovascular properties of a new non-barbiturate intravenous anesthetic agent with those of thiopental. Anesthesiology 17: 103–111

Lundy J S 1954a Will there be an era of analgesia? (Editorial.) Journal Lancet 74:155

Lundy J S 1954b Hope for an age of analgesia. Journal of the American Association of Nurse Anesthesiologists 22:225

Lundy J S 1955a Development of analgesia after a century of anesthesia. Journal of the American Medical Association 157:1399

Lundy J S 1955b Pediatric anesthesia. Journal of the American Association of Nurse Anesthesiologists 23:79

Lundy J S 1955c Progress in analgesia: a new note on an old theme. Texas State Journal of Medicine 51:301

Lundy J S 1955d Recent progress in the conquest of pain. Journal Lancet 75:320

Seldon T H 1940 The effect of general anaesthetic agents on small blood vessels. Thesis, University of Minnesota Graduate School

Thompson C R, Smith J D, Werner H W 1954 Pharmacology of 5-ethy-6-phenyl-m-thiazane-2, 4-dione, Federation Proceedings 13:411

Wyant G M, Kilduff C J, Merriman J E, Dobkin A B 1956 Evaluation of Dolitrone. Canadian Anaesthetists' Society Journal 3:291

METHAQUALONE

This non-barbiturate hypnotic is widely used in its oral form and Saxena *et al.* (1972) have given it intravenously to 40 patients. Because of low water solubility a 10 per cent solution in propylene glycol was used, which was slightly viscous, requiring a large bore needle for injection. Rapid loss of conciouness followed intravenous injection of adequate doses, but transient generalised muscle spasm followed the onset of sleep, after which there was muscle relaxation. Methaqualone appears to be fairly non-toxic in doses of 20 mg kg^{-1} and the authors of the only clincial report suggest that its use as an induction agent and as a muscle relaxant during laparotomy should be explored further.

Saxena R C, Bhatnagar N, Misra S C, Bhargave K P 1972 Intravenous methaqualone: a new non-barbiturate anaesthesia British Journal of Anaesthesia 44: 83–85

BARBITURATES

It is difficult to ascertain whether all of the drugs in Figure 5.2 are still in clinical use. Although no longer available in the developed countries, one of the authors recently encountered some clinical use of hexobarbitone in Central Africa. This drug is discussed briefly in Chapter 8. Thialbarbitone, although no longer manufactured was, until recently, in use in South America. It is almost half as potent as thiopentone and when the 10% solution was used clinically there were some solubility problems and its distinctive sulphur-like odour was very persistent on one's hands and clothes. Otherwise its action is similar to thiopentone.

Methitural

By introducing a methyl-thioethyl group in the side chain of mehitural it was hoped to accelerate breakdown and at the same time liberate methionine which would protect the liver from its toxic effects (Zima et al, 1954). Early clinical reports (Boone et al, 1956; Fitzpatrick et al, 1956) supported this view which, however, has not stood up to careful clinical examination. There is less variation in recovery time with methitural than with equipotent doses of thiopentone (O'Herlihy et al, 1956; Gale, 1957) but in view of the high incidence of excitatory and respiratory side effects with methitural this is of more academic than practical importance.

Thiohexital

(dl-5-(l-methyl-2-pentynyl)-5-allyl-2-thiobarbiturate) is chemically very similar to methohexitone, being its thioderivative, but without the methyl side chain. It is more highly bound (88 to 90%) to plasma proteins than either thiopentone or methohexitone and its location in fat is intermediate between thiopentone and methohexitone. This drug, which is the most rapidly metabolised intravenous barbiturate, has not been used extensively in man, but the impression was gained (Mark et al, 1968) that subjects receiving it awakened more promptly and were more alert than those receiving comparable doses of methohexitone. Although it is not used, thiohexital was an interesting compound because of its rapid metabolism, but not even this drug could be classed as 'ultra-short acting'.

Isopropylallyl-methylbarbiturate (Narconumal)

This was once popular in Continental Europe (Thalheimer, 1937). This is a methylated oxybarbiturate which, in clinical doses causes a high incidence of excitatory effects, particularly in unpremedicated patients (Barron, 1962). A number of workers have noted hypotension as an additional induction complication (Johnston, 1950; Jorgensen, 1953). This drug could not compete with other induction agents.

Methyl thiobarbiturates

The methylated forms of thiopentone and buthalitone have also been studied. In dogs, recovery from the former was more rapid than from thiopentone (Papper et al, 1955), while in man the latter was followed by an unacceptably high incidence of excitatory phenomena (Barron & Dundee, 1961b).

Spirobarbiturates and spirothiobarbiturates

These have also been investigated for their potential use as general anaesthetics (Swanson et al, 1950; Volpitto, 1951), but the lack of subsequent data suggests that these must have proved unsatisfactory for use in man.

Another group of compounds, bearing the letters JL, have been studied by continental workers (Kopp & Tchoubar, 1951; Buchel & Levy, 1951; Buchel et al, 1953). These have one very long side chain of five to eight carbon atoms. While it is claimed that recovery from these is extremely rapid, again a lack of subsequent clinical data shows that they have not proved satisfactory for continued use.

For details of other barbiturates the reader is referred to the reviews of Adams (1944), Richards & Taylor (1956), Barron & Dundee (1961a), Dundee & Barron (1962) and Mark (1963), and the original paper on sulphur-containing barbiturate hypnotics by Tabern & Volwiler (1935).

REFERENCES

Adams R C 1944 Intravenous anesthesia, lst edn. Hoeber, New York and London.

Barron D W 1962 Clinical studies of Induction Agents II: A comparison of the incidence of induction complications with two methylated oxybarbiturates, Narconumal and Narcodorm. British Journal of Anaesthesia 34: 391–394

Barron D W, Dundee J W 1961a The recently introduced rapidly acting barbiturates: a review and critical appraisal in relation to thiopentone. British Journal of Anaesthesia 33: 81–91

Barron D W, Dundee J W 1961b Further experiences with methylated thiobarbiturates. British Journal of Anaesthesia 33: 130–131

Boone J D, Rafael M, Dillon J B 1956 Nerval Sodium: a new ultra-short acting thiobarbiturate: preliminary clinical investigations. Anesthesiology 17: 284–287

Buchel L, Levy J 1951 Sur deux nouvelle substances de la serie des barbituriques et thiobarbituriques. Anesthesie et analgesie (Paris) 8: 433–437

Buchel L, Levy J, Tchoubar B 1953 Rapport entre la constitution et l'action dans la serie des barbituriques et des thiobarbituriques porteurs de raidcaux alcoyles ramifies en alpha. Anesthesie et analgesie (Paris) 10: 343–350

Dundee J W, Barron D W 1962 The Barbiturates. British Journal of Anaesthesia 34: 240–246

Fitzpatrick L J, Clarie, D'A C, Mersch M M 1956 Methitural sodium: new ultra-short acting intravenous anesthesia. Anesthesiology 17: 684–689

Gale A S 1957 Recovery from thiopental and methitural nitrous oxide anesthesia for a standard short procedure. Anesthesiology 81: 573–582

Johnson A S R 1950 Cardiovascular changes during various types of anaesthesia. Proceedings of lst Congress of Scandinavian Society of Anaesthetists 49

Jorgensen G 1953 Experimental investigations of the venous pressure with special reference to the regulation of the circulation. MD Thesis, University of Copenhagen

Kopp M, Tchoubar B 1951 1: Sur une methode avantageuse d'obtension des malonylurees et malonylthiourees a radicaux alcoyles ramifies. Bulletin de la Societe Chimique de France 18: 30–31

Mark L C 1963 Thiobarbiturates. In: Papper E M, Kitz R J (eds) Uptake and distribution of anesthetic agents. McGraw-Hill, New York, ch 23

Mark L C, Perel J M, Brand L, Dayton P G 1968 Studies with thiohexital, an anesthetic barbiturate metabolised with unusual rapidity in man. Anesthesiology 29: 1159–1166

O'Herlihy D B, Nishimura N, Little D Jr, Tovell R M 1956 The clinical use of Neraval. Canadian Anaesthetists' Society Journal 3: 326–334

Papper E M, Peterson R C, Burns J J, Bernstein E, Lief P, Brodie B B 1955 Physiological disposition of certain n-alkyl thiobarbiturates. Anesthesiology 16: 544–550

Richards R K, Taylor J D 1956 Some factors influencing distribution, metabolism and action of barbiturates: a review. Anesthesiology 17: 414–458

Swanson E E, Mueller L B, Henderson F G, Chen K K 1950 Pharmacology of spiro-barbituric and spiro-thiobarbituric acids. Current Researches in Anesthesia 29: 89–96

Tabern D L, Volwiler E H 1935 N-alkyl and N-aryl substituted barbituric acid. Journal of the American Chemical Society 57:1961 and 58:1354

Thalheimer M 1937 Anesthesia by intravenous injection of l-methyl-5,5-allyl-Isopropyl barbituric acid. Anesthesia and Analgesia, Current Researches 16: 61–65

Volpitto P V 1951 Experiences with ultra-short acting intravenous barbiturates combined with decamethonium bromide for endotracheal intubation. Anesthesiology 12: 648–655

Zima O, von Werder F, Hotovy R 1954 Methylthioathyl l pentyl thiobarbitursaures natrium (Thiogenal) ein neues Kurznarcoticum. Anaesthesist 3: 244–245

ALCOHOL

Alcohol has been known since the earliest days of recorded history and there is a graphic description of its soporific action in the Old Testament (Genesis 9:21). Along with crude opium, cannabis indica and mandragora, alcohol was one of the preparations which was taken by mouth by the ancients to relieve the pain of operations, but there are no authentic reports of its efficacy, whether given alone or with other ingredients. Keys (1945) alludes to the use of alcohol for anaesthetic purposes during subsequent centuries and at about the time of Christopher Wren's experiments with the injection of opium, Lausitz inebriated dogs by the intravenous administration of wine.

Alcohol does not appear, however, to have been used systemically in humans until Behan (1920) used it as a postoperative sedative and in the following year Nakagawa explored the possibility of inducing surgical anaesthesia by intravenous alcohol combined with chloroform or diethyl ether. Sporadic reports thereafter appeared in the literature (Constatin, 1929; 1930; Fohl, 1931), but it was not until 1945 that a preliminary study by

Moore & Karp reported an analysis of 150 patients given 5 to 10% alcohol in the operative or postoperative period; later Karp & Sokol (1951) recorded their experiences on about 2000 patients. In 1965 Schnelle reported another series of patients in which 5% alcohol had been used either as a basal narcotic or as an induction agent and analgesic during anaesthesia. He found the combination of alcohol, thiopentone and nitrous oxide unsatisfactory, although it was well-tolerated in debilitated poor-risk patients. The only major controlled study of alcohol as an induction agent (500 patients) was reported by Dundee et al (1969). To this study we owe most of the clinical pharmacology known about this agent although it indicated that alcohol is unsuitable as a routine induction agent. However, 0.8 to 1.0 g kg^{-1} alcohol infused over 4 to 6 min will provide rapid induction of anaesthesia without obvious delay in the onset of the hypnotic effect, 8% w/v (equivalent to 10% v/v) being the most suitable for routine clinical use. Delirium was often encountered immediately upon loss of consciousness and was the most severe disadvantage of this method. Intravenous alcohol causes remarkably little effect on the cardiovascular system, but it is a respiratory depressant and can cause a fall in arterial oxygen tension (Dundee et al, 1972).

The incidence of emergence delirium after alcohol was high, particularly in the absence of depressant premedication. Its incidence can be reduced by heavy premedication and the simultaneous administration of diazepam. Few patients have any memory of this recovery delirium. Hangover is a frequent occurrence, being manifested by headache, a flushed feeling, dizziness, thirst, vomiting and nausea, all being related to the amount of alcohol used. They too can be reduced but not abolished by appropriate premedication. These clinical studies have been reviewed in full in the first edition of this book (ch. 13).

Although it is difficult to see any use for alcohol as an induction agent, it has useful analgesic properties and dilute solutions can be used as adjunct to general anaesthesia or in the immediate postoperative period. Its most useful application is in alcoholic patients as it will prevent withdrawal symptoms in these individuals. Hewer (1964) has used intravenous alcohol extensively in hypothermia to facilitate skin cooling and suggests that it reduces the incidence of cardiac arrhythmias but this is not standard practice.

As far as the effect on the body is concerned, the infusion of ethanol is accompanied by a rise in plasma catecholamines. In the absence of hypoxia no deleterious effect on liver function has been demonstrated following doses of 25 to 44 g given for induction of anaesthesia (Isaac, 1970). The well-known diuretic action of alcohol has been shown to be due to reduced tubular reabsorption of water, mediated by its action on the osmoreceptors and the release of ADH from the posterior pituitary gland (Van Dyke & Ames, 1951). There is a great variation in the blood alcohol levels at which consciousness is lost after rapid intravenous infusion, even in individuals who are not habitual drinkers.

The only drugs with noticeable impact on the effectiveness of alcohol were found to be pentobarbitone 100 to 200 mg, sleep occurring with a significantly lower blood alcohol content and chlordiazepoxide 100 to 140 mg, which engendered acute resistance to alcohol (Dundee & Isaac, 1970). This antagonism of chloridazepoxide on the action of alcohol on the central nervous system has also been reported by Goldberg (1968) and by Benor & Ditman (1967).

Intravenous alcohol, while rarely used, still retains a measure of usefulness as an adjuvant during induction and maintenance of or emergence from anaesthesia.

Behan R J 1920 Ethyl Alcohol intravenously as postoperative sedative. American Journal of Surgery 69: 227–229

Benor D, Ditman K S 1967 Tranquillisers in the management of alcoholics: A review of literature to 1964. Part II. Journal of Clinical Pharmacology 1: 17–25

Constantin J D 1929 General anaesthesia by the intravenous injection of ethyl alcohol. Lancet 1:1247

Constantin J D 1930 General anaesthesia by the intravenous injection of ethyl alconol. Lancet 1: 1393–1395

Dundee J W, Isaac 1970 Interaction between intravenous alcohol and some sedatives and tranquillisers. British Journal of Pharmacology 39: 199–200

Dundee J W, Isaac M, Clarke R S J 1969 Alcohol in anesthetic practice. Anesthesia and Analgesia, Current Researches 38: 665–669

Dundee J W, Issac M, Davis E A, Sheridan B 1972 Effects of rapid infusion of ethanol on some factors controlling blood sugar levels in man. Quarterly Journal of Studies of Alcohol 33: 722–733

Fohl T 1931 Der Athylalkohol als Narkoticum and

Therapeuticum bei intravenoser Dorreichung. Archiv fur klinische Chirurgie, 165: 641–711
Goldberg L 1966 Behavioral and physiological effects of alcohol on man. Psychosomatic Medicine 28: 570–595
Hewer A J H 1964 Hypothermia for Neurosurgery. International Anesthesiology Clinics 2: 919–939
Isaac M 1970 Hepatic function following intravenous ethanol anaesthesia. Anaesthesia 25: 198–201
Karp M, Sokol J K 1951 Intravenous use of alcohol in the surgical patient. Journal of the American Medical Association 146: 21–23
Keys T E 1945 The History of Surgical Anesthesia. New York: Dover Publications Inc
Moore D C, Karp M 1945 Intravenous alcohol in surgery patient: preliminary report. Surgery, Gynecology and Obstetrics 80: 523–525
Schnelle N 1965 Alcohol given intravenously for general anaesthesia. Surgical Clinics of North America 45: 1041–1049
Van Dyke H B, Ames R G 1951 Alcohol diuresis. Acta Endocrinologica (Copehhagen) 7: 110–121

CHLORMETHIAZOLE

In 1957, Charonnat et al demonstrated that the thiazole fraction of thiamine (vitamin B_1) has hypnotic and sedative properties and in the same year Laborit and his colleagues reported favourably on its use in anaesthesia. In the following year Dundee used SCTZ as it was then called (it was later known as Heminevrin) in a 2% solution as an induction agent. He found many complications and was unable to confirm the favourable findings of the French workers. Large volumes of solution (40 to 100 ml) were required for induction and there was a delay of about half a minute before a soporific effect was observed. The drug was not suitable for use as a sole agent for minor operations, but could be used with nitrous oxide-oxygen and with a long-acting relaxant for major operations.

Anticonvulsant properties have been ascribed to chlormethiazole (Gastager et al, 1969) and it has been used in the treatment of patients with pre-eclampsia and eclampsia during labour (Duffus et al, 1968). This and sporadic use in status epilepticus are at present the only major applications for this agent. However, occasional reference is still being made to its use as an adjuvant to anaesthesia, especially to provide sedation during regional analgesia (Seow et al, 1984a, b) and most recently Sinclair et al (1985) have reported that sedation with an infusion of chlormethiazole at the rate of 30–40 ml min^{-1} has no clinically adverse cardiovascular effects during operations carried out under extradural analgesia.

Charonnat R, Lechat P, Chareton J 1957 Sur les proprietes pharmacodynamiques d'un derive thiazolique lere note. Therapie 12: 68–71
Dundee J W 1958 SCTZ — A new intravenous anaesthetic? British Journal of Anaesthesia 30:409
Duffus G M, Tunstall M E, Condie R G, McGillivary I 1969 Chlormethiazole in the prevention of eclampsia and the reduction of perinatal mortality. Journal of Obstetrics and Gynaecology of the British Commonwealth 76: 645–651
Gastager H, Haas I, Weinkamer E 1964 Erfahrungsbericht uber anwendung von distraneurin in der psychiatrie. Wiener klinische Wochenschrift 76: 639–644
Seow L T, Mather I E, Cousins M J 1984 Failure of L V atropine to abolish nasal irritation caused by chlormethiazole used in elderly patients undergoing spinal anaesthesia. Anesthesia & Intensive Care 12: 127–130
Seow L T, Mather I E, Cousins M J 1984 Chlormethiazole used in elderly patients undergoing spinal anaesthesia (letter) British Journal of Anaesthesia 56: 666–668
Sinclair C J, Fagan D, Scott D B 1985 Cardiovascular effects of chlormethiazole infusion in combination with extradural anaesthesia 57: 587–590

SODIUM GAMMA-HYDROXYBUTYRATE

Sodium gamma-hydroxybutyrate (Gamma-OH) has the unique distinction of being the only anaesthetic closely related to normal constituents of body metabolism. Butyric acid (CH3-CH2-CH2-COOH), a saturated fatty acid is a natural product of lipid metabolism and is known to have the capacity of inducing sleep accompanied by some muscle relaxation. Since, however, the administration of butyric acid in amounts sufficient to produce anaesthesia leads to the formation of ketone bodies, Laborit and his associates (1960) synthesised hydroxybutyric acid in the attempt to forestall that complication.

Gamma-OH is a derivative of gamma-aminobutyric acid (GABA) which has been isolated from human nervous tissue and is known to inhibit the passage of impulses across synapses. It is believed that its site of action in the brain is cortical, and in the spinal cord is on the internuncial neurones. There is some evidence that the activity of Gamma-OH is related to that of GABA although the exact mechanism is not known (Helrich et al, 1964). It appears to be a very safe drug since in acute experiments in animals the LD_{50} has been 5–15 times the dose necessary to produce coma. There appear to have been no deaths due to acute toxicity of the agent.

The recommended dose for induction of anaesthesia is 40 to 50 mg kg^{-1} but up to 70 mg kg^{-1} has been administered. In the lower dose ranges the first effects of the drug are noted in 5 to 15 min and manifest themselves by drowsiness followed later by sleep from which the individual can be roused. If the upper ranges are administered, proper anaesthesia is induced, lasting from one to two hours or longer. Induction might take up to 45 min to complete. Agitation has been known to be associated with the administration of smaller doses and transient mental disturbances have occurred on awakening. The onset of anaesthesia has been associated at times with muscular movements, often extrapyramidal in nature, but patients are not aware of these.

Administration of Gamma-OH is often associated with bradycardia and with a moderate fall in cardiac output. Both can be controlled by the administration of atropine. A mild elevation of blood pressure might be seen after induction, attributed by Virtue et al (1966) to vasoconstriction secondary to lack of analgesia. Respiration is little affected by the administration of Gamma-OH and spontaneous respiration is easily maintained (Lund et al, 1965). The jaw is well relaxed, permitting tracheal intubation in a spontaneously breathing patient, at a depth before stimulation is tolerated. Extensive manipulation of the upper airway and epiglottis is possible without coughing or bucking and the establishment of controlled ventilation is facilitated (Blumenfeld et al, 1962). Despite earlier contentions to the contrary, electrolyte balance is not adversely influenced (Madjidi, 1967). No abnormality in liver and kidney functions have been reported and oxygen consumption remains unchanged.

Gamma-hydroxybutyrate has not been advocated as a sole anaesthetic agent but rather has it been considered a basal agent upon which general anaesthesia may be superimposed. The preliminary injection of Gamma-OH has served to reduce quite markedly the need for additional analgesics. Use of this agent has been advocated for a wide range of general surgical, neurosurgical, orthopaediac, ophthalmological and endoscopic procedures, especially those of long duration.

Its main drawback lies in the uncertainty of control because of the long period of latency, its weak analgesic action and long recovery period. It is this lack of analgesic which, according to Solway & Sadove (1965) is implicated in the occasional emergence delirium. Again this agent has not achieved a lasting place in anaesthesia and its use has been virtually abandoned.

For a more complete survey, the reader is referred to the review by Vickers (1969).

Blumenfeld M, Suntay R A, Harmel M H 1962 Sodium gamma-hydroxybutyric acid: a new anesthetic adjuvant. Anesthesia and Analgesia, Current Researches 41: 721–726

Helrich M, McAslan T C, Skolnik S, Bessman S P 1964 Correction of blood levels of 4-hydroxybutyrate with state of consciousness. Anesthesiology 25: 771–775

Laborit H, Savany J M, Gerard J, Fabiani F 1960 Generalites concernant l'etude experimentale de l'emploi clinique du gamma hydroxybutyrate de Na. Agressology 1:407

Lund L O, Humphries J H, Virtue R W 1956 Sodium gamma hydroxybutyrate: Laboratory and clinical studies. Canadian Anaesthetist' Society Journal 12: 379–385

Madjidi A 1967 y-Hydroxybutyrat, ein neues intravenoses narkoticum. Anaesthesist 16:6

Solway J, Sadove M S 1965 4-hydroxybutyrate: a clinical study. Anesthesia and Analgesia, Current Researches 44: 532–539

Vickers M D 1969 Gammahydroxybutric Acid. In Newer Intravenous Anesthetics. Edited by R S J Clarke. International Anesthesiology Clinics 7: 75–89

Virtue R W, Lund L O, Belkwitt H J, Vogel J H K 1966 Cardiovascular reactions to gamma hydroxybutyrate in man. Canadian Anaesthetists' Society Journal 13: 119–123

PROPANIDID

Propanidid (Epontol, Fabontal) is the only eugenol derivative which has found clinical application and was at one time commercially available in Europe, but has now been largely abandoned. It was never marketed in North America. Two other eugenols had been prepared: one known as G 29505 was marketed for a short time in Germany under the trade name of Estil. Only one study from Japan has been published on the other, named Propinal (Nishimura, 1962).

Propanidid shares with all substances in this group the disadvantage of being insoluble in water and hence it has to be dissolved in Cremophor EL. This solvent has been implicated as the source of anaphylactic reactions. Studies of its onset of action place propanidid into a category similar to thiopentone and methohexitone, being around 8–11 s. While some comparative studies have given the ratio of the dose of thiopentone to propanidid as 1:1 (Dundee & Clarke, 1964; Howells et al, 1964), others have found that much larger doses are needed (Howells et al, 1964; Wyant & Zoerb, 1965).

Some early reports scarcely mention involuntary muscle movements (Horatz et al, 1965; Harrfeldt, 1965), while Wyant & Zoerb (1965) reported a very high incidence of side effects and Wynands & Burfoot (1965) were prepared to accept the few muscle movements and hiccoughs which occurred. The effect of the speed of injection increases the incidence of side effects with propanidid as with methohexitone (Barron, 1968).

Hypotension is not a significant problem in man provided low dosages are used. Dundee & Clarke (1964) found that its incidence was similar to that of equipotent low doses of thiopentone or methohexitone, but it is relatively more toxic in higher doses. Cardiac output and myocardial function are depressed and Soga and his colleagues (1973) actually found that propanidid was the more depressant. On the other hand respiratory stimulation is a striking feature of propanidid anaesthesia and there is some evidence (Gordh, 1973) that propanidid stimulates the carotid chemoreceptors leading to reflex increase in ventilation.

Since propanidid is broken down through the enzymatic action of pseudocholinesterase, it prolongs the effect of suxamethonium and reduces the incidence and severity of post-relaxation myalgia (Clarke et al, 1964; Clarke et al, 1967).

Propanidid was the first anaesthetic agent in which hypersensitivity and histamine release were demonstrated to be significant side effects. This subject is discussed in greater detail in Chapter 14. Few, if any, other general toxic reactions have been attributed to the drug. The recovery from anaesthesia after propanidid is both rapid (Fig. 6.9) and smooth, likely due to the fact that it is broken down rapidly in the body, in contradistinction to the redistribution of the barbiturates. The incidence of nausea and vomiting after propanidid is high (Dundee & Clarke, 1964; Wyant & Zoerb, 1965; Dundee et al, 1965). Limited studies have failed to show damage following the intra-arterial injection of propanidid (Liebegott, 1965), and, while it causes a slightly higher incidence of venous sequelae than thiopentone, these are of a degree which is clinically acceptable.

Summarising the advantages and disadvantages of propanidid, one can say that the brevity of action with rapid clear-headed recovery, its availability in solution, and its safety in porphyria (Dean, 1969) are definite advantages, whereas cardiovascular and excitatory side effects, the viscid properties of the solution, the high incidence of vomiting and the prolongation of the action of suxamethonium are cited as disadvantages. There may be considerable difficulty when one attempts to follow an induction dose of propanidid with an inhalation technique since the effect of the induction agent tends to have worn off before adequate levels of inhalation anaesthesia have been achieved. The main indication for this agent seemed to lie with relatively minor surgical procedures, such as very limited tooth extractions, minor gynaecological procedures and the like.

For a fuller review of propanidid, the reader is referred to the lst edition of this book (Ch. 8).

Barron D W 1968 Clinical studies of induction agents. XXII: Effect of rate of injection of incidence of side effects with thiopental and methohexital. Anesthesia and Analgesia, Current Researches 47: 171–173

Clarke R S J, Dundee J W, Daw R S 1964 Clinical studies of induction agents. XI: The influence of some intravenous anaesthetics on the respiratory effects and sequelae of suxamethonium. British Journal of Anaesthesia 36: 307–313

Clarke R S J, Dundee J W, Hamilton R C 1967 Interactions between induction agents and muscle relaxants: clinical observations. Anaesthesia 22: 235–248

Dean G 1969 A report on propanidid, an intravenous anaesthetic in porphyria variegata. South African Medical Journal South African Medical Journal 43: 227–229

Dundee J W, Clarke R S J 1964 Clinical studies of induction agents. IX: A comparative study of a new eugenol derivative, FBA 1420, with G 29,505 and standard barbiturates. British Journal of Anaesthesia 36: 100–105

Dundee J W, Kirwan M J, Clarke R S J 1965 Anaesthesia and premedication as factors in postoperative vomiting. Acta Anaesthesiologica Scandinavica 9: 223–231

Gordh T 1973 Analysis of hyperventilation in propanidid anaesthesia. In Anaesthesiology und Wiederbelebung, pp. 131–136. Edited by R Frey, F.Kern and O Mayrhofer. Berlin: Springer-Verlag

Harrfeldt H P 1965 Technik und Erfahrungen bei 2700 Kurznarkosen mit Propanidid. In Die intravenose Kurznarkose mit dem neuen Phenoxyessigsaurederivat Propanidid (Epontol), pp. 182–202. Edited by K Horatz, R Frey and M Zindler. Berlin: Springer-Verlag

Horatz K, Frey R, Zindler M Editors 1965 Die intravenose

Kurznarkose Hurznarkose mit dem neuen Phenoxyessigsaurederivat Propanidid (Epontol). Berlin: Springer-Verlag

Howells T H, Harnik E, Kellner G A, Rosenoer V M 1967 Propanidid and methohexitone: their comparative potency and narcotic action. British Journal of Anaesthesia 39: 31–34

Howells T H, Odell J R, Hawkins T J, Steane P A. 1964 An introduction to FBA. 1420: a new non-barbiturate intravenous anaesthetic. British Journal of Anaesthesia 36: 295–301

Liebegott G 1965 Pathologische-anatomische Befunde nach Anwendung von Kurznarkotika. in Die intravenose Kurznarkose mit dem neuen Phenoxyessigsaurederivat Propanidid (Epontol), pp. 125–154. Edited by K Horatz, F Frey, and M Zindler. Berlin: Springer-Verlag

Nishimura N 1962 On Propinal (2-M-4-P) a new intravenous, nonbarbiturate anesthetic agent. Anesthesia and Analgesia, Current Researches 41: 265–271

Soga D, Beer R, Andrae J, Bader R 1973a Die Beeinflussung des linksventrikularen Myokardkontraktiltat und Haemodynamick durch Propanidid beim Hund, pp. 27–39. Edited by R Frey, F Kern, O Mayrhofer. Berlin: Springer-Verlag. In: Anaesthesiologie und Wiederbelebung

Wyant G M, Zoerb D L 1965 Propanidid — a new non-barbiturate intravenous anaesthetic. Canadian. Anaesthetists' Society Journal 12: 569–586

Wynands J E, Burfoot M F 1965 A clinical study of propanidid (FBA 1420). Canadian Anaesthetists' Society Journal 12: 587–594

STEROIDS

The hypnotic properties of steroids have been known for over 30 years since Selye (1941) reported the occurrence of reversible unconsciousness in rats following the intraperitoneal injection of large quantities of several steroid hormones. More than a decade was to pass before any practical development of this work emerged when P'An et al (1955) reported their observations in animals of experiments with *hydroxydione* (Viadril, Presuren). Although this had a wider safety margin than thiopentone, there was a delay in onset of action, it was rather too long-lasting and it was followed by an unacceptably high incidence of thrombophlebitis. Some anaesthetists continued to use this drug for a short time mainly on the grounds that it was the first clinically acceptable non-barbiturate induction agent (Galley & Rooms, 1956; Lerman, 1956) but it was eventually abandoned in clinical practice.

Although it was difficult to find specific advantages of hydroxydione several workers claimed it caused less respiratory and cardiovascular depression than the barbiturates and that anaesthesia was followed by mild euphoria. These advantages were sufficient for the pharmaceutical industry to retain some interest in steroid anaesthesia but it was obvious that the delayed onset of action would have to be overcome. It was suggested (Robertson & Wynn Williams, 1961) that some metabolites of hydroxydione might be responsible for its anaesthetic activity: in clinical practice one noted a very prolonged onset of action in cases of liver dysfunction and jaundice and, although this supports the above claim, it was never fully documented.

A number of other steroids were studied, based on the pregnane nucleus, but it was some time before one had a clearer understanding of the relationship between structure and anaesthetic activity of this group of drugs (Sutton, 1972). It had become clear that rapid induction and high potency were associated with the presence of a free 3 -hydroxy group in the steroid molecule. All attempts, however, to achieve solubility of such steroids by esterification produced compounds with reduced potency or increased induction time (Davis & Pearce, 1972).

Althesin

In continuing research it became apparent that GR 2/234 (alphaxalone) showed promise as an anaesthetic having a rapid onset of action, high potency, and a wide safety margin. Problems of solubility were not entirely solved by the use of the non ionic surface active agent, Cremophor EL (polyoxyethylated castor oil). Fortunately, the addition of a small amount of a related steroid (alphadolone acetate) increased the solubility of alphaxalone in Cremophor EL more than threefold. Alphadolone has anaesthetic properties similar to alphaxalone but half as potent and it is merely additive as a hypnotic. This mixture, known originally as CT 1341, never had an official name and was known in Britain as *Althesin* and in some other countries as *Alfathesin*. The formulation of the commercially available ampoules was:

Alphaxalone	0.90 g
Alphadolone acetate	0.30 g
Poloxyethylated castor oil	20.00 g
Sodium chloride	0.25 g
Water for injection BP	to 100 ml

Thus each ml of Althesin contains 9 mg of alphaxalone and 3 mg of alphadolone acetate. It has a pH of about 7 and is isotonic with blood. As with all solutions made up in cremophor, it is slightly viscid and has a tendency to be frothy when drawn into the syringe.

Althesin possessed many of the properties of an ideal anaesthetic, having a rapid onset of action, comparable to thiopentone, being consistent in its action and not causing a high incidence of extraneous muscle movements although not as good as thiopentone in this respect. Recovery from equivalent doses is slightly shorter than that of thiopentone but longer than methohexitone. Perhaps more important is the fact that within a few hours after operation, patients given the steroid do not experience the hangover which is common with the barbiturates. In clinical practice one usually referred to the dose of Althesin in ml rather than mg and Clarke et al (1972) estimated that 60 μl kg^{-1} Althesin was equivalent to 4 mg kg^{-1} thiopentone, 1.2 mg kg^{-1} methohexitone and 4.2 mg kg^{-1} propanidid although 'depth of sleep' produced by the four drugs was very different. Some workers commented on the slower onset of action of Althesin when injected over 60 s (Scott & Virden, 1972) but this may have been due to the greater difficulty in injecting the 'oily' solution and in controlled studies no difference in onset time could be detected between the steroid and thiopentone.

As with other intravenous anaesthetics, the induction dose was reduced by opiate premedication which also reduced the incidence of muscle movement or tremor. As one might have expected from the animal pharmacology (Child et al, 1971; 1972) the 'dose toxicity' curve for Althesin was better than that from the barbiturates and up to 100 μg kg^{-1} could be given without any marked increase in the incidence of side effects. There is little to choose between the respiratory depression and hypotension with Althesin and with the equivalent doses of thiopentone and the steroid produced less tachycardia than methohexitone (Clarke et al, 1971). A number of workers (Prys-Roberts et al, 1972; Lyons & Clarke, 1972) found little to choose between the cardiodepressant effects of Althesin and thiopentone in hypotensive or cardiac patients and many people used these drugs interchangeably.

The withdrawal of Althesin from clinical use and its relation to hypersensitivity reactions and the use of the Cremophor solvent is discussed in Chapter 14. However, note should be made of Althesin infusions, for which an acceptable substitute has not yet been found. Its effect on cerebral perfusion, cerebral metabolism and intracranial pressure was very useful. Animal experiments (Pickerodt et al, 1972) showed a reduction in oxygen consumption and this metabolic depression led to a secondary fall in cerebral blood flow and cerebrospinal fluid pressure. This reduction in intracranial pressure which made the drug an ideal anaesthetic for use in neurosurgery is unlikely to have been due solely to arterial hypotension and in subsequent studies workers from Leeds (Turner et al, 1973) reported its use with controlled ventilation in patients undergoing neurosurgery. A number of workers subsequently confirmed its value in this field (Takahashi et al, 1973; Sari et al, 1976) and this appeared to be a real use for a preparation with these excellent neurological properties. Zorab & Baskett (1977) recommended its use as the induction agent of choice in patients with head injury. In this latter field, although infusions of Althesin have been used to maintain a low intracranial pressure in patients with head injuries, no severe reactions have been reported although the numbers involved are small. It could be given either directly from a time-control syringe or diluted and given as an infusion. It is this use of Althesin which was badly missed when the drug was withdrawn from clinical practice.

Minaxolone citrate

Minaxolone was a water-soluble steroid developed by Glaxo Group Research which underwent clinical trials in 1978–79 but was withdrawn from clinical use for toxicological reasons after 1250 administrations. This drug was interesting in that it showed the ability of the pharmaceutical industry to overcome the solubility problems which occurred with Althesin.

The early evaluation of minaxolone was promising and confirmed its rapid onset of action (Aveling et al, 1979; Dundee et al, 1980; McNeill et al, 1979a). Some early studies commented on the high incidence of excitatory effects (involun-

Table 18.1 A comparative evaluation of the properties of hydroxydione, Althesin, minaxolone and thiopentone.

	Hydroxydione	*Althesin*	*Minaxolone*	*Thiopentone*
Water solubility	High	Poor	High	High
Available in	Powder	Liquid	Liquid	Powder
Volume required	Large	Small	Variable	Variable
Onset of anaesthesia	Slow	Rapid	Rapid	Rapid
Safety margin	High	Very high	—	Acceptable
Recovery time	Prolonged	Acceptable	Prolonged	Acceptable
Incidence of venous thrombosis	High	Low	Acceptable	Low

tary muscle movement) and hypertonus (McNeill et al, 1979b; Dunn et al, 1980). Short term recovery following minaxolone was significantly slower than after Althesin (Sear et al, 1980) and this proved to be a problem when the drug was given by intermittent injection with nitrous oxide-oxygen.

It is interesting to review two 'Obituary Notices' which appeared about the time when minaxolone was withdrawn. Hope (1981) commented on the high incidence of excitatory effects and questioned whether clinical workers had been given all the known information on these by the pharmaceutical companies. He commented that although one might be able to 'tame' this agent with other drugs such as narcotics this is not the answer for coping with its untoward effects. He also pointed out that data on baboons may be directly comparable with expected effects in man. Dundee (1981) reviewing the clinical reports to date commented that although induction was not always as smooth as desired and anaesthesia may be longer than one would desire for short procedures, there was a need for collaboration between a number of centres in the area of studies of induction of anaesthesia with new drugs and he looked forward to the day when we might have a water soluble analogue of Althesin. This latter hope has not been fulfilled.

Table 18.1 summarises some of the important properties of these steroids and compares them with thiopentone.

REFERENCES

Aveling W, Sear J W, Fitch W, Chang H, Waters A, Cooper G M, Simpson P, Savege T M, Prys-Roberts C, Campbell D 1979 Early clinical evaluation of minaxolone: a new intravenous steroid anaesthetic agent. Lancet 2: 71–73

Child K J, Currie J P, Davis B, Dodds M G, Pearce D R, Twissell, D J 1971 The pharmacological properties in animals of CT 1341 — a new steroid anaesthetic agent. British Journal of Anaesthesia 43:2

Child K J, Davis B, Dodds M G, Twissell D J (1972) Anaesthetic, cardiovascular and respiratory effects of the new steroidal agent CT 1341: a comparison with other intravenous anaesthetic drugs in the unrestrained cat. British Journal of Pharmacology 46: 189–200

Clarke R S J, Dundee J W, Carson I W 1972 Some aspects of the clinical pharmacology of Althesin. Postgraduate Medical Journal, Supplement 2, 48: 62–65

Clarke R S J, Montgomery S J, Dundee J W, Bovill J G 1971 Clinical studies of induction agents. XXXIX: CT 1341, a new steroid anaesthetic. British Journal of Anaesthesia 43: 947–952

Davis B, Pearce D R 1972 An introduction to Althesin (CT 1341). Postgraduate Medical Journal, Supplement 2, 48: 17–24

Dundee J W 1981 Editorial: Minaxolone and beyond. Anaesthesia 36: 579–581

Dundee J W, Clarke R S J, McNeill H G 1980 Minaxolone: a preliminary communication. Trends in Intravenous Anaesthesia, 259–265

Dunn G L, Morison D , McChesney J, Pine W 1980 An early clinical assessment of the steroid anaesthetic minaxolone. Canadian Anaesthetists' Society Journal 27: 140–145

Galley A H, Rooms M (1956) Intravenous steroid anaesthetic: experiences with viadril. Lancet 1: 990–994

Hope C E 1981 Editorial: Clinical trial — the minaxolone story. Canadian Anaesthetists' Society Journal 28: 1–5

Lerman L H 1956 Viadril: new steroid anaesthetic. Preliminary communication. British Medical Journal ii: 129–132

Lyons S M, Clarke R S J 1972 A comparison of different drugs for anaesthesia in cardiac surgical patients. British Journal of Anaesthesia 44: 575–583

McNeill H G, Clarke R S J, Dundee J W 1979a Minaxolone: a new water-soluble steroid anaesthetic. Lancet, 2:73

McNeill H G, Clarke R S J, Dundee J W, Briggs L P 1979b The influence of dosage and premedication on induction of anesthesia with minaxolone. Acta Anaesthesiologica Belgica 30: Suppl, 169–173

P'an S Y, Gardocki J F, Hutcheon D E, Rudel H, Kodet M J, Laubach G D 1955 General anaesthetic and other pharmacological properties of a soluble steroid,

21-hydroxypregnanedione sodium succinate. Journal of Pharmacology and Experimental Therapeutics 115: 432–411

Pickerodt V W A, McDowall D G, Coroneos N J, Keaney N P 1972 Effect of Althesin on cerebral perfusion, cerebral metabolism and intracranial pressure in the anaesthetised baboon. British Journal of Anaesthesia 44: 751–757

Prys-Roberts C, Foex P, Biro G P 1972 Cardiovascular responses of hypertensive patients to induction of anaesthesia with Althesin. Postgraduate Medical Journal, Supplement 2, 48: 80–85

Robertson J D, Wynn Williams A 1961 Studies on clinical and pathological effects of hydroxydione. Anaesthesia 16: 389–409

Sari A, Maekawa T, Tohjo M, Okuda Y, Takeshita H 1976 Effects of Althesin on cerebral blood flow and oxygen consumption in man. British Journal of Anaesthesia 48: 545–550

Scott D F, Virden S 1972 Comparison of the effect of Althesin with other induction agents on electroencephalographic patterns. Postgraduate Medical Journal, Supplement 2, 48: 93–96

Sear J W, Cooper G M, Williams N B, Simpson P J, Prys-Roberts C 1980 Minaxolone or Althesin supplemented by nitrous oxide. A study in anaesthesia for short operative procedures. Anaesthesia 35: 119–120

Selye H 1941 Anaesthetic effects of steroid hormones. Proceedings of the Society of Experimental Biology and Medicine 46: 116–121

Sutton J A 1972 A brief history of steroid anaesthesia before Althesin (CT 1341). Postgraduate Medical Journal, Supplement 2, 48: 9–13

Takahashi T, Takasaki M, Namiki A, Dohi S 1973 Effects of Althesin on cerebrospinal fluid pressure. British Journal of Anaesthesia 45: 179–184

Turner J M, Coroneos N J, Gibson R M, Powell D, Ness M A, McDowall D G 1973 The effect of Althesin on intracranial pressure in man. British Journal of Anaesthesia 45: 168–172

Zorab J S M, Baskett P J F 1977 Immediate Care. W B Saunders, London

Additional references

Davis B, Dodds M G, Dolamore P G, Gardner C J, Sawyer P R, Twissell D J, Vallance D K 1979 Minaxolone: a new water-soluble steroid anaesthetic. British Journal of Anaesthesia 51:564P

Dechene J P 1977 Alfathesin by continuous infusion supplemented with intermittent pentazocine. Canadian Anaesthetists' Society Journal 24: 702–706

Dixon R A, Atkinson R W, Kenyon C, Lamb D, Thornton J A, Woodhead S 1976 Subanaesthetic dosage of Althesin as a sedative for conservative dentistry. British Journal of Anaesthesia 48: 431–439

Hannington-Kiff J G 1972 Comparative recovery rates following induction of anaesthesia with Althesin and methohexitone. Postgraduate Medical Journal, Supplement 2, 48: 116–120

Healy T E J, Birmingham A T, Chatterjee S C 1972 A comparison of the effect of induction of anaesthesia by thiopentone or Althesin on the duration of action of suxamethonium. Postgraduate Medical Journal, Supplement 2, 48: 90–93

Heinonen J, Orko R, Louhija A 1973 Anaesthesia for cardioversion: a comparison of Althesin and thiopentone. British Journal of Anaesthesia 45: 49–54

Keep P J, Manford M L M 1974 A comparison of Althesin and methohexitone in paediatric anaesthesia. British Journal of Anaesthesia 46: 685–686

Saarnivaara L 1974 Comparison of Althesin and thiopentone in anaesthesia for paediatric outpatient otology. British Journal of Anaesthesia 46: 268–272

Savege T M 1973 A new steroid anaesthetic, Althesin. Proceedings of the Royal Society of Medicine 66: 1029–1038

Tammisto T, Takki S, Tigerstedt I, Kauste A 1973 A comparison of Althesin and thiopentone in induction of anaesthesia. British Journal of Anaesthesia 45: 100–107

COMMENT

Two lessons appear in relation to drugs which have been introduced and not found acceptable in clinical anaesthesia. The first, and fairly obvious one, is that ideally one wants new drugs to be freely soluble in water. Whether one could ever get a stable solution of these is not important: for years anaesthetists made up solutions of thiopentone without complaint. This comment can be coupled with the fact that the solutions must not cause pain on injection or venous thrombosis. It is too early to assess whether an emulsion form of the drug will be equally acceptable clinically as an aqueous solution. Clearly there is no place for drugs which are solubilised in cremophor and similar compounds and only on rare occasions should one have to resort to organic solvents such as polyethylene or propylene glycol.

The second point, which has not always been fully appreciated, is that while one can reduce muscle movements and hiccough by the use of suitable premedication or pretreatment with a short-acting opioid, this may remove some of the advantages of the drug. Although the latter will decrease the 'induction' dose (thus minimising the cardiovascular effects), these opioids can cause their own problems; this practice is very acceptable with drugs such as etomidate and methohexitone which have advantages in specific fields. If one is going to introduce a compound with a high incidence of these complications, such as occurred with minaxolone, then the advantages of other aspects of its action must be very great indeed.

19

Intravenous regional analgesia

In 1908 August Bier described a technique of so-called 'venous anaesthesia' by which was meant the intravenous injection of procaine into an exsanguinated limb. He had carried out the procedure in 134 patients. Apart from a number of reports the following year and a description by Adams (1944) in his textbook on intravenous anaesthesia, little was heard of this technique until Holmes reintroduced it in 1963 as a means of producing local analgesia in a limb.

SITE AND MODE OF ACTION

There has been a good deal of speculation regarding the site of action of local anaesthetics administered by the intravenous route in the presence of a tourniquet. Miles et al (1964) have shown that lignocaine appears to affect a peripheral portion of the neurone and might act by blocking acetylcholine production and also by opposing its action at the neuromuscular junction. They have also shown that there is an action on the sensory nerve endings which accounts for the diminished pain sensation in the presence of a recordable sensory nerve action potential. They have differentiated between the effect of ischaemia produced by the tourniquet and the effects of lignocaine in the presence of the tourniquet. According to their findings the action potential latency in muscle is increased 55 per cent by ischaemia alone, but 180 per cent by ischaemia with lignocaine. There is also a similar effect on the sensory action potential in the median nerve. These observations have been confirmed by Shanks and McLeod (1970) who, using a serial nerve conduction technique, concluded that lignocaine and ischaemia produced analgesia and impairment of conduction at a faster rate than ischaemia alone. Of interest is the further observation by Miles et al (1964) that excitability after lignocaine injection recovers more slowly than after ischaemia alone, which is likely due to the fact that the washout of drugs is gradual after an initial fast release of approximately 30 per cent of the dose. Thirty minutes after deflation of the cuff half the dose still remains in the extremity (Tucker and Boas, 1971). These findings explain the experiences of Brown and Weissman (1966) that a second intravenous regional anaesthetic infused immediately upon return of sensation requires only half the original dose and that a third block thereafter can be accomplished with only one-quarter of the original dose.

By using ^{14}C-labelled lignocaine in dogs, Cotev and Robin (1966) have demonstrated a significant selective pick-up by nerve tissue without, however, being able to pinpoint the exact site of action. Shanks and McLeod (1970) observed that 1 per cent lignocaine caused a block in conduction of the nerve trunks at the site of maximal concentration. They concluded that the proximal sites of blockade might be of value in practice when the peripheral sensory nerve endings in the region of the operation site cannot be perfused adequately. Fleming and co-workers (1966) studied the site of action by means of lignocaine containing Hypaque as a radio-opaque medium. X-ray pictures of the injected limb showed that analgesia existed only in those areas where the radio-opaque medium could actually be demonstrated in the tissues and analgesia spread as the material penetrated into further tissue. This was interpreted as showing that intravenous lignocaine injected distal to a tourniquet acts at the tissue level on the nerve endings. This would explain the clinical observation that areas of analgesia and of complete preservation of sensation can exist in the distribution of the same nerve. Adriani (1968) states that the drug diffuses slowly from the endothelium of the vessels into the tissues of the isolated limb. It is probably 'fixed' to the nerve tissues and synapses, and stored in the tissue spaces. The nerve trunks themselves are not anaesthetised: only the nerve endings are affected. He concludes that this therefore is actually just another infiltration technique and that the designation of 'intravenous regional block' is not strictly accurate. Diffusion, fixation and the absorption of the drug by the tissues reduces the danger of the procedure since smaller quantities of the drug remain in the vessels to be carried into the systemic circulation at the end of the procedure when the tourniquet is released, or should the tourniquet inadvertently slip during the procedure. Other factors which suggest a peripheral site of action (such as on nerve endings) are the rapid onset of and recovery from analgesia and also that if a tourniquet is applied also at the wrist in addition to the upper arm, analgesia only occurs between the two tourniquets, leaving the hand unaffected (Atkinson, Modell and Moya, 1965). Yet Prithvi Raj and coworkers (1972), also using a mixture of lignocaine 0.5% and Renografin-60 concluded that the local anaesthetic acts on the main nerve trunks, and this was confirmed by Magora, Stern and Magora (1980) who found their block to begin at a proximal point of a nerve, the median being affected before the ulnar nerve; no explanation for this observation is given.

TECHNIQUE

After proper cleansing of the skin a needle of the Gordh or similar variety or a plastic cannula is inserted into the most peripheral vein available and is secured into position. Cox (1964), Harris, Slater and Bell (1965) and Dunbar and Mazze (1967) recommend positioning the needle close to the site of operation, but failures certainly are more frequent when the cubital fossa is used as the injection site (Sorbie and Chacha, 1965). Unless contraindicated by a fracture or other painful lesion, an Esmarch bandage is applied and the limb is thoroughly exsanguinated. Great care must be taken that the needle is well secured so that is cannot be dislodged during exsanguination. From this point of view a cannula is preferable to a needle. Long venous catheters, on the other hand, should be avoided so as to minimise the chance of its free end projecting proximally beyond the tourniquet lest the local anaesthetic be injected direct into the bloodstream (Clinical Anesthesia Conference, 1966). As an alternative to total exsanguination, the limb may be elevated for a matter of a few minutes to drain as much blood as possible before inflation of the tourniquet (Dawkins et al, 1964).

Jago (1977) has modified this further by suggesting manual occlusion of the brachial artery during the period of elevation. Winnie and Ramamurthy (1970) and later Finlay (1977) have described the use of an inflatable arm splint intended for the immobilisation of fractures, to achieve exsanguination in circumstances where application of an Esmarch bandage would be too painful. Lack of proper exsanguination in our experience is likely to result in spotty or inadequate analgesia apart from being accompanied by annoying back-bleeding from the operative site. However, there are those who contend that total exsanguination is not essential for success (Dawkins et al, 1964; Eriksson, 1966 and 1969; Trias, 1969; Thorn-Alquist, 1971).

A tourniquet previously applied proximal to the site of operation is now inflated to approximately 250 mmHg for the arm and even higher for the leg, or at least to well above systolic arterial pressure. In fact Lawes and associates (1984) have shown that the anaesthetic solution can enter the general circulation even when the tourniquet is properly inflated if the venous pressure is high as can happen when the injection is made particularly fast. It is concluded that the tourniquet ought to be inflated in excess of 50 mmHg above systolic pressure and the injection made over a period of not less than 60 seconds. Care should be taken to avoid nerve damage by correctly positioning the cuff (Arteaga and Russell, 1968) and by applying it over a layer of surgical wool (Monty and Deller, 1965). The Esmarch bandage is removed once the tourniquet has been inflated. A suitable local anaesthetic solution can now be injected into the previously placed needle or cannula, and analgesia will supervene within a matter of five to 15 minutes followed by loss of motor function.

A 0.5 per cent concentration of lignocaine, mepivacaine or prilocaine need rarely be exceeded, dosages for the upper extremity being in the region of 200 mg and for the lower extremity 350 mg or more, depending upon muscle mass; the dose is usually determined on the basis of clinical impression. Little is gained by calculating the dose on the basis of mg kg^{-1} body weight as suggested by some (Dunbar and Mazze, 1967; Harris, 1969; Rupp and Reid, 1969). The optimal amount for bupivacaine 0.25% is considered 200 mg; it is thought to be safe for prolonged regional analgesia (Magora, Stern and Magora, 1980). In order to avoid toxic reactions it is advisable not to deflate the tourniquet within less than 20 minutes after administration of the drug, and then only intermittently.

A second tourniquet is usually applied distal to the original one and inflated when analgesia has become established. The first one is then released. This will minimise the incidence and severity of tourniquet pain, since the second cuff is now applied over an already analgesic area. Hoyle (1964) has described a two-compartment tourniquet to serve the same purpose and many of these are now in clinical use. Motor power and sensation return within 5 to 10 minutes after release of the tourniquet, the time depending somewhat upon the total duration of the procedure and the nature, dose and concentration of the anaesthetic used.

Since the introduction of bupivacaine several studies have been reported in which that newer anaesthetic has been compared to the more established lidocaine. There has been little unanimity, as will be seen. Ware (1981) in a double-blind clinical study found both onset of analgesia and recovery times to be identical for the two agents and Magora, Stern and Magora (1980) moreover found the onset to be dose-related. Enright, Smith and Wyant (1980) also in a double-blind study, but on volunteers, failed to identify a difference of duration of analgesia between the two agents after release of the tourniquet and this observation was confirmed later also by Goolds (1982). However, the observations of Magora et al (1980) are somewhat at variance with these findings, as they reported persistent limb numbness up to 20 hours after tourniquet release; motor nerve conduction block persisted as long as three hours with up to 300 mg of bupivacaine, but none of these prolonged effects were seen if the total dose was kept at 150 mg. Evans at al (1974) were able to relate the duration of the residual block to the duration of the particular agent in other clinical situations which would indeed support the longer duration of bupivacaine. Like Enright, Smith and Wyant they found the residual analgesia to be patchy. Watson, Brown and Reich (1970) also concur with those who found the onset of regression of analgesia after bupivacaine increased over lignocaine. As far as the quality of analgesia is concerned, Ware (1981) found that from bupivacaine superior to lignocaine.

TOXICITY

Intravenous regional analgesia properly executed, has proven to be a safe and efficient method of producing regional analgesia in a limb. Hargrove and associates (1966) have been unable to find any lignocaine in the general circulation before deflation of the tourniquet, while after deflation the mean blood concentration never exceeded 1.95 $\mu g\ ml^{-1}$.

Cotev and Robin (1966) confirmed these findings by measuring the blood levels of ^{14}C-labelled lignocaine in the venous outflow of the limb after the removal of the tourniquet, when they found peak levels beneath the concentrations considered to be dangerous in clinical practice. Mazze and Dunbar (1966) showed that plasma concentrations of lignocaine determined chromatographically were lower with intravenous regional analgesia (1.5 μg ml$\pm$ 0.2) than with either axillary block or lumbar epidural analgesia. Also pulse rate, blood pressure and electrocardiographic changes were absent with intravenous regional analgesia and he concluded that intravenous lignocaine 3 mg kg^{-1} of a 0.5 per cent solution provides safe, effective analgesia when injected into an exsanguinated extremity. Toxic reactions from bupivacaine are unlikely unless the plasma concentration exceeds 4.0 $\mu g\ kg^{-1}$ (Moore, Balfour and Fitzgibbons, 1979). Magora et al (1980) observed three instances of toxic reactions after high doses of bupivacaine and having released the tourniquet in one step. In his comparative study Ware (1981) saw toxic reactions only after lignocaine and never after bupivacaine. Yet Davies, Gill and Weber (1981) were able to report 14 cases of bupivacaine toxicity with one fatality.

More recent information has called into question the safety of bupivacaine for intravenous regional analgesia. An article in the *Sunday Times* of 31 July 1983 lists six patients who died during operations carried out while bupivacaine was used with that technique. In each case tourniquet failure allowed the anaesthetic to enter the general circulation, resulting in convulsions and cardiac arrest. An editorial in the *Pharmaceutical Journal* the following month concluded that bupivacaine ought not to be used in intravenous regional analgesia. Unfortunately neither article gives details as to the amounts and concentrations used, thus making intelligent assessment difficult. Only time will tell whether such general condemnation is warranted in light of the several advantages of bupivacaine over other local anaesthetics, but it can be said with certainty that the 0.75% concentration is neither needed nor indicated.

Tucker and Boas (1971) found that after cuff release peak plasma levels of lignocaine, as determined by gas chromatography, were 20 to 80 per cent lower than those found when the same dose was injected directly into a vein over three minutes. They reported peak levels after release of the cuff to be inversely proportional to tourniquet time and were lower with a 0.5 per cent solution than after one per cent, identical total amounts of active drug having been injected.

It is safe, therefore, to conclude that only a small proportion of local anaesthetic is released into the circulation and that the remainder is slowly absorbed from the tissues. The amount released from the tissues, however, is raised by movement of the limb, presumably by milking out the local anaesthetic still stored within the tissues. Nevertheless, most authors advocate the slow release of the tourniquet or, indeed, intermittent release. On the other hand Kennedy and associates (1965) found an unacceptably high incidence of side effects including unconsciousness, hypotension, bradycardia, and cardiac arrhythmias with one case of asystole. It would seem that this high incidence might have been due to a combination of relatively large doses, up to 350 mg lignocaine, for operations on the hand with release of the tourniquet after an average of only 26.5 minutes. Merrifield and Carter (1965) corroborate the necessity of keeping the concentration of lignocaine to 0.5 per cent if complications are to be avoided with a dose range between 3.5 and 4.5 $mg\ kg^{-1}$. This dose range can be further reduced to 1.5 $mg\ kg^{-1}$ provided injection has been preceded by 20 minutes of ischaemia (Harris, Slater and Bell, 1965), a technique, however, which is not recommended.

If tourniquet time is likely to be short, thought might be given to the use of one of the faster hydrolised drugs like 2-choro-procaine, rather than the amines which are broken down much more slowly.

While lignocaine and bupivacaine are the preferred local anaesthetics for intravenous regional analgesia any local anaesthetic drug may be used for the purpose. Indeed mepivacaine 0.5 per cent might impart a certain additional degree of safety since milligram for milligram the drug has a lower systemic toxicity. Mazze (1968) recommends prilocaine and has shown that with an average of 3 $mg\ kg^{-1}$ of an 0.5 per cent concentration, methaemoglobinaemia is no problem. Harris and co-workers (1968) found that even with 5 $mg\ kg^{-1}$ prilocaine intravenously there was no discernible cyanosis although there was a moderate increase in methaemoglobin after tourniquet release. There was a significant decrease in oxygen content if venous Po_2 was below 30 mmHg or methaemoglobin levels exceeded 0.8 g per cent, while the difference in oxygen content was not significant when venous Po_2 exceeded 30 mmHg. They concluded that the magnitude of these changes does not contraindicate the use of prilocaine for intravenous regional analgesia in normal subjects, but might be important if coronary or cerebral oxygen transport were already compromised. Kerr (1967) in a double blind trial found that neurological symptoms were significantly more frequent after the use of lignocaine than after prilocaine for intravenous regional analgesia. The lower toxicity of prilocaine as related to lignocaine has been corroborated by others (Englesson *et al.*, 1964; Scott, 1965). Hooper (1964) confirmed that prilocaine provides adequate analgesia and has a good margin of safety even as a 1 per cent solution.

Absence of complications is largely dependent upon a meticulous technique and despite its simplicity, the procedure should never be carried out by anyone who does not have a thorough knowledge of the pharmacology of local anaesthetics or is not experienced in resuscitation. The most common serious complications arise from overdose or direct injection into the venous circulation, in other words are determined by the concentration and amount of local anaesthetic which might find its way into the systemic circulation.

CLINICAL APPLICATIONS

Intravenous regional analgesia has its greatest usefulness in the manipulation of fractures, repair of tendons, minor amputations, suture of lacerations, excision of ganglia and operations of a similar nature. By and large it is more often used in the upper extremity, primarily because of the larger amounts of local anaesthetic required for successful analgesia in the lower limbs. These larger amounts carry with them an increased risk of toxic reactions. Also, because of the more precarious venous circulation in the lower extremities it is generally preferable to avoid injecting extraneous substances there, and this is especially true where there is evidence of impaired venous circulation, as for instance in varicose veins. Although intravenous regional analgesia has been maintained for up to six hours without ill-effect (Ishibabi 1966), it would seem wise to restrict ischaemia time to the generally accepted one and a half hours, lest permanent hypoxaemic changes ensue. Acceptance of this principle places certain limitations upon the magnitude of the operative procedures which may be undertaken. It must also be remembered that as the tourniquet time increases, so does the incidence of tourniquet pain. Thorn-Alquist (1971) observed that intravenous regional analgesia gives complete muscle relaxation provided sufficient time is allowed for the local anaesthetic to exert its full effect. Ware (1975, 1981) found relaxation with bupivacaine invariably adequate for the setting of fractures and superior to that obtained with lignocaine. Such relaxation is in contrast to ischaemia alone in which the latent period is longer and is in line with observations on muscle action potentials discussed earlier in this chapter. Also relaxation under conditions of ischaemia alone is invariably accompanied by pain.

The *advantages* of intravenous regional analgesia lie in its simplicity, its rapidity of onset and disappearance. When compared with nerve blocks, not only is less local anaesthetic solution needed, but also no single nerve can escape. The technique is particularly useful in outpatients since they may be allowed to leave the hospital after a minimum of observation following the operation, and it may be used in patients who are less than adequately prepared for other forms of anaesthesia. Compared to brachial plexus block the possibility of pneumothorax and injury to the plexus itself is eliminated.

Under *disadvantages* one must mention the inability to deflate the tourniquet as long as analgesia is required, thus making it impossible for the surgeon to test haemostasis. Postoperative analgesia is not provided and application of an Esmarch bandage might be precluded by the pain this procedure engenders. However, alternative methods are available to produce ischaemia, and total exsanguination is not absolutely mandatory. The possibility of cardiovascular and neurological complications upon release of the tourniquet must always be borne in mind but the incidence of this complication can be minimised by attention to detail, all of which have been described in this chapter.

There are few *contraindications* to the method. Like other regional techniques intravenous analgesia is contraindicated in uncooperative patients and those who give a history of unfavourable reactions to the injection of local anaesthetics. Extensive tissue lesions may lead to loss of the local anaesthetic thus rendering the technique unsatisfactory. It goes without saying that inavailability of peripheral veins or pathology of the venous system in the limbs to be anaesthetised contraindicates this form of analgesia as do all conditions incompatible with the placement of a tourniquet.

INTRAVENOUS GENERAL ANALGESIA

Although not directly related to intravenous regional anaesthesia, no description of the intravenous use of local anaesthetics to provide relief from pain would be complete without reference to intravenous analgesia described by Gordon in 1943. It was used for the relief of pruritus associated with jaundice and to provide pain relief for burn dressings. To achieve this end, a slow drip infusion of 0.2 per cent procaine in 5 or 10 per cent glucose in saline is infused at a rate sufficient to provide analgesia, yet slow enough to prevent twitching, convulsions, or any other toxic local anaesthetic effects. The period of infusion varies from one to one and a half hours during which time up to 1 g of procaine has been administered. Pain relief lasts from two to twelve hours.

This topic has been fully reviewed by Graubard and Peterson (1950). With more modern methods and drugs this technique is largely of historical interest only yet one of the authors has recently seen it in use in China.

REFERENCES

Adams R C 1944. Intravenous Anasthesia: Intravenous Local Anesthesia, p. 111. New York and London: P B Hoeber, Inc

Adriani J 1968 Appraisal of Current Concepts of Anesthesiology. Venous Regional Block: Technique for Induction, 4: 184–190. St Louis: Mosby

Arteaga L F, Russell P H 1968 Intravenous regional anaesthesia. Medical Annals of the District of Columbia, 133:134

Atkinson D I, Modell J, Moya F 1965 Intravenous regional anesthesia. Anesthesia and Analgesia, Current Researches, 44: 313–317

Bier A 1908 Ueber einen neuen Weg Localanaesthesia an den Gliedmassen zu erzeugen. Archiv für klinische Chirurgie, vereinigt mit Deutsche Zeitschrift für Chirurgie, 86:1007

Brown E M Weissman F 1966 A case report: Prolonged intravenous regional anesthesia. Anesthesia and Analgesia, Current Researches, 45: 319–321

Clinical Anaesthesia Conference 1966: Complications of intravenous regional anesthesia. New York State Journal of Medicine, 66: 1344–1345

Cotev S, Robin G C 1966 Experimental studies on intravenous regional anaesthesia using radio-active lignocaine. British Journal of Anaesthesia, 38: 936–939

Cox J M R 1964 Intravenous regional anesthesia. Canadian Anaesthetists' Society Journal, 11: 503–508

Davies J A H, Gill S S, Weber J C P 1981 Intravenous regional analgesia using bupivacaine. Anaesthesia, 36:331

Dawkins O S, Russell E S, Adams A K, Hooper R L, Odiakosa O A, Fleming S A 1964 Intravenous regional anaesthesia. Canadian Anaesthetists' Society Journal, 11: 243–246

Dunbar R W, Mazze R I 1967 Intravenous regional anesthesia. Anesthesia and Analgesia, Current Researches, 46: 806–811

Editorial 1983. Anaesthetists caution on bupivacaine. Pharmaceutical Journal, 231:161

Englesson S, Eriksson E, Wahlgrist S, Ortengren B 1962 Difference in tolerance to intravenous Xylocaine and Citanest. A double blind study in man. First European Congress of Anaesthesiology, Vienna, 2:206

Enright A C, Smith G G, Wyant G M 1980 Comparison of bupivacaine and lidocaine for intravenous regional analgesia. Canadian Anaesthetists' Society Journal; 27: 553–555

Eriksson E 1966 Prilocaine, an experimental study in man of a new local anaesthetic with special regards to efficacy, toxicity and excretion. Acta Chirurgica Scandinavica, Supplement, 358: 37–46

Eriksson E 1969 The effects of intravenous local anaesthetic agents on the central nervous system. Acta Anaesthesiologica Scandinavica, Supplement, 36: 79–102

Evans C J, Dewar J A, Boyes R N, Scott D B 1974 Residual nerve block following intravenous regional anaesthesia. British Journal of Anaesthesia; 46: 668–670

Finlay H 1977 A modification of Bier's intravenous analgesia. Use of the pneumatic splint. Anaesthesia, 32: 357–358

Fleming S A, Veiga-Pires J A, McCutcheon R M, Emanual C 1966 A demonstration of the site of action of intravenous lignocaine. Canadian Anaesthetists' Society Journal, 13: 21–27

Goolds J E 1982 Intravenous regional analgesia with bupivacaine. Anaesthesia; 37:604

Gordon R A 1943 Intravenous novocaine for analgesia in burns (preliminary report). Canadian Medical Association Journal, 49: 478–481

Graubard D J, Peterson M C 1950 Clinical Uses of Intravenous Procaine. Springfield, Illinois: C C Thomas; Oxford: Blackwell Scientific Publications

Hargrove R I, Hoyle J R, Parker F B R, Beckett A H, Beyes R N 1966 Blood lignocaine levels following intravenous regional analgesia. Anaesthesia, 21: 37–41

Harris W H, Slater E M, Bell H M 1965 Regional anesthesia by the intravenous route. Journal of the American medical Association, 194–1273–1276

Harris W H, Cole D W, Mital M, Laver M B 1968 Methemoglobin formation and oxygen transport following intravenous regional anesthesia using prilocaine. Anesthesiology, 29: 65–69

Harris W J 1969 Choice of anesthetic agents for intravenous regional anaesthesia. Acta anaesthesiologica Scandinavica, Supplement, 36: 47–52

Holmes C McK 1963 Intravenous regional analgesia. A useful method of producing analgesia of the limbs. Lancet, i: 245–247

Hooper R L 1964 Intravenous regional anaesthesia: A report on a new local anaesthetic agent. Canadian Anaesthetists' Society Journal, 11: 247–251

Hoyle J R 1964 Tourniquet for intravenous regional analgesia. Anaesthesia, 19: 294–295

Ishibabi T 1966 Japanese Journal of Anaesthesiology, 15:239

Jago R H 1977 Exsanguination of the limb in Bier's intravenous analgesia. Anaesthesia, 32:811

Kennedy B R, Dutchie A M, Parbrook G D, Carr T L 1965 Intravenous regional analgesia: An appraisal. British Medical Journal, i: 954–956

Kerr J H 1967 Intravenous regional analgesia: A clinical comparison of lignocaine and prilocaine. Anaesthesia, 22: 562–567

Lawes E G, Johnson T, Pritchard P, Robbins P 1984 Venous pressures during simulated Bier's Block. Anaesthesia 39: 147–149

Magora F, Stern L, Magora A 1980 Motor nerve conduction in intravenous regional anaesthesia with bupivacaine hydrochloride. British Journal of Anaesthesia, 52: 1123–1129

Magora F, Stern L, Zylber-Katz E, Olshwang D, Donchin Y, Magora A 1980 Prolonged effect of bupivacaine hydrocloride after cuff release in i.v. regional anaesthesia. British Journal of Anaesthesia, 52: 1131–1136

Mazze R I, Dunbar R W 1966 Plasma lidocaine concentrations after caudal, lumbar epidural, axillary block, and intravenous regional anesthesia. Anesthesiology, 27: 574–579

Mazze R I 1968 Methemoglobin concentrations following intravenous regional anesthesia. Anesthesia and Analgesia, Current Researches, 47: 122–124

Merrifield A J, Carter S S 1965 Intravenous regional analgesia: lignocaine blood levels. Anaesthesia, 20: 287–293

Miles D W, James J L, Clark D E, Whitwam J G 1964 Site of action of intravenous regional anaesthesia, Journal of Neurology, Neurosurgery and Psychiatry, 27: 574–576

Monty C P, Deller C R 1965 Experiences with intravenous regional anaesthesia. Proceedings of the Royal Society of Medicine, 58: 338–340

Moore D C, Balfour R I, Fitzgibbons D 1979 Convulsive arterial plasma levels of bupivacaine and the response to diazepam therapy. Anesthesiology, 50: 454–456

Prithvi Raj P, Garcia C E, Burleson J W, Jenkins M T 1972 The site of action of intravenous regional anesthesia. Anesthesia and Analgesia, Current Researches, 51: 776–785

Rupp R F, Reid R L 1969 Intravenous regional anaesthesia. Military Medicine, 134:127

Shanks C A, McLeod J G 1970 Nerve conduction studies in regional intravenous analgesia using 1 per cent lignocaine. British Journal of Anaesthesia, 42: 1060–1065

Sorbie C, Chacha P 1965 Regional anaesthesia by the intravenous route. British Medical Journal, i: 957–960

Scott D B 1965 Toxicity and clinical use of prilocaine. Proceedings of the Royal Society of Medicine, 58: 420–422

Thorn-Alquist A M 1971 Intravenous regional anaesthesia. Acta Anaesthesiologica Scandinavica, Supplement, 40: 7–35

Trias A 1969 The use of intravenous regional anaesthesia in orthopedic surgery. Acta anaesthesiologica Scandinavica, Supplement, 36: 35–37

Tucker G T, Boas R A 1971 Pharmacokinetic aspects of intravenous regional anesthesia. Anesthesiology, 34: 538–549

Ware R J 1975 Intravenous regional analgesia using bupivacaine. Anaesthesia, 30: 817–822

Ware R J 1981 Intravenous regional analgesia using bupivacaine. Anaesthesia, 34: 231–235

Watson R L, Brown P W, Reich M P 1970 Venous and arterial bupivacaine concentrations after intravenous regional anesthesia. Anesthesia and Analgesia, Current Researches, 49: 300–304

Winnie A P, Ramamurthy S 1970 Pneumatic exsanguination for intravenous regional anesthesia. Anesthesiology, 33: 664–665

Appendix 1

Synthesis of barbiturates

There are two standard methods for making thiobarbiturates such as thiopentone:

1. By the malonate route
2. By the cyanacetate route.

Both are used for commercial manufacture and have certain features in common.

1 The malonate route

(*a*) Diethyl malonate is mono-alkylated at the 2-position with ethyl bromide in the presence of sodium ethoxide:

$$\begin{matrix} COOC_2H_5 \\ | \\ CH_2 \\ | \\ COOC_2H_5 \end{matrix} \quad \underset{Na}{-C_2H_5Br} \rightarrow \begin{matrix} COOC_2H_5 \\ \diagdown \\ HC \cdot C_2H_5 \\ \diagup \\ COOC_2H_5 \end{matrix} + NaBr$$

(*b*) The diethyl ethyl malonate is then alkylated with 2-bromopentane under conditions similar to those described under (*a*) above:

$$\begin{matrix} COOC_2H_5 \\ \diagdown \\ HC \cdot C_2H_5 \\ \diagup \\ COOC_2H_5 \end{matrix} \quad \underset{Na}{-CH_3CH_2CH_2\overset{CH_3}{CHBr}} \rightarrow \begin{matrix} CH_3 \quad COOC_2H_5 \\ \diagdown \quad | \\ C_3H_7-CH-C-C_2H_5 \\ | \\ COOC_2H_5 \end{matrix} + NaBr$$

(*c*) The purified 1.3 diethyl 2-(l-methylbutyl-ethyl) malonate is condensed with thio-urea in the presence of sodium ethoxide:

$$\begin{matrix} CH_3 \quad COOC_2H_5 \\ \diagdown \quad | \\ C_3H_7 \cdot CH-C-C_2H_5 \\ | \\ COOC_2H_5 \end{matrix} + \begin{matrix} NH_2 \\ | \\ CS \\ | \\ NH_2 \end{matrix} \quad \underset{}{-Na} \rightarrow \begin{matrix} CH_3 \qquad CO-NH \\ \diagdown \quad \diagup \qquad \diagdown \\ C_3H_7 \cdot CH-C \qquad\qquad CS \\ \diagup \diagdown \qquad \diagup \\ C_2H_5 \; CO-NH \end{matrix}$$

The pure acid is precipitated from an aqueous solution of the reaction mixture by the addition of mineral acid, filtered off and dried.

(*d*) The dried acid is dissolved in alcohol containing the appropriate quantity of sodium to form a solution of the sodium salt. This is precipitated by the addition of a suitable solvent, filtered off, dried and mixed in the ratio of 100:6 with sodium carbonate.

2 The cyanacetate route

(*a*) and (*b*) The first two stages are analogous to the malonate route, leading to ethyl l-methylbutyl ethylcyanacetate.

(*c*) Condensation with thio-urea in the presence of sodium ethoxide in this case gives an imide:

$$\begin{matrix} CH_3 \qquad\qquad CN \\ \diagdown \qquad \diagup \\ C_3H_7 \cdot CH-C \\ \diagup \quad \diagdown \\ CH_2H_5 \qquad COOC_2H_5 \end{matrix} + \begin{matrix} NH_2 \\ | \\ CS \\ | \\ NH_2 \end{matrix} \rightarrow \begin{matrix} CH_3 \qquad NH \\ \diagdown \qquad \| \\ C_3H_7 \cdot CH \quad C \cdot NH \\ \diagdown \; \diagup \qquad \diagdown \\ C \qquad\qquad CS \\ \diagup \; \diagdown \qquad \diagup \\ C_2H_5 \quad CO \cdot NH \end{matrix}$$

(*d*) This imide is suspended in dilute mineral acid and heated, to give the same end product as in 1 (c).

(*e*) The preparation of the product for injection is exactly as described in 1 (*d*).

Appendix 2

Metabolism of the barbiturates

There is an enormous published literature on the breakdown of barbiturates, and while all known routes of metabolism will be listed, detailed discussion will be limited to those aspects which are of direct clinical interest. It will be appreciated that not all available drugs have been studied to the same extent.

There are at least six chemical reactions involved in the metabolism of the barbiturates (Maynert and van Dyke, 1949, 1950a, b; Maynert and Dawson, 1952; Raventos, 1954; Mark, 1963):

1. Oxidation of substituents in position 5 of the barbiturate ring, with the formation of keto, hydroxy and carboxy barbiturate radicals.
2. Loss of an alkyl group attached to the carbon atom in position 5.
3. Desulphuration of thiobarbiturates.
4. Hydrolytic opening of the barbiturate ring.
5. Loss of alkyl groups attached to the nitrogen atom.
6. Addition of a methyl group to one of the nitrogen atoms.

5-demethylation has not been demonstrated after any of the intravenous drugs although Cochin and Daly (1963) have identified a diallylated barbiturate in the urine of man after the administration of quinalbarbitone. There is little evidence that N- methylation occurs in man and it has not been demonstrated with any of the anaesthetic barbiturates.

While there is no doubt that hydrolytic opening of the barbiturates ring structure occurs in man, it appears to play a minor part in the breakdown of thiobarbiturates in the body. It is one of the methods of destruction of amylobarbitone and pentobarbitone, but it may not be the primary mechanism of inactivation of these drugs, but rather a means of removing pharmacologically inert debris from the body (Shonle et al, 1933). Ring splitting has been demonstrated to occur, to a very small extent, with thiopentone in rats (Taylor et al, 1953), and with thialbarbitone (Raventos, 1954) and hexobarbitone (Tsukamoto et al, 1956) in rabbits. Thiourea (NH_2-CS-NH_2) has also been demonstrated in the urine after thialbarbitone.

N-dealkylation could only apply to drugs such as hexobarbitone and methohexitone. It has not been demonstrated to any significant degree with the latter but does occur with hexobarbitone in dogs (Bush et al, 1953) and rabbits (Tsukamoto et al, 1958). There is no evidence that it is a metabolic pathway of either methylbarbiturates or methylthiobarbiturates in humans. Even if it were to occur, it would not necessarily produce a compound with lesser hypnotic action.

This also applies to desulphuration of thiobarbiturates which undoubtedly occurs in both man and animals. Under some circumstances pentobarbitone has been identified after incubation of

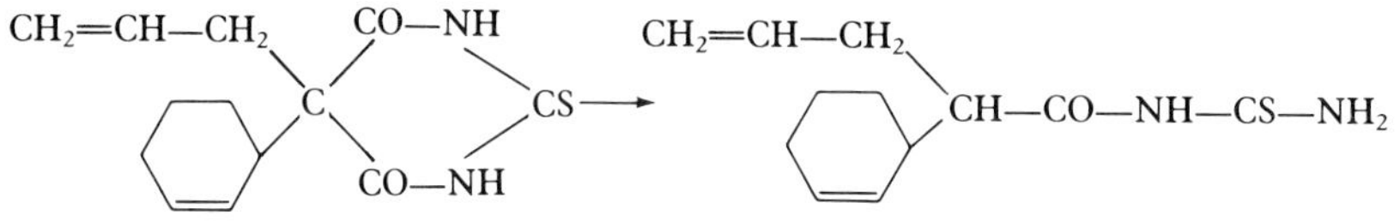

CH_2=CH—CH_2 / CO—NH / C / CS → / CO—NH; CH_2=CH—CH_2 / CH—CO—NH—CS—NH_2

Thialbarbitone → Allylcyclohexenylacetylthiourea

thiopentone with liver slices (Winters et al, 1955), but not in the presence of oxygen and triphosphopyridine where side chain oxidation occurs (Cooper and Brodie, 1957). With the addition of magnesium ions, Spector and Shideman (1959) converted 10 per cent of the thiopentone to pentobarbitone. Of more importance is the demonstration of pentobarbitone in the blood of dogs (Frey et al, 1961) and humans (Furano and Greene, 1963) after thiopentone. Furano and Greene carried out gas chromatographic analysis of serum 15 minutes after the administration of clinical doses of thiopentone, and found that pentobarbitone was present in such small quantities that it was unlikely to contribute to central nervous system depression. However, both pentobarbitone (Soehring and Dietz, 1956; Cochin and Daly, 1963) and the alcoholic metabolite of pentobarbitone (Winters, 1957) have been demonstrated in the urine following thiopentone and, after appropriate doses, the oxybarbiturate could well contribute to the post-anaesthetic hangover. The accumulation of appreciable quantities of pentobarbitone, amounting to 10% of the parent drug, has been demonstrated following the infusion of very large doses of thiopentone in cerebral resuscitation (p. 74) and this is presumed to be due to saturation of hepatic enzymes which metabolise the drug (Stanski et al, 1980). Frey et al (1961) made similar observations with thiobutobarbitone, finding the blood levels of butobarbitone to be higher than those of its thio equivalent at 8 and 24 h after induction of anaesthesia.

Desulphuration of thiamylal (Spector and Shideman, 1959; Cochin and Daly, 1963) methitural (Frey et al, 1961) and thialbarbitone (Carrington and Raventos, 1946) has also been shown to occur.

This leaves 5 side chain oxidation as the major mechanism in the metabolism of the barbiturates, since the derivatives produced are usually hypnotically inert. Although all the clinically useful drugs possess two substituents in this position, apparently only the longer of these is involved in oxidative chemical changes.

Oxidation to a ketone: Methitural has been shown to undergo an interesting ketone-like oxidation of the sulphur atom of the methylthioethyl side chain. Methitural sulphoxide (5-1(methylbutyl)-5-(2-methyl-sulphoxethyl)-2-thiobarbituric acid) had been demonstrated by Dietz and Soehring (1957) in the urine of man following methitural.

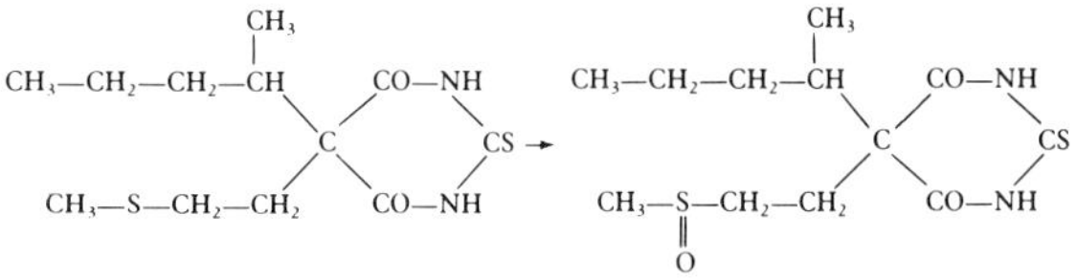

Using paper chromatography, Frey and his associates (1961) have demonstrated two isomers of ketohexobarbitone in the urine of man following hexobarbitone. They also isolated norhexobarbitone (de-methylated) and one isomer of ketonorhexobarbitone. Ketothialbarbitone has been demonstrated in the urine following the administration of thialbarbitone to the rabbit (Raventos, 1954).

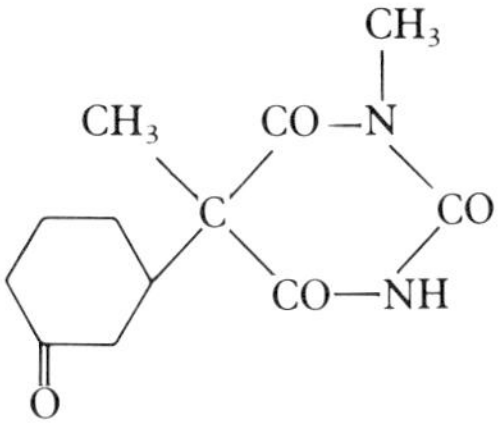

Ketohexobarbitone I

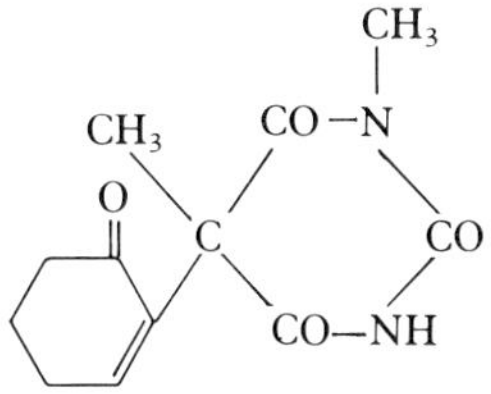

Ketohexobarbitone II

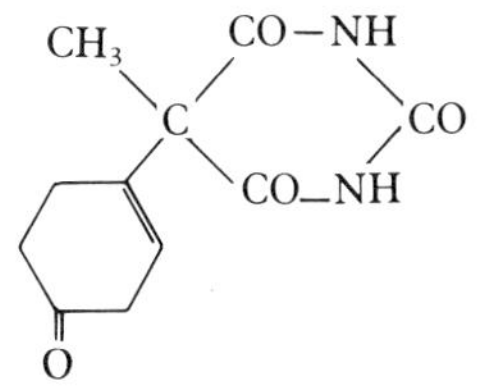

Ketonorhexobarbitone

Oxidation to an alcohol: This has been demonstrated as a route of metabolism of methohexitone (Welles, McMahon and Doran, 1963) as well as of pentobarbitone, quinalbarbitone and other barbiturates, but there is no evidence to show that it applies in man to thiobarbiturates.

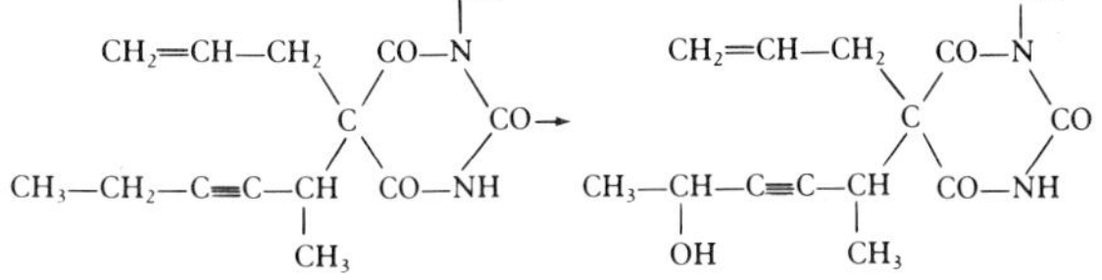

Oxidation to a carboxylic acid: Cooper and Brodie (1957) found that while rat liver homogenates convert thiopentone mainly to carboxylic acid a small amount of hydroxylated metabolite (corresponding to pentobarbitone alcohol) is also formed. While side chain oxidation of thiopentone to form carboxylic acid was demonstrated in man by Brodie and his associates in 1950, the exact position of the carboxyl group was not established until Wood and Horing (1953) determined the structure of the metabolite as 5-ethyl-5-(3-carboxy-1-methyl propyl) thiobarbituric acid.

```
            CH3—CH2   CO—NH                     CH3—CH2   CO—NH
                   \  /      \                         \  /      \
                    C         CS →                      C         CS
                   / \       /                         / \       /
CH3—CH2—CH2—CH      CO—NH       COOH—CH2—CH2—CH      CO—NH
             |                                |
             CH3                              CH3
```

Thiopentone — Thiopentone carboxylic acid

REFERENCES

Brodie B B, Mark L C, Papper E M, Lief P A, Bernstein E, Rovenstine E A 1950 Fate of thiopental in man and method for its estimation in biologic material. Journal of Pharmacology and Experimental Therapeutics 98: 85–96

Bush M T, Butler T C, Dickinson H L 1953 The metabolic fate of 5-(1-cyclo-hexon-1-yl)-1,5-dimethyl-barbityuric acid (hexobarbital, Evipal) and of 5-(1-cyclohexen-1-yl)-5-methylbarbituric acid ('nor-Evipal'). Journal of Pharmacology and Experimental Therapeutics 108: 104–111

Carrington H C, Raventos J 1946 Kemithal: a new intravenous anaesthetic. British Journal of Pharmacology 1: 215–224

Cochin J, Daly J W 1963 The use of thin-layer chromatography for the analysis of drugs, isolation and identification of barbiturates and non-barbiturate hypnotics from urine, blood and tissues. Journal of Pharmacology and Experimental Therapeutics 139: 154–159

Cooper J R, Brodie B B 1955 Enzymatic oxidation of pentobarbital and thiopental. Journal of Pharmacology and Experimental Therapeutics 120: 75–83

Dietz W, Soehring K 1957 Experimentelle Beitrage zum Nachweiss von Thiobarbitursauren aus dem Harn mit Hilfe der Papierchromatographie. Naunyn-Schmiedeberg's Archiv fur experimentelle Pathologie und Pharmakologie (Berlin) 290: 80–97

Frey H H, Doenicke A, Jager C 1961 Quantitativ Bedeutung der Desulfurierung im Stoffwechsel von thiobarbiturates. Medicina experimentalis 4: 243–250

Furano E S, Greene N M 1963 Metabolic breakdown of thiopental in man determined by gas chromatographic analysis of serum barbiturate levels. Anesthesiology 24: 796–800

Mark L C 1963 Thiobarbiturates. In: Papper E M, Kitz R J (eds) Uptake and Distribution of Anesthetic Agents, McGraw-Hill, New York. ch 23

Maynert E W, Dawson J M 1952 Ethyl (3-hydroxy-1-methylbutyl) barbituric acids as metabolites of pentobarbital. Journal of Biological Chemistry 195: 389–395

Maynert E W, van Dyke H B 1949 Metabolism of barbiturates. Pharmacological Reviews 1: 217–242

Maynert E W, van Dyke H B 1950a The metabolic fate of pentobarbital. Isotope dilution experiments with urine after administration of labelled pentobarbital. Journal of Pharmacology and Experimental Therapeutics 98: 174–179

Maynert E W, van Dyke H B 1950b The metabolism of Amytal labelled with N^{15} in dogs. Journal of Pharmacology and Experimental Therapeutics 98: 180–183

Raventos J 1954 The distribution in the body and metabolic fate of barbiturates. Journal of Pharmacy and Pharmacology 6: 217–235

Shonle H A, Keltch A K, Kempf G F, Swanson E E 1933 Question of elimination of barbituric acid (sodium amytal) and 1-methyl-butyl barbituric acid (pentobarbital sodium). Journal of Pharmacology and Experimental Therapeutics 49: 393–407

Soehring K, Dietz W 1956 Pentobarbital — ein Abbauprodukt von thiopental. Klinische Wochenschrift 34: 705–706

Spector E, Shideman F E 1959 Metabolism of thiopyrimidine derivatives: thiamylal, thiopental and thiouracil. Biochemical Pharmacology 2: 182–196

Stanski D R, Mihm F G, Rosenthal M H, Kalman S M 1980 Pharmacokinetics of high dose thiopental used in cerebral resuscitation. Anesthesiology 35: 169–171

Taylor J D, Richards R K, Tabern D L 1953 Metabolism of s^{35} thiopental (Pentothal). Chemical and paper chromatographic studies of S^{35} excretion by the rat and monkey. Journal of Pharmacology and Experimental Therapeutics 104: 93–101

Tsukamoto H, Yoshimura H, Toki S 1956 Metabolism of drugs. VII: the metabolic fate of methylhexabital (5-cyclohexenyl-3,5-dimethylbarbituric acid). (3) Isolation, characterisation and identification of metabolic products of methylhexabital. Chemical and Pharmaceutical Bulletin 3: 368–371

Tsukamoto H, Yoshimura H, Toki S 1958 Metabolism of drugs. XVIII: The metabolic fate of methylhexabital (5-cyclohexenyl-3,5-dimethylbarbituric acid). (8) The quantitative determination of main biotransformation products of methylhexabital in the urine of rabbits by ultraviolet spectrophotometry. Chemical and Pharmaceutical Bulletin 6: 88–91

Welles J S, McMahon R E, Doran W J 1963 The metabolism and excretion of methohexital in the rat and dog. Journal of Pharmacology and Experimental Therapeutics 139: 166–171

Winters W D 1957 Urinary metabolites of thiopental in rat, dog and man. Federation Proceedings 16: 347–348

Winters W D, Spector E, Wallach D P, Shideman F E 1955 Metabolism of thiopental S^{35} and thiopental-2-C^{14} by a rat liver mince and identification of pentobarbital as a major metabolite. Journal of Pharmacology and Experimental Therapeutics 114: 343–357

Wood H B J R, Horing E C 1953 Ethyl-5(1-methyl-3-carboxypropyl)-2-barbituric acid and its thioanalog. Metabolites from pentobarbital and thiopental. Journal of the American Chemical Society 75: 5511–5513

Measurement of thiopentone in biological materials

Barbiturates can be detected and estimated quantitatively by colorimetric methods, by ultra-violet light spectrophotometry (Brodie et al, 1950) or by physical methods such as thin layer chromatography (TLC), gas-liquid chromatography (GLC) (Van Hamme & Ghoneim, 1978) or more recently by high performance liquid chromatography (HPLC) (Toner et al, 1979). Colorimetric, ultra-violet spectrophotometry and thin layer methods are no longer considered to be sufficiently specific or accurate and have been superseded by GLC and latterly by HPLC.

An EMIT immunoassay, available from Syva* Laboratories can be used as a screening/semi-quantitative method for analysis in patients with barbiturate overdose. It is designed to measure quinalbarbitone within the range 3.0–6.0 μg ml^{-1} and to detect the presence of other barbiturates producing a response equivalent to 3 to 6 μg ml^{-1} quinalbarbitone. While this is a useful screening test which only uses 50 μl plasma or serum and can be done in a few minutes it does not differentiate between barbiturates and is only semi-quantitative. Similarly ultra-violet photometric methods which can be used in an emergency overdose case in hospital laboratories are not as specific as chromatographic methods. Flanagan & Berry (1977) reported on a method for screening and quantification of poisoning case samples using GLC with a flame ionization detector. None of these is sufficiently sensitive for pharmacokinetic or pharmacodynamic studies during anaesthesia.

* Syva UK, Syntex House, St Ives Road, Maidenhead, Berks SL6 IRD, UK

Becker (1976) described a GLC method for the measurement of thiopentone in plasma. This required on-column methylation of the thiopentone to improve peak resolution and a flame ionization detector. This gave a sensitivity of 200 ng ml^{-1}. Van Hamme and Ghoneim (1978) also reported a GLC method for the assay of thiopentone in plasma which did not require methylation and was sensitive to 25 ng ml^{-1}. Jung et al (1981) used a nitrogen specific detector and phenobarbitone as the internal standard which produced a sensitivity of 25 ng ml^{-1}.

The polarity of thiopentone and methohexitone and their ability to be extracted easily from plasma, make HPLC an acceptable method of analysis using a variable wavelength ultra-violet light detector. The maximum ultra-violet light spectrum for thiopentone is 290 nm in an acid medium and 305 nm in an alkaline medium: methohexitone has a maximum spectrum of 228 nm in an acid and 250 nm in an alkaline medium.

Blackman & Jordon (1978) assayed thiopentone levels by the direct injection of the plasma sample into an HPLC system using an ultra-violet light detector at a wavelength of 290 nm. This required a pre-column between injection port and the analytical column to remove particulate matter from the sample. The lower limit of detection was 500 ng ml^{-1} and only about fifty 10 μl injections of untreated plasma could pass through the pre-column before it had to be replaced. This could be expensive if a large number of samples had to be analysed but is extremely useful if an emergency screening is required. Christensen & Andreasen (1979) precipitated the proteins in serum with 96% ethanol, centrifuged the solution twice and injected 20 μl of the supernatant liquid into an HPLC system with a wavelength of 280 nm. This gave a detection limit of 90 ng ml^{-1}.

Because of the need to analyse a large number of samples in a short time Toner et al (1979) developed an HPLC method using a single stage ether extraction with methohexitone as the internal standard and using a wavelength of 254 nm. This gave an analysis time of 2 minutes per sample and a sensitivity down to 500 ng ml^{-1}. Salvadori et al (1981) extracted their samples with ethyl acetate and used carbamazepine as the internal standard; this gave a sensitivity down to 200 ng ml^{-1}. The method currently used is a modification of that of Toner et al (1979).

Method

Apparatus

Pye variable wavelength ultra-violet light detector with wavelength set at 290 nm.

Column of stainless steel tubing 25 cm long with an internal diameter of 2 mm packed with Spheresorb ODS 10 and fitted with zero volume (ZDV) unions.

Connecting tubing of stainless steel with lengths kept to a minimum to minimise the degree of adsorption.

Rheodyne 7125 syringe loading valve fitted with a 25 μl sample loop.

Solvent consists of 1000 ml double distilled water, 1150 ml methanol and 6.8 g sodium acetate mixed together and degassed in an ultrasonic bath for 15 min.

Attenuation of the detector is set at 0.16 AUFS.

Measurement

To 1 ml plasma in an extraction tube add 20 μl of a 0.5 mg ml^{-1} solution of thialbarbitone (internal standard) and 3 ml diethyl ether.

Cap the tubes and place in a rotary mixer for 15 min to allow extraction of drugs into ether.

Centrifuge for 5 min in a Chilspin at 4000 rpm. Transfer diethyl ether into an evaporating tube and dry off in a heating block.

Reconstitute samples in 50 μl of methanol. Inject 5 μl into the valve.

With each batch of patient samples, extract and chromatograph a set of known standards to cover the expected range. This gives a calibration curve against which the sample can be compared.

Under the above conditions the lower level of sensitivity is 25 ng ml^{-1}. If the amount of plasma extracted or the amount injected is increased it is possible to measure 10 ng ml^{-1}.

Methohexitone concentrations in plasma can be measured by an HPLC method very similar to that for thiopentone. The internal standard and extraction procedure are the same and chromatography is carried out using a Sperisorb 10 ODS column, 25 cm in length, and a solvent phase of 500 ml distilled water and 575 ml methanol. Detection is by ultra-violet light at 299 nm. The retention times for internal standard and methohexitone are 108 s and 156 s respectively.

The within-batch coefficients of variation for samples spiked with 1 μg ml^{-1}, 10 μg ml^{-1} and 20 μg ml^{-1} are 3.14%, 3.99% and 4.47% respectively. The between-batch coefficients of variation for samples spiked with 2 μg ml^{-1}, 10 μg ml^{-1} and 20 μg ml^{-1} are 4.07%, 6.10% and 3.17% respectively.

REFERENCES

Becker K E 1976 Gas chromatographic assay for free and total plasma levels of thiopental. Anesthesiology 45: 656–660

Blackman G L, Jordon G J 1978 Analysis of thiopentone in human plasma by high performance liquid chromatography. Journal of Chromatography 145: 492–495

Brodie B B, Mark L C, Papper E M, Lief P A, Bernstein E, Rovenstine E A 1950 The fate of thiopental in man and a method for its estimation in biological material. Journal of Pharmacology and Experimental Therapeutics 98: 85–96

Christensen J H, Andreasen F 1979 Determination of thiopental by high pressure liquid chromatography. Acta Pharmacologica et Toxicologica 44: 260–263

Flanagan R J, Berry D J 1977 Routine analysis of barbiturates and some other hypnotic drugs in blood plasma as an aid to the diagnosis of acute poisoning. Journal of Chromatography 131: 131–146

Jung G, Mayersohn M, Perrier D 1981 Gas chromatographic assay for thiopental in plasma, with use of a nitrogen specific detector. Clinical Chemistry 27: 113–115.

Salvadori C, Farinotti R, Duvaldestin P H, Dauphin A 1981 Liquid chromatography determination of thiopentone in human plasma. Therapeutic Drug Monitoring 3: 171–176

Toner W, Howard P J, Dundee J W, McIlroy P D A 1979 Estimation of plasma thiopentone by High Performance Liquid Chromatography and an ether extraction. Anaesthesia 34: 657–660

Van Hamme M J, Ghoneim M M 1978 A sensitive gas chromatographic assay for thiopentone in plasma. British Journal of Anaesthesia 50: 143–145

Appendix 4

P J Howard and E McClean

Measurement of benzodiazepines in biological fluids

A number of analytical procedures have been employed for the qualitative and quantitative analysis of benzodiazepines and their metabolites in biological fluids. Their relative usefulness depends on their sensitivity, the ability to differentiate between a parent drug and its metabolites and their ease of operation. These include:

1. Radioactively labelling;
2. Thin layer chromatography;
3. Radioimmunoassay;
4. Ultra-violet assay and HPLC;
5. Gas chromatography.

Radioactively labelling

Schwartz et al (1965) describe the preparation of labelled diazepam using H^3 labelled benzoic acid (Sternbach & Reeder, 1961; Sternbach et al, 1962). Following the administration of the labelled diazepam to man they were able to measure the total radioactivity emitted from the blood, urine and faeces using a liquid scintillation counter and quantify the concentration of diazepam in various tissues and organs. To distinguish between diazepam and its metabolites it was necessary to combine this method with thin layer chromatography.

Thin layer chromatography

Schwartz et al (1965) and de Silva et al (1966) have described the separation of diazepam and seven analogues of diazepam by two dimensional thin layer chromatography using Silica-Gel G and various solvents. This method is useful for identifying diazepam and metabolites but is unsuitable for quantitative analysis.

Radioimmunoassay

This relatively new technique has been developed in recent years and applied to the assay of diazepam and N-desmethyldiazepam by Peskar & Spector (1973). It involves the production of immunogens which are analogues of diazepam. Injection of these immunogens into rabbits produces sera with antibodies to diazepam and N-desmethyldiazepam. Using this antiserum, it is possible to detect 1 ng ml^{-1} diazepam in ether extracts of whole blood.

Ultra-violet assay

Ultra-violet light detectors used in conjunction with high performance liquid chromatography have been used for the estimation of benzodiazepines but have not been able in general to match the sensitivity of GLC.

Gas-liquid chromatography (GLC)

GLC is the most acceptable method for measurement of benzodiazepines in biological fluids. Described by de Silva et al (1964) for use with diazepam, with the proper choice of column and chromatographic conditions it is possible to estimate most benzodiazepines by this method.

Before analysis of benzodiazepines in biological fluids by GLC the drug must first be extracted into a suitable solvent. The method of extraction depends on a number of factors:

1. the necessity to distinguish between the drug and its metabolites;
2. the stationary phase used;
3. the expected concentration of the drug;
4. the detector.

de Silva et al (1964) used diethyl ether as their extracting solvent and acid hydrolysis to obtain aminobenzophenone derivatives which were then separated by GLC. Marcucci et al (1968) described a method whereby diazepam and its metabolites were extracted and chromatographed without chemical manipulation. Garattini et al (1969) pointed out that if an electron capture detector is to be used there must be sufficient purification of the samples.

The method used by a number of workers (de Silva & Puglisi, 1970; Van der Kleijn et al 1971; Kaplan et al, 1973) is a multi-stage extraction and clean up procedure which is time-consuming.

Berlin et al (1972) described single stage benzene extraction using 0.1 ml plasma and 4 ml benzene. This is a useful method for repeat analysis in infants.

By modifying the method of Berlin et al (1972) Gamble et al (1975) were able to measure accurately 5 ng ml^{-1} diazepam and 20 ng ml^{-1} N-desmethyldiazepam. Griseofulvin was the internal standard as this allowed the estimation of both diazepam and its N-desmethyl metabolite at the same time. The retention time for diazepam was 2 minutes, N-desmethyldiazepam 3 min 10 s and griseofluvin 7 min 20 s. This method has been modified by using flunitrazepam as the internal standard in place of griseofluvin which is difficult to obtain.

Method

Diazepam and N-desmethyl diazepam

To 0.5 ml of plasma in an extraction tube, add 0.5 ml of a saturated solution of potassium chloride and 20 μl (5 μg ml^{-1} solution) of flurazepam and 3 ml of the extracting solvent (double distilled benzene).

Stopper the tubes, mix on a whirlimixer for 15 min, and centrifuge in a Chilspin centrifuge for 5 min.

Transfer the benzene layer to small tubes and evaporate to dryness.

Reconstitute the sample in 50 μl benzene and inject 5 μl into the chromatograph.

The original chromatographic conditions were:

Chromatograph	Perkin Elmer F33 with ECD
Column	5 ft borosilicate glass with an internal diameter of 4 mm packed with 3% OV17 on 100–120 mesh Gas Chrom Q
Oven temperature	250°C
Injection temperature	300°C
Detector temperature	300°C
Gas pressure	450 kNm^2
Amplifier range	1
Amplifier attenuation	128

Under these conditions the retention time for diazepam is 2 min, N-desmethyldiazepam 3 min and flunitrazepam 3.8 min.

Lorazepam (Howard et al, 1977; 1978)

As it was necessary for a particular study to measure lorazepam levels in neonates, a method was developed that needed only small amounts of plasma.

To 0.1 ml plasma, add 0.1 ml of a saturated solution of potassium chloride, 25 μl flunitrazepam (91 ng ml^{-1} solution) — the internal standard — and 2 ml benzene in an extraction tube.

Stopper the tubes and mix for 15 min, centrifuge for 5 min, remove 1.5 ml of the benzene layer, and evaporate to dryness.

Reconstitute the sample in 50 μl benzene and inject 2.5 μl into the chromatograph.

The original chromatographic conditions were:

Chromatograph	Perkin Elmer F33 with ECD
Column	5 ft borosilicate glass with an internal diameter of 4 mm packed with 3% OV17 on 100–120 mesh Gas Chrom Q
Oven temperature	240°C
Injection temperature	300°C
Detector temperature	300°C
Gas pressure	350 kNm^2
Amplifier range	1
Amplifier attenuation	32

Under these conditions the retention time for lorazepam is 1.9 min and flunitrazepam 3.6 min with a sensitivity down to 5 ng ml^{-1}.

Midazolam (Howard et al, 1985)

To 0.5 ml of plasma, add 30 μl of a 5 μg ml^{-1} solution of diazepam (internal standard) and 4 ml benzene in an extraction tube.

Stopper the tubes and mix for 15 min; and centrifuge in a Chilspin for 5 min.

Transfer the benzene layer to small tubes and evaporated to dryness.

Reconstitute the sample in 50 μl benzene and inject 5 μl into the chromatograph.

The original chromatograph conditions were:

Chromatograph	Perkin Elmer F33 with ECD
Column	5 ft borosilicate glass with an internal diameter of 4 mm packed with 3% OV17 on 100–120 mesh Gas Chrom Q
Oven temperature	250°C
Injection temperature	300°C
Detector temperature	300°C
Gas pressure	450 kNm^2
Amplifier range	1
Amplifier attenuation	256

Under these conditions the retention time for midazolam is 3.25 min and diazepam 2 min with a sensitivity down to 5 ng ml^{-1}.

Temazepam

Before temazepam can be estimated by GLC it has to be derivatised. There are a number of derivatising agents available; a 10% solution of bis-trimethyl silylacetamide in toluene is the most suitable. To avoid the possibility of the drug adhering all glassware is silanised with a 5% solution of hexamethyl di-silazene in acetone.

To 0.1 plasma in silanised extraction tubes, add 10 μl of a 125 ng ml^{-1} solution of 1 methyl temazepam (internal standard) and vortex-mix for 3 s; add 3 ml of toluene and vortex-mix the tubes for 3 s. Shake the resulting mixture on a rotary mixer at 45 rpm for 15 min and centrifuge in a Chilspin at 4000 rpm for 5 min. Transfer 2 ml of the organic layer to silanised evaporation tubes and evaporate to dryness. Reconstitute the samples in 100 μl 10% bis-trimethyl silylacetamide in toluene, stopper the tubes and place in a dark cupboard to react overnight. On the next day inject 1 μl into the chromatograph.

Our chromatograph conditions were:

Chromatograph	Pye 304 with ECD and auto sample injector
Column	5 ft borosilicate glass with an internal diameter of 4 mm packed with 3% OV17 on 100–120 mesh Gas Chrom Q
Oven temperature	260°C
Injection temperature	300°C
Detector temperature	300°C
Gas pressure	
Amplifier range	1
Amplifier attenuation	256

Under these conditions the retention time for temazepam is 5.7 min and for 1 methyltemazepam 7.3 min. The lower level of reliable detection is 25 ng ml^{-1}; this can be improved upon by using a bigger volume of plasma.

In all of these methods a set of standard solutions to cover the expected range of the analysis should be prepared and extracted with every batch of patient samples. This gives a calibration curve against which the patient samples can be compared.

As with all analytical methods the precision should be tested by inclusion of 'spiked' samples in all batches.

REFERENCES

Berlin A, Siwers B, Agurell S, Hiort A, Sjoqvist F, Strom S 1972 Determination of bioactivity of diazepam in various formulations from steady state plasma concentration data. Clinical Pharmacology and Therapeutics 13: 733–744

de Silva J A F, d'Arconte L, Kaplan S A 1964 The determination of blood levels and the placental transfer of diazepam in humans. Current Therapeutic Research 6: 115–121

de Silva J A F Koechlin B A, Bader G 1966 Blood level distribution patterns of diazepam and its major metabolites in man. Journal of Pharmaceutical Science 55: 692–702

de Silva J A F, Puglisi C V 1970 Determination of medazepam (Nobrium), diazepam (Valium) and their major biotransformation products in blood and urine by electron capture gas liquid chromatography. Analytical Chemistry 42: 1725–1736

Gamble J A S, Assaf R A E, Mackay J S, Kennedy M S, Howard P J 1975 Estimation of plasma diazepam. Anaesthesia 30: 159–163

Garattini S, Marcussi F, Mussini E 1969 Gas chromatographic analysis of benzodiazepines. In: Porter R (ed) Gas chromatography in biology and medicine. J & A Churchill Ltd, London, p 161–172

Howard P J, Lilburn J K, Dundee J W, Toner W, McIlroy P D A 1977 Estimation of plasma lorazepam by gas–liquid chromatography and a benzene extraction. Anaesthesia 32: 767–770

Howard P J, Lilburn J K, Dundee J W, Toner W, McIlroy P D A 1978 Estimation of plasma lorazepam by gas–liquid chromatography and a benzene extraction: modification of original method. Anaesthesia 33: 67–68

Howard P J, McClean E, Dundee J W 1985 The estimation

of midazolam, a water-soluble benzodiazepine, by gas liquid chromatography. Anaesthesia 40: 664–668

Kaplan S A, Jack M L, Alexander K, Weinfeld R W 1973 Pharmacokinetic profile of diazepam in man following single intravenous and oral and chronic oral administrations. Journal of Pharmaceutical Science 62: 1789–1796

Marcucci F, Fanelli R, Mussini E 1968 A method for gas chromatographic determination of benzodiazepines. Journal of Chromatography 37: 318–320

Peskar B, Spector S 1973 Quantitative determination of diazepam in blood by radioimmunoassay. Journal of Pharmacology and Experimental Therapeutics 186: 167–172

Schwartz M A, Koechlin B A, Postma E, Palmer S, Krol G 1965 Metabolism of diazepam in rat, dog and man. Journal of Pharmacology 149: 423–435

Sternbach L H, Fryer R I, Metlesics W, Reeder E, Sach G, Saucy G, Stempel A 1962 Quinazolines and 1,4-benzodiazepines. VI: halo-methyl-, and methoxy-substituted 1-3-dihydro-5-phenyl-2H-1,4-benzodiazepines-2-ones. Journal of Organic Chemistry 27: 3788–3792

Sternbach L H, Reeder E 1961 Quinazolines and 1 4-benzodiazepines. IV: Transformation of 7-chloro-2-methylamine-5-phenyl-3H-1,4 benzodiazepine 4 oxide. Journal of Organic Chemistry 26: 4936–4939

Van der Kleijn E, Beelem G C, Frederick M A 1971 Determination of tranquillizers by GLC in biological fluids. Clinica Chimica Acta 34: 345–356

Appendix 5

Barbiturates and porphyria

The term 'porphyria' covers a number of diseases which fall into three distinct groups (Leading Article, 1985), although as many as nine types have been described. The complicated biochemical changes are described in the papers or reviews of Sunderman & Sunderman (1955), Dean (1960, 1963), Watson (1960), Eales & Saunders (1962), Eales et al (1963, 1966), Eales & Dowdle (1968) and Schmid (1971).

Animal studies by Goldberg (1954) show that only barbiturates with an allyl group cause an increase in the porphyrin in the urine, and this only with prolonged administration of sublethal doses. Porphobilinogen could not be demonstrated, except in very small quantities of doubtful significance and only after diallylbarbituric acid. In man, With (1957) examined the urine of 25 patients with acute and 25 with chronic barbiturate poisoning and found no rise in level of porphyrins and no porphobilinogen. The danger with the intravenous barbiturates lies not in their effects on porphyrin metabolism in normal subjects but in the fact that in susceptible patients they may precipitate an attack, or if given during an attack they may aggravate it and induce total paralysis.

The three main groups discussed below are from the classification of Waldenstrom (1937, 1957). Some overlapping occurs between groups and some place the South African type in a separate group. There is also confusion in the names used by different writers. It will be appreciated that many of the older descriptions of porphyria do not specify the class of disease and the South African type has only been described in recent years.

PORPHYRIA CONGENITA

Also known as erythropoietic porphyria, the basic defect in this very rare condition probably occurs at an early stage of fetal development. The condition, more common in males, is characterised by an excessive tissue and skeletal content of porphyrin, causing profound photosensitivity as a result of which scarring and mutilations occur. There are no abdominal symptoms or disturbances of the nervous system and porphobilinogen is not present in the urine. Barbiturates do not affect the course of the disease.

PORPHYRIA CUTANEA TARDA

Occurring later in life, this condition is not hereditary. It is characterised by photosensitivity and excretion of porphyrins in the urine. A tendency to scleroderma is present, but the disease is distinguished from the congenital type by the absence of gross mutilations. While periodic attacks of colic may occur, the disease differs from the acute intermittent type by the absence of serious nervous disorders. Barbiturates have not been found to have any effect on the condition. Porphobilinogen is not excreted in the urine when the attack is of the cutaneous type (Macgregor et al, 1952).

PORPHYRIA VARIEGATA

Porphyria variegata, or South African genetic porphyria, is a mixed form of the disease, first described by Dean and Barnes (1955). This is a hereditary disease in which cutaneous lesions are associated with abdominal and nervous symptoms. This form is very rare in most of Northern Europe but occurs frequently in South Africa and the Baltic States. In America it accounts for about 5 per cent of the total cases of porphyria. Porphobilinogen is present in the urine only during the acute stage of the disease and the administration of a barbiturate may precipitate neurological symptoms. It is interesting to note that Dean claims that all the South African cases can be traced back to one ancestor who was married at the Cape in 1688.

ACUTE INTERMITTENT PORPHYRIA

This is an intermittent illness affecting persons in whom the synthesis of porphyrin pigment is persistently deranged and who generally excrete porphobilinogen in the urine. It is distinguished from the other main forms of porphyria by the absence of photosensitivity and the presence of porphobilinogen in the urine. It is not as rare as was once supposed but there is a marked geographical distribution in its incidence, being more common in the Scandinavian countries and South Africa.

Gibson and Goldberg (1956) have shown that the significant lesions of the disease are multiple segmental scattered areas of demyelination of the autonomic nerves which leads to abdominal pain and bowel upset. The involvement of the peripheral motor and sensory nerves leads to paralysis and sensory loss and involvement of the cranial nerves, especially the vagus, is common. The central nervous system does not escape. Chromatolysis of the motor nerve cells in the spinal cord and medulla is frequent, while in the cerebellum, foci of demyelination of the white matter with slight shrinking of the Purkinje cells is seen. In the cerebrum, areas of demyelination, especially centred around blood vessels, are present most often in the parietal lobes but sometimes occur also in the temporal and occipital lobes. Because of these lesions psychiatric symptoms occur in 60 per cent of cases.

Porphobilinogen or porphyrins in general are not increased around these areas of degeneration. Consequently the demyelination is probably not directly due to these substances. Peters et al, (1958) have suggested that the symptoms are due to zinc, copper, or other cationic blocks of several metallo-enzyme systems. This results in exhaustion of certain portions of the body's natural chelative defences, subsequently leading to depletion of porphyrins for purposes of chelation. In consequence, the metabolism is impoverished, affecting the maintenance of myelin and the cytochrome systems which in turn interrelate with the porphyrin pool. The liver is probably the site of the deranged synthesis of the porphyrins. During acute phases the liver shows central lobular necrosis, but liver failure is not common (Gibson et al, 1957).

Acute intermittent porphyria can exist in different forms:

1. The latent form: there are no symptoms or signs, but porphobilinogen has been demonstrated in the urine on at least one occasion.
2. The abdominal form: purely abdominal symptoms are present with no involvement of the nervous system.
3. The neurological form: there are only neurological symptoms with none referable to the abdomen.
4. The mixed abdominal and neurological form.
5. The terminal comatose form.

The disease can in any one patient change from one group to the other in different episodes or in the course of a single acute exacerbation.

ROLE OF BARBITURATES

These were introduced into clinical medicine in 1903 and in 1906 a typical case of acute porphyria was described in a patient after the prolonged administration of diethyl barbituric acid (Dobrachansky, 1906). Subsequent writers mentioned the harmful effects of these drugs (Prunty, 1946; Goldberg and Rimington, 1955; Whittaker and Whitehead, 1956) but it was not until Dean (1963) focused attention on it and emphasised the potential dangers of thiopentone that anaesthetists began to be aware of them. The first detailed survey in an anaesthetic journal was by Dundee and Riding (1955). This and two other surveys are summarised in Table A5.1. The discrepancy between the findings of Ward (1965) and those of the other two reports is not unexpected. Dundee and Riding (1955) and Eales (1966, 1967) discussed the outcome of patients admitted to hospital in acute attacks while Ward surveyed the course of the disease in all known porphyrias admitted to one hospital.

In addition to these, Dean (1960) noted that in 1958, eight patients at the Provincial Hospital, Port Elizabeth, were known to have developed acute porphyria following thiopentone anaesthesia and three died. These patients all suffered from porphyria variegata. Dundee et al (1962) reported deaths in two out of three patients after thiopentone, the course of the disease being typical of acute intermittent porphyria. Dundee has details of two further deaths following acute intermittent porphyria, in each of whom thiopentone could be incriminated.

Table A5.1: Synopsis of three clinical surveys of the outcome of acute porphyria, particularly in association with anaesthesia

Dundee and Riding (1955)
SURVEY OF CASES REPORTED IN *British Medical Journal* AND *Lancet* 1948–1953
Types not stated.
37 attacks of acute porphyria in 32 patients (two-thirds were women and two-thirds were aged 31–50)
Paralysis occurred in 30 and proved fatal in ten instances
15 operations, 13 administrations of thiopentone, all of which developed paralysis and five died
Ward (1965)
ELEVEN YEAR SURVEY OF HOSPITAL ADMISSIONS IN SEATTLE, WASHINGTON
66 proven cases (type not stated) of porphyria — 163 hospital admissions
21 received a total of 44 anaesthetics of which 36 were induced with a barbiturate
These 36 received barbiturates of some kind on 110 occasions;
Two serious complications possibly due to barbiturates;
None developed paralysis
(Two cases of barbiturate-induced respiratory paralysis occurred in adjacent hospitals)
Eales (1966, 1967)
EXPERIENCE IN SOUTH AFRICA OVER THE PERIOD 1955–1965
82 attacks in 76 patients (68 with porphyria variegata and eight with acute intermittent porphyria)
22 patients had acute episodes in close association with thiopentone anaesthesia
19 peripheral neuritis, 11 severe quadriplegia with bulbar paralysis, three deaths
These 76 patients had previously undergone 26 operations — five with postoperative disability compatible with acute porphyria (14 were known to have had thiopentone)
An additional 69 other cases of porphyria variegata had purely cutaneous or biochemical manifestations; 26 of these had undergone 41 operations; 22 had thiopentone with 11 instances of severe postoperative disability

Other barbiturates involved in reported cases are phenobarbitone, butobarbitone, quinalbarbitone, pentobarbitone and amylobarbitone (Eales & Linder, 1962), while Dundee knows of one patient in whom thialbarbitone was involved and one with thiobutobarbitone. Although Goldberg (1959) has suggested that barbiturates which possess an allyl group, e.g. quinalbarbitone or thiamylal, are particularly dangerous in porphyria, subsequent clinical experience does not support this view.

Acute attack

There are some minor differences in the symptoms of the two types of disease which are affected by barbiturates, but the general course is one of progressive acute demyelination of nerves with signs and symptoms depending on which nerves are most affected. Table A5.2 compares the clinical picture in four reported series of cases (Eales and Linder, 1962). For further details the reader is referred to the above paper and to those of Dundee, McCleery and McLoughlin (1962) and Eales and Dowdle (1968).

The classical case presents with colicky abdominal pain, muscular weakness and paralysis, psychiatric manifestations and red-coloured urine. This description is often of little assistance in diagnosing the early stages of the disease, since the onset of an acute attack is frequently gradual, unless hastened by the administration of barbiturates. The patient may complain of nothing more than feeling 'off colour' and, apart from indefinite mental changes, objective symptoms may be absent. Insomnia is a frequent symptom and may prompt the administration of a barbiturate.

The abdominal pain when present is predominantly colicky but there may be periods of hours or even days when it is constant. It may occur in any part of the abdomen but it is most often in

A5.2 A comparison of the percentage incidence of the clinical features of an acute attack of porphyria. (Eales and Linder, 1962)

	Waldenstrom (233)	*Goldberg (50)*	*Markovitz (69)*	*Eales and Linder (80)**
Males (%)	40	38	39	30
Females (%)	60	62	61	70
Abdominal pain	85	94	95	90
Vomiting	59	78	52	80
Mental changes	55	56	80	55
Constipation	48	74	46	80
Paralysis	42	68	72	53
Hypertension	40	56	49	55
Pyrexia	37	14	36	38
Tachycardia	28	64	51	83
Seizures	10	18	—	12
Sensory loss	9	38	24	15
Diarrhoea	9	12	11	8
Azotaemia	9	?	67	69
Proteinuria	9	14	—	8
Leucocytosis	7	24	48	20
Amaurosis	4	3	—	3
Cranial nerves	?	29	51	9
EEG abnormalities	?	44	47	23

* 107 attacks in 80 patients

the right iliac fossa, or in the epigastrium. It may be deep-seated and cause great distress. All patients show some abdominal tenderness on examination but less than would be expected from the severity of the pain. Rigidity is generally absent and vomiting may occur either before or after the onset of abdominal pain. Constipation is severe and impaction of faeces common.

Many patients are subjected to an unnecessary laparotomy, and the combination of operation and thiopentone may exacerbate the acute disease at this stage.

BIOCHEMISTRY

Uroporphyrins are often present in the urine in acute porphyria, and they may be found in large quantities in other conditions also, or may be absent during acute exacerbations of this disease. Porphobilinogen, on the other hand, is always present during acute exacerbations. During latent periods the excretion may be intermittent and the urine must be tested on several occasions before a positive result is obtained. Porphobilinogen is probably a normal intermediary in haemopoiesis, consisting of one pyrrole ring. It is colourless in the urine, but this may be coloured by other porphyrin derivatives, mainly uroporphyrins.

When first voided, the urine containing porphobilinogen is usually normal in colour and darkens only when left in daylight for a few hours. This simple test can be used in the absence of laboratory facilities (Whittaker and Whitehead, 1956). A more refined version of it is to heat some of the urine in a water bath for 10 minutes and compare with the unheated specimen. This simple test demonstrates the presence of derivatives of porphobilinogen but not porphobilinogen itself. A false positive may be obtained after blood transfusion.

The laboratory test described by Watson and Schwartz (1941) is generally used: 2 ml of urine and 2 ml of Ehrlich's aldehyde reagent (0.7 g of p-dimethyl-amino benzaldehyde in 250 ml of 6 N hydrochloric acid) are mixed and allowed to stand for two minutes and compared with a mixture of 2 ml of urine and 2 ml of 6 N hydrochloric acid. (This safeguards against artefacts due to certain ingested foodstuffs.) A red colour develops in two to three minutes in the presence of porphobilinogen or urobilinogen. These two can be distinguished by the addition of 4 ml of amyl alcohol; urobilinogen dissolves in the alcohol while porphobilinogen remains in the aqueous solution. Sunderman and Sunderman (1955) consider amyl alcohol to be a better solvent than chloroform as porphobilinogen is more soluble in it. The Watson Schwartz test cannot be used for detecting quiescent porphyria variegata but details of suitable tests have been published by Dean (1960).

Eales (1967) includes two rarer varieties of porphyria — symptomatic porphyria and hereditary copro-porphyria — among those affected by drugs. Symptomatic porphyria occurs frequently in South Africa, especially among the non-white population and is usually associated with an excessive ingestion of alcohol (Hickman et al, 1967). Fungal contamination of prepared food may be another precipitating factor (Keen et al, 1966). In hereditary copro-porphyria the clinical syndrome somewhat resembles acute intermittent porphyria and the patients are similarly sensitive to barbiturates but porphobilinogen is absent from the urine. Coproporphyrin III is, however, detectable in abnormal amounts in the faeces.

In addition to barbiturates, many other drugs aggravate porphyria. These include sulphonamides, dichloraphenazone, meprobamate, glutethamide, tolbutamide, griseofulvin, methyldopa and the contraceptive pill. All these have one factor in common — in experimental animals they are inducers of hepatic gamma-aminolaevulinic acid synthetase (ALA synthetase). This enzyme limits the rate of synthesis of haem and porphyrin and is increased in all types of hepatic porphyria. Thus these drugs compound the metabolic defect which is an important component of the disease process (Leading Article, 1972). Goldberg (1959) has shown that there is also an increased susceptibility to acute attacks of porphyria in the first trimester of pregnancy.

There is a risk of inducing acute porphyria with etomidate (p. 168), but there are no data on the use of ketamine. Inhalational or local anaesthetics appear to have no deleterious effects on the disease.

REFERENCES

Dean G 1960 Routine testing for porphyria variegata. South African Medical Journal 34: 745–751

Dean G 1963 The porphyrias. Pitman, London

Dean G, Barnes H D 1955 The inheritance of porphyria. British Medical Journal ii: 89–94

Dobraschansky M 1906 Einiges uber malonal. Wiener medizinische Presse 47: 2145–2151

Dundee J W, McCleery W N C, McLoughlin G 1962 The hazard of thiopental anesthesia in porphyria. Anesthesia and Analgesia, Current Researches 41: 567–574

Dundee J W, Riding J E 1955 Barbiturate narcosis in porphyria. Anaesthesia 10:55

Eales L 1966 Porphyria and thiopentone. Anesthesiology 27: 703–704

Eales L 1967 Drugs and the porphyrias: acute porphyria. South African Medical Journal 41:566

Eales L, Dowdle E B 1968 Clinical aspects of importance in the porphyrias. British Journal of Clinical Practice 22: 505–515

Eales L, Dowdle E B, Saunders S J, Sweeney G D 1963 Presentation of patients with porphyria. South African Journal of Laboratory and Clinical Medicine 9: 162–176

Eales L, Levey M J, Sweeney G D 1966 The place of screening tests and quantitative investigations in the diagnosis of the porphyrias, with particular reference to variegate and symptomatic porphyria. South African Medical Journal 40: 63–71

Eales L, Linder G C 1962 Porphyria — the acute attack: an analysis of 80 cases. South African Medical Journal 36: 284–292

Eales L, Saunders S J 1962 The diagnostic importance of faecal porphyrins in the differentiation of the porphyrias. I: Values in normal subjects and in patients with non-porphyric disorders. South African Journal of Laboratory and Clinical Medicine 8: 127–138

Gibson J B, Goldberg A 1956 The neuropathology of acute porphyria. Journal of Pathology and Bacteriology 71:495

Gibson J B, Parkes W E, Brennan C F 1957 Acute porphyria with observations on liver lesions and on porphobilinogenuria. Irish Journal of Medical Science 6th series: No. 375: 127–139

Goldberg A 1954 Effect of certain barbiturates on porphyrin metabolism in rabbits. Biochemical Journal 57:55

Goldberg A 1959 Acute intermittent porphyria. Quarterly Journal of Medicine 28: 183–210

Goldberg A, Rimington C 1955 Experimentally produced porphyria in animals. Proceedings of the Royal Society of Medicine 143: 257–280

Hickman R, Saunders S J, Eales L 1967 Treatment of symptomatic porphyria in venesection. South African Medical Journal 41: 456–460

Keen G A, Saunders S J, Eales L 1966 Porphyrin production in liver cells by aspergillus fumigatus. Lancet i: 798–799

Leading Article 1972 The pill and porphyria. British Medical Journal 3:603

Leading Article 1985 Latent acute hepatic porphyria. Lancet 1: 197–198

Macgregor A G, Nicholas R E H, Rimington C 1952 Porphyria cutanea tarda. Archives of Internal Medicine 90:483

Peters H A, Eichman P L, Reese H H 1958 Therapy of acute, chronic and mixed hepatic porphyria in patients with chelating agents. Neurology 8:621

Prunty F T G 1946 Acute porphyria: investigations on pathology of porphyrins and identification of excretion of uroporphyrin I. Archives of Internal Medicine 77: 623–642

Schmid R 1971 Porphyria. In Cecil & Loeb Textbook of Medicine, 13th ed, Beeson P B, McDermott W (eds) 1704–1709

Sunderman F W Jr, Sunderman F W 1955 Practical consideration of diseases of porphyria metabolism, porphyria and porphyrinuria. American Journal of Clinical Pathology 25:123

Waldenstrom J 1937 Studien uber Porphyria. Acta Medica Scandinavica, Suppl 82, 1–254

Waldenstrom J 1957 The porphyrias as inborn errors of metabolism. American Journal of Medicine 22: 758–773

Ward R J 1965 Porphyria and its relation to anesthesia. Anesthesiology 26: 212–215

Watson C J 1960 The problem of porphyria — some facts and questions. New England Journal of Medicine 263: 1205–1215

Watson C J, Schwartz S 1941 Simple tests for urinary porphobilinogen. Proceedings of the Society for Experimental Biology and Medicine 47: 393–394

Whittaker S R F, Whitehead T P 1956 Acute and latent porphyria. Lancet i: 547–551

With T K 1957 Porphyrin metabolism and barbiturate poisoning. Journal of Clinical Pathology 10:165

Index